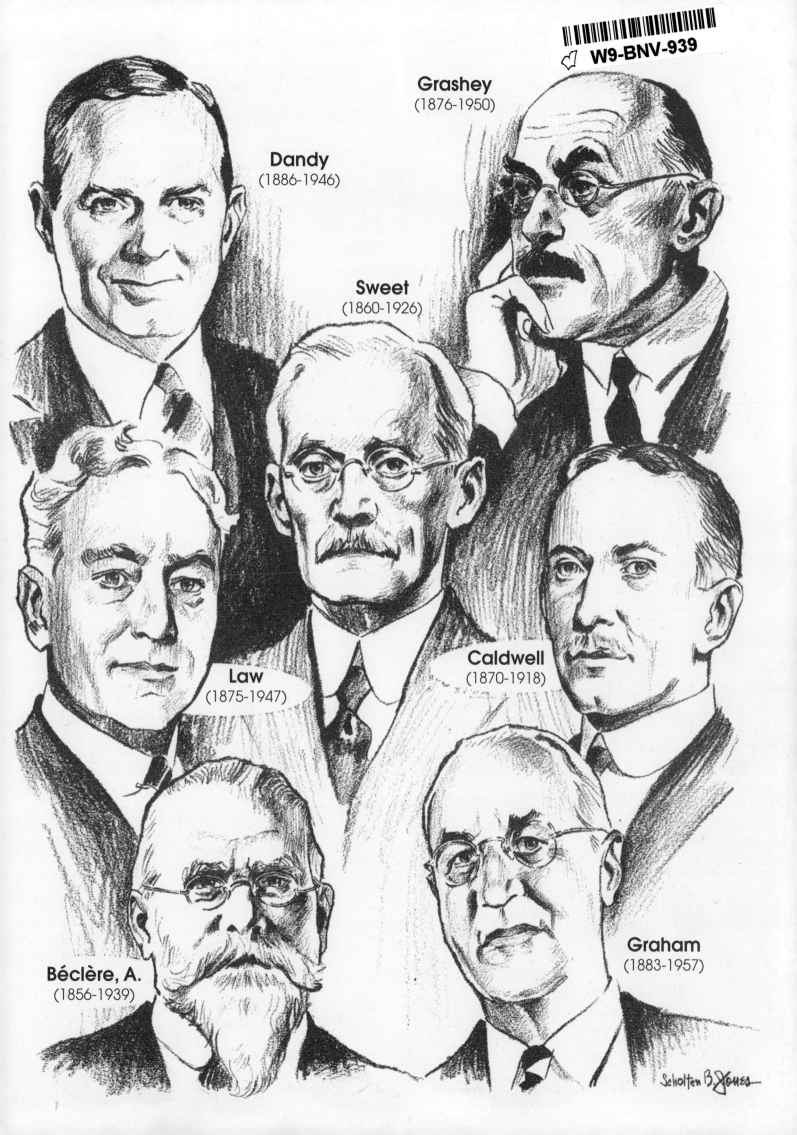

Grashey
(1876-1950)

Dandy
(1886-1946)

Sweet
(1860-1926)

Law
(1875-1947)

Caldwell
(1870-1918)

Béclère, A.
(1856-1939)

Graham
(1883-1957)

Scholten B. Jones

MERRILL'S ATLAS

of

RADIOGRAPHIC POSITIONS

and

RADIOLOGIC PROCEDURES

VOLUME ONE

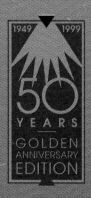

1949 — 1999

50 YEARS

GOLDEN
ANNIVERSARY
EDITION

MERRILL'S ATLAS

of

RADIOGRAPHIC POSITIONS and RADIOLOGIC PROCEDURES

VOLUME ONE

NINTH EDITION

Philip W. Ballinger,
MS, RT(R), FAERS

Assistant Professor Emeritus
Radiologic Technology Division
School of Allied Medical Professions
The Ohio State University
Columbus, Ohio

Eugene D. Frank,
MA, RT(R), FASRT

Director, Mayo Radiography Program
Department of Diagnostic Radiology
Mayo Clinic/Foundation
Assistant Professor of Radiology
Mayo Medical School
Rochester, Minnesota

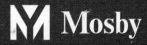

St. Louis Baltimore Boston Carlsbad Chicago Minneapolis New York Philadelphia Portland
London Milan Sydney Tokyo Toronto

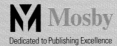
Dedicated to Publishing Excellence

Publisher: Don E. Ladig
Executive Editor: Jeanne Rowland
Developmental Editor: Carole Glauser
Project Manager: Linda McKinley
Production Editors: René Spencer Saller, Cathy Comer, Barrett Schroeder
Designer: Renée Duenow
Manufacturing Manager: Betty Mueller

NINTH EDITION
Copyright © 1999 by Mosby, Inc.

Previous editions copyrighted 1949, 1959, 1967, 1975, 1982, 1986, 1991, 1995

Composition and lithography by Graphic World, Inc.
Printing/binding by R.R. Donnelly & Sons Company

Mosby, Inc.
11830 Westline Industrial Drive
St. Louis, Missouri 63146

Library of Congress Cataloging in Publication Data

Ballinger, Philip W.
   Merrill's atlas of radiographic positions and radiologic
procedures. — 9th ed. / Philip W. Ballinger, Eugene D. Frank.
      p.   cm.
   Includes bibliographical references and index.
   ISBN 0-8151-2651-4 (alk. paper). — ISBN 0-8151-2652-2 (pbk.   :
alk. paper). — ISBN 0-8151-2653-0
   1. Radiography, Medical—Positioning—Atlases.   I.   Frank, Eugene
D.   II.   Merrill, Vinita, 1905-   Atlas of roentgenographic positions
and standard radiologic procedures.   III.   Title.   IV.   Title: Atlas
of radiographic positions and radiologic procedures.   V.   Title:
Radiographic positions and radiologic procedures.
   [DNLM: 1.   Technology, Radiologic atlases.   2.   Diagnostic Imaging
atlases.   WN 17 B192m   1999]
RC78.4.B35   1999
616.07'572—dc21
DNLM/DLC
for Library of Congress

International Standard Book Number (Set): **0-8151-2650-6**
99   00   01   02   03   /   9   8   7   6   5   4   3   2   1

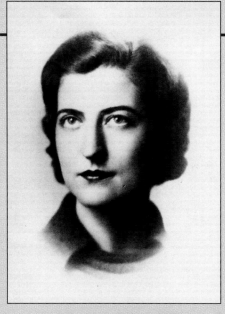

Vinita Merrill
1905-1977

Vinita Merrill had the foresight, talent, and knowledge to write the first edition
of this atlas in 1949. The text she wrote became known as *Merrill's Atlas* in honor
of the significant contribution she made to the profession of radiography
and in acknowledgment of the benefit of her work to generations of students
and practitioners.

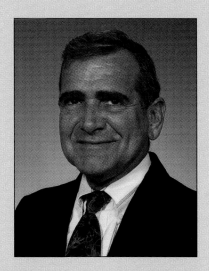

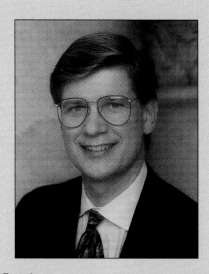

Philip Ballinger is now Assistant Professor Emeritus in
the Radiologic Technology Division of the School of
Allied Medical Professions at The Ohio State University
in Columbus, Ohio. In 1995, he retired after a 25-year ca-
reer as Radiography Program Director at The Ohio State
University. Since his retirement, he has become more
involved than ever in professional activities, such as
speaking engagements at state, national, and
international professional meetings. He began working
on *Merrill's Atlas* in its fifth edition,which was published
in 1982. The Golden Anniversary Edition is Phil's fifth
as author of the atlas.

Eugene Frank is currently in his twenty-eighth year in
radiography at the Mayo Clinic/Foundation in Rochester,
Minnesota. For the last 8 years, he has been Director
of the Mayo Radiography Program and Assistant
Professor of Radiology in the Mayo Medical School.
He frequently presents at professional gatherings throughout the world and has held leadership positions in state,
national, and international professional organizations. He
joins Philip Ballinger as co-author on this ninth edition of
Merrill's Atlas.

ADVISORY BOARD

This edition of Merrill's benefits from the expertise of a special advisory board. The following board members have provided professional input and advice and have helped the authors make decisions about atlas content throughout the preparation of the ninth edition:

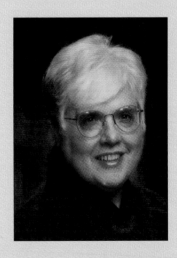

Joyce Ortego, MS, RT(R)
Program Coordinator,
  Radiologic Technology
Dona Ana Community
  College
Las Cruces, New Mexico

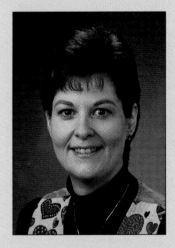

Rita M. Oswald, BS, RT(R) (CV)
Clinical Instructor,
  Radiography Program
Mayo Clinic/Foundation
Rochester, Minnesota

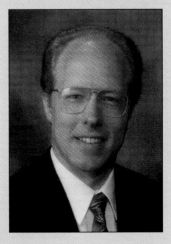

Curt L. Serbus, MEd, RT(R)
Radiologic Technology
  Educational Consultant
Indianapolis, Indiana

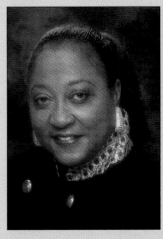

Bettye Greene Wilson, MA-Ed, RT(R)(CT), RDMS
Associate Professor,
  Division of Medical
  Imaging and Therapy
School of Health Related
  Professions
University of
  Alabama-Birmingham
Birmingham, Alabama

CONTRIBUTORS

Albert Aziza, BSc, MRT(R)
Hospital for Sick Children
Diagnostic Imaging
Toronto, Canada

Michael R. Bloyd, BSN, RN, RT(R)
Director of Educational Services
Taylor County Hospital
Greensburg, Kentucky

Barbara A. Blunt, MPH, RT(R), ARRT
Project Manager
Osteoporosis and Arthritis Research
    Group
University of California-San Francisco
San Francisco, California

Jeffrey A. Books, RT(R)
Director, Diagnostic Imaging
St Dominic-Jackson Memorial Hospital
Jackson, Mississippi

Michael G. Bruckner, BS, RT(R)(CV)
Angiographic Technologist and
    Clinical Instructor
The Ohio State University
Columbus, Ohio

Terri Bruckner, MA, RT(R)
Instructor, Radiologic Technology
    Division
The Ohio State University
Columbus, Ohio

**Stewart C. Bushong, ScD, FACR,
    FACMP**
Professor of Radiology
Baylor College of Medicine
Houston, Texas

Leila A. Bussman, BS, RT(R)(T)
Director, Radiation Therapy Program
Mayo Clinic/Foundation
Rochester, Minnesota

Luann J. Culbreth, MEd, RT(R)(MR)
MRI Manager
Baylor University Medical Center
Dallas, Texas

William F. Finney, MA, RT(R)
Assistant Professor, Radiography
    Program
The Ohio State University
Columbus, Ohio

**Sandra Hagen-Ansert, BA, RDMS,
    RDCS**
Program Director, Ultrasound
Baptist Memorial College of Health
    Science
Memphis, Tennessee

Richard D. Hichwa, PhD
Associate Professor
Director, PET Imaging Center
University of Iowa Hospitals
Iowa City, Iowa

Nancy L. Hockert, BS, ASCP, CNMT
Program Director, Nuclear Medicine
    Technology
Mayo Clinic/Foundation
Rochester, Minnesota

Jeffrey A. Huff, AS, RT(R)(CV), RCVT
Cardiac Catheterization Technologist
Kuakini Medical Center
Honolulu, Hawaii

Lorrie L. Kelley, MS, RT(R)(MR)(CT)
Associate Professor
Director CT/MRI Program
Boise State University
Boise, Idaho

Nina Kowalczyk, MS, RT(R)
Associate Director, Radiology
The Ohio State University
Columbus, Ohio

Deirdre Milne, MRT(R), ACR
ADAC Project Manager/Applications
    Specialist
Burlington, Ontario, Canada

Walter W. Peppler, PhD
Clinical Professor
University of Wisconsin-Madison
Madison, Wisconsin

Rex E. Profit, MA, RT(R)
Account Manager
Fuji Medical Systems, USA
Stamford, Connecticut

**Terese McShane Roth, MS,
    RT(R)(M)**
Assistant Professor, Radiology
Merritt College
Walnut Creek, California

**Jane A. Van Valkenburg, PhD,
    RT(R)(N), FASRT**
Department Chair, Radiologic
    Sciences
Weber State University
Ogden, Utah

Kari J. Wetterlin, MA, RT(R)
Unit Supervisor, Radiology
St. Mary's Hospital
Mayo Clinic/Foundation
Rochester, Minnesota

PREFACE

Welcome to the Golden Anniversary Edition of *Merrill's Atlas of Radiographic Positions and Radiologic Procedures*. The ninth edition continues the tradition of excellence begun in 1949, when Vinita Merrill wrote the first edition of what has become a classic text. Over the last 50 years, *Merrill's Atlas* has provided a strong foundation in anatomy and positioning for thousands of students who have gone on to successful careers as imaging technologists. *Merrill's Atlas* is also a mainstay for everyday reference in imaging departments all over the world. As the co-authors of this Golden Anniversary Edition, we are honored to follow in Vinita Merrill's footsteps.

Learning and Perfecting Positioning Skills

Merrill's Atlas has an established tradition of helping students learn and perfect their positioning skills. After covering preliminary steps in radiography, radiation protection, and terminology in introductory chapters, *Merrill's* then teaches anatomy and positioning in separate chapters for each bone group or organ system. The student learns to position the patient properly so that the resulting radiograph provides the information the physician needs to correctly diagnose the patient's problem. The atlas presents this information for commonly requested projections as well as those less commonly requested, making it the most comprehensive text and reference available.

The third volume of the atlas provides basic information about a variety of special imaging modalities, such as computed tomography, cardiac catheterization, magnetic resonance imaging, ultrasound, nuclear medicine technology, quality management, and radiation therapy.

Merrill's Atlas is not only a sound resource for students to learn from but also an indispensable reference as they move into the clinical environment and ultimately into their practice as imaging professionals.

New to This Edition

Since that first edition of *Merrill's Atlas* in 1949, many changes have occurred. This new edition incorporates many significant changes designed not only to reflect the technologic progress and advancements in the profession but also to meet the needs of today's radiography students. The major changes in this edition are highlighted below.

FULL COLOR THROUGHOUT!

The Golden Anniversary Edition of *Merrill's Atlas* will be the first-ever full-color anatomy and positioning text. As readers will quickly notice, full color greatly enhances the learning value of the anatomy illustrations and positioning photographs, making what has always been the best-illustrated anatomy and positioning text an even more effective learning tool.

NEW 3-D LINE ART

Over 45 three-dimensional line illustrations are new to this edition. Each is designed to clarify anatomy or projections that are difficult to visualize. New art appears in every chapter of Volumes 1 and 2.

NEW RADIOGRAPHS

Nearly every chapter contains new high-quality radiographs, including many that demonstrate pathology. With the addition of these new images, the ninth edition has the most comprehensive collection of high-quality radiographs available to students and practitioners in a text prepared for radiographers.

COMPUTED RADIOGRAPHY

Because of the rapid expansion and acceptance of computed radiography (CR), either selected positioning considerations and modifications or special instructions are indicated where necessary. A new icon

will alert the reader to CR notes. In addition, a newly revised chapter on CR (Chapter 33) will assist the reader in understanding the principles.

CLEARER TEXT WITH MORE BULLETED LISTS AND TABLES

The entire text has been carefully edited to present information, in particular descriptions of projections, more clearly and succinctly. Chapters 1 and 3 have been completely rewritten for clarity and the introduction of new material. More bulleted lists and tables than ever before help the reader organize information and focus quickly on the most important content.

NEW ORTHOPEDIC PROJECTIONS

New projections now commonly performed in imaging departments are presented for the first time in this edition. Among the new projections are the widely requested Robert projection of the thumb, the Rafert-Long scaphoid series, the Moore sternum, and standing projections of various joints.

SUMMARY OF PROJECTIONS

At the beginning of each procedural chapter is a new summary of all the projections described in the chapter. The projections and positions are organized by anatomic area. These summaries not only give a general overview of the chapter but also serve as a study guide for students.

ESSENTIAL PROJECTIONS

Essential projections are identified with the special icon shown here:

Essential projections are those most frequently performed and determined to be necessary for competency of entry-level practitioners. Of the over 400 projections described in this atlas, 192 have been identified as essential based on the results of two extensive surveys performed in the United States and Canada.[1]

OBSOLETE PROJECTIONS DELETED

Projections identified as obsolete by the authors and the advisory board have been deleted. A summary is provided at the beginning of any chapter containing deleted projections so that the reader may refer to previous editions for information.

NEW CHAPTERS AND CONTENT

An all-new, well-illustrated section on venipuncture (in Chapter 18) provides the theoretic basis and the procedural information needed to perform venipuncture.

Another entirely new chapter on mobile radiography (Chapter 30) describes the most frequently performed mobile projections, including for the first time anywhere detailed neonatal projections. The chapter includes an extensive introduction to mobile procedures and step-by-step instructions on how to perform each projection.

Also new to this edition is a chapter on bone mineral densitometry (Chapter 39), which discusses the relatively recent history, theoretic basis, equipment, and procedures for this technology. With the increased awareness and occurrence of osteoporosis and with radiographers performing these examinations in increasing numbers, this chapter is certainly a much-needed addition.

To reflect the continued rapid advancements in mammography, Chapter 24 has been entirely revised. It now includes all the American College of Radiology (ACR) recommended mammography projections along with all-new projection illustrations. This chapter, for the first time in radiologic technology, also details mammography as performed on the male patient. Chapter 42, on qual-

ity assurance, has also been expanded to include the latest ACR quality assurance procedures.

METRIC FILM SIZES

Because most radiographic film can no longer be purchased in English sizes, metric measurements are now used to state most film sizes. To ease the transition from English to metric, the English film size is parenthetically listed after the metric. For example, the traditional 14×17 inch film is now listed as 35×43 cm (14×17 in). Chapter 1 provides an introduction and discussion of the new metric sizes.

SUMMARY OF ANATOMY

At the beginning of each procedural chapter, the anatomic terms described and identified are succinctly summarized in a box. These boxes will enable readers, particularly students, to easily identify or study the anatomy described.

STANDARDIZED ANATOMY TERMINOLOGY

In the two previous editions of this atlas, the transition to new anatomic terminology was ongoing, with the more widely adopted anatomic term listed first, followed by the older term in parentheses (e.g., scaphoid [navicular]). In preparing this edition, we carefully reviewed the most widely used and adopted anatomy and physiology textbooks to identify the one anatomic term most commonly used in each case. After 8 years of printing dual anatomic terms, the secondary terms have been deleted from this edition.

Over 75 new anatomic terms have been introduced based on a comprehensive review of the widely used anatomy and physiology textbooks. The anatomy sections now present comprehensive anatomy equaling that of dedicated anatomy texts. An appendix at the end of volumes 1 and 2 contains a summary of the new and changed anatomic terms for this edition.

Learning Aids for the Student

POCKET GUIDE TO RADIOGRAPHY

A new edition of *Pocket Guide to Radiography* complements the revision of *Merrill's Atlas*. In addition to instruc-

tions for positioning the patient and the body part for all the essential projections, the new pocket guide includes information on computed radiography (CR) and automatic exposure control (AEC). Space is provided for writing department techniques specific to the user.

RADIOGRAPHIC ANATOMY, POSITIONING, AND PROCEDURES WORKBOOK BY STEVEN G. HAYES, SR.

The new edition of this two-volume workbook retains the features that made it so popular in its first edition: anatomy labeling exercises, positioning exercises, self-tests, and an answer key. The exercises include labeling of anatomy on drawings and radiographs, crossword puzzles, matching, short answers, and true/false. At the end of each chapter is a multiple-choice test to help students assess their comprehension of the whole chapter. New to this edition are more film evaluations to give students additional opportunities to evaluate images for proper positioning and more positioning questions to complement the workbook's strong anatomy review.

Teaching Aids for the Instructor

COMPUTERIZED TEST BANK BY EUGENE D. FRANK

An expanded, easy-to-use test bank of over 1200 questions, available electronically, facilitates test preparation. The test bank is on CD-ROM and can be used in both Mac and Windows environments.

MOSBY'S RADIOGRAPHIC INSTRUCTIONAL SERIES: RADIOGRAPHIC ANATOMY, POSITIONING, AND PROCEDURES

This multimedia program covers anatomy and the most commonly requested projections, with over 2200 images and over 20 hours of audio available in two formats: slides with audiotapes or CD-ROM for Windows. The program can be used for lecture support in the classroom or for self-directed learning and review by individual students in the media lab. The professionally recorded audio track discusses positioning of the patient and body part, central ray angle, and evaluation criteria.

[1]Ballinger PW, Glassner JL: Positioning competencies for radiography graduates, *Radiol Technol* 70:181-196, 1998.

RADIOGRAPHIC ANATOMY, POSITIONING, AND PROCEDURES INSTRUCTOR'S MANUAL REVISED BY CURT L. SERBUS, MEd, RT(R)

The Radiographic Anatomy, Positioning, and Procedures Instructor's Manual is available to help you enliven your teaching with *Merrill's Atlas* and the multimedia program, *Mosby's Radiographic Instructional Series: Radiographic Anatomy, Positioning, and Procedures.* The instructor's manual contains chapter outlines, teaching strategies, and a print version of the audio track from the multimedia program to aid in your planning.

We hope you will find this Golden Anniversary Edition of *Merrill's Atlas of Radiographic Positions and Radiologic Procedures* the best ever. Input from generations of readers has helped to keep the atlas strong through nine editions, and we welcome your comments and suggestions. We are constantly striving to build on Vinita Merrill's work, and we trust that she would be proud and pleased to know that the work she began 50 years ago is still so appreciated and valued by the imaging sciences community.

Philip W. Ballinger

Eugene D. Frank

ACKNOWLEDGMENTS

As with any publication or project, those identified as the authors could never accomplish all that needs to be done without the help and support of others. The Golden Anniversary Edition of the atlas is the result of the work of many, many individuals who provided assistance along the way.

Advisory Board

In preparing for the ninth edition, our advisory board continually provided professional expertise and aid in decision making on the revision of this edition. The advisory board members are listed on page vi. We are most grateful for their input and contributions to this edition of the atlas.

Anatomy Summaries

The design and content of the new anatomy summaries seen in each procedural chapter were completed by Ellen Collins, MS, RT(R)(M), and Paula Maramonte, MEd, RT(R).

Contributors: Past and Current Editions

We are pleased to identify and credit those who served as contributing authors or who submitted high-quality radiographic images that have been published in the text over the years. We extend our heartfelt thanks to all of them for their significant contributions. These individuals are identified in special sections on pages xv-xvi.

Reviewers

The group of radiography professionals listed below extensively reviewed this edition of the atlas and made many insightful suggestions for strengthening the atlas. We are most appreciative of their willingness to lend their expertise.

Janice M. Blanchard, RT(R)
Sharyn D. Gibson, EdD, RT(R)
Robin Jones, MS, RT(R)
David Lindsay, PhD
Cynthia Liotta, MS, RT(R)
Beckey Miller, MS, RT(R)
Marsha M. Sortor, MHE, RT(R)(N)(M)
O. Scott Staley, MS, RT(R)
Beverly J. Tupper, BS, RT(R)(CV)
Rhonda Stadt Wahl, PhD
P.W.B. and E.D.F.

Special Acknowledgments, P.W.B

I wish to extend special thanks to **Eugene D. Frank.** Your efforts made this ninth edition possible. Gene's involvement in the eighth edition set the stage for his becoming a co-author on the ninth. Gene, I am pleased to welcome you to *Merrill's Atlas.*

This edition includes many new illustrations and radiographs. I want to thank **Mr. Harry Condry,** who kept track of my many photography orders. To **Theron Ellinger,** thanks for printing numerous illustrations used to replace those from the eighth and earlier editions. Thanks also to **Jennifer Torbert,** senior medical photographer, for many of the new photographs in this edition.

I have had the privilege of working with Mosby for nearly 20 years and during that time, I have worked with several editors. To my first editor and now publisher, **Don Ladig,** I thank you for your continuous support for nearly 20 years. To **Jeanne Rowland,** Executive Editor, I also thank you for your work over two editions. Sometimes we've missed a deadline, but in the end, we've always published on schedule. To **Carole Glauser,** Developmental Editor, and **Jennifer Genett,** Editorial Assistant, and to **René Saller** and **Barrett Schroeder,** Production Editors, thank you for keeping the project continually moving in the right direction.

To my family, where do I commence to say thank you? Your love and support have been ever-present. To my father-in-law, **L. Neil Hathaway** and his wife **Ruth,** thank you for your continuing love, support, and affection. Your understanding and acceptance are certainly appreciated.

To my parents, **D. W.** and **Mildred Ballinger,** too many times I could not, or did not, take the time to provide assistance and show my appreciation and love. I publicly thank you and acknowledge your support, commencing when I first announced three decades ago that I was going into "x-ray." To my sister, **Ms. Sandra Jameson** and her husband **Tom,** thank you for always being there to lighten up the situation.

To my registered nurse son, **Eric,** and professional baker and pastry chef daughter, **Monica,** wow, you grew up too fast. Too many times I was not available because I was at a professional meeting, making a presentation, or working on "the book," as it is described in our house. I love you both, and thank you for making me proud with your recent graduations.

To my wife, **Nancy,** our nearly 30 years of marriage have been a real trip—yes, many times going too fast and in too many directions. While I was out on book-related matters, you were always available to support the family. You also responded to my asking innumerable times, "Hey, Nanc, got a minute?" You were, and still are, my source for proofreading, ideas, and conceptual advice. Since my 1995 health challenge, your love and affection have been more apparent than ever, and for that I am extremely grateful. Thank you, Nancy.

Special Acknowledgments, E.D.F.

Preparation of a comprehensive textbook such as *Merrill's Atlas* requires the support of numerous individuals. **Phil Ballinger** served as my mentor during the past 3½ years of revising over 1600 pages of text and nearly 3000 illustrations. With your direct guidance, Phil, this monumental task was eventually completed. Thank you for "teaching me the ropes."

It is with great pleasure that I acknowledge the significant contributions of the following individuals from various departments of the Mayo Clinic. **David A. Factor,** medical illustrator, designed and created over 45 new anatomic line drawings that enhance every aspect of this edition. **Joseph M. Kane,** professional photographer, produced over 150 new color figures, including all the photography in the venipuncture, mobile, and mammography chapters. **Merlin K. Schrieber,** photographic printer, hand printed over 50 new radiographic images, including many that took hours to get just right. **Nancy J. Baker,** medical secretary, typed, formatted, and organized hundreds of pages of new and revised text. She also meticulously managed a database of every anatomic term and projection in the entire atlas for the new anatomy and projection summaries. **Susan K. Cosgrove,** medical secretary, and **Kevin C. Seisler, BA, RT(R),** Assistant Director of the Mayo Radiography Program, supported this entire project by keeping various aspects of the Radiography Program here at Mayo operational during my absences. Faculty members **Beverly J. Tupper, BS, RT(R)(CV), Janice M. Blanchard, RT(R), S. Jo Dean, RT(R),** and **Kari W. Wetterlin, MA, RT(R),** gathered all the new radiographs that are included in every chapter of this edition. Thank you all.

Steven G. Hayes, MEd, RT(R), author of the accompanying workbook, played a significant role in suggesting items for revision and helping to standardize various aspects of the atlas.

I am greatly indebted to the Advisory Board members, **Joyce Ortego, MS, RT(R), Rita M. Oswald, BS, RT(R)(CV), Curt L. Serbus, MEd, RT(R),** and **Bettye Wilson, MA, RT(R)(CT), RDMS,** who assisted in the major decisions regarding new text, illustrations, critical editing, and new chapters. They tackled every challenge with enthusiasm and enjoyed every challenging query. Thanks to this highly talented and experienced group of radiography educators, this edition of the atlas is technically the best it can be.

Medical illustrators **Jeanne Robertson** and **Nadine Sokol** did an excellent job of accurately colorizing every line drawing in the atlas—a monumental task.

Linda Wendling, of Wordbench, assisted in the initial organization of all the chapters and figures. Linda's enthusiastic approach to her part of the work launched the developmental process on a positive note.

My close friend **Kenneth L. Bontrager, MA, RT(R),** assisted in standardizing many terms, central ray angles, positioning techniques, and other technical aspects in both of our textbooks. Our goal was to reduce discrepancies in our textbooks and make learning easier for students.

My wife, **Jane Frank,** and children, **Matthew** and **Jillian Frank,** supported and encouraged me as I worked many long hours preparing this edition. Thank you for your support of all my professional work.

Lastly, I extend special thanks to **Jeanne Rowland,** Executive Editor, who invited me to co-author the atlas. Along with Jeanne, **Cathy Comer, Renée Duenow, Carole Glauser, Jennifer Genett, Linda McKinley, René Saller,** and **Barrett Schroeder** played significant roles in producing the Golden Anniversary Edition of the atlas. My experience with the entire Mosby editorial and production team has been very enjoyable, rewarding, and interestingly, "fun."

Contributors to Past Editions

For this fiftieth anniversary edition, we want to give credit to all those who have contributed specialty chapters to the atlas over its first eight editions. Because of the contributions of the professionals listed below, the atlas has presented the most current information available in not only general radiography but all the special imaging modalities.

Mel Allen
Albert Aziza*
Thomas J. Beck
Dr. David L. Benninghoff
Mary J. Blome
Michael R. Bloyd*
Barbara A. Blunt*
Dr. Carl R. Bogardus, Jr.
Steven J. Bollin, Sr.
Jeffrey A. Books*
Michael G. Bruckner*
Terri Bruckner*
Dr. Stewart C. Bushong*
Leila A. Bussman*
John Michael Chudik
Dorothea F. Cook
Luann J. Culbreth*
Barbara M. Curcio
Chris Democko
Dr. John P. Dorst
Paul Early
Dr. James H. Ellis
William F. Finney*
Joseph Fodor, III
Dr. Atis K. Freimanis
Sandra Hagen-Ansert*
H. Dale Hamilton

Dr. Marcus W. Hedgcock
Dr. Richard D. Hichwa*
Nancy L. Hockert*
Jeffrey A. Huff*
Keith R. Johnson
Kenneth C. Johnson
Joseph W. Kaplan
Lorrie L. Kelley*
Nina Kowalczyk*
Dr. Robert A. Kruger
Dr. Richard G. Lester
Jack C. Malott
Charles E. Marschke
Philip R. Maynard
Deirdre Milne*
Stephen T. Montelli
Dr. John O. Olsen
Richard C. Paskiet, Jr.
Dr. Walter W. Peppler*
Rex E. Profit*
Sheila Rosenfeld
Dr. Ronald J. Ross
Terese McShane Roth*
Dr. Alan H. Rowberg
Ann Hrica Seglinski
William J. Setlak
Dr. William H. Shehadi
Dr. Roy D. Strand
Donald L. Sucher
Carole A. Sullivan
Dwayne J. Termaat
Dr. Michael E. Van Aman
Dr. Jane A. Van Valkenburg*
Rome V. Wadlington
Dr. Ronald D. Weinstein
Kari J. Wetterlin*
Joan A. Wodarski

*Ninth edition contributors

Radiograph Contributions

The authors would like to extend a special note of gratitude to all those who have contributed radiographs to *Merrill's Atlas* over its nine editions. Thanks to them, the collection of radiographs in the atlas is judged the finest of any radiography positioning textbook. Thousands of radiography students, radiologic technologists, and physicians around the world who regularly use the atlas are able to learn more effectively from the high-quality radiographs.

To our readers, we continue to extend an invitation to send us any radiographs that you feel could be used in the atlas or any that are of better quality than those that now appear in the book. Our goal is to provide our profession with the finest collection of radiographs for learning and reference purposes.

Sidney Alexander
Marek Anderson
April S. Apple
Kim Bailey
Lois Baird
Dr. David H. Baker
Annette Baldwin
Steve Bargiel
Karen J. Bauer
Dr. Joshua A. Becker
Dr. Javier Beltran
Dr. David L. Benninghoff
Dr. Walter E. Berdon
Dr. David Bloom
Steven J. Bollin, Sr.
Dr. Jacques Boreau
Frank J. Brewster
Dr. Michael Burman
Kalma Butler
Fayette Capik
Beth Changet
Patti Chapman
Dianna Childs
Dr. K. Y. Chynn
Roland Clements
Dr. Arthur R. Clemett
Sharon A. Coffey
Dr. Constantine Cope
Carol Corder
Sylvia L. Cousins
Karen Cox
Karen Cubler
Julianne M. Curtin
Jeannie M. Danker
Dr. Howard P. Daub

Barbara Davis
Laurie Davis
Peter DeGraaf
Betsy Delzeith
Michael DeSalu
Terry Doherty
Carol Drobik
Dr. Albert A. Dunn
Kimberly Edgar
Dr. Milton Elkin
Dr. Bernard S. Epstein
Dr. John A. Evans
Gail A. Fisher
Michael Franklin
Dr. Robert H. Freiberger
Laurie Funk
Heide Galli
Dr. Francis H. Ghiselin
Colleen Gillespie
Delores Goodwin
Dr. John A. Goree
Edward F. Gunson
Norma Harmon
Dr. Robert Harris
Colleen Harty
Dr. Herbert F. Hempel
Timothy Hill
Robbie F. Hockenberry
Jana Hoffman
Paul T. Ichino
Dr. Harold G. Jacobson
Angelique Jacopin
Emelda James
Eva M. James
Dr. James Jerele
Dr. John C. Johnson
David M. Jones
Darla Kaikis
Ann Kay
Marilyn Knight
Jane Kober
Nina Kowalczyk
D. Peter Kuum
Carmela Kvas
Dr. Roger W. Lambie
Dr. Oswald S. Lowsley
Marigold Marsh
Dr. Richard H. Marshak
Charles McCartly
Judy McLaughlin
Deborah Meeker
Dr. Alan C. Merchant
Tom Meridith
Jonathan Miller
Dr. Lawson E. Miller, Jr.
Randy Miller
Dr. Roscoe E. Miller
Betty Jo Mixon
Martha Montalvo

Leon Montgomery
Stephen G. Moon
Carrol Moore
Susan M. Orlando
Javier Pagan
Eric Parsels
Nancy Patfield
Sharon Peterson
Dr. Raymond Pfeiffer
Dr. Robert L. Pinck
Dr. Etta Pisano
W. William Pollino
Dr. Michael Portnoff
M. G. Rauckis
Lynn Rhatigan
Brenda J. Rogers
Jeffrey L. Rowe
Stephen Rusk
Ammar Saadeh
Valerie Sasson
Deborah Saunders
David R. Schumick
Dr. William B. Seaman
Dr. William H. Shehadi
Keith Shipman
Holly Simmons
Daphne Smith
Dr. John Spellmeyer
Dr. Ramsay Spillman
Theresa Spotts
Dr. William Z. Stern
Cheryl Stillberger
Dr. Harold L. Stitt
Dr. Marcy L. Sussman
Cindy Swords
John Syring
Joyce Tarzewski
Rinette Tavitri
Tracy Taylor
James B. Temme
Ellen S. Titen
Lyn Van Dervort
Cindy Wedel
Dr. Solve Welin
Annette Wendt
Thomas White
Jennifer Wilkes
Dr. A. Justin Williams
Linda Willman
Dr. Hudson J. Wilson, Jr.
Dr. Hugh M. Wilson
Deborah Wolfenberger
Dr. Ernest H. Wood
Ross J. Wright
Dr. Martin Yaffe
Dr. Judah Zizmor
Elizabeth Zuffuto

CONTENTS

MERRILL'S ATLAS

of

RADIOGRAPHIC POSITIONS

and

RADIOLOGIC PROCEDURES

VOLUME ONE

PRELIMINARY STEPS IN RADIOGRAPHY

RIGHT: Radiographic room from 1901, displayed in the Roentgen Museum, Lennep, Germany.

BELOW: Modern elevating radiographic table with chest unit.

(Courtesy Siemens Medical Systems, Inc.)

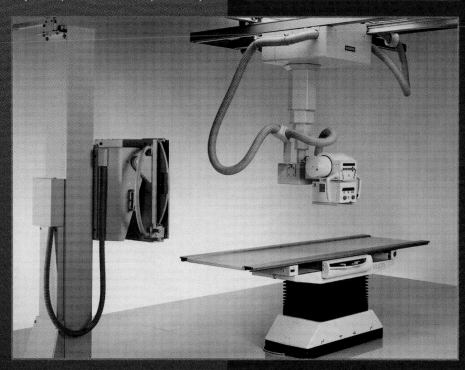

Ethics in Radiologic Technology

Ethics is the term applied to a health professional's moral responsibility and the science of appropriate conduct toward others. The work of the medical professional requires strict rules of conduct. The physician, who is responsible for the welfare of the patient, depends on the absolute honesty and integrity of all health care professionals to carry out orders and report mistakes.

The American Society of Radiologic Technologists (ASRT) developed the current code of ethics.[1] The Canadian Association of Medical Radiation Technologists (CAMRT) has also adopted a similar code of ethics.[2] All radiographers should familiarize themselves with these codes.

---

[1] Code of ethics, *Radiol Technol* 61:362,1990.
[2] CAMRT, *Personal communication,* Apr 1997.

ASRT CODE OF ETHICS

1. The radiologic technologist conducts himself or herself in a professional manner, responds to patient needs, and supports colleagues and associates in providing quality patient care.
2. The radiologic technologist acts to advance the principal objective of the profession to provide services to humanity with full respect for the dignity of mankind.
3. The radiologic technologist delivers patient care and service unrestricted by concerns of personal attributes or the nature of the disease or illness, and without discrimination, regardless of gender, race, creed, religion, or socioeconomic status.
4. The radiologic technologist practices technology founded on theoretic knowledge and concepts, utilizes equipment and accessories consistent with the purpose for which they have been designed, and employs procedures and techniques appropriately.
5. The radiologic technologist assesses situations; exercises care, discretion and judgment; assumes responsibility for professional decisions; and acts in the best interest of the patient.
6. The radiologic technologist acts as an agent through observation and communication to obtain pertinent information for the physician to aid in the diagnosis and treatment management of the patient, and recognizes that interpretation and diagnosis are outside the scope of practice for the profession.
7. The radiologic technologist utilizes equipment and accessories, employs techniques and procedures, performs services in accordance with an accepted standard of practice, and demonstrates expertise in minimizing the radiation exposure to the patient, self, and other members of the health care team.
8. The radiologic technologist practices ethical conduct appropriate to the profession and protects the patient's right to quality radiologic technology care.
9. The radiologic technologist respects confidence entrusted in the course of professional practice, respects the patient's right to privacy, and reveals confidential information only as required by law or to protect the welfare of the individual or the community.
10. The radiologic technologist continually strives to improve knowledge and skills by participating in educational and professional activities, sharing knowledge with colleagues, and investigating new and innovative aspects of professional practice. One means available to improve knowledge and skills is through professional continuing education.

CAMRT CODE OF ETHICS

The CAMRT recognizes its obligation to identify and promote professional standards of conduct and performance. The execution of such standards is the personal responsibility of each member.

The code of ethics, adopted in June 1991, requires every member to do the following:

- Provide service with dignity and respect to all people regardless of race, national or ethnic origin, color, gender, religion, age, type of illness, mental, or physical challenges.
- Encourage the trust and confidence of the public through high standards of professional competence, conduct, and appearance.
- Conduct all technical procedures with due regard to current radiation safety standards.
- Practice only those procedures for which the necessary qualifications are held unless such procedures have been properly delegated by an appropriate medical authority and for which the technologist has received adequate training to an acceptable level of competence.
- Practice only those disciplines of medical radiation technology for which he or she has been certified by the CAMRT and is currently competent.

- Be mindful that patients must seek diagnostic information from their treating physician. In those instances where a discreet comment to the appropriate authority may assist diagnosis or treatment, the technologist may feel morally obliged to provide one.
- Preserve and protect the confidentiality of any information, either medical or personal, acquired through professional contact with the patient. An exception may be appropriate when the disclosure of such information is necessary to the treatment of the patient, the safety of other patients and health care providers, or is a legal requirement.
- Cooperate with other health care providers.
- Advance the art and science of medical radiation technology through ongoing professional development.
- Recognize that the participation and support of our association is a professional responsibility.

Image Receptor

In radiography the *image receptor (IR)* is the device that receives the energy of the x-ray beam and forms the *image* of the body part. In diagnostic radiology, the IR will be one of the following three devices:

1. Cassette with film—First the film containing the image is removed from the cassette, requiring the use of a darkroom, and developed in a processor. Afterward the radiographic film image is ready for viewing on an illuminator.
2. Cassette with phosphor plate—First the phosphor plate stores the image. Next the cassette is inserted into a reader device, which does not require a darkroom. Then the radiographic image is converted to digital format and can be viewed on a computer monitor.
3. Fluoroscopic screen—The x-rays strike a fluoroscopic screen where the image is formed and the image of the body part is transmitted to a television monitor via a camera. This is a "real-time" device in which the body part is viewed live on a television.

Radiograph

Each step in performing a radiographic procedure must be completed accurately to ensure that the maximal amount of information is recorded on the image. The information that results from performing the radiographic examination generally demonstrates the presence or absence of abnormality or trauma. This information assists in the diagnosis and treatment of the patient. Accuracy and attention to detail are essential in every radiologic examination.

The radiographer must be thoroughly familiar with the radiographic densities cast by normal anatomy structures. To develop the ability to analyze radiographs properly and to correct or prevent errors in performing the examination, the radiographer should study radiographs from the following standpoints:

1. Superimposition—The relationship of the anatomic superimpositions to size, shape, position, and angulation must be reviewed.

2. Adjacent structures—Each anatomic structure must be compared with that of adjacent structures and reviewed to ensure that the structure is present and properly shown.

3. Optical density (OD)—Also known as the *degree of film blackening,* the optical density of the radiograph must be within a diagnostic range. If a radiograph is too light or dark, an accurate diagnosis becomes difficult or impossible (Fig. 1-1). If a change in technique is necessary, each of the following primary factors controlling density must be considered:
    * Milliamperage (mA)
    * Exposure time (second)
    * Milliampere-second (mAs)

4. Contrast—The contrast, or the difference in density between any two areas on a radiograph, must be sufficient to allow radiographic distinction of adjacent structures with different tissue densities. A wide range of contrast levels is produced among the variety of radiographic examinations performed (Fig. 1-2). A low-contrast image displays many density levels, and a high-contrast image displays few density levels. The primary controlling factor of radiographic contrast is kilovoltage peak (kVp).

5. Recorded detail—The recorded detail, or the ability to visualize small structures, must be sufficient to clearly demonstrate the desired anatomic part (Fig. 1-3). Recorded detail is primarily controlled by the following:
    * Geometry
    * Film
    * Distance
    * Screen
    * Focal spot size
    * Motion

A   B   C

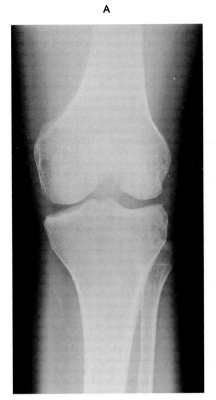 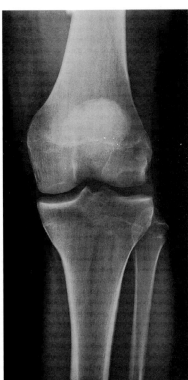 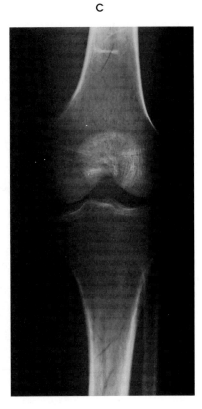

Fig. 1-1 Sufficient radiographic density is needed to make a diagnosis. **A,** Radiograph of the knee with insufficient density. It is too light to make a diagnosis and a repeat radiograph is needed. **B,** Radiograph of the knee with proper density. All bony aspects of the knee are seen, including soft tissue detail around the bone. **C,** Radiograph of the knee with too much density—diagnosis could not be made and a repeat radiograph is needed.

6. Magnification—The magnification of the body part must be evaluated, taking into account the controlling factors of *object-to-image receptor distance (OID)*, or how far the body part is from the IR, and *source-to-image receptor distance (SID)*, or how far the x-ray tube is from the IR. All radiographs yield some degree of magnification because all body parts are three dimensional.

7. Shape Distortion—The shape distortion of the body part must be analyzed, and the following primary controlling factors must be studied:
   - Alignment
   - Central ray
   - Anatomic part
   - IR
   - Angulation

An example of shape distortion is when a bone is projected longer or shorter than it actually is. *Distortion* is the misrepresentation of the size or shape of any anatomic structure.

A strong knowledge of anatomy and the ability to analyze radiographs correctly are paramount—especially to radiographers who work without a radiologist in constant attendance. In this situation the patient's physician must be able to depend on the radiographer to perform the technical phase of examinations without assistance.

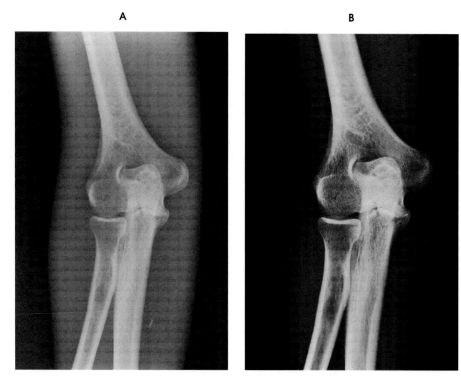

Fig. 1-2 Sufficient contrast is needed to make a diagnosis. Two different scales of contrast are shown on the elbow. **A,** Long scale (low contrast). **B,** Short scale (high contrast).

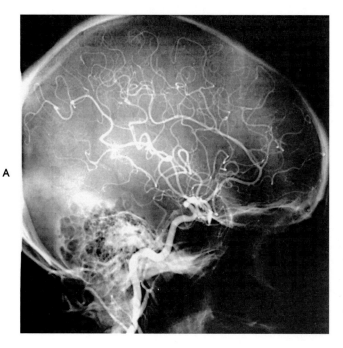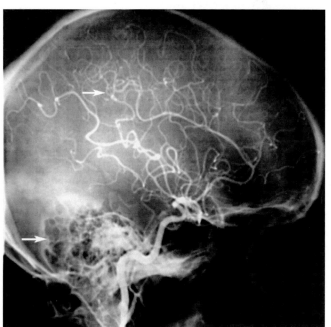

Fig. 1-3 Different levels of recorded detail. **A,** Excellent recorded detail is seen throughout this radiograph of the arteries in the head. **B,** Poor recorded detail. Note the fuzzy edges of the arteries and bony structures in this image *(arrows)*.

DISPLAY OF RADIOGRAPHS

Radiographs are generally displayed according to the preference of the interpreting physician. Because methods of displaying radiographic images have developed largely through custom, no fixed rules have been established. However, the radiologist, who is responsible for making a diagnosis based on the radiographic examination, and the radiographer, who performs the examination, follow traditional standards of practice regarding the placement of radiographs on the viewing device. In clinical practice, the viewing device is commonly called a *viewbox,* or *illuminator*.

ANATOMIC POSITION

Radiographs are usually placed on the illuminator and oriented so that the person looking at the image sees the body part placed in the anatomic position. The *anatomic position* refers to the patient standing erect with the face and eyes directed forward, arms extended by the sides with the palms of the hands facing forward, heels together, and toes pointing anteriorly (Fig. 1-4). When the radiograph is displayed in this manner, the patient's left side is on the viewer's right side and vice versa (Fig. 1-5). Professionals in medicine always describe the body, a body part, or a body movement as though it were in the anatomic position.

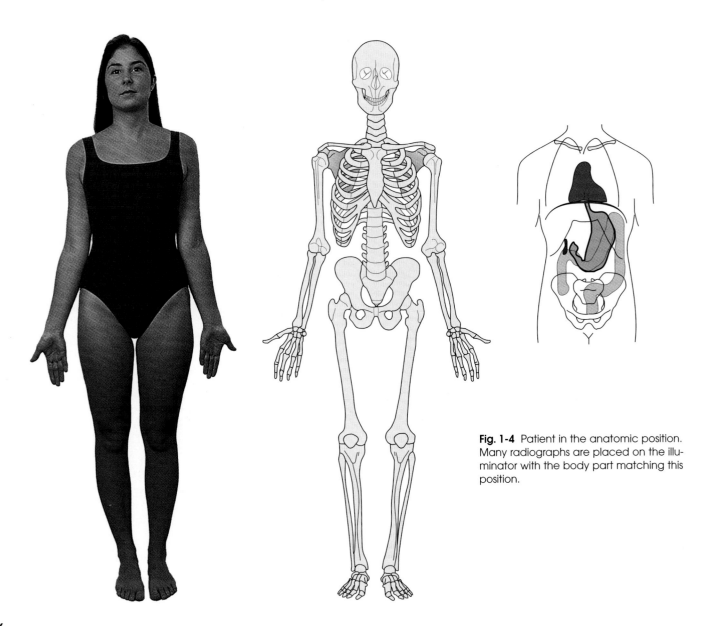

Fig. 1-4 Patient in the anatomic position. Many radiographs are placed on the illuminator with the body part matching this position.

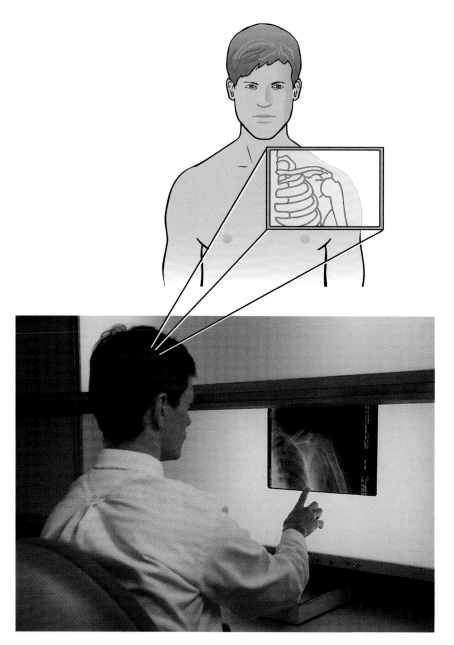

Fig. 1-5 A radiologist interpreting a radiograph of a patient's left shoulder. Note the radiograph is placed on the illuminator with the patient's left side on the viewer's right side. The radiologist spatially pictured the patient's anatomy in the anatomic position and then placed the radiograph on the illuminator in that position.

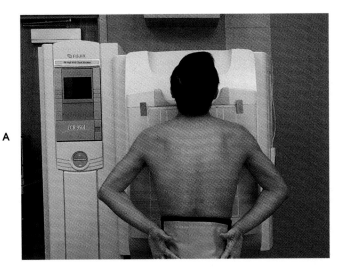
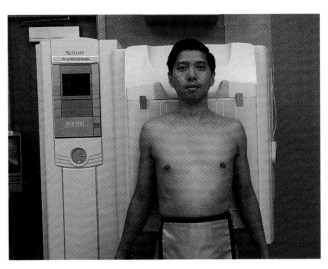

Fig. 1-6 A, A patient positioned for a posteroanterior (PA) projection of the chest. The anterior aspect of the chest is closest to the image receptor (IR). **B,** Patient positioned for an anteroposterior (AP) projection of the chest. The posterior aspect of the chest is closest to the IR.

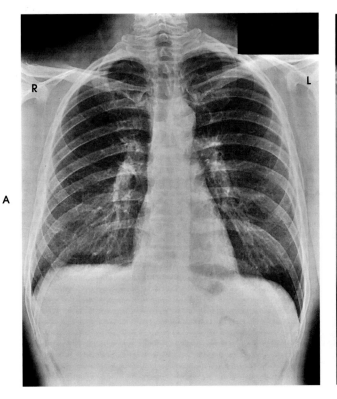
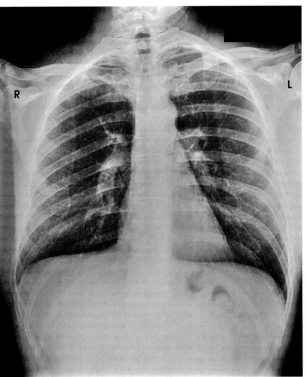

Fig. 1-7 A, Posteroanterior (PA) projection of the chest. **B,** Anteroposterior (AP) projection of the chest on the same patient as **A.** Both radiographs are correctly displayed with the anatomy in the anatomic position even though the patient was positioned differently. Note the patient's left side is on your right, as though the patient were facing you.

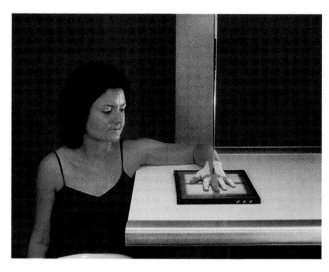

Fig. 1-8 Proper placement of patient and body part position for a posteroanterior (PA) projection of the left hand.

Posteroanterior and anteroposterior

Fig. 1-6, *A*, illustrates the anterior (front) aspect of the patient's chest placed closest to the IR for a posteroanterior (PA) projection. Fig. 1-6, *B*, illustrates the posterior (back) aspect of the patient's chest placed closest to the IR for an anteroposterior (AP) projection. Regardless of whether the anterior or posterior body surface is closest to the IR, the radiograph is usually placed in the anatomic position (Fig. 1-7). (Positioning terminology is fully described in Chapter 3.)

Exceptions to these guidelines include the hands, wrists, feet, and toes. Hand and wrist radiographs are routinely displayed with the digits (fingers) pointed to the ceiling. Foot and toe radiographs are also placed on the illuminator with the toes pointing to the ceiling. Hand, wrist, toe, and foot radiographs are viewed from the perspective of the x-ray tube, or exactly as the anatomy was projected onto the IR (Figs. 1-8 and 1-9). This perspective means that the individual looking at the radiograph is in the position of the x-ray tube.

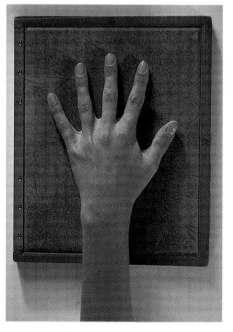

A

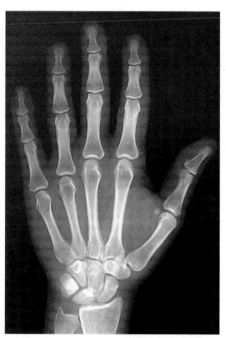

B

Fig. 1-9 A, Left hand positioned on IR. This view is from the perspective of the x-ray tube. **B,** Radiograph of the left hand is placed on the illuminator in the same manner, with the digits up.

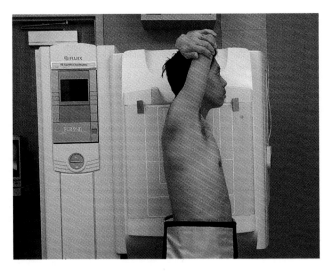

Fig. 1-10 Proper patient position for a left lateral chest. Note the left side of the patient is placed against the image receptor.

Lateral radiographs

Lateral radiographs are obtained with the patient's right or left side placed against the IR. They are generally placed on the illuminator in the same orientation as if the viewer were looking at the patient from the perspective of the x-ray tube at the side where the x-rays first enter the patient—exactly like radiographs of the hands, wrists, feet, and toes. Another way to describe this is to display the radiograph so that the side of the patient closest to the IR during the procedure is also the side in the image closest to the illuminator. For example, a patient positioned for a left lateral chest radiograph is depicted in Fig. 1-10. The resulting left lateral chest radiograph is placed on the illuminator as shown in Fig. 1-11. A right lateral chest position and its accompanying radiograph would be positioned and displayed the opposite of that shown in Figs. 1-10 and 1-11.

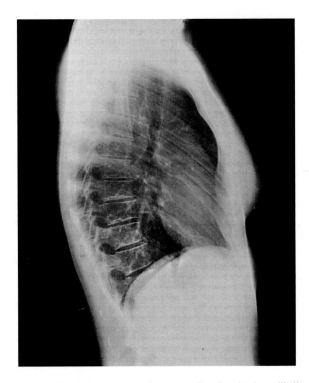

Fig. 1-11 Left lateral chest radiograph placed on the illuminator with the anatomy seen from the perspective of the x-ray tube.

Oblique radiographs

Oblique radiographs are obtained when the patient's body is rotated so that the projection obtained is not frontal, posterior, or lateral (Fig. 1-12). These radiographs are viewed with the patient's anatomy placed in the anatomic position (Fig. 1-13).

Other radiographs

Many other less commonly performed radiographic projections are described throughout this book. The most common method of displaying the radiograph that is used in the radiology department and most clinical practice areas is generally either in the anatomic position or from the perspective of the x-ray tube; however, exceptions do occur. Some physicians prefer to view all radiographs from the perspective of the x-ray tube rather than in the anatomic position. A neurosurgeon, for example, operates on the posterior aspect of the body and therefore does not display spine radiographs in the anatomic position or from the perspective of the x-ray tube. The radiographs are displayed with the patient's right side on the surgeon's right side as though looking at the posterior aspect of the patient. What the surgeon sees on the radiograph is exactly what is seen in the open body part during the surgery.

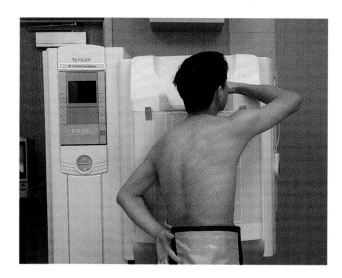

Fig. 1-12 A patient placed in the left anterior oblique (LAO) position for a posteroanterior (PA) oblique projection of the chest.

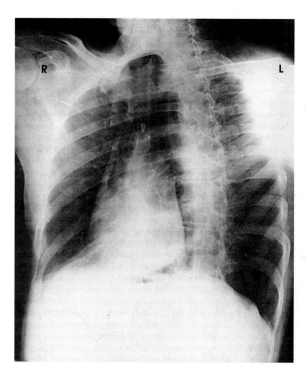

Fig. 1-13 Posteroanterior (PA) oblique chest radiograph is placed on the illuminator with the anatomy in the anatomic position. Note that the patient's left side is on your right, as though the patient were facing you.

Clinical History

The radiographer is responsible for performing radiographic examinations according to the standard department procedure except when contraindicated by the patient's condition. The radiologist is a physician who is board certified to read, or interpret, x-ray examinations. As the demand for the radiologist's time increases, less time is available to devote to the technical aspects of radiology. This situation makes the radiologist more dependent on the radiographer to perform the technical aspects of patient care. The additional responsibility makes it necessary for the radiographer to know the following:

- Normal anatomy and normal anatomic variations so that the patient can be accurately positioned
- The radiographic characteristics of numerous common abnormalities

Although the radiographer is not responsible for explaining the cause, diagnosis, or treatment of the disease, the radiographer's professional responsibility is to produce an image that makes the abnormality evident.

When the physician does not see the patient, the radiographer is responsible for obtaining the necessary clinical history and observing any apparent abnormality that might affect the radiographic result. Examples include noting jaundice in gallbladder examinations, body surface masses possibly casting a density that could be mistaken for internal changes, tattoos that contain ferrous pigment, surface scars that may be visible radiographically, and some decorative or ornamental tee shirts. The physician should give specific instructions about what information is needed if the radiographer assumes this responsibility.

The requisition received by the radiographer should clearly identify the exact region to be radiographed and the suspected or existing diagnosis. The patient must be positioned and the exposure factors selected according to the region involved and the radiographic characteristics of the existent abnormality. Radiographers must understand the rationale behind the examination; otherwise, radiographs of diagnostic value cannot be produced. Having the information in advance prevents delay, inconvenience, and much more important, the unnecessary radiation exposure to the patient.

Initial Examination

The radiographs obtained for the initial examination of each body part are based on the anatomy or function of the part and the type of abnormality indicated by the clinical history. The radiographs obtained for the initial examination are usually the minimum required to detect any demonstrable abnormality in the region. Supplemental studies for further investigation are then made as needed. This method saves time, eliminates unnecessary radiographs, and reduces patient exposure to radiation.

Diagnosis and the Radiographer

A patient is naturally anxious about examination results and will ask questions. The radiographer should tactfully advise the patient that the referring physician will receive the report as soon as the radiographs have been interpreted by the radiologist. Referring physicians may also ask the radiographer questions, and they should be instructed to contact the interpreting radiologist.

Care of the Radiographic Examining Room

The radiographic examining room should be as scrupulously clean as any other room used for medical purposes. The mechanical parts of the x-ray machine such as the table sides and the supporting structure and the collimator should be wiped with a clean, damp (not soaked) cloth every day. The metal parts of the machine should be periodically cleaned with a disinfectant. The overhead system, x-ray tube, and other parts that conduct electricity should be cleaned with alcohol or a clean, dry cloth. Water is never used to clean electrical parts.

The tabletop should be cleaned after each examination. Cones, collimators, compression devices, gonad shields, and other accessories should be cleaned daily and after any contact with a patient. Adhesive tape residue left on cassettes and cassette stands should be removed and the cassette disinfected. Cassettes should be protected from patients who are bleeding, and disposable protective covers should be manipulated so that they do not come in contact with ulcers or other discharging lesions. Use of stained or damaged cassettes is inexcusable and does not represent a professional atmosphere.

The radiographic room should be prepared for the examination before the patient arrives. The room should look clean and organized—not disarranged from the previous examination (Fig. 1-14). Fresh linen should be put on the table and pillow, and accessories needed during the examination should be placed nearby. Performing these preexamination steps requires only a few minutes but creates a positive, lasting impression on the patient; however, not performing these steps beforehand leaves a negative impression.

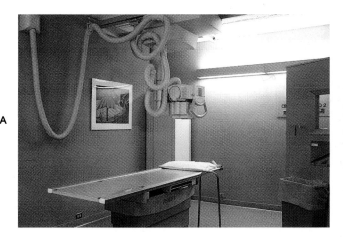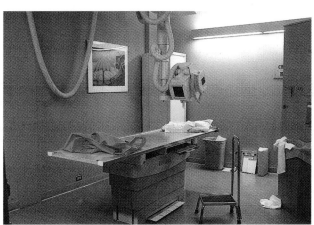

Fig. 1-14 A, The radiographic room should always be clean and straightened before beginning any examination begins. **B,** This room is not ready to receive a patient. Note devices stored on the floor and previous patient's gowns and towels laying on the table. Room does not present a welcoming sight for a patient.

Universal Precautions

Radiographers are engaged in caring for sick people and therefore should be thoroughly familiar with *universal precautions*. They should know the way to handle patients who are on isolation status without contaminating their hands, clothing, or apparatus, and radiographers must know the method of disinfecting these items when they become contaminated.

Hand washing is the easiest and most convenient method of preventing the spread of microorganisms. Radiographers should wash their hands before and after each patient. Hands must always be washed, without exception, in the following specific situations:

- After examining patients with known communicable diseases
- After coming in contact with blood or body fluids
- Before beginning invasive procedures
- Before touching patients who are at risk of infections

As one of the first steps in aseptic technique, radiographers' hands should be kept smooth and free from roughness or chapping by the frequent use of soothing lotions. All abrasions should be protected by bandages to prevent the entrance of bacteria.

For the protection of radiographers' and patients' health, the laws of asepsis and prophylaxis must be obeyed. Radiographers should practice scrupulous cleanliness when handling all patients, whether the patients are known to have an infectious disease or not. If a radiographer is to examine the patient's head, face, or teeth, the patient should ideally see the radiographer perform hand washing. If this is not possible, the radiographer should perform hand washing and then enter the room drying the hands with a fresh towel. If the patient's face is to come in contact with the IR front or table, the patient should see the radiographer clean the device with a disinfectant or cover it with a clean drape.

A sufficient supply of gowns and disposable gloves should be kept in the radiographic room to be used to care for infectious patients. After examining infectious patients, radiographers must wash their hands in warm, running water and soapsuds and rinse and dry them thoroughly. If the sink is not equipped with a knee control for the water supply, the radiographer opens the valve of the faucet with a paper towel. After proper hand washing, the radiographer closes the valve of the faucet with a paper towel.

Before bringing an isolation unit patient to the radiology department, the transporter should drape the stretcher or wheelchair with a clean sheet to prevent contamination of anything the patient might touch. When the patient must be transferred to the radiographic table, the table should be draped with a sheet. The edges of the sheet may then be folded back over the patient so that the radiographer can position the patient through the clean side of the sheet without becoming contaminated.

A folded sheet should be placed over the end of the stretcher or table to protect the IRs when a non-Bucky technique is used. The IR is then placed between the clean fold of the sheet, and with the hands between the clean fold, the radiographer can position the patient through the sheet. If the radiographer must handle the patient directly, an assistant should position the tube and operate the equipment to prevent contamination. If a patient has any moisture or body fluids on the body surface that could come in contact with the IR, a non–moisture-penetrable material must be used to cover the IR.

When the examination is finished, the contaminated linen should be folded with the clean side out and returned to the patient's room with the patient. There it will receive the special attention given to linen used for isolation unit patients or be disposed of according to the established policy of the institution.

Centers for Disease Control and Prevention

For the protection of health care workers, the Centers for Disease Control and Prevention (CDC) has issued recommendations for handling blood and other body fluids. According to the CDC, all human blood and certain body fluids should be treated as if they contain pathogenic microorganisms (Table 1-1). These precautions should apply to all contacts involving patients. Health care workers should wear gloves whenever they come into contact with blood, mucous membranes, wounds, and any surface or body fluid containing blood. For any procedure in which blood or other body fluids may be sprayed or splashed, the radiographer should wear a mask, protective eyewear (such as eye shields and goggles), and a gown.

Health care workers must be cautious to prevent needle stick injuries. Needles should never be recapped, bent, broken, or clipped. Instead, they should be placed in a puncture-proof container and properly discarded.

Disinfectants and Antiseptics

Chemical substances that kill pathogenic bacteria are classified as *germicides* and *disinfectants* (e.g., dilute bleach is sometimes used as a disinfectant). Disinfection is the process of killing only those microorganisms that are pathogenic. The objection to the use of many chemical disinfectants is that to be effective, they must be used in solutions so strong that they damage the material being disinfected. Chemical substances that inhibit the growth of without necessarily killing pathogenic microorganisms are called *antiseptics*. Alcohol, which is commonly used for medical or practical asepsis in medical facilities, has antiseptic but not disinfectant properties. Sterilization, which is usually performed by means of heat or chemicals, is the destruction of all microorganisms.

Operating Room

A radiographer who has not had extensive patient care education must exercise extreme caution to prevent contaminating sterile objects in the operating room. The radiographer should perform hand washing and wear scrub clothing, a scrub cap and a mask and should survey the particular setup in the operating room before taking in the x-ray equipment. By taking this precaution, the radiographer can ensure that sufficient space is available to do the work without the danger of contamination. If necessary, the radiographer should ask the circulating nurse to move any sterile items. Because of the danger of contamination of the sterile field, sterile supplies, and persons scrubbed for the procedure, the radiographer should never approach the operative side of the surgical table unless directed to do so.

After checking the room setup, the radiographer should thoroughly wipe the x-ray equipment with a damp (not soaked) cloth before taking it into the operating room. The radiographer moves the mobile machine, or C-arm unit, to the free side of the operating table—the side opposite the surgeon, scrub nurse, and sterile layout. The machine should be maneuvered into a general position that will make the final adjustments easy when the surgeon is ready to proceed with the examination.

The cassette is placed in a sterile covering, depending on the type of examination to be performed. The surgeon or one of the assistants holds the sterile case open while the radiographer gently drops the cassette into it while being careful not to touch the sterile case. The radiographer may then give directions for positioning and securing the cassette for the exposure.

The radiographer should make the necessary arrangements with the operating room supervisor when performing work that requires the use of a tunnel or other special equipment. When a cassette is being prepared for the patient, any tunnel or grid should be placed on the table with the tray opening to the side of the table opposite the sterile field. With the cooperation of the surgeon and operating room supervisor, a system can be developed for performing radiographic examinations accurately and quickly without moving the patient or endangering the sterile field.

TABLE 1-1

Body fluids that may contain pathogenic microorganisms

Blood	Synovial fluid
Any fluid containing blood	Cerebrospinal fluid
Amniotic fluid	Semen fluid
Pericardial fluid	Vaginal fluid
Pleural fluid	

Minor Surgical Procedures in the Radiology Department

Procedures that require a rigid aseptic technique, such as cystography, intravenous urography, spinal punctures, angiography, and angiocardiography, are performed in the radiology department (Fig. 1-15). Although the physician needs the assistance of a nurse in certain procedures, the radiographer can make the necessary preparations and provide assistance in many procedures.

For procedures that do not require a nurse, the radiographer should know which surgical instruments and supplies are needed and the way to prepare and sterilize them. Radiographers may make arrangements with the surgical supervisor to acquire the education necessary to perform these procedures.

Procedure Book

A procedure or protocol book covering every examination performed in the radiology department is essential. Under the appropriate heading, each procedure should be outlined and state the staff required and duties of each member of the team. A listing of sterile and nonsterile items should also be included. A copy of the sterile instrument requirements should be given to the supervisor of the central sterile supply department to facilitate preparation of the trays for each procedure.

Bowel Preparation

Radiologic examinations involving the abdomen often require that the entire colon be cleansed before the examination so that diagnostic quality radiographs can be obtained. The patient's colon may be cleansed by one or any combination of the following:

- Limited diet
- Laxatives
- Enemas

The technique used to cleanse the patient's colon generally is selected by the medical facility or physician. The patient should be questioned about any bowel preparation that may have been completed before an abdominal procedure is begun. For additional information on bowel preparation, see Chapter 17, Volume 2.

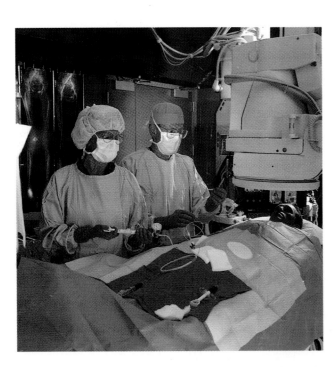

Fig. 1-15 Many radiographic procedures require strict aseptic technique, such as seen in this procedure involving passing a catheter into the patient's femoral artery.

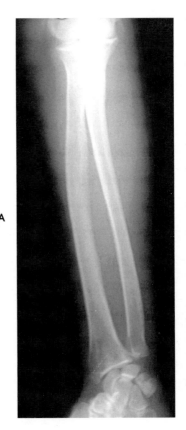
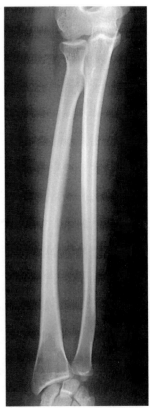

A

B

Fig. 1-16 A, Forearm radiograph of a patient who moved during the exposure. Note the fuzzy appearance of the edges of the bones. **B,** Radiograph of the patient without motion.

Motion and Its Control

Patient motion plays a large role in radiography (Fig. 1-16). Because motion is the result of muscle action, the radiographer needs to know some information about the functions of various muscles. The radiographer should use this knowledge to eliminate or control motion for the exposure time necessary to complete a satisfactory examination. The three types of muscular tissue that affect motion are the following:
- Smooth (involuntary)
- Cardiac (involuntary)
- Striated (voluntary)

INVOLUNTARY MUSCLES

The visceral (organ) muscles are composed of *smooth* muscular tissue and are controlled partially by the autonomic nervous system and the muscles' inherent characteristics of rhythmic contractility. By their rhythmic contraction and relaxation, these muscles perform the movement of the internal organs. The rhythmic action of the muscular tissue of the alimentary tract, called *peristalsis*, is normally more active in the stomach (about three or four waves per minute) and gradually diminishes along the intestine. The specialized *cardiac* muscular tissue functions by contracting the heart to pump blood into the arteries and expanding or relaxing to permit the heart to receive blood from the veins. The pulse rate of the heart varies with emotions, exercise, diet, size, age, and gender.

Involuntary motion is caused by the following:
- Heart pulsation
- Chill
- Peristalsis
- Tremor
- Spasm
- Pain

Involuntary muscle control

The primary method of reducing involuntary motion is to control the length of exposure time—the less exposure time to the patient, the better.

VOLUNTARY MUSCLES

The voluntary, or skeletal, muscles are composed of *striated* muscular tissue and are controlled by the central nervous system. These muscles perform the movements of the body initiated by the individual. In radiography the patient's body must be positioned in such a way that the skeletal muscles are relaxed. The patient's comfort level is a good guide to determine the success of the position.

Voluntary motion resulting from lack of control is caused by the following:
- Nervousness
- Discomfort
- Excitability
- Mental illness
- Fear
- Age
- Breathing

Voluntary muscle control

The radiographer can control voluntary patient motion by the following:
- Giving clear instructions
- Providing patient comfort
- Adjusting support devices
- Applying immobilization

Decreasing the length of exposure time is the best way to control voluntary motion that results from mental illness or the age of the patient. Immobilization for limb radiography can often be obtained for the duration of the exposure by having the patient phonate an *mmm* sound with the mouth closed or an *ahhh* sound with the mouth open. The radiographer should always be watching the patient during the exposure to ensure that the exposure is made during suspended respiration. Sponges and sandbags are commonly used as immobilization devices (Fig. 1-17).

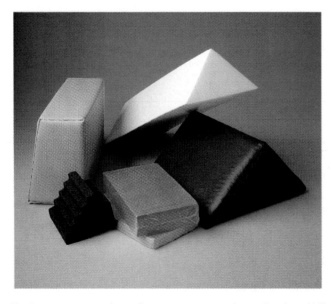

Fig. 1-17 Positioning sponges and sandbags are commonly used as immobilization devices.

Patient Instructions

When an examination requires preparation such as in kidney and gastrointestinal examinations, the radiographer must carefully instruct the patient. Although the particular examination or procedure may be repetitive to the radiographer, it is new to the patient. Frequently, what a radiographer interprets as patient stupidity results from lack of sufficiently explicit directions. The radiographer must be sure that the patient understands not only what to do but also why it has to be done. A patient is more likely to follow instructions correctly the reason for the instructions is clear. If the instructions are complicated, they should be written out and verbally reviewed with the patient if necessary. For example, few patients know the way to give themselves an enema correctly, so the radiographer should question the patient and, when necessary, take the time to explain the correct procedure. This approach often saves film, time, and radiation exposure to the patient.

Patient's Attire, Ornaments, and Surgical Dressings

The patient should be dressed in a gown that allows exposure of limited body regions under examination. A patient is never exposed unnecessarily; a sheet should be used when appropriate. If a region of the body needs to be exposed to complete the examination, only the area under examination should be uncovered while the rest of the patient's body is completely covered for warmth and privacy. When the radiographer is examining parts that must remain covered, disposable paper gowns or cotton cloth gowns without metal or plastic snaps are preferred (Fig. 1-18). If washable gowns are used, they should not be starched; starch is somewhat *radiopaque*, which means it cannot be penetrated easily by x-rays. Any folds in the cloth should be straightened to prevent confusing densities on the radiograph. The length of exposure should also be considered. Material that does not cast a density on a heavy exposure, such as that used on an adult abdomen, may show clearly on a light exposure, such as that used on a child's abdomen.

Any radiopaque object should be removed from the region to be radiographed. Zippers, necklaces, snaps, thick elastic, and buttons should be removed when radiographs of the chest and abdomen are produced (Fig. 1-19). When radiographing the skull, the radiographer must make sure that dentures, removable bridgework, earrings, necklaces, and all hairpins are removed.

When the abdomen, pelvis, or hips of an infant are radiographed, the diaper should be removed. Because some diaper rash ointments are somewhat radiopaque the area may need to be cleansed before the procedure.

Surgical dressings such as metallic salves and adhesive tape should be examined for radiopaque substances. If permission to remove the dressings has not been obtained or the radiographer does not know the way to remove them and the radiology department physician is not present, the surgeon or nurse should be asked to accompany the patient to the radiology department to remove the dressings. When dressings are removed, the radiographer should always make sure that a cover of sterile gauze adequately protects open wounds.

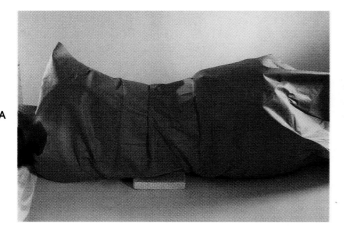 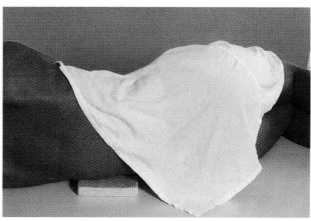

Fig. 1-18 A, A female patient wearing a disposable paper gown and positioned for a lateral projection of the lumbar spine. Private areas are completely covered. The gown is smoothed around the contour of the body for accurate positioning. **B,** The same patient wearing a traditional cloth hospital gown. The gown is positioned for maximal privacy.

Handling of Patients

Patients who are coherent and capable of understanding deserve an explanation of the procedure to be performed. Patients should understand exactly what is expected and be made comfortable. If patients are apprehensive about the examination, their fears should be alleviated. However, if the procedure will cause discomfort or be unpleasant, such as with cystoscopy and intravenous injections, the radiographer should calmly and truthfully explain the procedure. Patients should be told that it will cause some discomfort or be unpleasant, but because the procedure is a necessary part of the examination, full cooperation is needed. Patients usually respond favorably if they understand that all steps are being taken to alleviate discomfort.

Because the entire procedure may be a new experience, patients usually respond incorrectly when given more than one instruction at a time. For example, when instructed to get up on the table and lie on the abdomen, patients may get onto the table in the most awkward possible manner and lie on their backs. Instead of asking patients to get onto the table in a specific position, the radiographer should first have patients sit on the table and then give instructions on assuming the desired position. If patients sit on the table first, the position can be assumed with less strain and fewer awkward movements. The radiographer should never rush a patient. If patients feel hurried, they will be nervous and less able to cooperate. When moving and adjusting patients into position, the radiographer should manipulate the patients gently but firmly; a light touch can be as irritating as one that is too firm. Patients should be instructed and allowed to do as much of the moving as possible.

X-ray grids move under the radiographic table, and with floating or moving tabletops, patients may injure their fingers. To reduce the possibility of injury, the radiographer should inform patients to keep their fingers on top of the table at all times. Regardless of the part being examined, the patient's entire body must be adjusted with resultant motion or rotation to prevent muscle pull in the area of interest. When patients are in an oblique (angled) position, the radiographer should use support devices and adjust the patients to relieve any strain. Immobilization devices and compression bands should be used whenever necessary but not to the point of discomfort. The radiographer should be cautious when releasing a compression band over the abdomen and should perform the procedure slowly.

In making final adjustments on a patient's position, the radiographer should stand with the eyes in line with the position of the x-ray tube, visualize the internal structures, and adjust the part accordingly. Though few rules on positioning patients are few, many repeat examinations can be eliminated by following these guidelines.

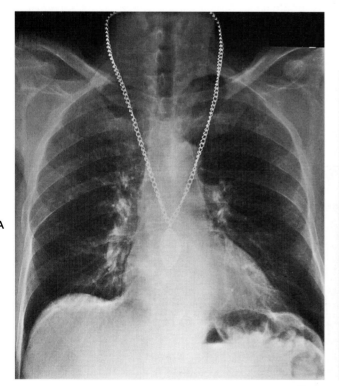

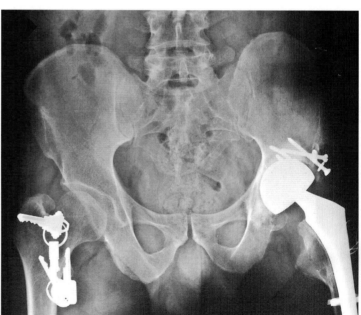

Fig. 1-19 A, A necklace was left on for this chest radiograph. **B,** Keys were left in the pocket of a lightweight hospital robe during the examination of this patient's pelvis. Both radiographs had to be repeated because the metal objects were not removed before the examination.

ILL OR INJURED PATIENTS

Great care must be exercised in handling trauma patients, particularly those with skull, spinal, and long bone injuries. A physician should perform any necessary manipulation to prevent the possibility of fragment displacement. The positioning technique should be adapted to each patient and necessitate as little movement as possible. If the tube-part-imaging plane relationship is maintained, the resultant projection will be the same regardless of the patient's position.

When a patient who is too sick to move alone must be moved, the following considerations should be kept in mind:

1. Move the patient as little as possible.
2. Never try to lift a helpless patient alone.
3. To prevent straining the back muscles when lifting a heavy patient, flex the knees, straighten the back, and bend from the hips.
4. When a patient's shoulders are lifted, the head should be supported. While holding the head with one hand, slide the opposite arm under the shoulders and grasp the axilla so that the head can rest on the bend of the elbow when the patient is raised.

5. When moving the patient's hips, first flex the patient's knees. In this position, patients may be able to raise themselves. If not, lifting the body when the patient's knees are bent is easier.
6. When helpless patients must be transferred to the radiographic table from a stretcher or bed, they should be moved on a sheet by at least four and preferably six people. The stretcher is placed parallel to and touching the table. Under ideal circumstances, at least three people should be stationed on the side of the stretcher and two on the far side of the radiographic table to grasp the sheet at the shoulder and hip levels. One person should support the patient's head and another the feet. When the signal is given, all six should smoothly and slowly lift and move the patient in unison (Fig. 1-20).

Many hospitals now have a specially equipped radiographic room adjoining the emergency department. These units often have special radiographic equipment and stretchers with radiolucent tops that allow severely injured patients to be examined on the stretcher and in the position in which they arrive. A mobile radiographic machine is often taken into the emergency department and radiographs are exposed there. Where this ideal emergency setup does not exist, trauma patients are often conveyed to the main radiology department. There they must be given precedence over nonemergency patients.

Preexposure Instructions

The radiographer should instruct the patient in breathing and have the patient practice until the needed actions are clearly understood. After the patient is in position but before the radiographer leaves to make the exposure, the radiographer should have the patient practice breathing once more. This step requires a few minutes, but it saves much time and the need for repeat radiographs.

Inspiration (inhalation) depresses the diaphragm and abdominal viscera, lengthens and expands the lung fields, elevates the sternum and pushes it anteriorly, and elevates the ribs and reduces their angle near the spine. *Expiration* (exhalation) elevates the diaphragm and abdominal viscera, shortens the lung fields, depresses the sternum, and lowers the ribs and increases their angle near the spine.

During trunk examinations the patient's phase of breathing is important. When exposures are to be made during shallow breathing, the patient should practice slow, even breathing, so that only the structures above the one being examined move. When lung motion and not rib motion is desired, the patient should practice slow, deep breathing after a compression band has been applied across the chest. (The correct *respiration phase* is printed in the positioning instructions for each projection in the text.)

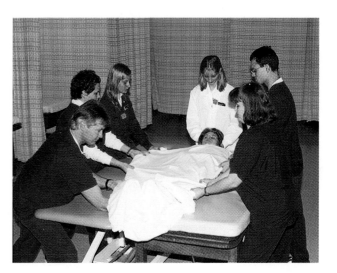

Fig. 1-20 Technique for a six-person transfer on a patient who is unable to move from a cart to the procedure table. Note the person holding and supporting the head.

Foundation Exposure Techniques and Charts

Specific exposure techniques are not included in this text; too many variable factors are involved, not only from one department to another but from one unit to another within the same department. A satisfactory technique can only be established by the radiographer's familiarity with the characteristics of the particular equipment and accessories used and the radiologist's preference in image quality. The following primary factors must be taken into account when the correct foundation technique is being established for each unit:

- Milliamperage (mA)
- Kilovolt (peak) (kVp)
- Exposure time (seconds)
- Automatic exposure controls (AEC)
- Source-to-image receptor distance (SID)
- Grid
- Film and screen speed number
- Electrical supply

With this information available, the exposure factors can be selected for each region of the body and balanced so that the best possible radiographic quality is obtained.

An exposure technique chart should be placed in every radiographic room and on mobile machines including those that use AEC and computed radiography (CR).[1-3] The chart should be organized to display all the radiographic projections performed in the room. The specific exposure factors for each projection should also be indicated (Fig. 1-21).

---

[1] Eastman TR: Digital systems require x-ray charts too, *Radiol Technol* 67:354, 1996.
[2] Gray JE et al: *Quality control in diagnostic imaging,* Rockville, Md, 1983, Aspen.
[3] Eastman TR: Get back to the basics of radiography, *Radiol Technol* 68:285, 1997.

Adaptation of Exposure Technique to Patient

The radiographer's responsibility is to select the combination of exposure factors that produces the desired quality of radiographs for each region of the body and to standardize this quality. Once the radiographer establishes this standard quality, deviation from the exposure factors should be minimal. These foundation factors should be adjusted for every patient's size to maintain uniform quality. However, the same definition on all subjects cannot be achieved because of congenital and developmental factors and age and pathologic changes. Some patients have fine, distinct bony trabecular markings; whereas others do not. Individual differences must be considered when the quality of the radiograph is judged.

Certain pathologic conditions require the radiographer to compensate when establishing an exposure technique. Selected conditions that require a decrease in technical factors include the following:

- Old age
- Pneumothorax
- Emphysema
- Emaciation
- Degenerative arthritis
- Atrophy

Some conditions require an increase in technical factors to penetrate the part to be examined, such as the following:

- Pneumonia
- Pleural effusion
- Hydrocephalus
- Enlarged heart
- Edema
- Ascites

ROUTINE RADIOGRAPHIC TECHNIQUE CHART

Examination	Time	mA	kVp	mAs	SID	Cassette
Skull All are Bucky or Grid						
AP and LAT (Adult)	.15	200	1/2	30.0	48"	24 x 30 cm
Towne (Adult)	.15	200	1/2	30.0	48"	24 x 30 cm
Shoulder						
Shoulder AP	.050	200	1/2	10.0	48"	24 x 30 cm
Neer View	.050	200	1/2	10.0	48"	24 x 30 cm
Axillary GRID	.050	200	1/2	10.0	48"	10 x 12 in
Scapula AP & LAT OBL	.080	200	1/2	16.0	48"	24 x 30 cm
Clavical	.050	200	1/2	10.0	48"	24 x 30 cm
Humerus	.050	200	1/2	10.0	48"	35 x 43 cm
West Point Dual 25° Angles NO GRID	.025	200	1/2	5.0	48"	24 x 30 cm
Dialysis Shoulder	.037	200	1/2	7.4	48"	24 x 30 cm
Stryker Notch 10° ↑	.15	200	1/2	30.0	48"	8 x 10 in

Fig. 1-21 Radiographic exposure technique chart showing the technical factors for the examinations identified.

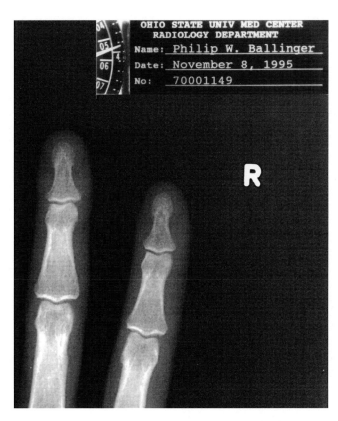

Fig. 1-22 All radiographs must be permanently identified and should contain a minimum of four identification markings.

Identification of Radiographs

All radiographs must to include the following information (Fig. 1-22):

• Date
• Patient's name or identification number
• Right or left marker
• Institution identity

Correct identification is paramount and should always be confirmed. Identification is vital in comparison studies, on follow-up examinations, and in medicolegal and compensation cases. Radiographers should develop the habit of rechecking the identification marker just before placing it on the IR. The CR systems introduced in recent years use a computer in the radiography room. The radiographer inputs the patient's identification and other data directly on each radiograph via the computer (Fig. 1-23).

Other patient identification markings may include the patient's age or date of birth, time of day, and the name of the radiographer or attending physician. For certain examinations, the radiograph should include such markings as cumulative time after introduction of contrast medium (e.g., 5 minute postinjection) and the level of the fulcrum (e.g., 9 cm) in tomography,. Other radiographs are marked to indicate the position of the patient (e.g., upright, decubitus) or other markings specified by the institution.

Numerous methods of marking films for identification are available. These methods include radiographing it along with the part, "flashing" it onto the film in the darkroom or examination room before development, writing it on the film after it has been processed, perforating the information on the film, or using the specialty cassette-marking systems designed for accurate and efficient operation.

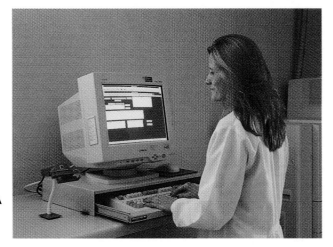

A

BALDWIN RADIOLOGY

0-000-000
FRANK EUGENE D   [M]
EXP:1997.11.14   SCALE:100% RT-0

B

Fig. 1-23 A, A radiographer using a computed radiography system and entering a patient's identification data into a computer in the radiography room. **B,** The resulting laser image showing the patient's information.

Image Receptor Placement

The part to be examined is usually centered to the center point of the IR or to the position where the angulation of the central ray will project it to the center. The IR should be adjusted so that its long axis lies parallel with the long axis of the part being examined. Although a long bone angled across the radiograph does not impair the diagnostic value of the image, such an arrangement can be aesthetically distracting.

Even though the lesion may be known to be at the midbody (central portion) of a long bone, an IR large enough to include at least one joint should be used on all long bone studies. This method is the only means of determining the precise position of the part and localizing the lesion. Many institutions require that both joints be demonstrated when a long bone is initially radiographed. For tall patients, two exposures may be required, one for the long bone and joint closest to the area of concern and a second to demonstrate the joint at the opposite end.

An IR just large enough to cover the region under examination should always be used. In addition to being extravagant, large IRs include extraneous parts that detract from the appearance of the radiograph and, more important, cause unnecessary radiation exposure to the patient.

A standard rule in radiography is to place the object as close to the IR as possible. For example, when obtaining lateral images of the middle and ring fingers, the radiographer increases the OID so that the part lies parallel with the IR. In some situations this rule is modified. Although magnification is greater, less distortion occurs. The radiographer can increase the SID to compensate for the increase in OID, thus reducing magnification. In certain instances, intentional magnification is desirable. It is obtained by positioning and supporting the object between the IR and the focal spot of the tube. This procedure is known as *magnification radiography*.

For ease of comparison, bilateral examinations of small body parts may be placed on one IR. However, exact duplication of the location of the images on the film is difficult if the IR is not marked accurately. Many IRs have permanent markings on the edges to assist the radiographer in equally spacing multiple images on one IR. Depending on the size and shape of the body part being radiographed, the IR can be divided in half either transversely or longitudinally. In some instances, the IR may be divided into thirds or fourths (Fig. 1-24).

However, body parts *must* always be identified by right or left side and placed on the IR in the same manner, either facing or backing each other, according to established routines. The radiographer plans the exposures so that the image identification marker will not interfere with the part of interest.

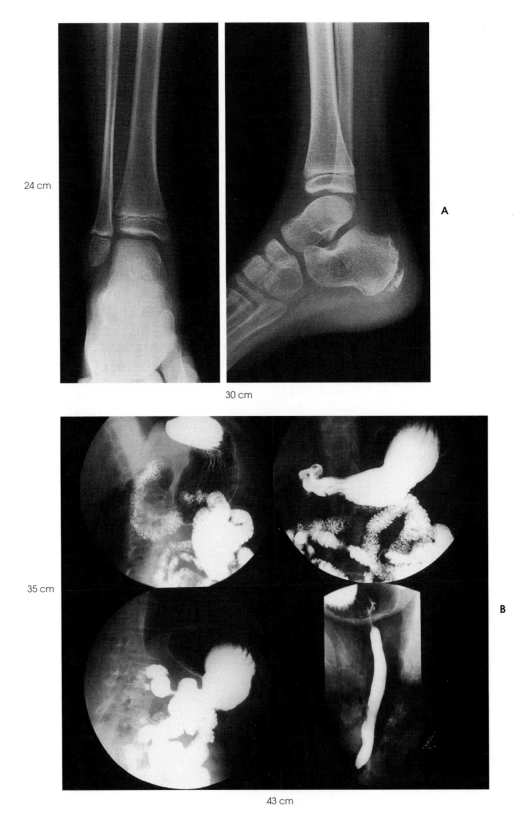

Fig. 1-24 Examples of multiple exposures on one film. **A,** AP and lateral projections of the ankle radiographically exposed side by side on a 24 x 30 cm film. **B,** Four projections of the stomach directly imaged on a 35 x 43 cm film.

English-Metric Conversion and Film Sizes

Measures are the standards used to determine size. People in the United States and a few other countries use standards that belong to the customary, or English, system of measurement. Although this system was developed in England, people in nearly all other countries, including England, now use the metric system of measurement.

In the past couple of decades, efforts have been made to convert all English measurements to the world standard metric system. These efforts have not been particularly effective. Nevertheless, total conversion to the metric system most likely will occur in the future.

The following information is provided to assist the radiographer in converting measurements from the English system to the metric system and vice versa:
- 1 inch = 2.54 centimeters (cm)
- 1 cm = 0.3937 inch
- 40 inch SID = 1 meter (m) (approximately)

Radiographic film is manufactured in both English and metric sizes. Most sizes used in the United States have recently been converted to metric. (Table 1-2 lists the most common film sizes used in radiology departments in the United States along with their general usage.) However, 4 of the 11 common sizes continue to be manufactured in an English size. The 24 × 30 cm size has replaced the 10 × 12 inch size. However, the 10 × 12 inch size continues to be manufactured for use in grid cassettes. Very few if any English sizes are used outside the United States. Four of the former English film sizes are no longer manufactured. Several additional film sizes are used routinely in departments outside the United States, including the 30 × 40 cm and 40 × 40 cm sizes.

FILM SIZES IN THIS ATLAS

During the continuing English-to-metric conversion of film sizes, both sizes will continue to be identified in this atlas. For sizes that have been converted to metric, the English size is identified in parentheses to facilitate the learning of the new sizes, for example, 35 × 43 cm (14 × 27 inches).

Direction of the Central Ray

The central or principal beam of rays, simply referred to as the *central ray*, is always centered to the IR unless receptor displacement is being used. The central ray is angled through the part of interest under the following conditions:
- When overlying or underlying structures must not be superimposed
- When a curved structure such as the sacrum or coccyx must not be stacked on itself
- When projection through angled joints such as the knee joint and lumbosacral junction is needed
- When projection through angled structures must be obtained without foreshortening or elongation, such as with a lateral image of the neck of the femur

The general goal is to place the central ray at right angles to the structure. Accurate positioning of the part and accurate centering of the central ray are of equal importance in obtaining a true structural projection.

TABLE 1-2

Most common radiology film sizes used in the United States*

Current film sizes*	Former film sizes†	Usage‡
18 x 24 cm		Mammography
8 x 10 inches		General examinations
24 x 24 cm	9 x 9 inches	Fluoroscopic spots
24 x 30 cm		General examinations and mammography
10 x 12 inches		General examinations (grid cassettes)
18 x 43 cm	7 x 17 inches	Forearms, legs
30 x 35 cm	11 x 14 inches	General examinations
35 x 35 cm		Fluoroscopic spots
35 x 43 cm	14 x 17 inches	General examinations
14 x 36 inches		Upright spine
14 x 51 inches		Upright hip-to-ankle

*In order of the smallest to largest size.
†English sizes no longer in use.
‡Most common uses in the United States. Outside the United States, usage may differ.

Source-to-Image Receptor Distance

SID is an important technical consideration in the production of radiographs of optimal quality. This distance is a critical component of each radiograph because it directly affects magnification of the body part and the recorded detail. The greater the SID, the less the body part is magnified and the greater the recorded detail will be. An SID of 40 inches (102 cm) traditionally has been used for most conventional examinations. In recent years, however, the SID has increased to 48 inches (122 cm) in some departments.[1-4] Technically, a greater SID requires a longer exposure time because the x-ray tube is farther from the IR. This could prompt motion on the image. However, with the use of faster film-screen systems and the flexibility of technical factors when using CR systems, short exposure times are commonplace with SIDs up to 48 inches (122 cm). An SID must be established for each radiographic projection, and it also must be indicated on the technique chart.

For some radiographic projections an SID less than 40 inches (102 cm) is desirable. For example, in certain skull examinations such as that of the paranasal sinuses, a short SID of 32 to 36 inches (81 to 91 cm) is used to magnify the opposite side of the skull, thereby prompting an increase in the recorded detail of the side being examined.

Conversely, a longer than standard SID is used for some radiographic projections. In chest radiography a 72-inch (183-cm) SID is the minimum distance, and in many departments a distance up to 120 inches (305 cm) is used. These long distances are necessary to ensure that the lungs fit onto the 14-inch (35-cm) width of the IR (via reduced magnification of the body part) and, most importantly, to ensure that the heart is not technically enlarged for diagnoses of cardiac enlargement.

SOURCE-TO-IMAGE RECEPTOR DISTANCE IN THIS ATLAS

An SID is not identified for projections in this atlas because of the wide variety of distances used in radiology departments. In addition, many specialized radiographic machines have a nonchangeable SID. However, when a specific SID is necessary for optimal image quality, it is identified on the specific projection's section.

SOURCE-TO-SKIN DISTANCE

The distance between the radiography tube and the skin of the patient is termed the *source-to-skin distance (SSD)*. This distance affects the dose to the patient and is regulated by the National Council on Radiation Protection (NCRP).

The current NCRP regulations state that the SSD *shall not* be less than 12 inches (30 cm) and *should not* be less than 15 inches (38 cm).[1]

[1]Eastman TR: Digital systems require x-ray charts too, *Radiol Technol* 67:354,1996.
[2]Eastman TR: X-ray film quality and national contracts, *Radiol Technol* 69:12,1997.
[3]Gray JE et al: *Quality control in diagnostic imaging,* Rockville, Md, 1983, Aspen.
[4]Kebart RC, James CD: Benefits of increasing focal film distance, *Radiol Technol* 62:434,1991.

[1]National Council on Radiation Protection: *NCRP Report 102,* Bethesda, Md, 1989, The Council.

Collimation of X-Ray Beam

The beam of radiation must be narrow enough to irradiate only the area under examination. This restriction of the x-ray beam serves two purposes. First, it minimizes the amount of radiation to the patient and reduces the amount of scatter radiation that can reach the IR. Second, it produces radiographs that demonstrate excellent recorded detail and increased radiographic contrast by reducing scatter radiation, thereby producing a shorter scale of contrast, and preventing secondary radiation from unnecessarily exposing surrounding tissues, with resultant image fogging (Fig. 1-25).

The area of the beam of radiation is reduced to the required size by using an *automatic collimator* or a specifically shaped diaphragm constructed of lead or other metal with high radiation absorption capability. Because of beam restriction, the peripheral radiation strikes and is absorbed by the collimator metal and only those x-rays in the exit aperture are transmitted to the exposure field. Because their effectiveness depends on their proximity to the x-ray source, extension cones and diaphragms can be attached to the collimator.

Fig. 1-25 Radiographs of the hip joint and acetabulum. **A,** Collimator inadvertently opened to size 35 × 43 cm. Note that scatter and secondary radiation have reduced the radiographic contrast and a poor-quality image results. **B,** Collimator set correctly to 18 × 24 cm, improving radiographic contrast and the visibility of detail.

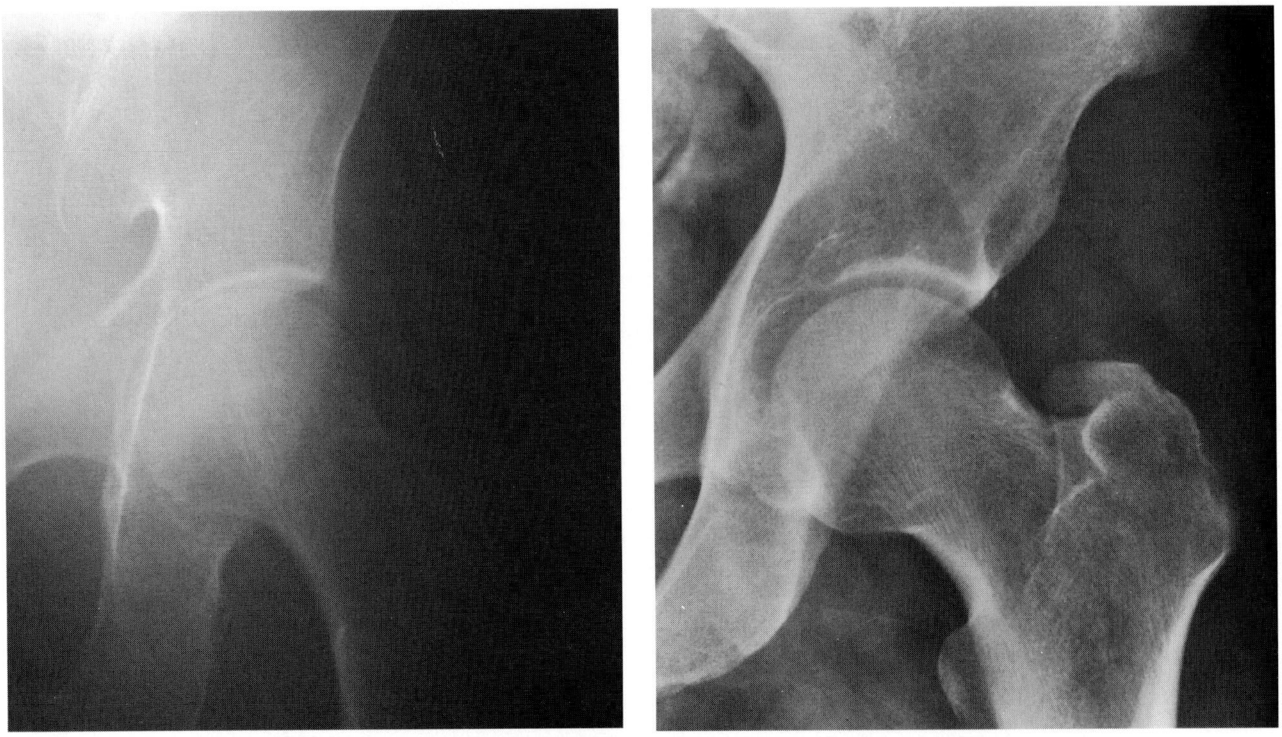

Gonad Shielding

The patient's gonads may be irradiated when radiographic examinations of the abdomen, pelvis, and hip areas are performed. When practical, gonad shielding should always be used to protect the patient. Contact, shadow, and large part area shields are used for radiography examinations (Figs. 1-26 through 1-28). The Center for Devices of Radiological Health has developed guidelines recommending gonad shielding in the following instances[1]:

- If the gonads lie within or close to the primary x-ray field (about 5 cm from) despite proper beam limitation
- If the clinical objective of the examination is not compromised
- If the patient has a reasonable reproductive potential

[1]Bureau of Radiological Health: *Gonad shielding in diagnostic radiology,* Pub No (FDA) 75-8024, Rockville, Md, 1975, The Bureau.

In addition, gonad shielding is often appropriate when limbs are radiographed with the patient seated at the end of the radiographic table (see Fig. 1-8). Finally, gonad shielding must be considered and used when requested by the patient unless it is contraindicated (see Chapter 2). Gonad shielding is included in selected illustrations in this text. For additional information on the rationale of gonad shielding see Chapter 2.

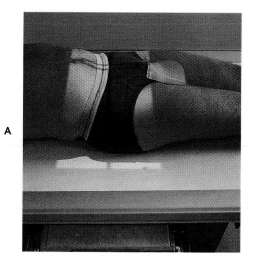 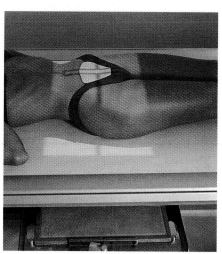

A   B

Fig. 1-26 A, Contact shield placed over the gonads of this male patient. **B,** Contact shield placed over the gonads of this female patient.

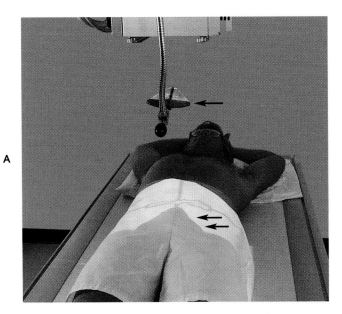

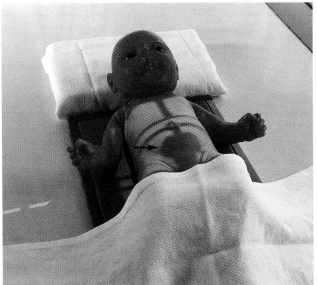

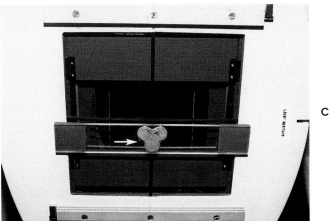

Fig. 1-27 A, Shadow shield used on male patient. The triangular lead device *(arrow)* is hung from the x-ray tube and positioned so its shadow falls on the gonads *(double arrows)*. **B,** Shadow shield used on female baby. The cloverleaf shield was positioned under the collimator with magnets, so its shadow falls over the gonads *(arrow)*. **C,** The cloverleaf-shaped shadow shield *(arrow)* positioned under the collimator with magnets.

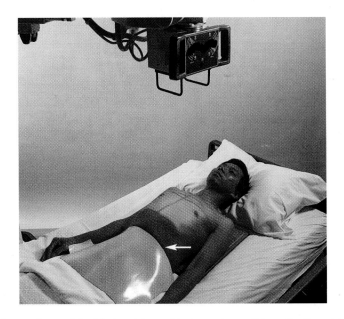

Fig. 1-28 A large piece of flexible lead *(arrow)* is draped over this patient's pelvis to protect the gonads during a mobile radiography examination of the chest.

31

Computed Radiography

Since the discovery of x-rays in 1895, computed radiography (CR) has prompted some of the most technically significant changes in the way radiographs are produced. Radiography departments worldwide are slowly converting to CR systems. In the future, all radiographs may eventually be done with CR or some other digital technology.

CR involves conventional radiographic projection radiography in which the latent image (the unseen image) is produced in digital format using computer technology. The CR system uses a conventional radiography machine and conventional positioning and technical factors. However, the image is acquired in a phosphor material plate inside a closed cassette rather than on a film in a light-tight cassette. After exposure the CR cassette is inserted into an image reader device (Fig. 1-29), where it is scanned by a laser beam and the final image appears on a computer monitor. The radiographer can either adjust the image for appropriate density and contrast and then print it on laser film or store the image in the computer to be read directly from the monitor by the radiologist (Fig. 1-30).

Attention to detail is paramount when the radiographer is using CR. The following sections address the technical considerations that are different from those used in conventional radiography (A more detailed description of CR is presented in Chapter 34.)

KILOVOLTAGE

Because of the somewhat wider dynamic range of CR, a specific kVp setting is not as critical as in conventional radiography. A broader range of kVp settings may be acceptable for a specific radiography projection. However, not using a kVp that is significantly low or high is crucial. Slightly overpenetrating the body part is better than underpenetrating it. An optimum kVp range should be posted on the technique chart for all CR projections. In addition, for body parts that have different thicknesses of structures and densities but must be imaged on one projection (e.g., a femur), the thickest part must be well penetrated.

PART CENTERING

The body part that is being radiographed must always be placed in or near the center area of the CR cassette. If the central ray is directed to a body part that is positioned at the periphery of the cassette (e.g., a finger placed near the edge), the computer may not be able to form the image properly. This also depends on whether the computer is in the autoprocessing or manual-processing mode. Cassettes can be split in half and used for two separate exposures because the image reader will note the two areas of exposure.

SPLIT CASSETTES

If a CR cassette is divided in half and used for two separate exposures, the side not receiving the exposure must always be covered with a lead shield. Storage phosphors in the CR cassette are hypersensitive to small levels of exposure and may show on the image if not properly shielded. Covering the unused half prevents scatter radiation from reaching the unexposed side of the CR cassette. Although this technique is practiced in conventional radiography, it is more critical with CR. Depending on the specific technical factors used, the images may not appear at all, may contain artifacts, or may display other image-processing failures. In addition, technical factors for the two exposures must be relatively close to each other.

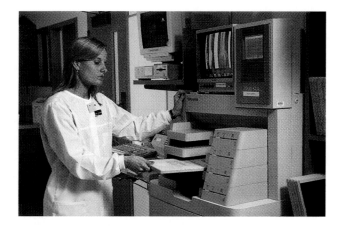

Fig. 1-29 Radiographer inserting a CR cassette into an image reader unit. The unit scans the plate with a laser beam and places the digitized image of the body part in a computer for reading on a monitor or, if necessary, for printing on a laser film.

OVEREXPOSURE AND UNDEREXPOSURE

A light or dark image on the CR monitor may not indicate that the body part was underexposed or overexposed with x-rays as in conventional radiography. A wide array of computer-related factors can cause a light or dark image when using CR. CR images are displayed with numbers that indicate the amount of the exposure reaching the plate. The determination of overexposure or underexposure is made by evaluating this number for the exposure and not the lightness or darkness of the initial image on the monitor.

COLLIMATION

As with conventional radiology the body part being radiographed must be collimated cautiously. With CR a collimated area that exposes the cassette to noncollimated radiation (e.g., a lateral lumbar spine) produces an unacceptable image or one that is very dark or light.

OPEN CASSETTES

Once an exposure is made on a cassette, it can be opened momentarily and exposed to light without compromising the image—a 15-second exposure will start the erasure process. Exposing the phosphor starts the erasure process, but the process is slow. With CR cassettes the latent image remains stored in the phosphors. The cassette is not designed to be light tight. The plate is designed to protect the image storage phosphors from dust, scratches, and other damage. This is different from conventional radiography, in which the film inside the cassette is ruined even if momentarily exposed to light.

GRIDS

The phosphors in CR cassettes are much more sensitive to scatter radiation. Some projections may require a grid if the kVp is above a certain level. For example, one manufacturer requires that a grid be used for any exposure above 90 kVp. This consideration is particularly important in mobile radiography where many projections are done without a grid.

COMPUTED RADIOGRAPHY IN THIS ATLAS

For most radiographic examinations, radiographic positioning does not markedly change with CR. However, for some projections the part centering, central ray, collimation, and other technical factors may be slightly different. When this occurs, a comment will be made and indicated under the following:

COMPUTED RADIOGRAPHY

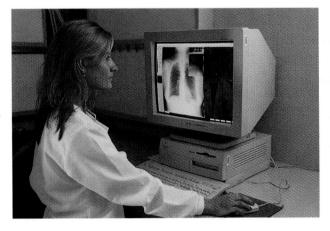
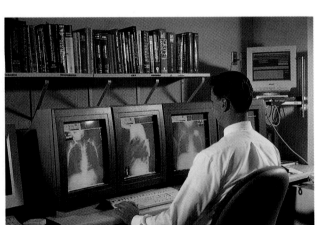

A

B

Fig. 1-30 A, The radiographer at the monitor uses the mouse to adjust the CR image of the body part to the proper size, density, and contrast before electronically sending the image for reading. **B,** The radiologist at the monitor is reading several CR images on one patient.

Technical Factors

The variation in power delivered by the x-ray tube permits the radiographer to control several prime technical factors: *milliamperage (mA), kilovolt (peak) (kVp),* and *exposure time* (seconds). The radiographer selects the specific factors required to produce a quality radiograph using the generator's control panel after consulting a technique chart. Manual and automatic exposure control systems (AEC) are used to set the factors.

Detailed aspects of each technical factor are presented in physics and imaging courses. Because of the variety of exposure factors and equipment used in clinical practice, specific technical factors are not presented in this atlas. However, the companion *Pocket Guide* is designed to allow students and radiographers to organize and write in the technical factors used in respective departments with the different equipment available.

MILLAMPERAGE IN THIS ATLAS

The mA setting controls the number or quantity of x-rays emitted from the x-ray tube. A variety of mA settings are used depending on the equipment type, x-ray examination, patient, and other factors. A specific or range of mA settings is cited in this atlas only when it directly affects the quality of an examination, such as when breathing techniques are used with long exposure times.

KILOVOLTAGE IN THIS ATLAS

The kVp setting is a critical factor that controls the energy and penetrating ability of the x-ray beam. A variety of kVp settings are used depending on whether single-phase, three-phase, or high-frequency x-ray generators are used, the type of grid used, and the contrast of the finish radiograph. For example, a 70-kVp technique with a three-phase generator requires 80 kVp with a single-phase generator to maintain the same contrast level.[1] A specific kVp is indicated in this atlas only when it directly affects the quality of an examination, such as a high kVp used in chest radiography or a very low kVp used in mammography.

[1]Cullinan AM, Cullinan JE: *Producing quality radiographs,* Philadelphia, 1994, Lippincott.

EXPOSURE TIME IN THIS ATLAS

The exposure time setting determines the total time of x-ray exposure. For most exposures this time is given in fractions of seconds. As with other prime factors, a variety of exposure time settings are used. A specific exposure time is indicated in this atlas only when it directly affects the quality of an examination, such as with a chest radiograph on a small child or for a breathing technique to blur anatomy.

AUTOMATIC EXPOSURE CONTROL IN THIS ATLAS

X-ray generators contain AEC systems that are very complex and require several settings for each exposure—kVp, mA, backup timer, density control, screen setting, and sensor selection. A number of factors, including the type of examination, tabletop or Bucky technique, patient cooperation, and cassette size, determine which settings are used. Because of the complexity and variations, no AEC factors are discussed in this atlas. Readers are urged to use the *Pocket Guide* to write in the specific AEC factors used in their departments for their equipment available.

RADIATION PROTECTION

STEWART C. BUSHONG

RIGHT The "latest" in radiation protection—a lead mask from about 1900.

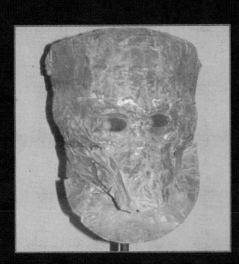

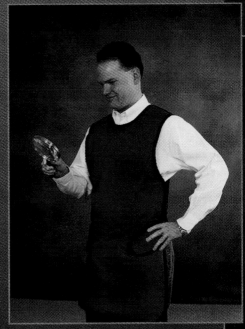

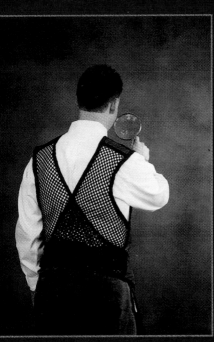

LEFT An example of modern radiation protection—a lightweight, mesh-backed protective lead apron.

(Courtesy Pro-Tech X-Ray, Inc.)

Introduction

EARLY INJURIES

Perhaps no other event in our technologic history caused as much feverish scientific activity by so many as the accidental discovery of x-rays by Wilhelm Roentgen in November 1895. Because Roentgen was so thorough in his investigations, within a few short weeks he was able to characterize the nature of x-rays to nearly the same level of understanding as we have today. This early work earned him the first Nobel Prize in physics in 1901. Roentgen immediately recognized the potential diagnostic medical applications of his new "X-light." He produced the first radiograph, which was of his wife's hand.

Throughout 1896, the first year after Roentgen's discovery, the world's scientific literature was flooded with reports of experiments with x-rays. Very soon thereafter associated cases of *radiodermatitis* (reddening of the skin caused by exposure to ionizing radiation), in some instances severe enough to require surgery, were reported. These reports had two immediate effects: (1) they accelerated the experimentation and application of x-rays in radiation therapy and (2) they suggested that radiation protection methods were necessary during diagnostic procedures to ensure the safety of both the operator and the patient. However, it took more than 30 years for even moderately consistent radiation protection measures to be universally applied.

By 1910 several hundred cases of severe x-ray burns, many leading to death, had been reported. To understand the magnitude of this tragedy among radiation pioneers, consider the case of Charles T. Dally, Thomas Edison's friend and principal assistant. Within a few days after the cable announcement of the discovery of x-rays, Edison was deeply involved in his own investigations, using x-ray apparatus that he had assembled. Within months several of his assistants experienced radiodermatitis. Dally's condition was mild at first but, because of continued exposure, deteriorated rapidly and resulted in several amputations. He died in 1904 and is considered the first radiation fatality in the United States. When Dally died, Edison discontinued his work with x-rays. He had already discovered *calcium tungstate* as an intensifying phosphor and developed the *fluoroscope*. Who knows what additional contributions Edison might have made to radiology had he continued his investigations.

PRESENT SUSPECTED RADIATION RESPONSES

In the 1930s a consensus was reached on the need for radiation protection devices and procedures. These activities were principally in response to the reported radiation injuries to early radiologists. In the 1950s scientific publications began to suggest that even the low levels of radiation exposure experienced in diagnostic radiology could be responsible for late radiation responses such as cancer and leukemia in patients. Current radiation protection practices are prompted by concern for *late effects* in patients and radiation workers.

After exposure to high doses of radiation, a number of acute early responses may appear. A whole-body radiation dose in excess of 200 rad (2 Gy) can result in death within weeks. Partial-body irradiation to any organ or tissue can cause atrophy (shrinking) and dysfunction (improper metabolism). A whole-body radiation dose as low as 25 rad (250 mGy) can produce measurable *hematologic depression* (reduction in the number of circulating blood cells), which may require months for recovery. These early effects result from high doses of radiation and therefore are of little concern in diagnostic radiology. Such effects are called *deterministic*; the severity of response is dose related and there is a dose threshold.

Concern today is for the late effects of radiation exposure. These effects are called *stochastic*; the incidence of response is dose related and there is no dose threshold. Such effects follow low-dose radiation exposures and may not occur for years. They fall into two categories: genetic effects and somatic effects. Genetic effects of radiation exposure are suspected; they have not been observed in humans. However, data from a considerable number of animal studies indicate that such effects may occur. Somatic effects refer to the response to radiation by all cells of the body except the genetic cells. The principal somatic effects after low-dose irradiation have been measured in humans by the use of rather sophisticated epidemiologic and statistical methods. No individual has ever been identified as a radiation victim after low-dose radiation exposure. A low dose is generally considered to be a whole-body radiation dose of less than about 25 rad (250 mGy). The low dose for partial-body irradiation is somewhat higher. Such effects

are detectable only when observations of thousands and even hundreds of thousands of irradiated individuals are made.

The shortening of life resulting from nonspecific premature aging was observed many years ago in American pioneer radiologists. This effect does not exist today because of improved radiation protection practices. Local tissues can also experience late radiation effects of a nonmalignant nature. The most prominent late effect is *radiation-induced cataracts*. However, this effect does not follow low-dose irradiation: it requires at least 200 rad (2 Gy) of exposure to the lens of the eye and that level is essentially impossible for patients or personnel to incur.

Radiation-induced malignant disease is the delayed somatic effect of primary concern. This cause of leukemia, solid-tumor neoplasia, and cancers of nearly every type involving almost every organ has been implicated by animal investigations and epidemiologic observations of humans.

Leukemia is more readily observed in a heavily irradiated population than cancer. The BEIR (Biologic Effects of Ionizing Radiation) Committee's estimate for the induction of leukemia by irradiation suggests that if 1 million persons received 1 rad (10 mGy) of radiation, up to 55 additional cases of leukemia would occur during the 25 years after irradiation. This equals approximately 2 cases/million persons/rad/yr. Without irradiation the incidence of leukemia is approximately 80 cases/million persons/yr.

Because cancer is not uncommon, radiation-induced cancer is difficult to detect. The 1990 report of the BEIR Committee— known as the BEIR-V Report—provides the most authoritative estimate of this radiation response. Although this report is exceedingly thorough, it can be summarized briefly by the data in Table 2-1.

The BEIR committee postulated three scenarios. The first assumes a once-in-a-lifetime dose of 10 rad (100 mGy), simulating an accidental exposure. The second assumes an annual dose of 1000 mrad/yr (10 mGy/yr). The third assumes an annual exposure of 100 mrad/yr, approprimating the dose received as occupational exposure. Of 100,000 unirradiated persons, nearly 20,000 will die of malignant disease. After a single 10-rad (100-mGy) accidental dose, an additional 800 malignant deaths might occur. After an assumed exposure of 1000 mrad/yr, an additional 3000 may die of malignant disease. With an occupational exposure of 100 mrad/yr for a 40-year working period, an additional 600 cases of malignant disease may be expected. The range of possible deaths in Table 2-1 results from adoption of a *relative risk* model of radiation response.

NEED FOR RADIATION PROTECTION

Radiographers receive approximately 60 mrad/yr (0.6 mGy/yr), nearly all during fluoroscopy and portable radiography when protective apparel is worn. Consequently, exposures, although identified as whole body on the exposure report, are actually partial-body exposures. Although exposure levels are low and the possibility of a late effect is remote, it is prudent to keep radiation exposure to radiographers and patients ALARA (*As Low As Reasonably Achievable*).

A recent survey of 143,000 radiographers by The American Registry of Radiologic Technologists yielded a large amount of statistical data about dose, demographics, and biologic effects. There was no indication that occupational radiation exposure caused any biologic effects. In fact, in all cases in which radiographers have been studied, no biologic effects have been observed. Nevertheless, late genetic and somatic effects of importance are considered possible.

There is no dose threshold for such effects. Should a dose threshold exist, all doses below the threshold would be absolutely safe. Even though the occupational exposures that radiographers experience result in a very small and indeterminate probability of producing such effects, an effective radiation protection program is required.

TABLE 2-1

Biologic Effects of Ionizing Radiation (BEIR) Committee: estimated excess mortality from malignant disease, cases per 100,000 persons

	Male	Female
Normal expectation	20,560	16,680
Excess cases		
Single exposure to 10 rad	770	810
Continuous exposure to 1000 mrad/yr	2880	3070
Continuous exposure to 100 mrad/yr	520	600

TABLE 2-2

Conventional radiation units, SI radiation units, and conversion factors

Quantity	Conventional unit	SI unit	Conversion factor
Exposure	roentgen (R)	C/kg	2.58×10^{-4} C/kg/R
Absorbed dose	rad	gray (Gy)	10^{-2} Gy/rad
Dose equivalent	rem	sievert (Sv)	10^{-2} Sv/rem
Activity	curie (Ci)	becquerel (Bq)	3.7×10^{10} Bq/Ci

SI, International System of units; *C/kg*, Coulomb per kilogram; *rad*, radiation absorbed dose; *rem*, roentgen equivalent, man.

Radiation Units

A special set of units is used to express the quantity of ionizing radiation. These units, the *roentgen*, the *rad*, and the *rem*, have been developed and defined over many years and are familiar to radiologic workers. However, those in educational programs and in professional practice must become familiar with a second set of radiation units derived from the International System (SI) of Units. The SI units associated with classical radiation units and the appropriate conversions are shown in Table 2-2. Although they are referred to only superficially in this chapter, radiographers should be aware that they exist and should be prepared to implement them. At this time the United States is the only developed country that has yet to fully adopt SI radiation units as a system of measure.

UNIT OF EXPOSURE

When an x-ray tube is energized, x-rays are emitted in a collimated beam in the same way light is emitted from a flashlight. This useful beam of x-rays *ionizes* the air through which it passes. This effect is called *exposure*, and the unit of exposure is the *roentgen (R)*. An exposure of 1 R will produce 2.08×10^9 ionizations in 1 cm^3 of air at standard temperature and pressure. The official definition of the roentgen is 2.58×10^{-4} coulombs per kilogram (C/kg) of air, and this quantity is equivalent to the previous quantity. The SI unit of radiation exposure has no special name; it is simply the C/kg. Because of many difficulties encountered with this unit, the radiologic community employs the *gray (Gy)* when expressing dose to air. For our purposes we may assume that 1 R = 10 mGy, although this quantity is not precisely correct.

UNIT OF RADIATION DOSE

When a radiation exposure occurs, the resulting ionizations deposit energy in the air. If an object such as a patient is present at the point of exposure, energy will be deposited in the patient. This deposition of energy by radiation exposure is called *radiation absorbed dose*, or simply *absorbed dose*, and it is measured in *rad*. One rad is equivalent to depositing 100 erg of energy in each gram of the irradiated object. The SI unit of absorbed dose is the *gray*, and 1 Gy = 100 rad = 1 J/kg. The *erg* and *joule* are units of energy.

UNIT OF DOSE EQUIVALENT

If the irradiated object is a radiographer or other radiation worker, then the radiation dose resulting from an occupational radiation exposure is said to result in a *radiation dose equivalent*. The dose equivalent is measured in *rem (radiation equivalent man)*, and 1 rem = 100 erg/g. The SI unit of dose equivalent is the *sievert (Sv)*, and 1 Sv = 1 J/kg. Note that the rad and rem (gray and sievert) are expressed in similar units. The basic difference between the rem and other radiation units is that the rem is used only for radiation protection purposes; it is the unit of occupational exposure.

In diagnostic radiology 1 R can be considered equal to 1 rad and to 1 rem. This simplifying assumption is accurate to within about 15% and therefore is sufficiently precise for nearly all considerations of exposure and dose in diagnostic radiology. Radiation workers in the nuclear power industry and in some other industrial and research activities may be exposed to different kinds of radiation, in which case this simplifying assumption does not apply.

APPLICATION OF RADIATION UNITS

Although roentgen, rad, and rem are used interchangeably in diagnostic radiology, such usage is incorrect because each unit has a precise application. Furthermore, 1 roentgen, 1 rad, and 1 rem are all rather large quantities. In practice, quantities 1000 times smaller are used: milliroentgen (mR), millirad (mrad), and millirem (mrem).

When a medical physicist evaluates the performance of a radiographic or fluoroscopic x-ray tube, the radiation intensity is expressed in mR. The radiation intensity is measured by any one of the various types of radiation detectors; output is expressed in mR or sometimes as mR/milliampere-seconds (mAs) at some given *kilovolt (peak) (kVp)*.

When a patient is irradiated during an examination and the amount of radiation received by the patient is of concern, the radiation dose is expressed in mrad. If a pregnant patient is irradiated, the fetal dose is also expressed in mrad. The radiation dose to any of the patient's organs would likewise be expressed in mrad. Often, however, the skin dose is expressed as an exposure in mR and is called an *entrance skin exposure (ESE)*.

Exposure received by radiographers is measured with a personnel radiation monitor. The source of their occupational exposure is nearly always scattered radiation from the patient (Fig. 2-1). The radiation monitor measures exposure; the radiation report indicates the dose equivalent in mrem. The mrem is reserved exclusively for use in radiation protection and therefore is a unit used not only to quantify occupational exposure but also sometimes to express the dose received by populations as the consequence of medical, industrial, and research applications of radiation.

Radiation Sources and Levels

We are exposed to ionizing radiation in our daily lives from multiple sources. The largest source is natural background radiation, something over which we have no control. Other sources are medical, diagnostic, and therapeutic procedures and radiation applications associated with industry, research, and consumer products. To place in perspective the radiation exposures and risks associated with being a radiographer, we need to know something about the radiation levels associated with these other sources (Table 2-3).

NATURAL BACKGROUND

Human beings have inhabited Earth for hundreds of thousands of years and have evolved in the presence of a constant radiation exposure called *natural background radiation*. Natural background radiation comes from three principal sources: (1) terrestrial radiation resulting from naturally occurring radionuclides in the earth, (2) cosmic radiation resulting from principally the sun but also sources outside our solar system and galaxy, and (3) internal exposure from radionuclides naturally deposited in the human body, principally potassium -40 (^{40}K). In the United States these sources produce a whole-body dose of 50 to 300 mrad/yr (0.5 to 3 mGy/yr), depending on location and diet. Table 2-3 includes these components of the natural background radiation.

TABLE 2-3

Estimated average annual whole-body radiation dose (mrem) in the United States from various sources

Radiation source	Annual dose (mrem)
Natural sources	
Internal radionuclides, principally ^{40}K	39
Terrestrial radionuclides, principally ^{220,222}R, ^{226,228}Ra, ^{14}C	29
Cosmic rays	29
Radon (dose to lungs only)	198
TOTAL	295
Human sources	
Diagnostic x-rays	40
Nuclear medicine	14
Consumer products	10
Other	1
TOTAL	65
COMBINED TOTAL	360

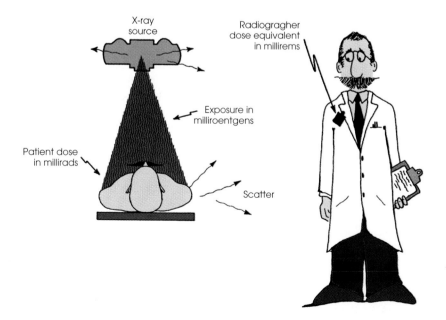

Fig. 2-1 The useful x-ray beam is measured in milliroentgen, the patient dose is expressed in millirad, and occupational exposure is measured in millirem.

Terrestrial radiation

At the time of Earth's formation 4 billion years ago, some radioactive elements (principally uranium and thorium) were created that have radioactive half-lives equally as long. As these radionuclides decay, they emit radiation, which contributes to the total natural background radiation level.

This *terrestrial radiation* level is very dependent on geographic location and on the type of soil or rock present. Along the Atlantic and Gulf coasts, the terrestrial radiation dose ranges from 15 to 35 mrem/yr (0.15 to 0.35 mSv/yr). In the northeastern, central, and far western portions of the United States, the terrestrial radiation dose ranges from 35 to 75 mrem/yr (0.35 to 0.75 mSv/yr). Along the Colorado plateau, this dose ranges from 75 to 140 mrem/yr (0.75 to 1.4 mSv/yr).

With the application of the appropriate terrestrial radiation dose rate to the resident population, the average U.S. rate is estimated to be 29 mrem/yr (0.29 mSv/yr). This figure does not include the dose from radon, a radioactive gas that emanates from the earth and earthlike building materials such as concrete and bricks. As a gas, radon contributes only to the dose to lungs—an estimated 198 mrem/yr (2 mSv/yr).

Cosmic radiation

Cosmic radiation consists of x-rays, gamma rays, and particles that are emitted by the sun and by sources outside of our solar system—even outside our galaxy. When this radiation is incident on Earth, its intensity is reduced by the shielding of the overlying atmosphere and is altered by Earth's magnetic field. In general, radiation intensity increases with latitude toward the North Pole because of the deflection of solar flare protons by Earth's magnetic field. The intensity also increases with altitude. One mile above Earth's surface the cosmic radiation intensity is approximately twice that at sea level. When all of these influences are considered, the U.S. population receives an estimated 29 mrem/yr (0.29 mSv/yr) from cosmic radiation exposure.

Internally deposited radionuclides

The air we breathe, the water we drink, and the food we eat all contain small quantities of naturally occurring radionuclides. Some of these radionuclides are metabolized and incorporated permanently into the tissues of the body. The radionuclides of principal importance are ^{3}H, ^{14}C, ^{40}K, ^{226}Ra, and ^{210}Po. Collectively, these internally deposited radionuclides result in an average estimated annual dose of 39 mrem (0.4 mSv).

MEDICAL RADIATION EXPOSURE

Patients receive radiation exposure from radiographic examinations, fluoroscopic procedures, dental diagnostic procedures, radioisotope procedures, and radiation oncologic procedures. By far, the greatest amount of man-made radiation exposure is received from medical x-ray procedures. Approximately 65% of the U.S. population is exposed to radiation each year for medical purposes.

Two measures of patient dose are important in assessing the extent of medical radiation exposure on the population: the *genetically significant dose (GSD)* and the *mean marrow dose (MMD)*. The GSD is a genetic dose index. It is the gonad dose that, if received by every member of the population, would be expected to produce the sum total effect on the population as the sum of the individual doses actually received. At this time in the United States the GSD is estimated to be 20 mrem/yr (0.2 mSv/yr). The GSD indicates nothing about possible or probable genetic effects. It is only an attempt to estimate the dose received by the population gene pool.

The MMD is a similar index for somatic effects; it too is expressed in mrem/yr. The MMD to the U.S. population is currently estimated to be 77 mrem/yr (0.77 mSv/yr). Like the GSD, the MMD is an average weighted over the entire population, including those who are and those who are not medically irradiated. It takes into account the fraction of bone marrow irradiated as a function of each type of examination and averages this fraction over the total bone marrow. Because bone marrow irradiation is considered to be responsible for radiation-induced leukemia, the MMD is a somatic dose index. The MMD is a measure of radiation dose and not of radiation effect.

INDUSTRIAL APPLICATIONS

Industrial applications of ionizing radiation result in average occupational exposures of up to several hundred millirem per year in some groups such as nuclear power plant workers. Occupational radiation exposure is also received by others employed in the mining, refining, and fabrication of nuclear fuel, industrial radiography, and in the handling of radio-isotopes for a large number of industrial applications. Included in these industrial applications is the transportation of radioactive material, particularly air freight of nuclear medicine radiopharmaceutical products. When prorated over the entire U.S. population, these industrial activities add approximately 0.2 mrem/yr (2 μSv/yr) of radiation exposure.

RESEARCH APPLICATIONS

Research applications of ionizing radiation include particle accelerators, other radiation-producing machines, and radionuclides. Particle accelerators, such as cyclotrons, synchrocyclotrons, and linear accelerators, are employed in university and industrial research laboratories. Although these machines can generate intense fields of radiation, they are always shielded and protected.

X-ray diffraction units and electron microscopes are common research tools used to investigate the structure of matter. The x-ray diffraction unit generates an intense field of highly collimated and low-energy radiation. It does not normally represent a whole-body hazard, but it can present a danger to hands if they are accidentally placed in the useful beam. Electron microscopes likewise produce low-energy x-rays, but these devices are well shielded and do not represent a significant occupational radiation hazard or a radiation hazard to the population.

Many research activities employ radionuclides, mostly low-energy, beta-emitting radionuclides such as ^{3}H and ^{14}C. Although a small occupational hazard is associated with the use of these materials, the population exposure is nil. Collectively, these research applications contribute no more than 1 mrem/yr (10 μSv/yr) to the population dose.

CONSUMER PRODUCTS

Many consumer products incorporate x-ray devices or radioactive material. Television receivers, video display terminals, and airport surveillance systems are three devices that produce x-rays. The first two produce x-rays of a very low energy and intensity and pose no hazard to the consumer because these low-energy x-rays are absorbed completely by the glass envelope of the video tube. Surveillance systems likewise emit low levels of x-rays, and these units are well shielded and are provided with adequate safety interlocks.

Radioactive material is incorporated into various luminous products, such as instrument gauges, clocks, and exit signs. Radioactive material is also incorporated into such devices as check sources, static eliminators, and smoke detectors. Collectively, these devices may contribute an additional 4 mrem/yr (40 μSv/yr) to the population dose. Natural radioactive materials are present in many consumer products, such as tobacco, building materials, highway and road construction materials, combustible fuels, glass, and ceramics. Under some circumstances the use of these naturally occurring materials can enhance the existing natural background radiation dose by as much as 6 mrem/yr (60 μSv/yr).

Radiation Protection Guidelines

Most radiation biology research dealing with experimental animals or observations of humans has been devoted to describing the quantitative relationship between radiation dose and biologic effect. Such *dose-response relationships* have been described with great precision for the early effects of radiation following high doses. Most early effects, such as skin erythema, hematologic depression, and lethality, exhibit a *threshold*-type dose-response relationship. Such a dose threshold indicates that there is a dose below which that response will not occur.

This is not true for the late effects of low-level radiation exposure. Late effects are considered to have no dose threshold

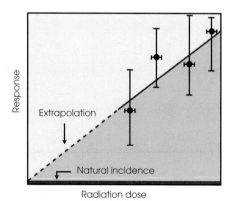

Fig. 2-2 A dose-response relationship is produced by extrapolating high-dose experimental data to low doses.

and to increase in incidence with increasing dose (Fig. 2-2). This type of dose-response relationship suggests that no radiation dose, regardless how small, is considered absolutely safe. At zero dose a small but measurable response may be observed. This response represents the natural incidence of the effect.

BASIS FOR RADIATION PROTECTION STANDARDS

The linear, nonthreshold type of dose-response relationship is the basis for radiation protection standards. The late effects of principal concern are leukemia and cancer, and they have been shown with reasonable accuracy to follow this dose-response model.

This basis for radiation protection guidance in the United States was first enunciated in 1932 when the National Council for Radiation Protection and Measurements (NCRP) recommended a whole-body dose limit of 50 rem/yr (500 mSv/yr). Over the years the dose limit has been revised downward several times and is now 5 rem/yr (50 mSv/yr). Thousands of occupationally exposed persons have been observed, and very few have been exposed to a dose that exceeded this present dose limit. For instance, in diagnostic radiology radiographers receive less than 100 mrem/yr (1 mSv/yr). The observations of occupationally exposed radiographers have not resulted in a single observed case of radiation effect.

It should be clear that any attempt to establish a dose-limiting recommendation is highly subjective and requires value assessments beyond the realm of science. The present recommended dose limits have been in effect for more than 20 years and remain prudent and safe levels.

The development of recommended dose limits and other radiation protection guides acknowledges that some risk is involved in radiation exposure. The task is to set these standards at a level of radiation exposure associated with an acceptable risk. Of course, this means recognizing that what may be an acceptable risk for one individual is unacceptable for another. The recommended dose limits are considered to be an acceptable exposure for all radiation workers. Therefore it is that dose which, if received each year for a 40-year working lifetime, would not be expected to produce any significant effect.

The term *recommended dose limit* replaces earlier terms such as *maximum permissible dose, tolerance dose,* or *allowable dose.* In addition, radiation protection programs must be consistent with the ALARA concept, as previously defined.

SPECIFIC RADIATION PROTECTION CONCEPTS

In addition to the specification of a whole-body recommended dose limit for occupationally exposed persons and for the population at large, several tissues and organs of the body have been given special consideration for their individual radiosensitivity. Specific individuals in the population are likewise accorded attention in specifying a recommended dose limit.

In 1987 the NCRP revised its long-standing recommendations, which are summarized in Table 2-4. These newer recommendations have now been adopted by state and federal regulatory agencies and are law in all states. Note that only SI units are used and the units relate to limits of *dose equivalent.*

The effective dose equivalent for the whole body remains the same—50 mSv/yr. This is the prospective annual effective dose equivalent. The cumulative effective dose equivalent is now 10 mSv × N, where N is the age of the worker. This dose limit is a considerable reduction from the previous level of 50 mSv (N = 18).

Effective dose equivalent is the sum of the weighted dose equivalents for irradiated tissues or organs. It takes into account the different mortality risks from cancer and the risk of severe hereditary effects in the first two generations associated with irradiation of different organs and tissues.

Effective dose equivalent is expressed symbolically as

$$H_E = (w_T H_T)$$

where w_T is the tissue-weighting factor representing the proportionate risk of tissue *(T)* and H_T is the average dose received by tissue *(T)*. The tissue-weighting factor, w_T, accounts for the relative radiosensitivity of various tissues and organs. Values for w_T are given in Table 2-5.

A good radiation protection program must recognize not only the prospective effective dose equivalent but also the long-term cumulative effective dose equivalent. The cumulative figure restricts an individual's lifetime exposure to no more than 10 mSv multiplied by the worker's age. Use of the terms *prospective dose equivalent* and *cumulative* dose *equivalent* serves to emphasize that these figures are guidelines only and that exceeding a numerical recommended dose limit may be acceptable under some circumstances.

Other regions of the body have different recommended dose limits. The dose limit for the skin is 500 mSv/yr. This dose limitation applies to exposure to nonpenetrating radiation such as electrons and low-energy x-rays. In diagnostic radiology, mammography is the only type of procedure in which exposure of the radiographer's skin can reach its limit before the whole-body limit becomes applicable.

During fluoroscopy it is often necessary for the hands or forearms of the radiographer to be near the useful beam. Usually these parts are protected by lead gloves. However, during certain procedures the use of such protective apparel is not possible. The dose limit for the hands is 500 mSv/yr. The recommended dose limit for the lens of the eye is now 150 mSv/yr, a threefold increase over the previous level.

The unborn child is known to be particularly sensitive to the effects of ionizing radiation; consequently, a dose limit of 5 mSv/9 mo is applied (the same as the previous recommendation). This dose limit presents a special problem in diagnostic radiology. In the case of the pregnant radiographer, it is unlikely that this recommended dose limit for the fetus would ever be approached, much less exceeded, because of the use of protective apparel during fluoroscopy and portable radiography. Nevertheless, rigorous radiation protection methods may be required during pregnancy. In recognizing this special concern, the NCRP has added the additional dose limit of 0.5 mSv/mo once the pregnancy is *declared*.

Under some circumstances students may be exposed to radiation during educational experiences. In such cases they are given a separate dose limit of 1 mSv/yr. This dose limit is directed particularly to high school and college students of any age but also to radiography students under age 18.

Although many of the current NCRP recommended dose limits represent an increase, the dose limit for the general public is a fivefold reduction to 1 mSv/yr. If applied without modification, this reduced dose limit means that future radiologic suites will require considerably more shielding than before.

Even more changes in recommended dose limits are on the way. The changes are not made because of fear that current limits are dangerous or even harmful; they are made in keeping with the principle of ALARA. The changes also acknowledge that we can function efficiently, even with these more restrictive recommended dose limits. In 1991 the International Commission on Radiological Protection (ICRP) issued a number of recommendations, including an annual prospective effective dose equivalent of 20 mSv. Such a reduction is currently under consideration in the United States. Fig. 2-3 summarizes the history of radiation protection guidelines over the past century.

TABLE 2-4

Natural Council for Radiation Protection and Measurements (NCRP): Recommended dose limits

Occupational exposure (annual)	
Effective dose equivalent limit (stochastic effects)	50 mSv
Dose equivalent limits for tissues and organs	
lens of eye	150 mSv
all others (e.g., red bone marrow, breast, lung, gonads, thyroid skin and extremities)	500 mSv
Cumulative dose equivalent	10 mSv × N
Public exposure (annual)	1 mSv
Education and training exposure (annual)	1 mSv
Embryo-fetus exposure	
Total dose equivalent limit	5 mSv
Dose equivalent limit in a month	0.5 mSv

N, Age of the worker.
From NCRP Report No. 91, 1986.

TABLE 2-5

Recommended values of tissue weighting factors (w_T) for calculating effective dose equivalent

Tissue (T)	Risk coefficient	w_T
Gonads	40×10^{-4} Sv^{-1}	0.25
Breast	25×10^{-4} Sv^{-1}	0.15
Red bone marrow	20×10^{-4} SV^{-1}	0.12
Lung	20×10^{-4} Sv^{-1}	0.12
Thyroid	5×10^{-4} Sv^{-1}	0.03
Bone surfaces	5×10^{-4} Sv^{-1}	0.03
Remainder	50×10^{-4} Sv^{-1}	0.30
TOTAL	165×10^{-4} Sv^{-1}	1.00

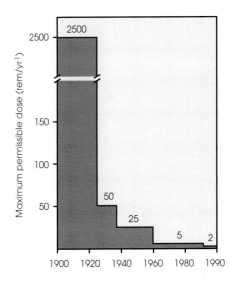

Fig. 2-3 Dose limits have decreased over the past century.

Medical Radiation Dose and Exposure

The output x-ray intensity from any given radiographic or fluoroscopic imager can vary widely depending on the type of equipment and technique employed. There may even be a sizable variation among x-ray imagers of the same manufacture and model when identical techniques are used. The output x-ray intensity, of course, determines the radiation dose to not only the patient but also the radiographer. Consequently, several methods are used to determine x-ray output to estimate the dose to patient and radiographer.

The *tabletop output intensity* during fluoroscopy is difficult to estimate by computation with even moderate precision; it must be measured. Modern fluoroscopes have beam intensities limited to 10 R/min (100 mGy/min) at the tabletop. Experience has shown that, when operated at approximately 90 kVp, most fluoroscopes produce tabletop exposure of 4 to 7 R/min (40 to 70 mGy/min).

Radiographic x-ray intensity is also difficult to estimate by computation unless at least a single measurement is available. For a properly calibrated radiographic im-ager, the x-ray intensity varies directly with the mAs and the square kVp. It also varies inversely as the square of the distance from the source. Mathematically this is represented as follows:

$$\text{x-ray intensity} = k(mAs)\,(kVp)^2/d^2$$

where k is the empirically determined constant, *mAs* is the x-ray tube current multiplied by the exposure time, *kVp* is the tube potential, and d is the distance from the source to the entrance surface of the patient (SSD).

Using this formulation and one measurement of k, a reasonably accurate estimate of radiographic x-ray intensity can be determined for any technique. Usually this one measurement is made at 70 kVp and is expressed in mR/mAs at a source-to-image receptor distance (SID) of 100 cm. Experience shows that this value ranges from about 2 to 8 mR/mAs (20 to 80 μGy/mAs), depending on the age, manufacture, and filtration of the x-ray beam. With this measured value the x-ray output intensity at any other radiographic technique can be computed using the following expression:

$$\text{Output intensity (mR)} = (3)\,k(mR/mAs)\,(mAs^*)\,(kVp^*/70)^2\,(100\ cm/d^*)^2$$

where k is the measured value at 70 kVp/100 cm SID, *mAs** and *kVp** are the desired technique, and $d^* = $ SSD.

For example, the medical physics report shows the radiographic intensity to be 4.8 mR/mAs at 70 kVp/100 cm SID. The technique chart calls for 76 kVp/80 mAs for a kidney, ureter, and bladder examination. If the SSD is 80 cm, the ESE is as follows:

$$\text{ESE} = (4.8\ mR/mAs)\,(80\ mAs)\,(76/70)^2\,(100/80)^2 = 707\ mR$$

Some investigators have produced nomograms for ease in estimating radiographic output intensity (Fig. 2-4).

PATIENT DOSE

The dose received by patients during diagnostic radiologic examinations is usually expressed in one of three ways: ESE, *organ dose*, or *fetal dose*. Each has a specific application in assessing the risk to the patient, but ESE is the easiest to estimate.

Entrance skin exposure

The ESE to the entrance surface of the patient during any radiographic examination can be measured directly or estimated by using the techniques previously described. ESE during fluoroscopy usually must be measured although it too can be estimated from a tabletop exposure measurement at the technique under investigation.

Two methods generally are used to measure ESE. Small ion chambers or solid state diodes can be placed on the entrance surface of the patient and exposed during any clinical procedure. Ion chambers and solid-state diodes have a sufficiently wide range and are sensitive and accurate. However, they are difficult to position and use, and therefore their application is limited.

Most current estimates of ESE are made with *thermoluminescent dosimeters (TLDs)*. TLDs are as sensitive and precise as ion chambers and solid-state diodes, and they have a much wider range of response. Furthermore, they are easy to use, and because of their small size, they can easily be positioned on the skin. TLDs are nearly tissue equivalent and therefore will not be imaged except at a very low kVp.

In recent years some government agencies have attempted to restrict patients' radiation exposure during commonly performed radiographic examinations. It is also recognized that too low a radiation exposure can be just as hazardous as an excessive radiation exposure because an inadequate image is produced making diagnosis less precise and necessitating repeat radiologic examinations. Table 2-6 shows acceptable ranges for several radiographic examinations. These ranges are rather generous, reflecting the techniques and image receptors currently used.

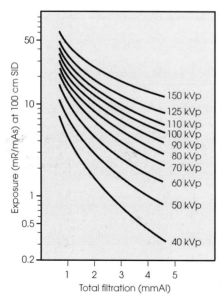

Fig. 2-4 A nomogram estimates the radiation intensity from a single-phase radiographic unit.

Organ dose

Sometimes the radiation dose received by a specific organ or tissue is significant. Of course, organ dose usually cannot be measured directly but must be estimated. The breast, for example, is a tissue of primary concern because of the high utilization of x-ray mammography and the potential for radiation-induced breast cancer. Table 2-7 shows the approximate ESE and glandular dose received by the breast as a function of the type of examination employed. The glandular dose is that which is used to evaluate radiation carcinogenesis.

Another organ of particular concern is the bone marrow. Bone marrow dose is used to estimate the population *mean marrow dose (MMD)* as an index of the somatic effect of radiation exposure. Table 2-8 relates the MMD associated with various radiographic examinations. Each of these doses results from partial-body exposure and is averaged over the entire body.

Exposure of the gonads to radiation during diagnostic radiology is of concern because of the possible genetic effects of ionizing radiation. Table 2-9 indicates average gonad doses received during various procedures. The large difference between males and females results from the shielding of the ovaries by overlying tissue. The weighted average gonad dose to the general population is used to estimate the GSD.

TABLE 2-6

Range of acceptable entrance skin exposures (ESE) for selected radiographic examinations

Examination	ESE per projection (mR)
Chest (PA)	12 to 26
Skull (lateral)	105 to 240
Abdomen (AP)	375 to 698
Retrograde pyelogram	475 to 829
Cervical spine (AP)	35 to 165
Thoracic spine (AP)	295 to 485
Extremity	8 to 327
Dental (bite-wing and periapical)	227 to 425

PA, posteroanterior; *AP,* anteroposterior.

TABLE 2-7

Representative entrance skin exposure (ESE) and glandular dose for mammography

Examination	ESE per projection (mR) per projection (mrad)	Approximate glandular dose
Screen-film (nongrid)	800	100
Screen-film (4:1 grid)	1200	150
Magnification (2×)	1600	200

TABLE 2-8

Representative bone marrow dose for selected radiographic examinations

Examination	Mean marrow dose (mrad)
Skull	10
Cervical spine	20
Chest	2
Stomach and upper gastrointestinal tract	100
Gallbladder	80
Lumbar spine	60
Intravenous urography	25
Abdomen	30
Pelvis	20
Extremity	2

TABLE 2-9

Approximate gonad dose resulting from various radiographic examinations

Examination	Gonad dose (mrad)	
	Male	Female
Skull	<1	<1
Cervical spine	<1	<1
Full-mouth dental	>1	<1
Chest	<1	<1
Stomach and upper gastrointestinal tract	<2	40
Gallbladder	1	20
Lumbar spine	175	400
Intravenous urography	150	300
Abdomen	100	200
Pelvis	300	150
Extremity	<1	<1

Fetal dose

Like most organ doses, fetal dose cannot be measured; it must be estimated. This estimate is usually obtained from phantom measurements or computer-generated calculations. Table 2-10 shows the results of an analysis by the U.S. Center for Devices and Radiological Health and reports fetal dose as a function of the normalized ESE. Before this table can be used, the ESE for the type of examination in question must be measured. The fetal dose is given in mrad/R ESE. Obviously the fetal dose is highest when the uterus is in the useful beam, such as during abdominal and pelvic examinations of the mother. During examination of distal parts of the mother's body, the fetal dose is very low, often not exceeding 1 mrad.

RADIOGRAPHER EXPOSURE

The radiographer receives at least 95% of occupational exposure during fluoroscopy and portable radiography. However, because the radiographer wears protective apparel while performing these examinations, only part of the body is exposed.

For the field adjacent to the examination table, exposure rates may approach 500 mR/hr (5 mGy/hr). The protective curtain draping the image intensifier tower usually reduces the exposure to less than 5 mR/hr (50 µGy/hr). The radiographer exposure can be estimated by assuming a position near the table and determining the x-ray beam on-time. For example, if a barium enema requires 3 minutes of x-ray tube on-time and the radiographer is positioned in a 100 mR/hr (1 mGy/hr) field, the occupational exposure to the unshielded part of the radiographer would be as follows:

$$100 \text{ mR/hr} \times 3/60 \text{ hr} = 5 \text{ mR}$$

Protective apparel usually provides an exposure reduction factor of at least one tenth. Therefore in the above example the exposure to the trunk of the body of the radiographer would be less than 1 mR (10 µGy).

During conventional radiography the radiographer is positioned behind a protective barrier, which often may be a secondary barrier. In this situation the useful beam is never directed at the radiographer. A helpful way to estimate exposure to the radiographer during radiography is to apply the following rule of thumb: the exposure 1 meter laterally from the patient is approximately 0.1% of the ESE. For example, in Fig. 2-1 the radiographer is positioned 2 meters from the patient. If the examination were of the chest, the ESE would be approximately 20 mR (200 µGy). The scatter radiation intensity 1 meter laterally would be 0.1% of the ESE or 0.02 mR (0.2 µGy). According to the inverse square law, at 2 meters the scatter radiation intensity would be 0.005 mR or 5 µR (0.05 µGy).

Protection of the Patient

The patient is protected from unnecessary radiation during diagnostic x-ray examinations by certain design features of x-ray equipment and specially fabricated auxiliary apparatus. Special administrative procedures also help to avoid unnecessary patient dose.

EQUIPMENT AND APPARATUS DESIGN

Usually the features of radiographic and fluoroscopic equipment that are designed to reduce patient dose also reduce exposure to the radiographer. This aspect of radiation control should be kept in mind when patient protection is considered.

Filtration

A minimum of 2.5 mm aluminum equivalent total filtration is required on all fluoroscopic x-ray tubes and for radiographic tubes operating above 70 kVp. The patient couch is considered part of the fluoroscopic filtration. The purpose of filtration is to reduce the amount of low-energy x-rays reaching the patient. Because only higher energy x-rays are useful in producing an image, low-energy x-rays are absorbed in the patient and contribute only to patient dose and not to the radiographic or fluoroscopic image. In general, the higher the total filtration, the lower the patient dose.

Collimation

Collimation is the restriction of the useful x-ray beam to the body part being examined, thereby sparing adjacent tissue from unnecessary exposure. This factor is extremely important in patient protection. The x-ray beam should always be collimated to the anatomic region of interest. The larger the useful x-ray beam, the higher the patient dose. Restricting the x-ray beam by collimation reduces not only the volume of tissue irradiated but also the absolute dose at any point because of the accompanying reduction in scatter radiation. Reduction of scatter radiation also increases image quality by improving image contrast.

TABLE 2-10

Approximate fetal dose as a function of entrance skin exposure

Examination	Fetal dose (mrad/R)
Skull	<0.01
Cervical spine	<0.01
Full-mouth dental	<0.01
Chest	2
Stomach and upper gastrointestinal tract	25
Gallbladder	3
Lumbar spine	250
Intravenous urography	265
Abdomen	265
Pelvis	265
Extremity	<0.01

Specific area shielding

Often only part of the primary beam needs to be absorbed during the examination, and thus those areas of the body that lie in or near the useful beam but do not need to be imaged can be shielded. Gonad shielding is a good example of such *specific area shielding* and can be applied with either shadow or contact shields. Shadow shields are attached to the radiographic tube head and are positioned with the aid of the light localizer between the x-ray tube and the patient. Contact shields are usually fabricated of vinyl lead cut into various shapes and are simply laid on the patient.

Gonad shields should be used in the following situations: (1) when a patient is of reproductive age, (2) when the gonads lie in or near the useful beam, and (3) when the use of such shielding will not compromise the required diagnostic information. The use of gonad shields reduces the gonad dose to near zero.

Image receptors

The speed of an image receptor can greatly influence patient dose. Rare-earth screens developed in conjunction with matched photographic emulsions show relative speeds of up to 12 times those of a conventional calcium tungstate screen-film combination. Rare-earth screen-film combinations that will reduce patient dose to one fourth can be used with no loss of diagnostic information. Higher patient-dose reductions are possible, but the quality of the image may be compromised somewhat by radiographic noise.

Today's fluoroscopic image intensifiers also incorporate more efficient input phosphors that can reduce patient dose by 25% to 50%. Digital fluoroscopy incorporating pulsed x-ray beams and image-hold techniques results in a large reduction in patient dose. Use of these newer imaging modalities has been responsible for the significant reduction in patient dose in recent years.

Radiographic technique

Radiographic technique not only is important in the production of a quality image but also greatly influences patient dose. Ideally, the higher the kVp, the lower the patient dose, because a large reduction in mAs must accompany an increase in kVp. However, as kVp is raised, image contrast is reduced, and for some examinations this reduction in contrast may be unacceptable. For example, mammography could be performed at far lower patient doses if the operating kVp were increased. However, the radiographic contrast would be very poor and the image would contain less diagnostic information. In general, the highest practicable kVp with an appropriate mAs should be used in all examinations.

ADMINISTRATIVE PROCEDURES

Patient selection and examination selection are two areas in which radiographers can contribute to reducing unnecessary patient dose.

Pregnancy

Safeguards against accidental fetal irradiation are particularly critical during the first 2 months of pregnancy. In those early weeks, a pregnancy may not be suspected and the fetus could be exposed unknowingly; the first-trimester fetus is particularly sensitive to radiation exposure. After a couple of months' gestation, the risk of irradiating an undetected fetus becomes small because the patient is generally aware of her condition.

The radiographer should never knowingly conduct a radiologic examination on a pregnant patient unless a documented decision has been made to do so. When such an examination does proceed, all of the previously discussed techniques for minimizing patient dose should be employed.

For many years, radiologists subscribed to the *10-day rule*. This rule was first stated in 1970 by the ICRP. It recommended that all x-ray examinations of the abdomen or pelvis of fertile women be performed only during the 10 days following the onset of menstruation. In the 1980s both the American College of Radiology (ACR) and the ICRP published thoughtful documents showing why the 10-day rule should be abandoned. The 1983 statement of the ICRP reads:

In the first 10 days following the onset of a menstrual period, there can be no risk to any conceptus, since no conception will have occurred. The risk to a child who had previously been irradiated in utero during the remainder of the 4-week period following the onset of menstruation is likely to be so small that there need be no special limitation on exposures required within these 4 weeks.

The risk of injury following irradiation in utero is small and the usual benefit is so great that if the examination is clinically indicated, it should be performed. Many studies have shown that delay in scheduling such an examination is more harmful to the patient than the x-ray exposure.

Fetal doses during radiographic exposure rarely exceed a few hundred millirad. However, if the examination is a high-dose procedure of the pelvis, such as a computed tomographic scan or a fluoroscopic examination, special attention may be appropriate if the patient suspects pregnancy. If the examination is necessary at that time, it should be conducted. When a pregnant patient must be examined, the examination should be performed with precisely collimated beams and carefully positioned specific area shields. Use of a high-kVp technique is most appropriate in such situations.

Radiographers fulfill their responsibility to potentially pregnant patients by posting caution signs in the waiting room and in each examining room. Such signs warn patients about the importance of informing the radiographer or radiologist that pregnancy is a possibility. Fig. 2-5 shows a helpful poster available from the National Center for Devices and Radiological Health that provides this message.

Patient and examination selection

Precautions against unnecessary patient dose are generally the responsibility of the radiologist, not the radiographer. Patient selection and examination selection are two such situations.

Patients selected for x-ray examination fall into two categories: those who have symptoms and those who do not. Patients with symptoms usually require x-ray examinations to evaluate any previous clinical management and to provide the physician with information to plan the patient's future clinical management. Patients without symptoms usually are referred for x-ray examination to provide baseline information for possible future problems or to satisfy certain legal, insurance, or employment requirements. Screening mammography is one such example.

When accepting a patient with symptoms for x-ray examination, the radiologist must be certain that the type of examination prescribed can provide the information necessary for proper medical management of that patient. Furthermore, even if the findings of the examination are negative or normal, the performance of the examination should be beneficial and should significantly influence the course of patient management. For example, a skull series following trauma should be carefully evaluated by the radiologist and clinician. Several investigational series have reported that skull examinations influence the medical management of less than 10% of patients.

Selection of patients without symptoms for an x-ray examination involves mass screening with selected routine procedures, many of which may not be medically justified. Routine x-ray examinations should not be performed when there is no precise medical indication. Substantial evidence shows that some such examinations are of little benefit because the disease detection rate is very low. Examples of such unacceptable screening programs follow:

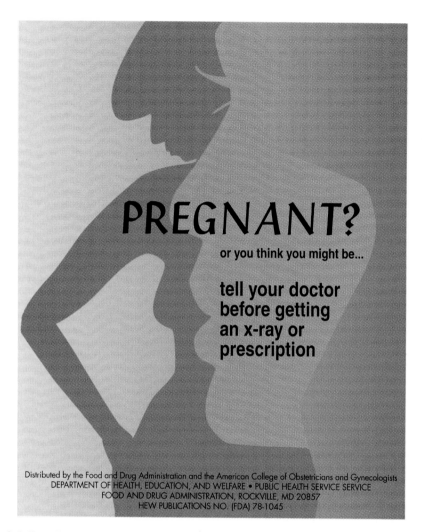

Fig. 2-5 Signs like this one alert patients to the possibility that radiation can harm an unknown pregnancy.

1. Tuberculosis—Mass general screening has not been found effective; better methods of tuberculosis testing are now available. Some x-ray screening in high-risk groups (e.g., medical and paramedical personnel) and in personnel posing a potential community hazard (e.g., miners and workers having contact with beryllium, asbestos, glass, or silica) may be appropriate.
2. Hospital admissions—Chest x-ray examination for routine hospital admission should not be performed in patients with no clinical indication of chest disease. Patients who would be candidates for such examinations include those admitted to the pulmonary or thoracic surgical service and elderly patients.
3. Preemployment physicals—Chest and lower back x-ray examinations are not justified because no knowledge is gained about previous injury or disease.
4. Periodic health examinations—Many physicians debate the frequency of a general physical examination as a preventive medicine protocol. Certainly, the physical evaluation of an asymptomatic patient should not include x-ray examination, especially fluoroscopy.

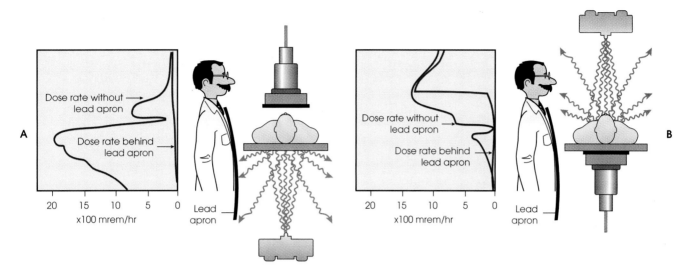

Fig. 2-6 Scatter radiation during mobile fluoroscopy is low when the x-ray tube is under the table **(A)** and more intense when the x-ray tube is over the patient **(B).**

Protection of the Radiographer

EQUIPMENT AND APPARATUS DESIGN

For the radiographer, radiation exposure is most likely to occur during fluoroscopy (Fig. 2-6) or mobile radiography. Consequently, particular care and attention should be exercised during these examinations.

Protective apparel should always be worn for both fluoroscopic and mobile radiographic procedures. Table 2-11 shows the degree of protection provided by the principal sizes of the available protective lead aprons. Most radiographers find the 0.5-mm lead apron perfectly adequate. Thicker aprons may be too heavy for some radiographers engaged in a heavy fluoroscopy schedule. Each mobile x-ray unit should have a protective apron assigned to it, and the apron should remain with the unit at all times.

Protective barriers

During conventional radiography the radiographer is positioned behind the control console barrier or other fixed protective barrier. Mobile protective screens should be avoided whenever possible. Although most protective barriers consist of a certain thickness of lead, not all do; nor is it necessary for all barriers to contain lead. Table 2-12 shows the British, metric, and construction equivalencies of common thicknesses of lead employed in diagnostic radiology. Rarely is it necessary to exceed 1.6 mm of lead.

Newer x-ray equipment and faster image receptors are significantly reducing the intensity of radiation during diagnostic x-ray procedures; therefore the amount of shielding required today is not what it was in years past. Although the radiographer does not need to know how to compute barrier thickness, some of the considerations that enter into that computation should be understood.

TABLE 2-11

X-ray attenuation values for the common lead (Pb) equivalent thicknesses of protective aprons

Equivalent thickness (mm Pb)	X-ray attenuation (%)			
	60 kVp	80 kVp	100 kVp	120 kVp
0.3	99	97	94	92
0.5	99	99	96	95
1.0	99	99	98	97

TABLE 2-12

British, metric, and construction equivalencies of common thicknesses of lead used in diagnostic radiology*

British (inch)	Metric (mm)	Construction (lb/ft²)
1/64	0.4	1
1/32	0.8	2
3/64	1.2	3
1/16	1.6	4
5/64	2.0	5
3/32	2.4	6

*Protective lead shielding is usually computed in metric units, but it is given to the constructor in pounds per square foot.

Primary and secondary barriers

A *primary barrier* is any barrier that intercepts the useful, or primary, x-ray beam. A *secondary barrier* is one that intercepts only *leakage* and *scatter radiation*. The floor is almost always considered a primary barrier; from one to four walls may also be primary barriers. The ceiling is always considered a secondary barrier.

The control console barrier is usually considered a secondary barrier. *Thus the useful beam should never be directed at the control console barrier.* During fluoroscopy all fixed barriers are considered secondary because the image intensifier is designed as a built-in primary barrier.

Dose-limiting recommendations

The effective dose equivalent expressed as a weekly intensity is determined for each barrier on the basis of the use of the area being protected. If the adjacent area, such as another x-ray examination room or the darkroom, is to be occupied only by radiation workers and patients, it is identified as a *controlled area*. The dose limit for a controlled area is 1 μSv/wk. If the adjacent area is a laboratory, office, or area occupied by persons in the general population, it is called an *uncontrolled area*, and the dose limit is 20 μSv/wk.

Distance

The distance from the x-ray tube to the area being protected is important because the radiation intensity decreases rapidly according to the *inverse square law*. If the barrier is designated as a primary barrier, the distance is seldom less than 1 meter and is usually much more. The distance to a secondary barrier is often shorter. Obviously, for larger examination rooms, the respective distances will be larger and the required shielding will be less.

Workload

Workload is an expression of the total intensity of radiation employed during any week. It is described in units of milliampere-minutes per week (mA-min/wk) and takes into account the number of patients examined, the number of images per patient, and the average milliampere seconds per image. The radiographic workload of a busy room rarely exceeds 500 mA-min/wk. Special-purpose radiographic units may have considerably lower workloads. Less shielding is required for low-workload facilities.

CARDINAL PRINCIPLES OF RADIATION PROTECTION: TIME, DISTANCE, AND SHIELDING

1. Keep your time of exposure to radiation to a minimum.
2. Stay as far from the source of radiation (the patient during fluoroscopy) as possible.
3. Use the provided protective apparel.

Use factor

Under normal conditions, a radiographic tube is pointed toward the floor for most of the time that it is energized. During some fraction of its beam on-time, the tube may be pointed toward any vertical barrier. The relative amount of time that the useful x-ray beam is directed toward a given barrier is the use factor. The floor is generally assigned a use factor of 1, and each wall is given a use factor of 0.05 to 0.25. The use factor is 1 for all secondary barriers because at all times that the x-ray tube is energized, scatter and leakage radiation is generated.

Time of occupancy factor

The time of occupancy factor is the extent to which the area being protected is occupied. Obviously an area that is always occupied will require more shielding than one that is rarely occupied. The recommended occupancy factors range from *full* occupancy for an adjacent office or laboratory to *partial* occupancy for a hallway or restroom to *occasional* occupancy for outside areas, elevators, and stairwells.

• • •

All of these factors are considered when the required protective barrier thickness is computed. Although lead is the usual shielding material for most diagnostic x-ray applications, other types of building material may be acceptable, particularly for secondary barriers. Brick, concrete block, gypsum board, and conventional plate glass are sometimes suitable. Frequently, multiple thicknesses of gypsum board may be used instead of lead-lined gypsum board. Plate glass that is $\frac{1}{2}$ to 1 inch thick may sometimes be substituted for leaded glass in, for example, the viewing window of a control console barrier.

A block, brick, or concrete wall often satisfies the requirements for a primary barrier. Likewise, a 4-inch-thick concrete slab floor usually provides adequate protection as a primary barrier. If the slab is thin, it is sometimes permissible to position additional protective lead under the examination table with an appropriate overhang. If the x-ray room is located on ground level, the earth serves as a primary barrier and no additional shielding is necessary.

ADMINISTRATIVE PROCEDURES

Every radiographer should be familiar with the cardinal principles of radiation protection—time, distance, and shielding (box):

1. The *time* of exposure to a radiation source should be kept to a minimum.
2. The *distance* between the radiation source and the radiographer should be as great as possible.
3. When appropriate and practicable, protective *shielding* material should be positioned between the radiation source and the radiographer.

A prime example of these cardinal principles occurs during fluoroscopy. As shown in Fig. 2-6, the maximum exposure rate in a fluoroscopic examination exists in the field adjacent to the table. Because the primary beam is emitted by the under-table tube and intercepts the patient, the patient becomes the radiation source because of scatter radiation.

The radiologist must *minimize the exposure time* by activating the foot or hand control intermittently for minimum x-ray beam on-time. The radiographer can help by making certain that the 5-minute fluoroscopic reset timer is functioning and is used properly. The radiographer can minimize occupational exposure by *taking one step back* from the edge of the fluoroscopic table when it is not absolutely essential to remain there. During fluoroscopy the radiologist and radiographer must wear *protective lead apparel*, which is the most effective method for reducing occupational exposure.

Personnel monitoring

Perhaps the single most important aspect of a radiation control program in diagnostic radiology is a properly designed personnel radiation monitoring program. Three types of radiation measuring devices are used as personnel monitors: pocket ionization chambers, film badges, and thermoluminescent dosimetry badges.

Pocket ionization chambers can be used for personnel monitoring, although they seldom are used in diagnostic radiology. The singular advantage to these devices is that they can be evaluated daily. However, pocket chamber dosimeters require a great deal of record keeping; thus their use in diagnostic radiology is generally restricted to monitoring occasional visitors.

Photographic film in the form of a *film badge* has been the principal personnel radiation monitor for years. The design of the film badge has undergone many refinements, such as integral metal filters that enable it to measure not only the quantity of radiation but also the type of radiation, approximate energy, and direction. Consequently, this type of monitor must be handled and worn properly.

Thermoluminescent dosimetry (TLD) badges are used as personnel radiation monitors and have many of the same performance characteristics as film badges. The TLD-sensitive material is reusable. Although the initial cost is high, the long-term expense is comparable to that of film badges. The TLD badge can be used for lengths of time exceeding the monthly interval limits placed on film badges. Under some circumstances it is not only permissible but advisable to monitor x-ray workers for calendar-quarter intervals rather than monthly or biweekly intervals. The principal advantage to this mode of radiation monitoring is the reduced record keeping that is required.

Regardless of the type of monitor employed, a successful personnel radiation monitoring program has certain important requirements. Each shipment of personnel monitors should be accompanied by a *control badge*. The control badge should normally be stored in a location distant from any radiation source, such as in the office of the director of radiology.

Individual radiation monitors should not leave the hospital. A rack or other holding device should be available on which radiographers can store their badges at the end of the day. This system helps to ensure that the monitors are not inadvertently damaged or exposed to environmental elements outside the hospital. Of course, the holding rack should be positioned away from any radiation source.

Radiographers receive most of their occupational exposure during fluoroscopy and portable radiography, but they wear protective apparel for these procedures. Therefore the anatomic position of the personnel monitor is important. The monitor should be worn unshielded (outside the protective apron) at the collar region. This region of the body will receive at least 10 times the radiation exposure of the protected trunk of the body. Therefore it is prudent to monitor the collar region because this provides a way to estimate thyroid and eye lens dose as a means of estimating effective dose equivalent and as the most realistic means of monitoring the radiation environment. Furthermore, most state regulations require the monitor to be worn at the collar position. Regardless of the position of the personnel radiation monitor, a notation of where the device is worn should be included in each radiation monitoring report and in department rules and regulations.

The orientation of the monitor is also important. The front of the monitor must face the radiation source. If the orientation of the monitor is reversed, the filters in the monitor will not be in the correct position and the readings may be false.

A personnel monitoring program is not complete unless proper documentation is provided. Most commercial vendors of personnel radiation monitors will provide the user with a periodic computer-generated report containing all of the required information. For this report to be complete, all of the requested information on each individual must be supplied, including name, social security number, date of birth, gender, and previous radiation exposure. Quantification of previous radiation exposure may sometimes be difficult to obtain. Documentation of efforts to obtain this information must be generated and filed.

Pregnant radiographers

Special administrative procedures are required for pregnant radiographers. It is the responsibility of each female radiographer to inform her supervisor when she discovers or suspects that she is pregnant. This situation then becomes a *declared pregnancy* and new rules take effect. A supervisor should then consult with the pregnant radiographer and review completely the ongoing radiation control program of the department.

Under normal circumstances a radiographer receives less than 5 mSv annually, as recorded by the personnel monitor. The exposure under the protective apron should not exceed 0.5 mSv annually, and the resulting fetal dose should not exceed 0.25 mSv. Because the dose limitation to the fetus is 5 mSv for the gestation period, under most circumstances additional radiation protective measures may not be necessary.

To comply with current NCRP recommendations, management must deliberately review each radiation monitoring report to ensure that the occupational fetal dose does not exceed 0.5 mSv in any month. The collar-positioned monitor can be used to estimate fetal dose by multiplying the reported result by 0.1. Better yet, a second monitor may be positioned at waist level under the protective apron.

When a second monitor is provided, the two monitors must consistently be worn at the assigned positions. To avoid confusion, the second monitor should be labeled "baby badge" or "fetal monitor" with the label colored a "baby" blue or yellow for "belly." The exposure reported on the baby badge should be maintained on a separate record and identified as exposure to the mother's pelvis. The fetal dose will be 25% to 50% of this value, depending on the time during the pregnancy.

Summary of Procedures

For radiographers, nearly all occupational radiation exposure occurs during fluoroscopy and mobile radiography. The following procedures will help to reduce this occupational exposure:

- During radiography, always remain behind the control console barrier.
- Never enter a fluoroscopic procedure without a protective apron.
- Always position your radiation monitor on your collar.
- Review your monthly radiation monitoring report.
- Wear a protective apron during mobile radiography, and stand on the opposite side of the operating console from the patient.
- During C-arm fluoroscopy, be sure the x-ray tube is below the patient.
- If you become pregnant, inform your supervisor so that additional radiation protection procedures can be implemented.

The following procedures will help to reduce patient radiation dose. However, remember that a quality image is more important than reduced patient radiation dose.

- Use high kVp technique for radiography.
- Record the fluoroscopic x-ray beam on-time if it is expected to exceed 20 minutes.
- Use gonad shields when such use will not interfere with the examination.
- Make sure the patient is properly prepared so that repeat examination is not necessary.
- If the patient thinks she may be pregnant, consult the radiologist before continuing the examination.

Observing these essentials of radiation protection will ensure that your exposure and that of your patient is ALARA—*as low as reasonably achievable* (Fig 2-7).

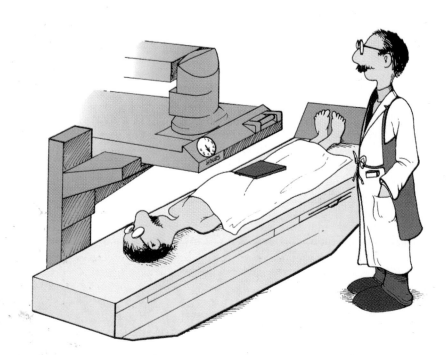

Fig. 2-7 What is *wrong* with this scene?
1. Radiation monitor is positioned improperly
2. Gonad shield is in wrong place
3. Protective apron is not worn properly
4. There is too much x-ray beam on-time
   a. 1 and 3 only are correct.
   b. 2 and 4 only are correct.
   c. 1, 2, and 3 only are correct.
   d. 1, 2, 3, and 4 are correct.

GENERAL ANATOMY AND RADIOGRAPHIC POSITIONING TERMINOLOGY

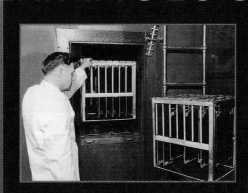

RIGHT Hand processing tanks, 1950. Wet films were placed in a dryer for 30 minutes before being read. An hour or more was required to produce a readable film.

(Courtesy Mayo Clinic/Foundation.)

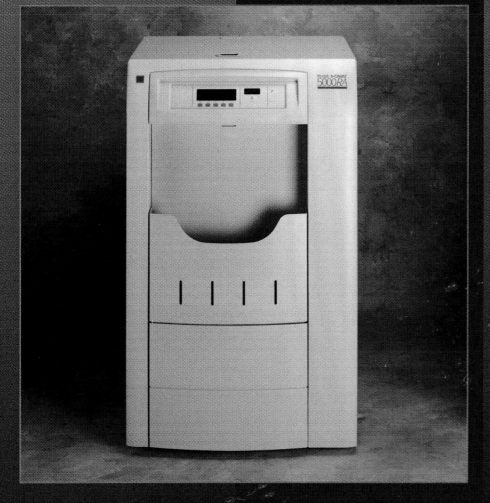

LEFT Kodak X-Omat 5000 RA processor with keypad-selectable cycles and room-light-handling option. With a 45-second cycle, this processor produces 483 films per hour.

(Courtesy Eastman Kodak Co.)

General Anatomy

Radiographers must possess a thorough knowledge of anatomy, physiology, and osteology to obtain radiographs that demonstrate the desired body part. *Anatomy* is the term applied to the science of the structure of the body. *Physiology* is the study of the function of the body organs. *Osteology* is the detailed study of the body of knowledge relating to the bones of the body.

Radiographers also must have a general understanding of all body systems and their functions. Particular attention must be given to thoroughly understanding the skeletal system and the surface landmarks used to locate different body parts. The radiographer must be able to mentally visualize the internal structures that are to be radiographed. By using external landmarks, the radiographer should properly position body parts to obtain the best diagnostic radiographs possible.

BODY PLANES

The full dimension of the human body as viewed in the *anatomic position* (see Chapter 1) can be effectively subdivided through the use of imaginary body planes. These planes slice through the body at designated levels from all directions. The following four fundamental body planes referred to in radiography are illustrated in Fig. 3-1, *A:*

- Sagittal
- Coronal
- Horizontal
- Oblique

Sagittal plane

A sagittal plane divides the entire body or a body part into right and left segments. The plane passes vertically through the body from front to back (Fig. 3-1, *A* and *B*). The *midsagittal plane* is a specific sagittal plane that passes through the midline of the body and divides it into equal right and left halves (Fig. 3-1, *C*).

Coronal plane

A coronal plane divides the entire body or a body part into anterior and posterior segments. The plane passes through the body vertically from one side to the other (see Fig. 3-1, *A* and *B*). The midcoronal plane is a specific coronal plane that passes through the midline of the body, dividing it into equal anterior and posterior halves (see Fig. 3-1, *C*). This plane is often referred to as the *midaxillary plane.*

Horizontal plane

A horizontal plane passes crosswise through the body or a body part at right angles to the longitudinal axis. It is positioned at a right angle to the sagittal and coronal planes. This plane divides the body into superior and inferior portions. Often it is referred to as a *transverse* or *axial plane* (Fig. 3-1, *A*).

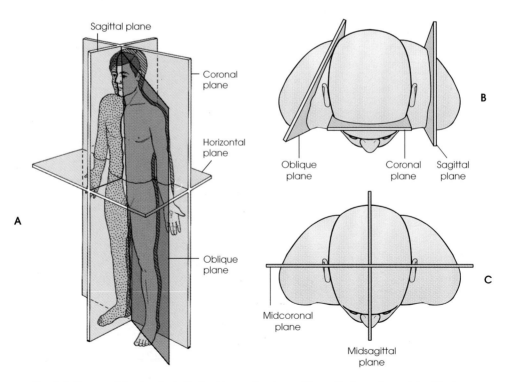

Fig. 3-1 Planes of the body. **A,** Patient in anatomic position with four planes identified. **B,** Top-down perspective of patient's body showing a sagittal plane through the left shoulder, a coronal plane through the anterior head, and an oblique plane through the right shoulder. **C,** Midsagittal plane dividing the body equally into right and left halves and midcoronal plane dividing the body equally into anterior and posterior halves. Note that sagittal, coronal, and horizontal planes are always at right angles to one another.

Oblique plane

An oblique plane can pass through a body part at any angle between the three planes discussed earlier (see Fig. 3-1, *A* and *B*).

Planes are used in radiographic positioning to center a body part to the image receptor (IR) or central ray and to ensure that the body part is properly oriented and aligned with the IR. For example, the midsagittal plane may be centered and perpendicular to the IR with the long axis of the IR parallel to the same plane. Planes can also be used to guide projections of the central ray. The central ray for an anteroposterior (AP) projection, for example, passes through the body part parallel to the sagittal plane and perpendicular to the coronal plane. Quality imaging requires attention to all relationships among body planes, the IR, and the central ray.

Body planes are used in computed tomography (CT), magnetic resonance imaging (MRI), and ultrasound (US) to identify the orientation of anatomic *cuts* or *slices* demonstrated in the procedure. Imaging in several planes is often used to demonstrate a body part (Fig. 3-2).

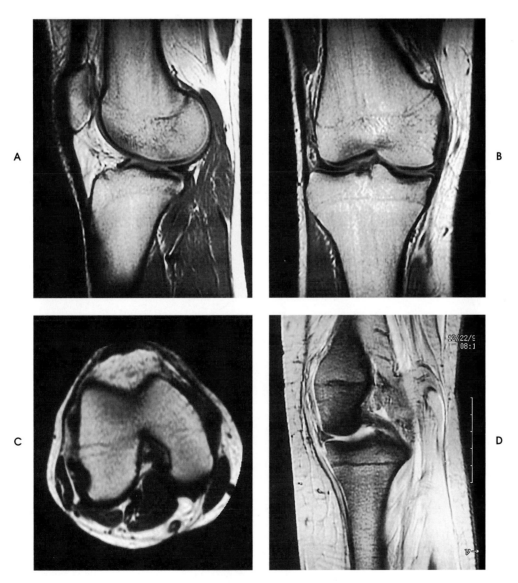

Fig. 3-2 Magnetic resonance images of the knee in four planes. **A,** Sagittal. **B,** Coronal. **C,** Horizontal. **D,** Oblique, 45 degrees.

BODY CAVITIES

The two great cavities of the torso are the *thoracic* and *abdominal cavities* (Fig. 3-3). The thoracic cavity is subdivided into a pericardial segment and two pleural portions. Although the abdominal cavity has no intervening partition, the lower portion is called the *pelvic cavity*. Some anatomists combine the abdominal and pelvic cavities and refer to them as the *abdominopelvic cavity*. The principal structures located in the cavities follow.

Thoracic cavity
- Pleural membranes
- Lungs
- Trachea
- Esophagus
- Pericardium
- Heart and great vessels

Abdominal cavity
- Peritoneum
- Liver
- Gallbladder
- Pancreas
- Spleen
- Stomach
- Intestines
- Kidneys
- Ureters
- Major blood vessels
- Pelvic portion: rectum, urinary bladder, and parts of the reproductive system

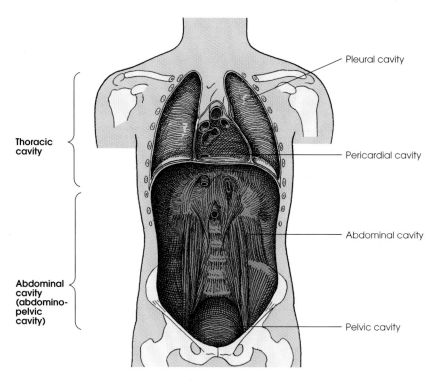

Pleural cavity

Pericardial cavity

Abdominal cavity

Pelvic cavity

Thoracic cavity

Abdominal cavity (abdomino-pelvic cavity)

Fig. 3-3 Anterior view of the torso showing the two great cavities: thoracic and abdominal

DIVISIONS OF THE ABDOMEN

The abdomen is the portion of the trunk that is bordered superiorly by the diaphragm and inferiorly by the superior pelvic aperture (pelvic inlet). The location of organs or an anatomic area can be described by dividing the abdomen according to one of two methods: four quadrants or nine regions.

Quadrants

The abdomen is often divided into four clinical divisions called *quadrants* (Fig. 3-4). The midsagittal plane and a horizontal plane intersect at the umbilicus and create the boundaries. The quadrants are named as follows:

- Right upper quadrant (RUQ)
- Right lower quadrant (RLQ)
- Left upper quadrant (LUQ)
- Left lower quadrant (LLQ)

Dividing the abdomen into four quadrants is useful for describing the location of the various abdominal organs. For example, the spleen can be described as being located in the left upper quadrant.

Regions

Some anatomists divide the abdomen into nine regions by using four planes (Fig. 3-5). These anatomic divisions are not used as often as quadrants in clinical practice. The nine regions of the body, divided into three groups, are named as follows.

Superior

- Right hypochondrium
- Epigastrium
- Left hypochondrium

Middle

- Right lateral
- Umbilical
- Left lateral

Inferior

- Right inguinal
- Hypogastrium
- Left inguinal

In the clinical setting a patient could be described as having "epigastric" pain. A patient with discomfort in the right lower abdomen could be described as having "RLQ" pain. Sometimes a quadrant term is used and sometimes a region term.

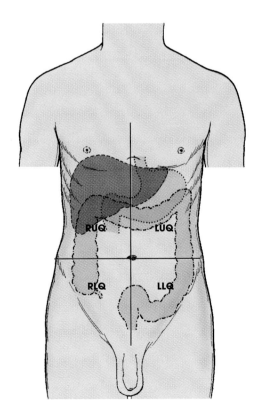

Fig. 3-4 Four quadrants of the abdomen.

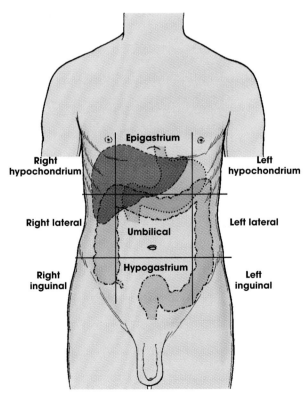

Fig. 3-5 Nine regions of the abdomen.

TABLE 3-1

External landmarks related to body structures at the same level

Body structures	External landmarks
Cervical area (see Fig. 3-6)	
C1	Mastoid tip
C2, C3	Gonion (angle of mandible)
C3, C4	Hyoid bone
C5	Thyroid cartilage
C7, T1	Vertebra prominens
Thoracic area	
T1	Approximately 2 in (5 cm) above level of jugular notch
T2, T3	Level of jugular notch
T4, T5	Level of sternal angle
T7	Level of inferior angles of scapulae
T9, T10	Level of xiphoid process
Lumbar area	
L2, L3	Inferior costal margin
L4, L5	Level of most superior aspect of crests of ilia
Sacrum and pelvic area	
S1, S2	Level of anterior superior iliac spines (ASIS)
Coccyx	Level of pubic symphysis and greater trochanters

SURFACE LANDMARKS

Most anatomic structures cannot be visualized directly; therefore the radiographer must use various protuberances, tuberosities, and other external indicators to accurately position the patient. These surface landmarks enable the radiographer to consistently obtain radiographs of optimal quality for a wide variety of body types. If surface landmarks are not used for radiographic positioning or if they are used incorrectly, the chance of having to repeat the radiograph greatly increases.

Many of the commonly used landmarks are listed in Table 3-1 and diagrammed in Fig. 3-6. However, these landmarks are accepted averages for the majority of patients and should be used only as guidelines. Variations in anatomic build or pathologic conditions may warrant positioning compensation on an individual basis. The ability to compensate is gained through experience.

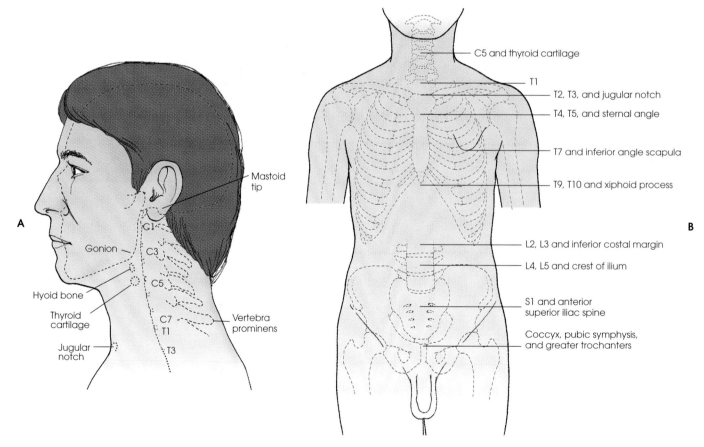

Fig. 3-6 Surface landmarks. **A,** Head and neck. **B,** Torso.

BODY HABITUS

The common variations in the shape of the human body are termed the *body habitus*. Mills[1] determined the primary classifications of body habitus based on his study of 1000 patients. The specific type of body habitus is important in radiography because it determines the size, shape, and position of the organs of the thoracic and abdominal cavities.

[1]Mills WR: The relation of bodily habitus to visceral form, position, tonus, and motility, *AJR* 4:155, 1917.

Body habitus directly affects the location of the following:
• Heart
• Lungs
• Diaphragm
• Stomach
• Colon
• Gallbladder

An organ such as the gallbladder may vary in position by as much as 8 inches, depending on the body habitus. The stomach may be positioned horizontally, high, and in the center of the abdomen for one type of habitus and positioned vertically, low, and to the side of the midline in another type. Fig. 3-7 shows an example of the placement, shape, and size of the lungs, heart, and diaphragm in patients with four different body habitus types.

Body habitus and the placement of the thoracic and abdominal organs are also important in the determination of technical and exposure factors for the appropriate radiographic density and contrast and the radiation doses. For example, contrast medium in the gallbladder may affect the automatic exposure control detector. For one type of habitus the gallbladder may lie directly over the detector (which is not desirable); for another it may not even be near the detector. The standard placement and size of the IR may have to be changed because of body habitus. The selection of kilovolt (peak) and milliampere-second exposure factors may also be affected by the type of habitus because of wide variations in physical tissue density. These technical considerations are described in greater detail in radiography physics and imaging texts.

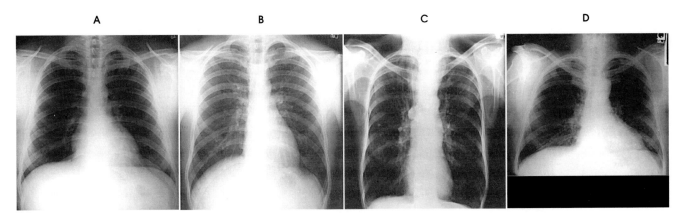

Fig. 3-7 Placement, shape, and size of the lungs, heart, and diaphragm in patients with four different body habitus types. **A,** Sthenic. **B,** Hyposthenic. **C,** Asthenic. **D,** Hypersthenic.

Table 3-2 describes specific characteristics of the four types of body habitus and outlines their general shapes and variations. The four major types of body habitus and their approximate frequency in the population are identified below.

- Sthenic, 50%
- Hyposthenic, 35%
- Asthenic, 10%
- Hypersthenic, 5%

More than 85% of the population has either a *sthenic* or *hyposthenic* body habitus. The sthenic type is considered the dominant type of habitus. The relative shape of patients with a sthenic or hyposthenic body habitus and the position of their organs are referred to in clinical practice as *ordinary* or *average.* All standard radiographic positioning and exposure techniques are based on these two groups. Therefore radiographers must become thoroughly familiar with the characteristics and organ placements of these two body types.

Radiographers must also become familiar with the two extreme habitus types: *asthenic* and *hypersthenic.* In these two small groups (15% of the population), the placement and size of the organs significantly affect positioning and the selection of exposure factors. Consequently, radiography of these patients can be challenging. Experience and professional judgment enable the radiographer to determine the correct body habitus and to judge the specific location of the organs.

Body habitus is not an indication of disease or other abnormality, and it is not determined by the body fat or physical condition of the patient. Habitus is simply a classification of the four general shapes of the trunk of the human body.

TABLE 3-2

Four types of body habitus: prevalence, organ placement, and characteristics*

Sthenic, 50%

Organs

Heart: moderately transverse
Lungs: moderate length
Diaphragm: moderately high
Stomach: high, upper left
Colon: spread evenly; slight dip in transverse colon
Gallbladder: centered on right side, upper abdomen

Characteristics

Build: moderately heavy
Abdomen: moderately long
Thorax: moderately short, broad, and deep
Pelvis: relatively small

Hyposthenic, 35%

The organs and characteristics for this habitus are intermediate between the sthenic and asthenic body habitus types. This habitus is the most difficult to classify.

Asthenic, 10%

Organs

Heart: nearly vertical and at midline
Lungs: long, apices above clavicles, may be broader above base
Diaphragm: low
Stomach: low and medial, in the pelvis when standing
Colon: low, folds on itself
Gallbladder: low and nearer the midline

Characteristics

Build: frail
Abdomen: short
Thorax: long, shallow
Pelvis: wide

Hypersthenic, 5%

Organs

Heart: axis nearly transverse
Lungs: short, apices at or near clavicles
Diaphragm: high
Stomach: high, transverse, and in the middle
Colon: around periphery of abdomen
Gallbladder: high, outside, lies more parallel

Characteristics

Build: massive
Abdomen: long
Thorax: short, broad, deep
Pelvis: narrow

*Note the significant differences between the two extreme habitus types (i.e., sthenic and hypersthenic). The differences between the sthenic and hyposthenic types are less distinct.

TABLE 3-3

Axial skeleton: 80 bones

Area	Bones	Number
Skull	Cranial	8
	Facial	14
	Auditory ossicles*	6
Neck	Hyoid	1
Thorax	Sternum	1
	Ribs	24
Vertebral column	Cervical	7
	Thoracic	12
	Lumbar	5
	Sacrum	1
	Coccyx	1

*Auditory ossicles are small bones in the ears. They are not considered official bones of the axial skeleton but are placed here for convenience.

TABLE 3-4

Appendicular skeleton: 126 bones

Area	Bones	Number
Shoulder girdle	Clavicles	2
	Scapulae	2
Upper limbs	Humeri	2
	Ulnae	2
	Radii	2
	Carpals	16
	Metacarpals	10
	Phalanges	28
Lower limbs	Femora	2
	Tibias	2
	Fibulae	2
	Patellae	2
	Tarsals	14
	Metatarsals	10
	Phalanges	28
Pelvic girdle	Hip bones	2

Osteology

The adult human skeleton is composed of 206 primary bones. Ligaments unite the bones of the skeleton. Bones provide the following:

- Attachment for muscles
- Mechanical basis for movement
- Protection of internal organs
- A frame to support the body
- Storage for calcium, phosphorus, and other salts
- Production of red and white blood cells

The 206 bones of the body are divided into two main groups:

- Axial skeleton
- Appendicular skeleton

The *axial skeleton* supports and protects the head and trunk with 80 bones (Table 3-3). The *appendicular skeleton* allows the body to move in various positions and from place to place with its 126 bones (Table 3-4). Fig. 3-8 identifies these two skeletal areas.

GENERAL BONE FEATURES

The general features of most bones are shown in Fig. 3-9. All bones are composed of a strong, dense outer layer called the *compact bone* and an inner portion of less dense *spongy bone*. The hard outer compact bone protects the bone and gives it strength for supporting the body. The softer spongy bone contains a speculated network of interconnecting spaces called the *trabeculae* (Fig. 3-10). The trabeculae are filled with red and yellow marrow. Red marrow produces red and white blood cells, and yellow marrow stores adipose (fat) cells. Long bones have a central cavity called the *medullary cavity,* which contains trabeculae filled with yellow marrow. In long bones the red marrow is concentrated at the ends of the bone and not in the medullary cavity.

A tough, fibrous connective tissue called the *periosteum* covers all bony surfaces except the articular surfaces, which are covered by the articular cartilage. The tissue lining the medullary cavity of bones is called the *endosteum*. Bones contain various knoblike projections called *tubercles* and *tuberosities,* which are covered by the periosteum. Muscles, tendons, and ligaments attach to the periosteum at these projections. Blood vessels and nerves enter and exit the bone through the periosteum.

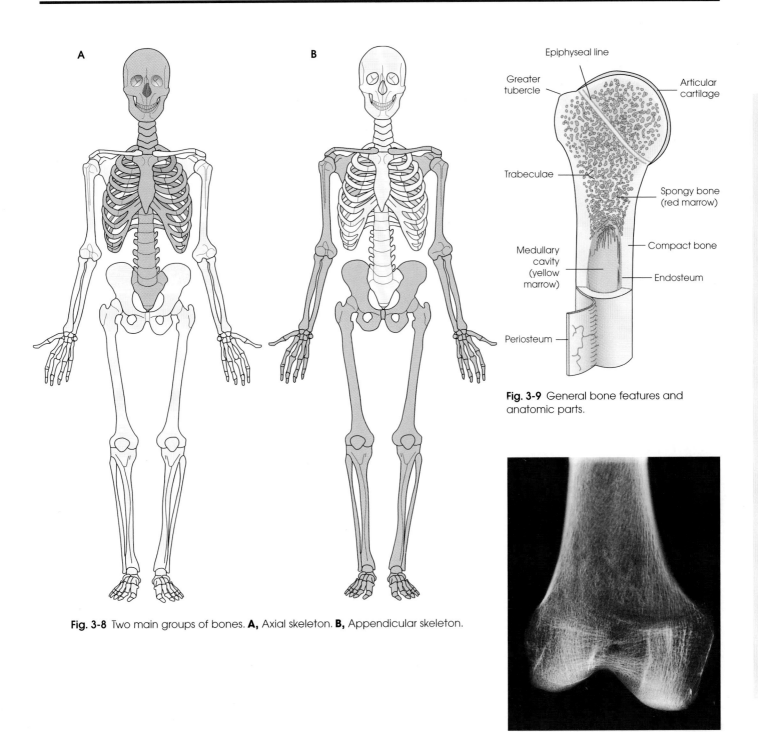

Fig. 3-8 Two main groups of bones. **A,** Axial skeleton. **B,** Appendicular skeleton.

Fig. 3-9 General bone features and anatomic parts.

Epiphyseal line

Greater tubercle

Articular cartilage

Trabeculae

Spongy bone (red marrow)

Medullary cavity (yellow marrow)

Compact bone

Endosteum

Periosteum

Fig. 3-10 Radiograph of the distal femur and condyles showing the bony trabeculae within the entire bone.

BONE VESSELS AND NERVES

Bones are live organs and must receive a blood supply for nourishment or they will die. Bones also contain a supply of nerves. Blood vessels and nerves enter and exit the bone at the same point, through openings called the *foramina*. Near the center of all long bones is an opening in the periosteum called the *nutrient foramen*. The nutrient artery of the bone passes into this opening and supplies the cancellous bone and marrow. The epiphyseal artery separately enters the ends of long bones to supply the area, and periosteal arteries enter at numerous points to supply the compact bone. Veins exiting the bones carry blood cells to the body (Fig. 3-11).

BONE DEVELOPMENT

Ossification is the term given to the development and formation of bones. Bones begin to develop in the second month of embryonic life. Ossification occurs separately by two distinct processes: *intermembranous ossification* and *endochondral ossification*.

Intermembranous ossification

Bones that develop from fibrous membranes in the embryo produce the flat bones such as those of the skull, clavicles, mandible, and sternum. Before birth these bones are not joined. As flat bones grow after birth, they join and form sutures. Other bones in this category merge together and create the various *joints* of the skeleton.

Endochondral ossification

Bones created by endochondral ossification develop from hyaline cartilage in the embryo and produce the short, irregular, and long bones. Endochondral ossification occurs from two distinct centers of development called the *primary* and *secondary centers of ossification*.

Primary ossification

Primary ossification begins before birth and forms the entire bulk of the short and irregular bones. This process forms the long central shaft in long bones. During development only, the long shaft of the bone is called the *diaphysis* (Fig. 3-12, *A*).

Secondary ossification

Secondary ossification occurs after birth when a separate bone begins to develop at both ends of every long bone. Each end is called the *epiphysis* (Fig. 3-12, *B*). At first the diaphysis and epiphysis are distinctly separate. As growth occurs, a plate of cartilage called the *epiphyseal plate* develops between the two areas (Fig. 3-12, *C*). This plate is seen on the long-bone radiographs of all pediatric patients (Fig. 3-13, *A*). The epiphyseal plate is important radiographically because it is a common site of fractures in pediatric patients. Near the age of 21, full ossification occurs and the two areas become completely joined; only a moderately visible epiphyseal line appears on the bone (Fig. 3-13, *B*).

CLASSIFICATION OF BONES

Bones are classified by shape, as follows (Fig. 3-14):
- Long
- Short
- Flat
- Irregular
- Sesamoid

Long bones

Long bones are found only in the limbs. They consist primarily of a long cylindric shaft called the *body* and two enlarged, rounded ends that contain a smooth, slippery articular surface. A layer of articular cartilage covers this surface. The ends of these bones all articulate with other long bones. The femur and humerus are typical long bones. The phalanges of the fingers and toes are also considered long bones. A primary function of long bones is to provide support.

Short bones

Short bones consist mainly of cancellous bone containing red marrow and have a thin outer layer of compact bone. The carpal bones of the wrist and the tarsal bones of the ankles are the only short bones. They are varied in shape and allow minimum flexibility of motion in a short distance.

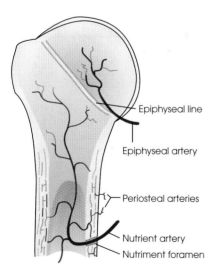

Fig. 3-11 Long bone end showing its rich arterial supply. Arteries, veins, and nerves enter and exit the bone at the same point.

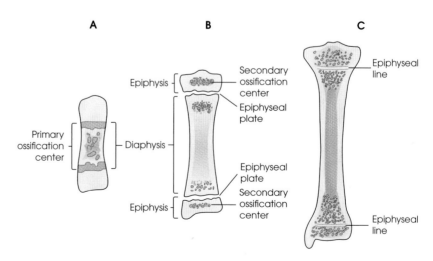

Fig. 3-12 Primary and secondary ossification of bone. **A,** Primary ossification of the tibia before birth. **B,** Secondary ossification, which forms the two *epiphyses* after birth. **C,** Full growth into a single bone, which occurs by the age of 21 years.

Flat bones

Flat bones consist largely of two tables of compact bone. The narrow space between the inner and outer tables contains cancellous bone and red marrow, or *diploe* as it is called in flat bones. The bones of the cranium, sternum, and scapula are examples of flat bones. The flat surfaces of these bones provide protection, and their broad surfaces allow muscle attachment.

Irregular bones

Irregular bones are so termed because their peculiar shapes and variety of forms do not place them in any other category. The vertebrae and the bones in the pelvis and face fall into this category. Like other bones, they have compact bone on the exterior and cancellous bone containing red marrow in the interior. Their shape serves many functions, including attachment for muscles, tendons, and ligaments, or they attach to other bones to create joints.

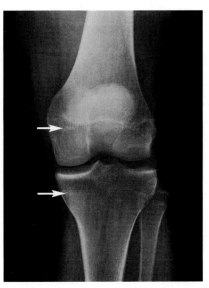
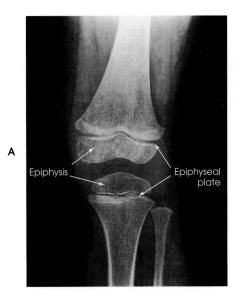

Fig. 3-13 A, Radiograph of 6-year-old child. Epiphysis and epiphyseal plate shown on a knee radiograph *(arrows).* **B,** Radiograph of the same area in a 21-year-old individual. Full ossification has occurred, and only subtle epiphyseal lines are seen *(arrows).*

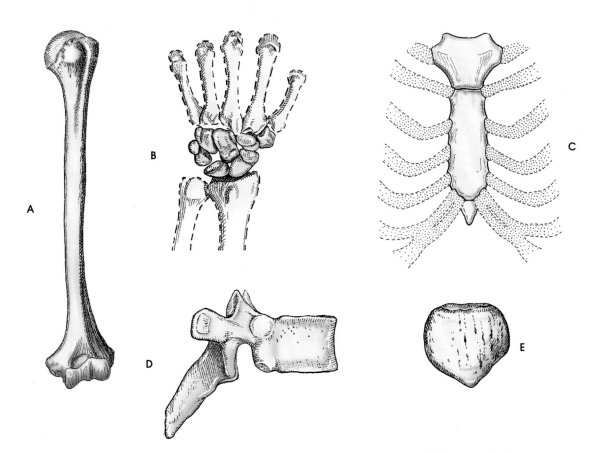

Fig. 3-14 Bones are classified by shape. **A,** The humerus is a long bone. **B,** The carpals of the wrist are short bones. **C,** The sternum is a flat bone. **D,** The vertebra is an irregular bone. **E,** The patella is a sesamoid bone.

TABLE 3-5

Structural classification of joints

Connective tissue	Classification	Movement
Fibrous	1. Syndesmosis	Slightly movable
	2. Suture	Immovable
	3. Gomphosis	Immovable
Cartilaginous	4. Symphysis	Slightly movable
	5. Synchondrosis	Immovable
Synovial	6. Gliding	Freely movable
	7. Hinge	Freely movable
	8. Pivot	Freely movable
	9. Ellipsoid	Freely movable
	10. Saddle	Freely movable
	11. Ball and socket	Freely movable

Sesamoid bones

Sesamoid bones are very small and oval. They develop inside and beside tendons. Their function is to protect the tendon from excessive wear. The largest sesamoid bone is the patella, or the kneecap. Other sesamoids are located beneath the first metatarsal of the foot and adjacent to the metacarpals of the hand. Two small but prominent sesamoids are located beneath the base of the large toe. Like all other bones, they can be fractured.

Arthrology

Arthrology is the study of the joints, or articulations between bones. Joints make it possible for bones to support the body, protect internal organs, and create movement. A variety of specialized articulations are needed for these functions to occur.

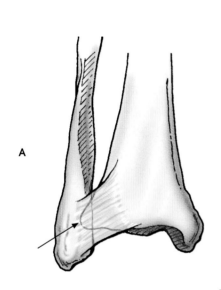

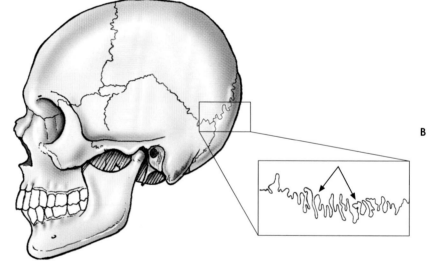

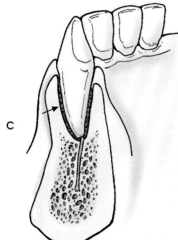

Fig. 3-15 Examples of the three types of fibrous joints. **A,** Syndesmosis: inferior tibiofibular joint. **B,** Suture: sutures of the skull. **C,** Gomphosis: roots of the teeth in the alveolus.

Anatomic Relationship Terms

Various terms are used to describe the relationship of parts of the body in the anatomic position. Radiographers should be thoroughly familiar with these terms, which are commonly used in clinical practice. Most of the following positioning and anatomic terms are paired as opposites. Fig. 3-20 illustrates two commonly used sets of terms.

anterior (ventral) Refers to forward or front part of the body or forward part of an organ

posterior (dorsal) Refers to back part of a body or organ. (Note, however, that the superior surface of the foot is referred to as the dorsal surface.)

caudad Refers to parts away from the head of the body

cephalad Refers to parts toward the head of the body

superior Refers to nearer the head or situated above

inferior Refers to nearer the feet or situated below

central Refers to midarea or main part of an organ

peripheral Refers to parts at or near the surface, edge, or outside of another body part

medial Refers to parts toward the median plane of the body or toward the middle of another body part

lateral Refers to parts away from the median plane of the body or away from the middle of another body part to the right or left

superficial Refers to parts near the skin or surface

deep Refers to parts far from the surface

distal Refers to parts farthest from the point of attachment, point of reference, origin, or beginning; away from center of body

proximal Refers to parts nearer the point of attachment, point of reference, origin, or beginning; toward the center of the body

external Refers to parts outside an organ or on the outside of the body

internal Refers to parts within or on the inside of an organ

parietal Refers to the wall or lining of a body cavity

visceral Refers to the covering of an organ

ipsilateral Refers to a part or parts on the same side of the body

contralateral Refers to a part or parts on the opposite side of the body

palmar Refers to the palm of the hand

plantar Refers to sole of the foot

Radiographic Positioning Terminology

Radiography is the process of recording an image of a body part using one or more types of image receptors (IRs) (cassette/film, cassette/phosphor plate, or fluoroscopic screen/ TV). The terminology used to position the patient and to obtain the radiograph was developed through convention. Attempts to analyze the usage often lead to confusion because the manner in which the terms are used does not follow one specific rule. During the preparation of this chapter, contact was maintained with the American Registry of Radiologic Technologists (ARRT) and the Canadian Association of Medical Radiation Technologists (CAMRT). The ARRT first distributed the "Standard Terminology for Positioning and Projection" in 1978[1]; it has not been substantially revised since initial distribution.[2] Despite its title, the ARRT document did not actually define selected positioning terms.[3] Terms not defined by the ARRT are defined in this text.

Approval of Canadian positioning terminology is the responsibility of the CAMRT Radiography Council on Education. This council provided information for the development of this chapter and clearly identified the terminology differences between the United States and Canada.[4]

---

[1] ARRT Educator's handbook, ed 3, 1990, ARRT.
[2] ARRT Conventions specific to the radiographic examinations, 1993, ARRT.
[3] ARRT, Personal communication and permission, May 1993.
[4] CAMRT, Radiography Council on Education, Personal communication, July 1993.

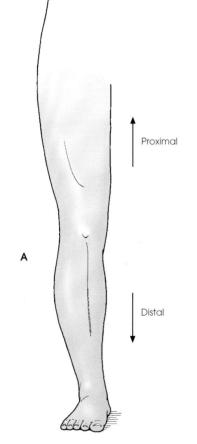

A

Proximal

Distal

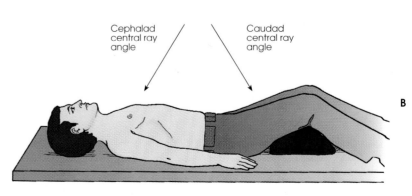

Cephalad central ray angle

Caudad central ray angle

B

Fig. 3-20 A, Use of the common radiology terms *proximal* and *distal*. **B,** Use of the common radiology terms *caudad angle* and *cephalad angle*.

TABLE 3-6

Primary x-ray projections and body positions

Projections	Positions
Anteroposterior (AP)	**General body positions**
Posteroanterior (PA)	Upright
Lateral	Seated
AP oblique	Supine
PA oblique	Prone
Axial	Recumbent
AP axial	Fowler's
PA axial	Trendelenburg
AP axial oblique	**Radiographic body positions**
PA axial oblique	Lateral
Axiolateral	Right
Axiolateral oblique	Left
Transthoracic	Oblique
Craniocaudal	Right posterior (RPO)
Tangential	Left posterior (LPO)
Inferosuperior	Right anterior (RAO)
Superoinferior	Left anterior (LAO)
Plantodorsal	Decubitus
Dorsoplantar	Right lateral
Lateromedial	Left lateral
Mediolateral	Ventral
Submento-vertical	Dorsal
Verticosubmental	Lordotic
Parietoacanthial	
Orbitoparietal	
Parieto-orbital	

The terminology used by the ARRT and CAMRT is consistent overall with that used in this text. The only difference is that the term *view* is commonly used in Canada for some projections and positions.

The following are the four positioning terms most commonly used in radiology:
- Projection
- Position
- View
- Method

PROJECTION

The term *projection* is defined as the path of the central ray as it exits the x-ray tube and goes through the patient to the IR. Most projections are defined by the entrance and exit points in the body and are based on the *anatomic position*. For example, when the central ray enters anywhere in the front (anterior) surface of the body and exits the back (posterior), an *anteroposterior (AP) projection* is obtained. Regardless of which body position the patient is in (e.g., supine, prone, upright, etc.), if the central ray enters the anterior body surface and exits the posterior body surface, the projection is termed an *AP projection* (Fig. 3-21).

Projections can also be defined by the relationship formed between the central ray and the body as the central ray passes through the entire body or body part. Examples include the *axial* and *tangential projections*.

All radiographic examinations described in this text are standardized and titled by their x-ray projection. It is the x-ray projection that accurately and concisely defines each image produced in radiography. A complete listing of the projection terms used in radiology is provided in Table 3-6. The essential radiographic projections follow.

AP projection

In Fig. 3-22 a perpendicular central ray enters the anterior body surface and exits the posterior body surface. This is an *AP projection*. The patient is shown in the supine or dorsal recumbent body position. AP projections can also be achieved with upright, seated, or lateral decubitus positions.

PA projection

In Fig. 3-23 a perpendicular central ray is shown entering the posterior body surface and exiting the anterior body surface. This illustrates a *posteroanterior (PA) projection* with the patient in the upright body position. PA projections can also be achieved with seated, prone (ventral recumbent), and lateral decubitus positions.

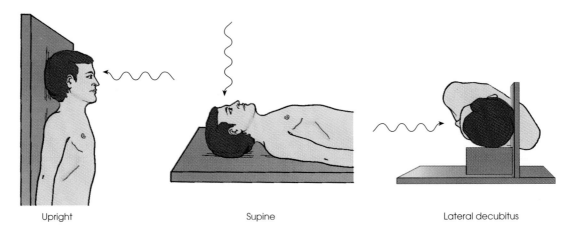

Upright	Supine	Lateral decubitus

Fig. 3-21 Patient's head placed in upright, supine, and lateral decubitus positions for a radiograph. All three body positions produce an AP projection of the skull.

Axial projection

In an axial projection (Fig. 3-24), there is *longitudinal angulation* of the central ray with the long axis of the body or a specific body part. This angulation is based on the anatomic position and is most often produced by angling the central ray cephalad or caudad. The longitudinal angulation in some examinations is achieved by angling the entire body or body part while maintaining the central ray perpendicular to the IR.

The term *axial,* as used in this text, refers to all projections in which the longitudinal angulation between the central ray and the long axis of the body part is *10 degrees or more.* When a range of central ray angles, such as 5 to 15 degrees, is recommended for a given projection, the term *axial* is used because the angulation could exceed 10 degrees. Axial projections are used in a wide variety of examinations and can be obtained with the patient in virtually any body position.

Tangential projection

Occasionally the central ray is directed toward the outer margin of a curved body surface to profile a body part just under the surface and project it free of superimposition. This is called a *tangential projection* because of the tangential relationship formed between the central ray and the entire body or body part (Fig. 3-25).

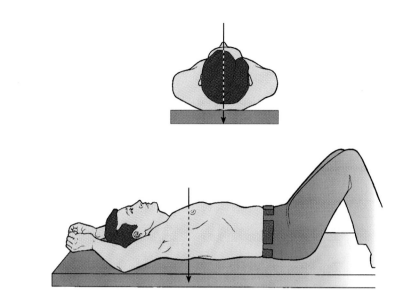

Fig. 3-22 AP projection of chest. The central ray enters the anterior aspect and exits the posterior.

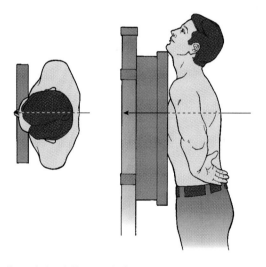

Fig. 3-23 PA projection of chest. The central ray enters the posterior aspect and exits the anterior aspect. Patient is in upright position.

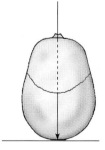 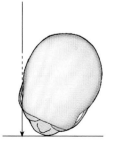

Fig. 3-24 AP axial projection of the skull. The central ray enters the anterior aspect at an angle and exits the posterior aspect.

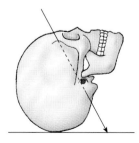 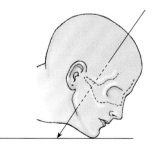

Fig. 3-25 Tangential projection of the zygomatic arch. The central ray skims the surface of the skull.

Lateral projection

For a lateral projection, a perpendicular central ray enters one side of the body or body part, passes transversely along the coronal plane, and exits on the opposite side. Lateral projections can enter from either side of the body or body part as needed for the examination. This can be determined by the patient's condition or ordered by the physician. When a lateral projection is used for head, chest, or abdominal radiography, the direction of the central ray is described with reference to the associated radiographic position. A left lateral position or right lateral position specifies the side of the body *closest to the IR* and corresponds with the side exited by the central ray (Fig. 3-26). Lateral projections of the limbs are further clarified by the terms *lateromedial* or *mediolateral* to indicate the sides entered and exited by the central ray (Fig. 3-27). The *transthoracic projection* is a unique lateral projection used for shoulder radiography and is described in Chapter 5 of this atlas.

Oblique projection

During an oblique projection the central ray enters the body or body part from a side angle following an oblique plane. Oblique projections may enter from either side of the body and from anterior or posterior surfaces. If the central ray enters the anterior surface and exits the opposite posterior surface, it is an *AP oblique projection;* if it enters the posterior surface and exits anteriorly, it is a *PA oblique projection* (Fig. 3-28).

Most oblique projections are achieved by rotating the patient with the central ray perpendicular to the IR. As in the lateral projection the direction of the central ray for oblique projections is described with reference to the associated radiographic position. A right posterior oblique position, for example, places the right posterior surface of the body closest to the IR and corresponds with an AP oblique projection exiting through the same side. This relationship is discussed later. Oblique projections can also be achieved for some examinations by angling the central ray diagonally along the horizontal plane rather than rotating the patient.

Complex projections

For additional clarity, projections may be defined by entrance and exit points and by the central ray relationship to the body at the same time. For example, in the PA axial projection the central ray enters the posterior body surface and exits the anterior body surface following an axial or angled trajectory relative to the entire body or body part. Axiolateral projections also use angulations of the central ray, but the ray enters and exits through lateral surfaces of the entire body or body part.

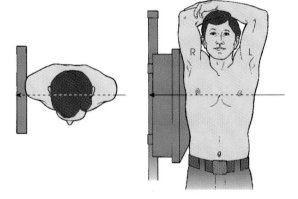

Fig. 3-26 Lateral projection of chest. The patient is placed in the right lateral position. The right side of chest is touching the image receptor. The central ray enters the left or opposite side of body.

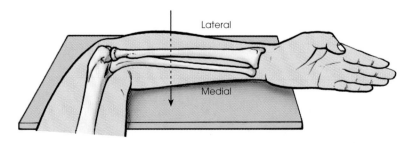

Fig. 3-27 Lateromedial projection of the forearm. The central ray enters the lateral aspect of the forearm and exits the medial aspect.

True projections[1]

The term *true* (true AP, true PA, and true lateral) is often used in clinical practice. True is used to specifically indicate that the body part must be placed exactly in the anatomic position.

A true AP or PA projection is obtained when the central ray is perpendicular to the coronal plane and parallel to the sagittal plane. A true lateral projection is obtained when the central ray is parallel to the normal plane and perpendicular to the sagittal plane. When a body part is rotated for an AP or PA oblique projection, a true AP or PA cannot be obtained. In this atlas the term *true* is used only when the body part is placed in the anatomic position.

---

[1]Bontrager KL. *Textbook of radiographic positioning,* ed 4, St Louis, 1997, Mosby.

POSITION

The term *position* is used in two ways in radiology. One way identifies the overall posture of the patient or the general body position. The patient may, for example, be described as upright, seated, or supine. The other use of *position* refers to the specific placement of the body part in relation to the radiographic table or IR during imaging. This is the radiographic position and may be a right lateral, left anterior oblique, or other position depending on the examination and anatomy of interest. A listing of all general body positions and radiographic positions is provided in Table 3-6.

During radiography, general body positions are combined with radiographic positions to produce the appropriate image. For clarification of the positioning for an examination, it is often necessary to include references to both because a particular radiographic position such as right lateral can be achieved in several general body positions (upright, supine, lateral recumbent, etc.) with differing image outcomes. Specific descriptions of general body positions and radiographic positions follow.

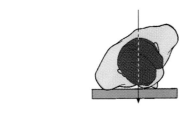

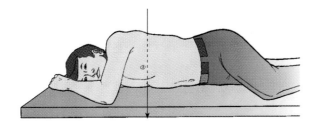

Fig. 3-28 PA oblique projection of the chest. The central ray enters the posterior aspect of the body (even though it is rotated) and exits the anterior aspect.

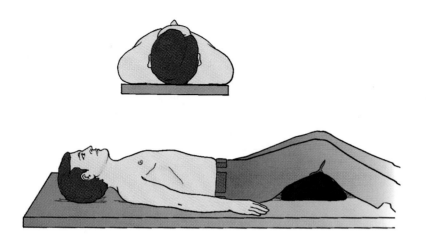

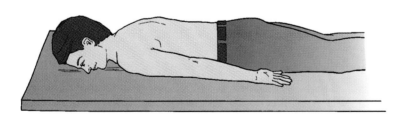

Fig. 3-29 Supine position of the body, also termed the *dorsal recumbent position*. The patient's knees are flexed for comfort.

General body positions

The following list describes the general body positions. All are commonly used in radiography practice.

upright   Erect or marked by a vertical position (Fig. 3-23)

seated   Upright position in which the patient is sitting on a chair or stool

recumbent   General term referring to lying down in any position, such as dorsal recumbent (Fig. 3-29), ventral recumbent (Fig. 3-30), or lateral recumbent (Fig. 3-31)

supine   Lying on the back (see Fig. 3-29)

prone   Lying face down (see Fig. 3-30)

Trendelenburg's position   Supine position with the head tilted downward (Fig. 3-32)

Fowler's position   Supine position with the head higher than the feet (Fig. 3-33)

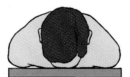

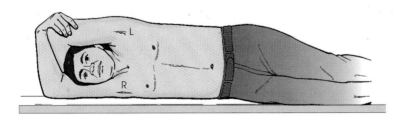

Fig. 3-30 Prone position of the body. It can also be termed the *ventral recumbent position*.

Fig. 3-31 Recumbent position of the body, specifically a *right lateral recumbent position*.

Lateral position

Lateral radiographic positions are always named according to the side of the patient that is placed closest to the IR (Figs. 3-34 and 3-35). In this text, the right or left lateral positions are indicated as subheadings for all lateral x-ray projections of the head, chest, and abdomen in which either the left or right side of the patient is placed adjacent to the IR. The specific side selected depends on the condition of the patient, the anatomic structure of clinical interest, and the purpose of the examination. Note that in Figs. 3-34 and 3-35 the x-ray projection for the positions indicated is lateral projection.

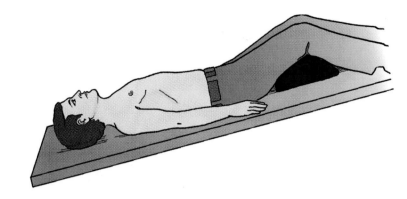

Fig. 3-32 Trendelenburg's position of the body. The feet are higher than the head.

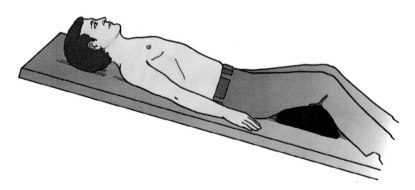

Fig. 3-33 Fowler's position of the body. The head is higher than the feet.

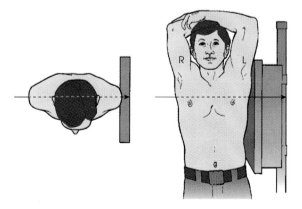

Fig. 3-34 Left lateral radiographic position of the chest results in a lateral projection.

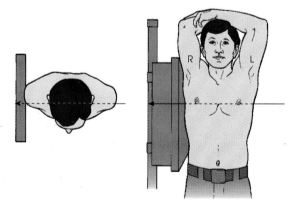

Fig. 3-35 Right lateral radiographic position of the chest results in a lateral projection.

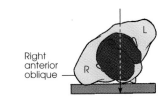

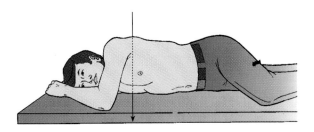

Fig. 3-36 RAO radiographic position of the chest results in a PA oblique projection.

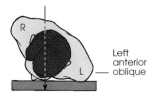

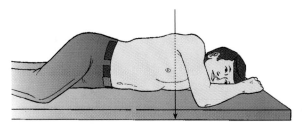

Fig. 3-37 LAO radiographic position of the chest results in a PA oblique projection.

Oblique position

An oblique radiographic position is achieved when the entire body or body part is rotated so that the coronal plane is not parallel with the radiographic table or IR. The angle of oblique rotation varies with the examination and structures to be demonstrated. In this atlas an angle is specified for each oblique position (e.g., rotated 45 degrees from the prone position).

Oblique positions, like lateral positions, are always named according to the side of the patient that is placed closest to the IR. In Fig. 3-36 the patient is rotated with the right anterior body surface in contact with the radiographic table. This is a *right anterior oblique (RAO) position* because the right side of the anterior body surface is closest to the IR. Fig. 3-37 shows the patient placed in a *left anterior oblique (LAO) position.*

The relationship between oblique position and oblique projection can be summarized simply. Anterior oblique positions result in PA oblique projections as shown in Figs. 3-36 and 3-37. Similarly, posterior oblique positions result in AP oblique projections as illustrated in Figs. 3-38 and 3-39.

The oblique positioning terminology used in this atlas has been standardized using the RAO and LAO or RPO and LPO positions along with the appropriate PA or AP oblique projection. For oblique positions of the limbs, the terms *medial rotation* and *lateral rotation* have been standardized to designate the direction in which the limbs have been turned from the anatomic position (Fig. 3-40).

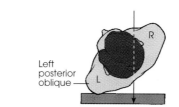

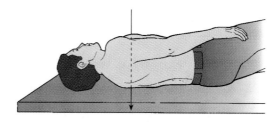

Fig. 3-38 LPO radiographic position of the chest results in an AP oblique projection.

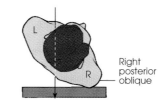

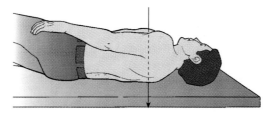

Fig. 3-39 RPO radiographic position of the chest results in an AP oblique projection.

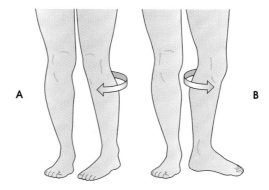

Fig. 3-40 A, Medial rotation of the knee. **B,** Lateral rotation of the knee.

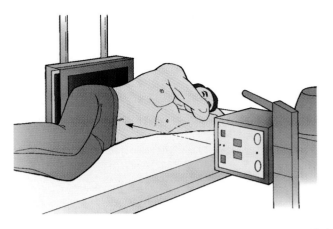

Fig. 3-41 Left lateral decubitus radiographic position of the abdomen results in an AP projection. Note the horizontal orientation of the central ray.

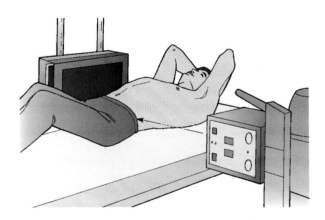

Fig. 3-42 Dorsal decubitus radiographic position of the abdomen results in a lateral projection. Note the horizontal orientation of the central ray.

Decubitus position

In radiographic positioning terminology, the term *decubitus* indicates that the patient is lying down and that the central ray is horizontal and parallel with the floor. Three primary decubitus positions are named according to the body surface on which the patient is lying: *lateral decubitus (left or right), dorsal decubitus,* and *ventral decubitus.* Of these, the lateral decubitus position is most often used to demonstrate the presence of air-fluid levels or free air in the chest and abdomen.

In Fig. 3-41 the patient is placed in the left lateral decubitus radiographic position with the back (posterior surface) closest to the IR. In this position a horizontal central ray provides an AP projection. Thus Fig. 3-41 is accurately described as an AP projection with the body in the left lateral decubitus position. Alternatively, the patient may be placed with the front of the body (anterior surface) facing the IR, resulting in a PA projection. This would be correctly described as a PA projection of the body in the left lateral decubitus position. Right lateral decubitus positions may be necessary with AP or PA projections, depending on the examination.

In Fig. 3-42 the patient is shown in a dorsal decubitus radiographic position with one side of the body next to the IR. The horizontal central ray provides a lateral projection. This is correctly described as a lateral projection with the patient placed in the dorsal decubitus position. Either side may face the IR, depending on the examination or the patient's condition.

The ventral decubitus radiographic position (Fig. 3-43) also places a side of the body adjacent to the IR, resulting in a lateral projection. Similar to the earlier examples, the accurate terminology is lateral projection with the patient in the ventral decubitus position. Once again, either side may face the IR.

Lordotic position

The lordotic position is achieved by having the patient lean backward while in the upright body position so that only the shoulders are in contact with the IR (Fig. 3-44). An angulation forms between the central ray and the long axis of the upper body, producing an AP axial projection. This position is used for the visualization of pulmonary apices (see Chapter 10) and clavicles (see Chapter 5).

Note to educators, students, and clinicians

In clinical practice the terms *position* and *projection* are interchangeably and incorrectly used. Incorrect use leads to confusion for the student who is attempting to learn the correct terminology of the profession. Educators and clinicians are encouraged to generally use the term *projection* when describing any examination performed. The word *projection* is the only term that accurately describes how the body part is being examined. The term *position* should be used only when referring to the placement of the patient's body. These are two distinct terms that should not be interchanged. A correct example is "We are going to perform a PA projection of the chest with the patient in the upright position."

VIEW

The term *view* is used to describe the body part as seen by the IR. Use of this term is restricted to the discussion of a finished radiograph or image. *View* and *projection* are exact opposites. The shadows cast on an IR by the x-rays projected through a body part are viewed on the resulting image from the opposite direction. Simply stated, the image "looks back" into the body from the side that was closest to the IR. For many years *view* and *projection* were often used interchangeably, which led to confusion. In the United States *projection* has replaced *view* as the preferred terminology for describing radiographic images. In Canada *view* remains an acceptable positioning term. For consistency, the atlas refers to all views as *images* or *radiographs*.

METHOD

Some radiographic projections and procedures are named after individuals (e.g., Waters or Towne) in recognition of their development of a method to demonstrate a specific anatomic part. Method, which was first described in the fifth edition of this atlas, describes the specific radiographic projection that the individual developed. The method specifies the x-ray projection and body position, and it may include specific items such as IR and central ray position. In this atlas, standard projection terminology is used first and a named method is listed secondarily (e.g., PA axial projection; Towne method). The ARRT and CAMRT use the standard anatomic projection terminology and list the originator in parentheses.

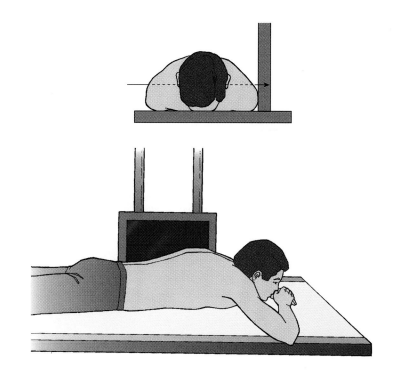

Fig. 3-43 Ventral decubitus radiographic position of the abdomen results in a lateral projection. Note the horizontal orientation of the central ray.

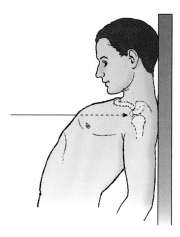

Fig. 3-44 Lordotic radiographic position of the chest results in an AP axial projection. Note that the central ray is not angled; however, it enters the chest axially as a result of body position.

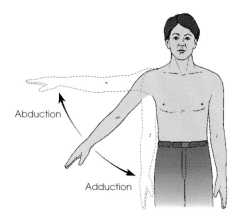

Fig. 3-45 Abduction and adduction of the arm.

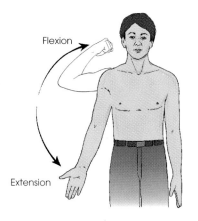

Fig. 3-46 Extension of the arm (anatomic position) and flexion (bending).

Body Movement Terminology

The following terms are used to describe movement related to the limbs. These terms are often used in positioning descriptions and in the patient history provided to the radiographer by the referring physician. They must, therefore, be studied thoroughly.

abduct or abduction Movement of a part away from the central axis of the body or body part

adduct or adduction Movement of a part toward the central axis of the body or body part (Fig. 3-45)

extension Straightening of a joint; When both elements of the joint are in the anatomic position; the normal position of a joint (Fig. 3-46).

flexion Act of bending a joint; the opposite of extension (Fig. 3-46)

hyperextension Forced or excessive extension of a limb or joints

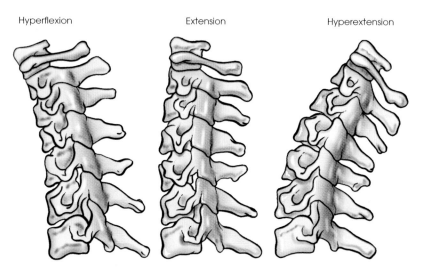

Fig. 3-47 Hyperextension, extension, and hyperflexion of the neck.

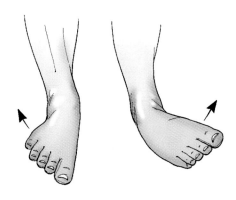

Fig. 3-48 Inversion and eversion of the foot at the ankle joint.

hyperflexion Forced overflexion of a limb or joints (Fig. 3-47)

evert/eversion Outward turning of the foot at the ankle

invert/inversion Inward turning of the foot at the ankle (Fig. 3-48)

pronate/pronation Rotation of the forearm so that the palm is down

supinate/supination Rotation of the forearm so that the palm is up (in the anatomic position) (Fig. 3-49)

rotate/rotation Turning or rotating of the body or a body part around its axis (Fig 3-50, *A*). Rotation of a limb will be either *medial* (toward the midline of the body from the anatomic position; Fig. 3-50, *B*) or *lateral* (away from the midline of the body from the anatomic position; Fig. 3-50, *C*)

circumduction Circular movement of a limb (Fig. 3-51)

tilt Tipping or slanting a body part slightly. The tilt is in relation to the long axis of the body (Fig. 3-52)

deviation A turning away from the regular standard or course (Fig. 3-53).

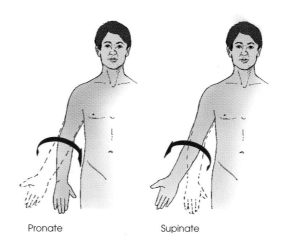

Pronate   Supinate

Fig. 3-49 Pronation and supination of the forearm.

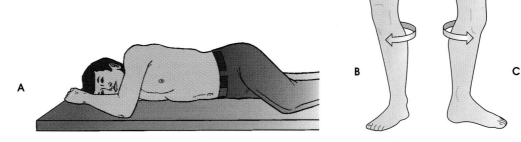

A   B   C

Fig. 3-50 A, Rotation of the chest and abdomen. The patient's arm and knee are flexed for comfort. **B,** Medial rotation of the left leg. **C,** Lateral rotation of the left leg.

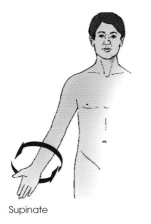

Supinate

Fig. 3-51 Circumduction of the arm.

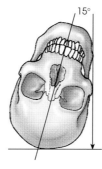

15°

Fig. 3-52 Tilt of the skull is 15 degrees from the long axis.

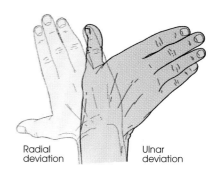

Radial deviation   Ulnar deviation

Fig. 3-53 Radial deviation of the hand (turned to the radial side) and ulnar deviation (turned to the ulnar side).

TABLE 3-7

Greek and Latin nouns: common singular and plural forms

Singular	Plural	Examples: singular—plural
-a	-ae	maxilla—maxillae
-ex	-ces	apex—apices
-is	-es	diagnosis—diagnoses
-ix	-ces	appendix—appendices
-ma	-mata	condyloma—condylomata
-on	-a	ganglion—ganglia
-um	-a	antrum—antra
-us	-i	ramus—rami

TABLE 3-8

Frequently misused single and plural word forms

Singular	Plural	Singular	Plural
adnexus	adnexa	mediastinum	mediastina
alveolus	alveoli	medulla	medullae
areola	areolae	meninx	meninges
bronchus	bronchi	meniscus	menisci
bursa	bursae	metastasis	metastases
calculus	calculi	mucosa	mucosae
coxa	coxae	omentum	omenta
diagnosis	diagnoses	paralysis	paralyses
diverticulum	diverticula	plexus	plexi
fossa	fossae	pleura	pleurae
gingiva	gingivae	pneumothorax	pneumothoraces
haustrum	haustra	ramus	rami
hilum	hila	ruga	rugae
ilium	ilia	sulcus	sulci
labium	labia	thrombus	thrombi
lamina	laminae	vertebra	vertebrae
lumen	lumina	viscus	viscera

Medical Terminology

Single and plural word endings for common Greek and Latin nouns are presented in Table 3-7. Single and plural word forms are often confused. Examples of commonly misused word forms are listed in Table 3-8. Generally the singular form is used when the plural form is intended.

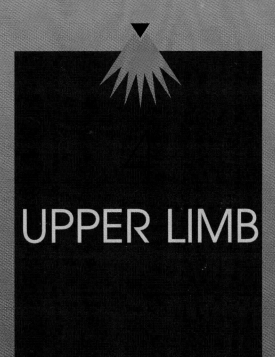

UPPER LIMB

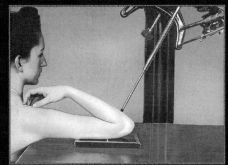

RIGHT Acute flexion elbow, 1949.

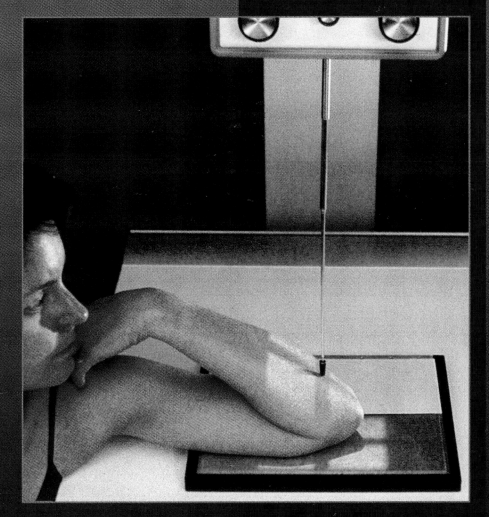

LEFT Acute flexion elbow 1999.

PROJECTIONS, POSITIONS & METHODS

Page	Essential	Anatomy	Projection	Position	Method
92	♠	Digits (second through fifth)	PA		
94	♠	Digits (second through fifth)	Lateral		
96	♠	Digits (second through fifth)	PA oblique	Lateral rotation	
98	♠	First digit (thumb)	AP		
98		First digit (thumb)	PA		
98	♠	First digit (thumb)	Lateral		
99	♠	First digit (thumb)	PA oblique		
100		First digit (thumb): *first carpometacarpal joint*	AP		ROBERT
102		First digit (thumb): *first carpometacarpal joint*	AP		BURMAN
104	♠	Hand	PA		
106	♠	Hand	PA oblique	Lateral rotation	
108	♠	Hand	Lateral	Extension and fan lateral	
110		Hand	Lateral	Flexion	
110		Hand	AP oblique	Medial rotation	NORGAARD
112	♠	Wrist	PA		
113		Wrist	AP		
114	♠	Wrist	Lateral		
116	♠	Wrist	PA oblique	Lateral rotation	
117		Wrist	AP oblique	Medial rotation	
118	♠	Wrist	PA	Ulnar deviation (flexion)	
119		Wrist	PA	Radial deviation (flexion)	
120	♠	Wrist: *scaphoid*	PA axial		STECHER
122		Wrist: *scaphoid series*	PA, PA axial	Ulnar deviation (flexion)	RAFERT-LONG
124		Wrist: *trapezium*	PA axial oblique		CLEMENTS-NAKAYAMA
125		Carpal bridge	Tangential		
126	♠	Carpal canal	Tangential		GAYNOR-HART
128	♠	Forearm	AP		
130	♠	Forearm	Lateral		
131	♠	Elbow	AP		
132	♠	Elbow	Lateral		
134	♠	Elbow	AP oblique	Medial rotation	
135	♠	Elbow	AP oblique	Lateral rotation	
136	♠	Elbow: *distal humerus*	AP	Partial flexion	
137	♠	Elbow: *proximal forearm*	AP	Partial flexion	
138		Elbow: *distal humerus*	AP	Acute flexion	
139		Elbow: *proximal forearm*	PA	Acute flexion	
140		Elbow: *radial head*	Lateral		
142		Distal humerus	PA axial		
143		Olecranon process	PA axial		
144	♠	Humerus	AP	Upright	
145	♠	Humerus	Lateral	Upright	
146	♠	Humerus	AP	Recumbent	
147	♠	Humerus	Lateral	Recumbent, lateral recumbent	
150	♠	Proximal humerus	Transthoracic lateral	R or L	LAWRENCE

The icons in the Essential column indicate projections frequently performed in the United States and Canada. Students should demonstrate competence in these projections.

Anatomists divide the bones of the upper limbs, or extremities, into the following main groups:
- Hand
- Forearm
- Arm
- Shoulder girdle

The proximal arm and shoulder girdle are discussed in Chapter 5.

Hand

The *hand* consists of 27 bones, which are subdivided into the following groups:
- Phalanges: bones of the digits (fingers and thumb)
- Metacarpals: bones of the palm
- Carpals: bones of the wrist (Fig. 4-1)

DIGITS

The *digits* are described by numbers and names; however, description by number is the more correct practice. Beginning at the lateral, or thumb, side of the hand the numbers and names are as follows:
- First digit (thumb)
- Second digit (index finger)
- Third digit (middle finger)
- Fourth digit (ring finger)
- Fifth digit (small finger)

The digits contain a total of 14 *phalanges* (*phalanx,* singular), which are long bones that consist of a cylindric body and articular ends. Nine digits have two articular ends. The first digit has two phalanges—the proximal and distal. The other digits have three phalanges—the proximal, middle, and distal. The proximal phalanges are the closest to the palm, and the distal phalanges are the farthest from the palm. The distal phalanges are small and flattened, with a roughened rim around their distal anterior end; this gives them a spatulalike appearance.

METACARPALS

Five *metacarpals,* which are cylindric in shape and slightly concave anteriorly, form the palm of the hand (see Fig. 4-1). They are long bones consisting of a *body* and two articular ends, the *head* distally and the *base* proximally. The metacarpal heads, commonly known as the *knuckles,* are located on the dorsal hand. The metacarpals are numbered one to five, beginning from the lateral side of the hand.

WRIST

The *wrist* has eight *carpal* bones, which are fitted closely together and arranged in two horizontal rows (see Fig. 4-1). The carpals are classified as short bones and are composed largely of cancellous tissue with an outer layer of compact bony tissue. These bones, with one exception, have two or three names; this book uses the preferred terms (see box). The proximal row of carpals, which is nearest the forearm, contains the scaphoid, lunate, triquetrum, and pisiform. The distal row includes the trapezium, trapezoid, capitate, and hamate.

Each carpal contains identifying characteristics. Beginning the proximal row of carpals on the lateral side, the *scaphoid,* the largest bone in the proximal carpal row, has a tubercle on the anterior and lateral aspect for muscle attachment and is palpable near the base of the thumb. The *lunate* articulates with the radius proximally and is easy to recognize because of its crescent shape. The *triquetrum* is roughly pyramidal and articulates anteriorly with the hamate. The *pisiform* is a pea-shaped bone situated anterior to the triquetrum and is easily palpated.

CARPAL TERMINOLOGY CONVERSION	
Preferred	**Synonyms**
Proximal row:	
Scaphoid	Navicular
Lunate	Semilunar
Triquetrum	Triquetral, cuneiform, or triangular
Pisiform	(none)
Distal row:	
Trapezium	Greater multangular
Trapezoid	Lesser multangular
Capitate	Os magnum
Hamate	Unciform

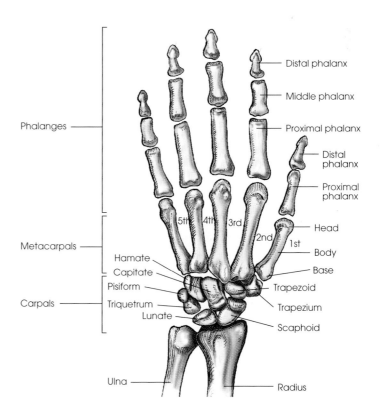

Fig. 4-1 Posterior aspect of right hand and wrist.

Beginning the distal row of carpals on the lateral side, the *trapezium* has a tubercle and groove on the anterior surface. The tubercles of the trapezium and scaphoid comprise the lateral margin of the carpal groove. The *trapezoid* has a smaller surface anteriorly than posteriorly. The *capitate* articulates with the base of the third metacarpal and is the largest and most centrally located carpal. The wedge-shaped *hamate* exhibits the prominent *hook of hamate,* which is located on the anterior surface. The hamate and the pisiform form the medial margin of the carpal groove.

A triangular depression is located on the posterior surface of the wrist and is visible when the thumb is abducted and extended. This depression, known as the *anatomic snuffbox*, is formed by the tendons of the two major muscles of the thumb. The anatomic snuffbox overlies the scaphoid bone and the radial artery, which carries blood to the dorsum of the hand. Tenderness in the snuffbox area is a clinical sign suggesting fracture of the scaphoid—the most commonly fractured carpal bone.

CARPAL SULCUS

The anterior or palmar surface of the wrist is concave from side to side and forms the *carpal sulcus* (Fig. 4-2). The *flexor retinaculum,* a strong fibrous band, attaches medially to the pisiform and hook of hamate and laterally to the tubercles of the scaphoid and trapezium. The *carpal tunnel* is the passageway created between the carpal sulcus and flexor retinaculum. The *median nerve* and the *flexor tendons* pass through the carpal canal. Carpal tunnel syndrome results from compression of the median nerve inside the carpal tunnel.

Forearm

The *forearm* contains two bones that lie parallel to each other—the *radius* and *ulna.* Like other long bones, they have of a body and two articular extremities. The radius is located on the lateral side of the forearm, and the ulna is on the medial side (Figs. 4-3 and 4-4).

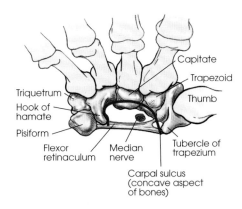

Fig. 4-2 Carpal sulcus.

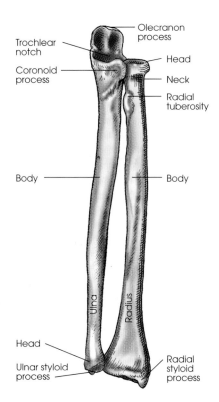

Fig. 4-3 Anterior aspect of left radius and ulna.

ULNA

The *body* of the ulna is long and slender and tapers inferiorly. The upper portion of the ulna is large and presents two beaklike processes and concave depressions (Fig. 4-5). The proximal process, or *olecranon process,* concaves anteriorly and slightly inferiorly and forms the proximal portion of the *trochlear notch.* The more distal *coronoid process* projects anteriorly from the anterior surface of the body and curves slightly superiorly. The process is triangular and forms the lower portion of the trochlear notch. A depression called the *radial notch* is located on the lateral aspect of the coronoid process.

The distal end of the ulna includes a rounded process on its lateral side called the *head* and a narrower conic projection on the posteromedial side called the *ulnar styloid process.* An articular disk separates the head of the ulna from the wrist joint.

RADIUS

The proximal end of the radius is small and presents a flat disklike *head* above a constricted area called the *neck.* Just inferior to the neck on the medial side of the *body* of the radius is a roughened process called the *radial tuberosity.* The distal end of the radius is broad and flattened and has a conic projection on its lateral surface called the *radial styloid process.*

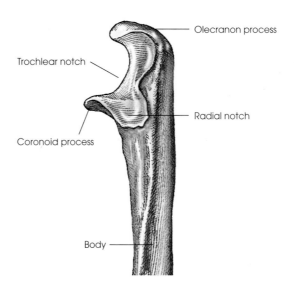

Fig. 4-5 Radial aspect of left proximal ulna.

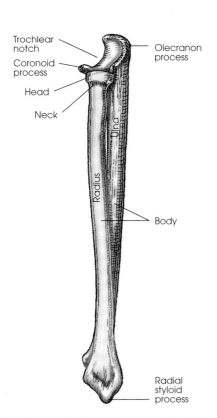

Fig. 4-4 Lateral aspect of left radius and ulna.

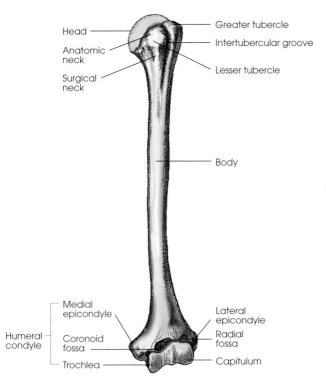

Fig. 4-6 Anterior aspect of left humerus.

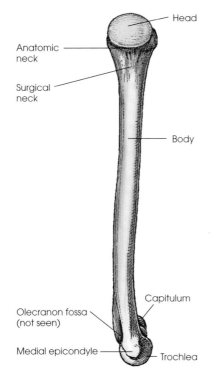

Fig. 4-7 Medial aspect of left humerus.

Arm

The arm has one bone called the *humerus,* which consists of a *body* and two articular ends (Figs. 4-6 and 4-7). The proximal part of the humerus articulates with the shoulder girdle and is described further in Chapter 5. The distal humerus is broad and flattened and presents numerous processes and depressions.

The distal end of the humerus is called the *humeral condyle* and includes two smooth elevations for articulation with the bones of the forearm—the *trochlea* on the medial side and the *capitulum* on the lateral side. The *medial* and *lateral epicondyles* are superior to the condyle and easily palpated. On the anterior surface superior to the trochlea, a shallow depression called the *coronoid fossa* receives the coronoid process when the elbow is flexed. The relatively small *radial fossa,* which receives the radial head when the elbow is flexed, is located lateral to the coronoid fossa and proximal to the capitulum. The *olecranon fossa* is a deep depression found immediately behind the coronoid fossa on the posterior surface and accommodates the olecranon process when the elbow is extended.

The proximal end of the humerus contains the *head,* which is large, smooth, and rounded and lies in an oblique plane on the superomedial side. Just below the head, lying in the same oblique plane, is the narrow, constricted *anatomic neck.* The constriction of the body just below the tubercles is called the *surgical neck,* which is the site of many fractures.

The *lesser tubercle* is situated on the anterior surface of the bone immediately below the anatomic neck. The tendon of the subscapularis muscle inserts at the lesser tubercle. The *greater tubercle* is located on the lateral surface of the bone just below the anatomic neck and is separated from the lesser tubercle by a deep depression called the *intertubercular groove.*

Upper Limb Articulations

Table 4-1 contains a summary of the joints of the upper limb. A detailed description of the upper limb articulations follows.

The *interphalangeal* articulations between the phalanges are *synovial hinge* type and allow only flexion and extension. The interphalangeal joints are named by location and are differentiated as either *proximal interphalangeal (PIP)* or *distal interphalangeal (DIP),* by the digit number, and by right or left hand (e.g., the PIP articulation of the fourth digit of the left hand) (Fig. 4-8, *A*). Because the first digit has only two phalanges, the joint between the two phalanges is simply called the *interphalangeal joint.*

The *metacarpals* articulate with the phalanges at their distal ends and the carpals at their proximal ends. The *metacarpophalangeal (MCP)* articulations are *synovial ellipsoidal* joints and have the movements of flexion, extension, abduction, adduction, and circumduction. Because of the less convex and wider surface of the MCP joint of the thumb, only limited abduction and adduction are possible.

TABLE 4-1
Joints of the upper limb

| Joint | Structural classification | | Movement |
	Tissue	Type	
Interphalangeal	Synovial	Hinge	Freely movable
Metacarpophalangeal	Synovial	Ellipsoidal	Freely movable
Carpometacarpal:			
First digit	Synovial	Saddle	Freely movable
Second to fifth digits	Synovial	Gliding	Freely movable
Intercarpal	Synovial	Gliding	Freely movable
Radiocarpal	Synovial	Ellipsoidal	Freely movable
Radioulnar:			
Proximal	Synovial	Pivot	Freely movable
Distal	Synovial	Pivot	Freely movable
Humeroulnar	Synovial	Hinge	Freely movable
Humeroradial	Synovial	Hinge	Freely movable

The carpals articulate with each other, the metacarpals, and the radius of the forearm. In the *carpometacarpal (CMC)* articulations the first metacarpal and trapezium form a *synovial saddle* joint, which permits the thumb to oppose the fingers (touch the fingertips). The articulations between the second, third, fourth, and fifth metacarpals and the trapezoid, capitate, and hamate form *synovial glid-* ing joints. The *intercarpal* articulations are also *synovial gliding* joints. The articulations between the lunate and scaphoid form a gliding joint. The *radiocarpal* articulation is a *synovial ellipsoidal* type. This joint is formed by the articulation of the scaphoid, lunate, and triquetrum, with the radius and the articular disk just distal to the ulna (Fig. 4-8, *B*).

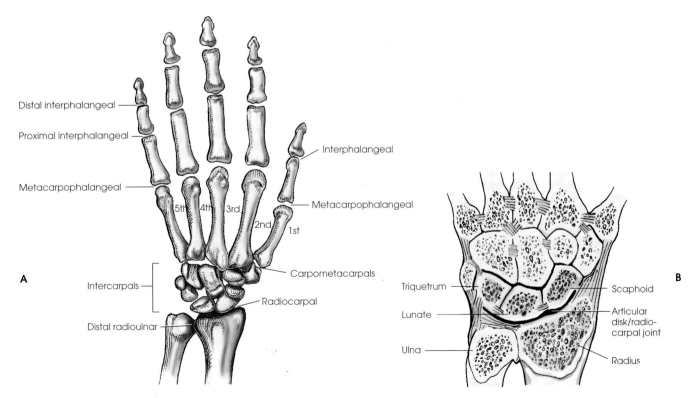

Fig. 4-8 A, Articulations of the hand and wrist. **B,** Radiocarpal articulation formed by the scaphoid, lunate, and triquetrum with the radius.

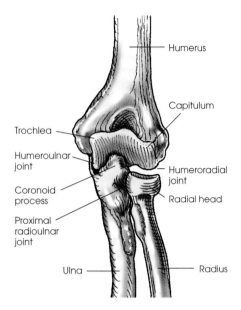

Fig. 4-9 Anterior aspect of left elbow joint.

The *distal* and *proximal radioulnar* articulations are *synovial pivot* joints. The distal ulna articulates with the ulnar notch of the distal radius. The proximal head of the radius articulates with the radial notch of the ulna at the medial side. The movements of supination and pronation of the forearm and hand largely result from the combined rotary action of these two joints. In pronation the radius turns medially and crosses over the ulna at its upper third and the ulna makes a slight counterrotation that rotates the humerus medially.

The elbow joint proper includes the proximal radioulnar articulation and the articulations between the humerus and the radius and ulna. The three joints are enclosed in a common capsule. The trochlea of the humerus articulates with the ulna at the trochlear notch. The capitulum of the humerus articulates with the flattened head of the radius. The *humeroulnar* and *humeroradial* articulations form a *synovial hinge* joint and allow only flexion and extension movement (Figs. 4-9 and 4-10, *A*). The proximal humerus and its articulations are described with the shoulder girdle in Chapter 5.

Fat Pads

The three areas of fat[1,2] associated with the elbow joint can be visualized only in the lateral projection (Fig. 4-10, *B*). The *posterior fat pad* covers the largest area and lies within the olecranon fossa of the posterior humerus. The superimposed coronoid and radial fat pads, which lie in the coronoid and radial fossae of the anterior humerus, form the *anterior fat pad*. The *supinator fat pad* is positioned anterior to and parallel with the anterior aspect of the proximal radius.

When the elbow is flexed 90 degrees for the lateral projection, only the anterior and supinator fat pads are visible and the posterior fat pad is depressed within the olecranon fossa. In a negative elbow the anterior fat pad somewhat resembles a teardrop and the supinator fat pad appears as shown in Fig. 4-10, *B*. The fat pads become significant radiographically when an elbow injury causes effusion and displaces the fat pads or alters their shape. Visualization of the posterior fat pad is a reliable indicator of elbow pathology. Exposure factors designed to demonstrate soft tissues are extremely important on lateral elbow radiographs because visualization of the fat pads may be the only evidence of injury.

[1]McQuillen-Martensen K: *Radiographic critique,* Philadelphia, 1996, WB Saunders.
[2]Griswold R: Elbow fat pads: a radiography perspective, *Radiol Technol* 53:303, 1982.

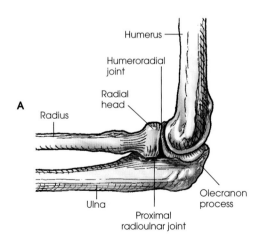

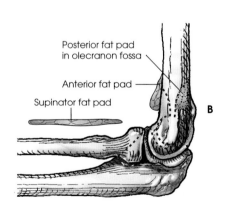

Fig. 4-10 A, Lateral aspect of elbow. **B,** Fat pads of elbow joint.

SUMMARY OF ANATOMY*

Hand
phalanges (bones of
 digits)
digits
metacarpals
carpals

Metacarpals
first to fifth
 metacarpals
body
head
base

Wrist
scaphoid
lunate
triquetrum
pisiform
trapezium
trapezoid
capitate
hamate
hook of hamate
anatomic snuffbox

Carpal sulcus
carpal tunnel
flexor retinaculum
median nerve
flexor tendons

Forearm
ulna
radius

Ulna
body
olecranon process
trochlear notch
coronoid process
radial notch
head
ulnar styloid process

Radius
head
neck
body
radial tuberosity
radial styloid process

Arm
humerus

Humerus
body
humeral condyle
trochlea
capitulum

medial condyle
lateral condyle
coronoid fossa
radial fossa
olecranon fossa
head
anatomic neck
surgical neck
lesser tubercle
greater tubercle
intertubercular
 groove

Articulations
interphalangeal
metacarpo-
 phalangeal
carpometacarpal
intercarpal
radiocarpal
radioulnar
humeroulnar
humeroradial

Fat pads
anterior fat pads
posterior fat pad
supinator fat pad

*See *Addendum* at the end of the volume for a summary of the changes in the
anatomic terms used in this edition.

General Procedures

When the upper limb is radiographed, the following steps should be initiated:

- Remove rings, watches, and other radiopaque objects, and place them in secure storage during the procedure.
- Seat the patient at the side or end of the table to avoid a strained or uncomfortable position.
- Place the cassette at a location and angle that allows the patient to be in the most comfortable position. Because the degree of immobilization (particularly of the hand and digits) is limited, the patient must be comfortable to promote relaxation and cooperation in maintaining the desired position.
- Unless otherwise specified, direct the central ray at a right angle to the midpoint of the cassette. Because the joint spaces of the limbs are narrow, accurate centering is essential to avoid obscuring the joint spaces.
- Radiograph each side *separately* when performing a bilateral examination of the hands or wrists. This prevents distortion, particularly of the joint spaces.
- *Shield gonads* from scattered radiation with a sheet of lead-impregnated rubber or a lead apron placed over the patient's pelvis (Fig. 4-11).
- Use close collimation. This technique is recommended for all upper limb radiographs.
- Placing multiple exposures on one cassette is a common practice. The side of the unexposed cassette should always be covered with lead, especially when the new computed radiography cassettes are used.
- Use right or left markers and all other vital identification markers when appropriate.

Digits (Second Through Fifth)

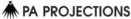 **PA PROJECTIONS**

Image receptor: 8 × 10 inch (18 × 24 cm) crosswise for two or more images on one cassette

Position of patient

- Seat the patient at the end of the radiographic table.

Position of part

When radiographing individual digits (except the first), take the following steps:

- Place the extended digit with the palmar surface down on the unmasked portion of the cassette.
- Separate the digits slightly, and center the digit under examination to the midline portion of the cassette.
- Center the PIP joint to the cassette (Figs. 4-12 to 4-15).
- *Shield gonads.*

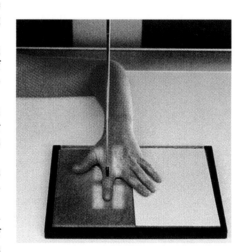

Fig. 4-12 PA second digit.

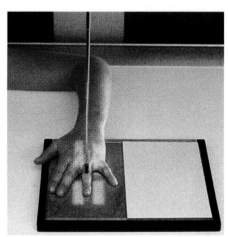

Fig. 4-14 PA fourth digit.

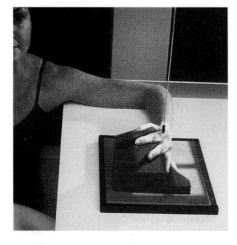

Fig. 4-11 Properly shielded patient.

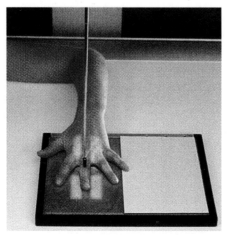

Fig. 4-13 PA third digit.

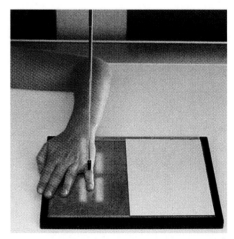

Fig. 4-15 PA fifth digit.

Upper limb

Digits (Second Through Fifth)

Central ray

- Perpendicular to the PIP joint of the affected digit.
- Collimate to the digit under examination.

COMPUTED RADIOGRAPHY

The digit must be placed in the central area of the cassette for all finger projections. Two or more images can be projected on one cassette; however, the finger must be placed in the central area, and the exposed and unexposed areas must be covered with lead.

Structures shown

A PA projection of the appropriate digit is visualized (Figs. 4-16 through 4-19).

EVALUATION CRITERIA

The following should be clearly demonstrated:

- No rotation of the digit:
  - □ Concavity of the phalangeal shafts and an equal amount of soft tissue on both sides of the phalanges
  - □ Fingernail, if visualized and normal, centered over the distal phalanx
- Entire digit from fingertip to distal portion of the adjoining metacarpal
- No soft tissue overlap from adjacent digits
- Open interphalangeal and MCP joint spaces without overlap of bones
- Soft tissue and bony trabeculation

NOTE: Digits that cannot be extended can be examined in small sections with dental films. When joint injury is suspected, an AP projection is recommended instead of a PA projection.

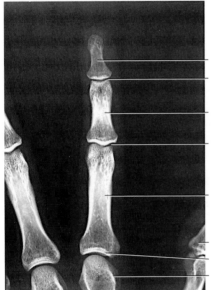

Distal phalanx
Distal interphalangeal joint
Middle phalanx
Proximal interphalangeal joint
Proximal phalanx
Thumb
Metacarpophalangeal joint
Head of metacarpal

Fig. 4-16 PA second digit.

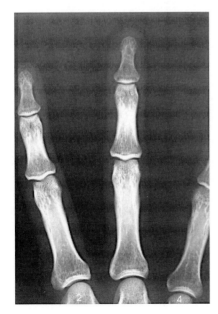

Fig. 4-17 PA third digit.

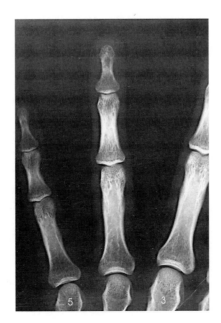

Fig. 4-18 PA fourth digit.

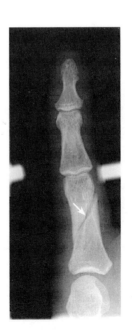

Fig. 4-19 Fractured fifth digit *(arrow)*.

▲ LATERAL PROJECTION
Lateromedial or mediolateral

Image receptor: 8×10 inch (18×24 cm) crosswise for two or more images on one cassette

Position of patient
- Seat the patient at the end of the radiographic table.

Position of part
- Because lateral digit positions are difficult to hold, tell the patient how the digit is adjusted on the cassette, and demonstrate with your own finger. Let the patient assume the most comfortable arm position.
- Ask the patient to extend the digit to be examined. Close the rest of the digits into a fist, and hold them in complete flexion with the thumb.
- Support the elbow on sandbags or provide other suitable support when the elbow must be elevated to bring the digit into position.
- With the digit under examination extended and other digits folded into a fist, have the patient's hand rest on the lateral, or radial, surface for the second or third digit (Figs. 4-20 and 4-21) or on the medial, or ulnar, surface for the fourth or fifth digit (Figs. 4-22 and 4-23).

- Before making the final adjustment of the digit position, place the cassette so that the midline of its unmasked portion is parallel with the long axis of the digit. Center the cassette to the PIP joint.
- Rest the second and fifth digits directly on the cassette, but for an accurate image of the bones and joints, elevate the third and fourth digits and place their long axes parallel with the plane of the cassette. A radiolucent sponge may be used to support the digits.
- Immobilize the extended digit by placing a strip of adhesive tape, a tongue depressor, or other support against its palmar surface. The patient can hold the support with the opposite hand.
- Adjust the anterior or posterior rotation of the hand to obtain a true lateral position of the digit.
- *Shield gonads.*

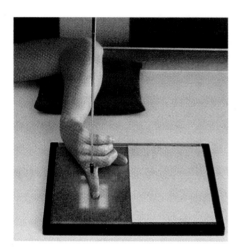

Fig. 4-20 Lateral second digit.

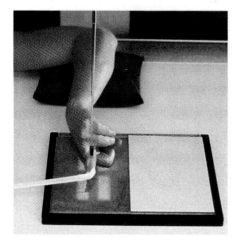

Fig. 4-21 Lateral third digit (adhesive tape).

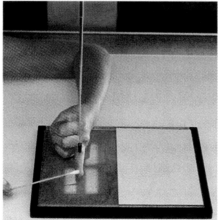

Fig. 4-22 Lateral fourth digit (cotton swab).

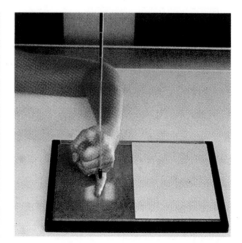

Fig. 4-23 Lateral fifth digit.

Digits (Second Through Fifth)

Central ray
- Perpendicular to the PIP joint of the affected digit.
- Collimate to the digit being examined.

Structures shown
A lateral projection of the affected digit is shown (Figs. 4-24 through 4-27).

EVALUATION CRITERIA
The following should be clearly demonstrated:
- Entire digit in a true lateral position:
  - ☐ Fingernail in profile, if visualized and normal
  - ☐ Concave, anterior surfaces of the phalanges
  - ☐ No rotation of the phalanges
- No obstruction of the proximal phalanx or MCP joint by adjacent digits
- Open interphalangeal and MCP joint spaces
- Soft tissue and bony trabeculation

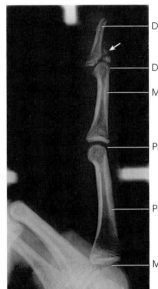

Distal phalanx
Distal interphalangeal joint
Middle phalanx
Proximal interphalangeal joint
Proximal phalanx
Metacarpophalangeal joint

Fig. 4-24 Lateral digit showing a chip fracture *(arrow)* and dislocation involving the distal interphalangeal joint of second digit *(arrow)*.

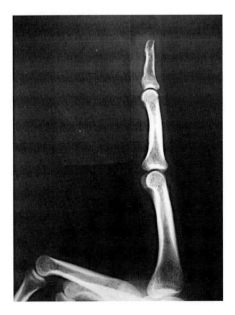

Fig. 4-25 Lateral third digit.

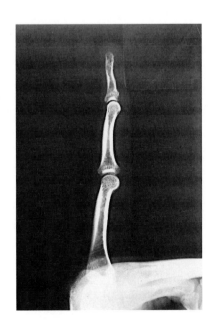

Fig. 4-26 Lateral fourth digit.

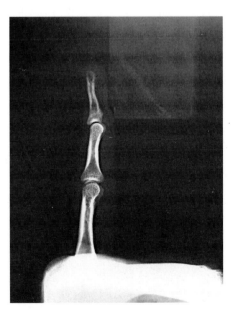

Fig. 4-27 Lateral fifth digit.

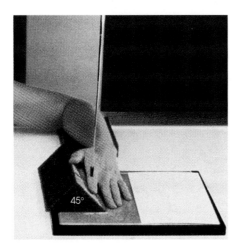

Fig. 4-28 PA oblique second digit.

♠ PA OBLIQUE PROJECTION
Lateral rotation

Image receptor: 8 × 10 inch (18 × 24 cm) crosswise for two or more images on one cassette

Position of patient
- Seat the patient at the end of the radiographic table.

Position of part
- Place the patient's forearm on the table with the hand pronated and the palm resting on the cassette.
- Center the cassette at the level of the PIP joint.
- Rotate the hand externally until the digits are separated and supported on a 45-degree foam wedge. The wedge supports the digits in a position parallel with the cassette plane (Figs. 4-28 through 4-31) so that the interphalangeal joint spaces are open.
- *Shield gonads.*

Central ray
- Perpendicular to the PIP joint of the affected digit.
- Collimate to the digit being examined.

Structures shown
The resultant image shows a PA oblique projection of the bones and soft tissue of the affected digit (Figs. 4-32 through 4-35).

EVALUATION CRITERIA

The following should be clearly demonstrated:
- Entire digit rotated at a 45-degree angle, including the distal portion of the adjoining metacarpal
- No superimposition of the adjacent digits over the proximal phalanx or MCP joint
- Open interphalangeal and MCP joint spaces
- Soft tissue and bony trabeculation

OPTION: Some radiographers rotate the second digit medially from the prone position (Fig. 4-36). The advantage of medially rotating the digit is that the part is closer to the cassette for improved recorded detail and increased ability to see certain fractures.[1]

---

[1]Street JM: Radiographs of phalangeal fractures: importance of the internally rotated oblique projection for diagnosis, *AJR* 160:575, 1993.

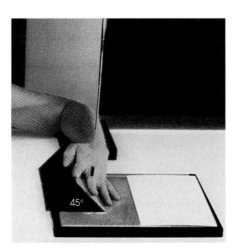

Fig. 4-29 PA oblique third digit.

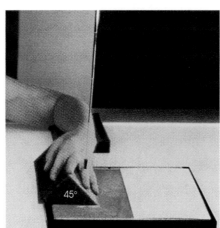

Fig. 4-30 PA oblique fourth digit.

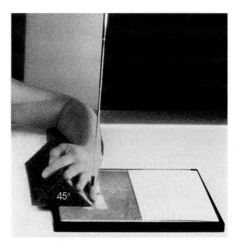

Fig. 4-31 PA oblique fifth digit.

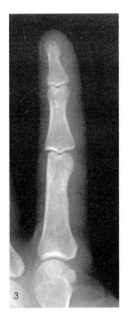

Fig. 4-32 PA oblique second digit.

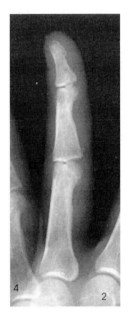

Fig. 4-33 PA oblique third digit.

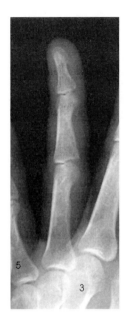

Fig. 4-34 PA oblique fourth digit.

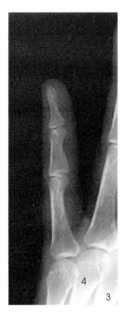

Fig. 4-35 PA oblique fifth digit.

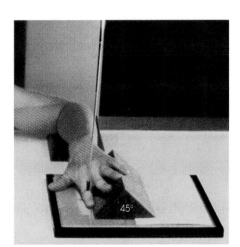

Fig. 4-36 PA oblique second digit (alternative method, medial rotation).

First Digit (Thumb)

AP, PA, LATERAL, AND PA OBLIQUE PROJECTIONS

Image receptor: 8 × 10 inch (18 × 24 cm) crosswise for two or more images on one cassette

✷ AP PROJECTION
Position of patient

- Seat the patient at the end of the radiographic table with the arm internally rotated.

Position of part

- Demonstrate how to avoid motion or rotation with the hand. By adjusting the body position on the chair, the patient can place the hand in the correct position with the least amount of strain on the arm.
- Put the patient's hand in a position of extreme internal rotation. Have the patient hold the extended digits back with tape or the opposite hand. Rest the thumb on the cassette. If the elbow is elevated, place a support under it and have the patient rest the opposite forearm against the table for support (Fig. 4-37).
- Center the long axis of the thumb parallel with the long axis of the cassette. Adjust the position of the hand to ensure a true AP projection of the thumb. Place the fifth metacarpal back far enough to avoid superimposition.
- Lewis[1] suggested directing the central ray 10 to 15 degrees along the long axis of the thumb toward the wrist to demonstrate the first metacarpal free of the soft tissue of the palm.
- *Shield gonads.*

---

[1] Lewis S: New angles on the radiographic examination of the hand—II, *Radiogr Today* 54:29, 1988.

PA PROJECTION

Position of patient

- Seat the patient at the end of the radiographic table with the hand resting on its medial surface.

Position of part

- If a PA projection of the first CMC joint and first digit is to be performed, place the hand in the lateral position. Rest the elevated and abducted thumb on a radiographic support, or hold it up with a radiolucent stick. Adjust the hand to place the dorsal surface of the digit parallel with the cassette. This position magnifies the part (Fig. 4-38).
- Center the MCP joint to the center of the cassette.
- *Shield gonads.*

LATERAL PROJECTION
Position of patient

- Seat the patient at the end of the radiographic table with the relaxed hand placed on the cassette.

Position of part

- Place the hand in its natural arched position with the palmar surface down and fingers flexed or resting on a sponge.
- Place the midline of the cassette parallel with the long axis of the digit. Center the cassette to the MCP joint.
- Adjust the arching of the hand until a true lateral position of the thumb is obtained (Fig. 4-39).

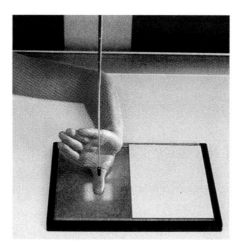

Fig. 4-37 AP first digit.

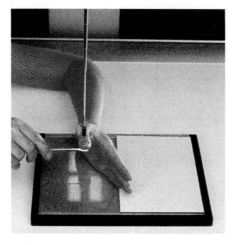

Fig. 4-38 PA first digit (cotton swab).

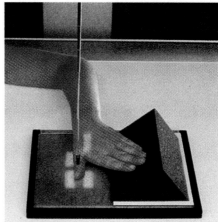

Fig. 4-39 Lateral first digit.

First Digit (Thumb)

☀ PA OBLIQUE PROJECTION

Position of patient

- Seat the patient at the end of the radiographic table with the palm of the hand resting on the cassette.

Position of part

- With the thumb abducted, place the palmar surface of the hand in contact with the cassette. Ulnar deviate the hand slightly. This relatively normal placement positions the thumb in the oblique position.
- Align the longitudinal axis of the thumb with the long axis of the cassette. Center the cassette to the MCP joint (Fig. 4-40).
- *Shield gonads.*

Central ray

- Perpendicular to the MCP joint for the AP, PA, lateral, and oblique projections.
- Collimate to include entire first digit.

Structures shown

AP, PA, lateral, and PA oblique projections of the thumb are demonstrated (Figs. 4-41 through 4-44).

EVALUATION CRITERIA

AP and PA thumb

The following should be clearly demonstrated:

- No rotation:
  - □ Concavity of the phalangeal and metacarpal shafts
  - □ Equal amount of soft tissue on both sides of the phalanges
  - □ Thumbnail, if visualized, in the center of the distal thumb
- Area from the distal tip of the thumb to the trapezium
- Open interphalangeal and MCP joint spaces without overlap of bones
- Overlap of soft tissue profile of the palm over the midshaft of the first metacarpal
- Soft tissue and bony trabeculation
- PA thumb projection magnified compared to AP projection

Lateral thumb

The following should be clearly demonstrated:

- First digit in a true lateral projection:
  - □ Thumbnail, if visualized and normal, in profile
  - □ Concave, anterior surface of the proximal phalanx
  - □ No rotation of the phalanges
- Area from the distal tip of the thumb to the trapezium
- Open interphalangeal and MCP joint spaces
- Soft tissue and bony trabeculation

Oblique thumb

The following should be clearly demonstrated:

- Proper rotation of phalanges, soft tissue, and first metacarpal
- Area from the distal tip of the thumb to the trapezium
- Open interphalangeal and MCP joint spaces
- Soft tissue and bony trabeculation

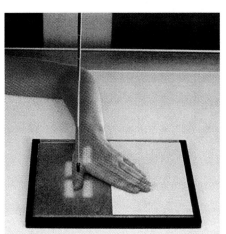

Fig. 4-40 PA oblique first digit.

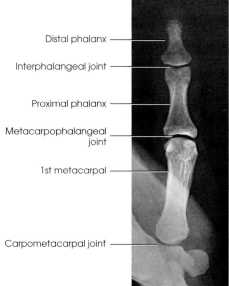

Distal phalanx —
Interphalangeal joint —
Proximal phalanx —
Metacarpophalangeal joint —
1st metacarpal —
Carpometacarpal joint —

Fig. 4-41 AP first digit.

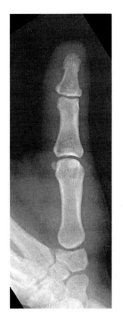

Fig. 4-42 PA first digit.

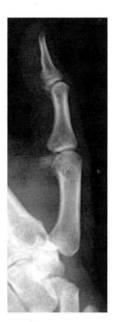

Fig. 4-43 Lateral first digit.

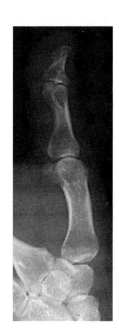

Fig. 4-44 PA oblique first digit.

Upper limb

First Carpometacarpal Joint
AP PROJECTION
ROBERT METHOD[1]

Robert[1] first described the radiographic projection of the first CMC joint in 1936. Lewis[2] modified the central ray for this projection in 1988, and Long and Rafert[3] further modified the central ray in 1995. This projection is commonly performed to demonstrate arthritic changes, fractures, displacement of the first CMC joint, and the Bennett's fracture. The Robert method does not replace the initial AP or PA thumb projection.

Image receptor: 8 × 10 inch (18 × 24 cm) lengthwise

---

[1]Robert M: X-ray of trapezo-metacarpal articulation: the arthroses of this joint, *Bulletins et memories de la Societe de Radiologie Medicale de France* 24:687, 1936.
[2]Lewis S: New angles on the radiographic examination of the hand—II, *Radiogr Today* 54:29, 1988.
[3]Long B, Rafert J: *Orthopaedic radiography,* Philadelphia, 1995, WB Saunders.

Position of patient
- Seat the patient sideways at the end of the radiographic table. The patient should be positioned low enough to place the shoulder, elbow, and wrist on the same plane. The entire limb *must* be on the same plane to prevent elevation of the carpal bones and closing of the first CMC joint (Fig. 4-45, *A*).

Position of part
- Extend the limb straight out on the radiographic table.
- Rotate the arm internally to place the posterior aspect of the thumb on the cassette with the thumbnail down (Fig. 4-45, *B*).

- Place the thumb in the center of the cassette.
- Hyperextend the hand so that the soft tissue over the ulnar aspect does not obscure the first CMC joint (Fig. 4-46). Ensure that the thumb is not oblique.
- Long and Rafert[1] state that the patient may hold the fingers back with the other hand.
- Steady the hand on a sponge if necessary.
- *Shield gonads.*

---

[1]Long B, Rafert J: *Orthopaedic radiography,* Philadelphia, 1995, WB Saunders.

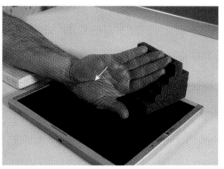
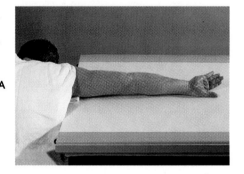

A   **B**

Fig. 4-45 A, Patient in position for AP thumb to demonstrate the first carpometacarpal joint: Robert method. The patient leans forward to place the entire arm on the same plane and for ease of maximum internal arm rotation. **B,** Thumb, hand, and wrist in correct position for AP of first carpometacarpal joint. Note the specific area of the wrist where the joint is located *(arrow).*

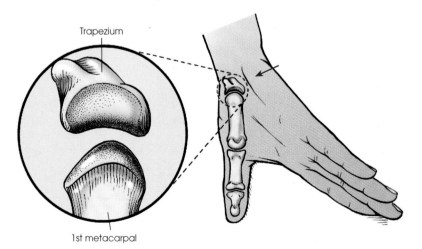

Trapezium

1st metacarpal

Fig. 4-46 Hyperextended hand and thumb position for AP projection of first carpometacarpal joint: Robert method. The soft tissue of the palm *(arrow)* is positioned out of the way so that the joint will be clearly shown. *Inset:* the first carpometacarpal joint is a saddle joint; the articular surfaces are shown.

Central ray (Fig. 4-47)

Robert method

- Perpendicular entering at the first CMC joint

Long and Rafert modification

- Angled 15 degrees proximally along the long axis of the thumb and entering the first CMC joint.
- Collimate to include the entire thumb.

Lewis modification

- Angled 10 to 15 degrees proximally along the long axis of the thumb and entering the first MCP joint

NOTE: Angulation of the central ray serves two purposes: (1) it may help project the soft tissue of the hand away from the first CMC joint, and (2) it can help open the joint space when the space is not shown with a perpendicular central ray.

Structures shown

This projection demonstrates the first CMC joint free of superimposition of the soft tissues of the hand (Fig. 4-48, *A*).

EVALUATION CRITERIA

The following should be clearly demonstrated:

- First CMC joint free of superimposition of the hand or other bony elements
- First metacarpal with the base in convex profile
- Trapezium

A

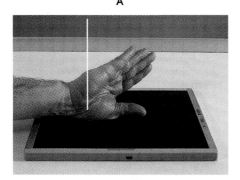

B

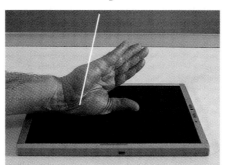

C

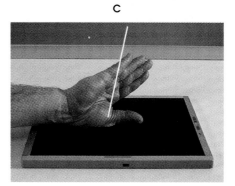

Fig. 4-47 Central ray angulation choices for demonstration of the first carpometacarpal joint. **A,** Robert method, 0 degrees to carpometacarpal joint. **B,** Long-Rafert modification, 15 degrees cephalad to carpometacarpal joint. **C,** Lewis modification, 10 to 15 degrees cephalad to the metacarpophalangeal joint.

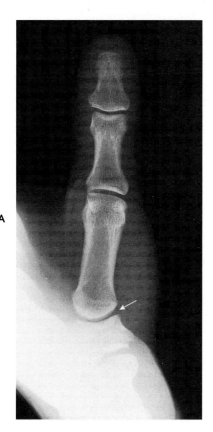

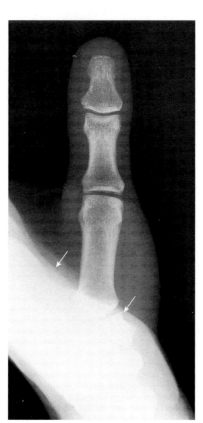

Fig. 4-48 A, Optimal radiograph of an AP first carpometacarpal joint *(arrow):* Robert method. **B,** Example of a typical repeat radiograph. Soft tissue of the palm *(arrows)* obscured first carpometacarpal joint. The Long-Rafert or Lewis modification of the central ray would help demonstrate the joint on this patient.

First Carpometacarpal Joint
AP PROJECTION
BURMAN METHOD[1]

When hyperextension of the wrist is not contraindicated, Burman[1] stated that this projection provides a clearer image of the first CMC joint than the standard AP projection.

Image receptor: 8 × 10 inch (18 × 24 cm) lengthwise

SID: The recommended distance is 18 inches. This produces a magnified image that creates a greater field of view of the concavoconvex aspect of this joint.

[1]Burman M: Anteroposterior projection of the carpometacarpal joint of the thumb by radial shift of the carpal tunnel view, *J Bone Joint Surg* 40A:1156, 1958.

Position of patient
- Seat the patient at the end of the radiographic table so that the forearm can be adjusted to lie approximately parallel with the long axis of the cassette.

Position of part
- Place the cassette under the wrist, and center the first CMC joint to the center of the cassette.
- Hyperextend the hand, and have the patient hold the position with the opposite hand or with a bandage looped around the digits.
- Rotate the hand internally, and abduct the thumb so that it is flat on the cassette (Fig. 4-49).
- *Shield gonads.*

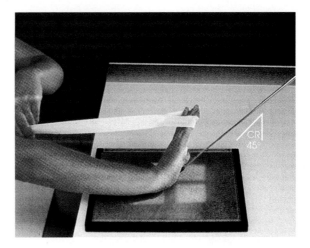

Fig. 4-49 Hyperextended hand and abducted thumb position for AP of the first carpometacarpal joint: Burman method.

First Digit (Thumb)

Central ray
- Through the first CMC joint at a 45-degree angle toward the elbow

Structures shown
This image shows a magnified concavo-convex outline of the first CMC joint (Fig. 4-50).

EVALUATION CRITERIA
The following should be clearly demonstrated:
- First metacarpal
- Trapezium in concave profile
- Base of the first metacarpal in convex profile
- First CMC joint, unobscured by adjacent carpals

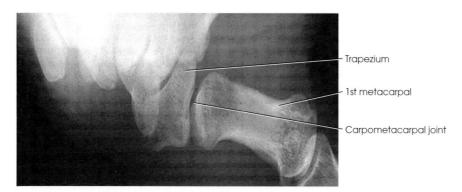

Trapezium

1st metacarpal

Carpometacarpal joint

Fig. 4-50 AP thumb to demonstrate the first carpometacarpal joint: Burman method.

(Courtesy Michael Burman)

PA PROJECTION

Image receptor: 8 × 10 inch (18 × 24 cm) for hand of average size or 24 × 30 cm (10 × 12 inch) crosswise for two images

Position of patient

- Seat the patient at the end of the radiographic table.
- Adjust the patient's height so that the forearm is resting on the table (Fig. 4-51).

Position of part

- Rest the patient's forearm on the table, and place the hand with the palmar surface down on the cassette .
- Center the cassette to the MCP joints, and adjust the long axis of the cassette parallel with the long axis of the hand and forearm.
- Spread the fingers slightly (Fig. 4-52).
- Ask the patient to relax the hand to avoid motion. Prevent involuntary movement with the use of adhesive tape or positioning sponges. A sandbag may be placed over the distal forearm.
- *Shield gonads.*

Central ray

- Perpendicular to the third MCP joint

Structures shown

PA projections of the carpals, metacarpals, phalanges (except the thumb), interarticulations of the hand, and distal radius and ulna are shown in Fig. 4-53. This image also demonstrates a PA oblique projection of the first digit.

EVALUATION CRITERIA

The following should be clearly demonstrated:

- No rotation of the hand:
  - ☐ Equal concavity of the metacarpal and phalangeal shafts on both sides
  - ☐ Equal amount of soft tissue on both sides of the phalanges
  - ☐ Fingernails, if visualized, in the center of each distal phalanx
- Open MCP and interphalangeal joints, indicating that the hand is placed flat on the cassette
- Slightly separate digits with no soft tissue overlap
- All anatomy distal to the radius and ulna
- Soft tissue and bony trabeculation

NOTE: When the MCP joints are under examination and the patient cannot extend the hand enough to place its palmar surface in contact with the cassette, the position of the hand can be reversed for an AP projection. This position is also used for the metacarpals when the hand cannot be extended because of an injury, a pathologic condition, or the use of dressings.

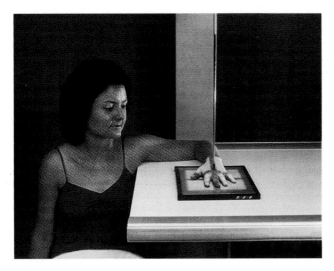

Fig. 4-51 Properly shielded patient in position for a PA hand.

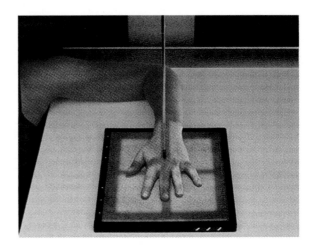

Fig. 4-52 PA hand.

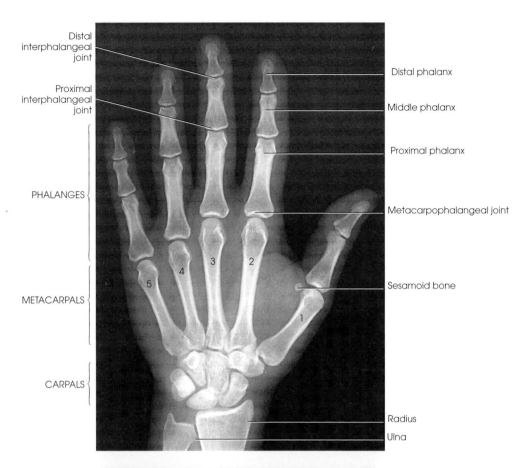

Distal interphalangeal joint

Proximal interphalangeal joint

PHALANGES

METACARPALS

CARPALS

Distal phalanx

Middle phalanx

Proximal phalanx

Metacarpophalangeal joint

Sesamoid bone

Radius

Ulna

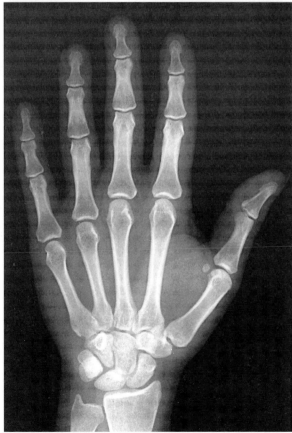

Fig. 4-53 PA hand.

🦅 PA OBLIQUE PROJECTION
Lateral rotation

Image receptor: 8 × 10 inch (18 × 24 cm) lengthwise or 24 × 30 cm (10 × 12 inch) crosswise for two images

Position of patient
- Seat the patient at the end of the radiographic table.
- Adjust the patient's height to rest the forearm on the table.

Position of part
- Rest the patient's forearm on the table with the hand pronated and the palm resting on the cassette.
- Adjust the obliquity of the hand so that the MCP joints form an angle of approximately 45 degrees with the cassette plane.
- Use a 45-degree foam wedge to support the fingers in the extended position to demonstrate the interphalangeal joints (Figs. 4-54 and 4-55).
- When examining the metacarpals, obtain a PA oblique projection of the hand by rotating the patient's hand laterally (externally) from the pronated position until the fingertips touch the cassette (Fig. 4-56).
- If it is not possible to obtain the correct position with all fingertips resting on the cassette, elevate the index finger and thumb on a suitable radiolucent material (see Fig. 4-55). Elevation opens the joint spaces and reduces the degree of foreshortening of the phalanges.
- For either approach, center the cassette to the MCP joints and adjust the midline to be parallel with the long axis of the hand and forearm.
- *Shield gonads.*

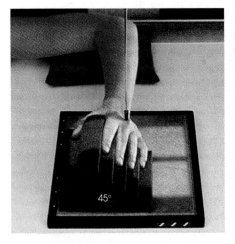

Fig. 4-54 PA oblique hand for demonstration of joint spaces.

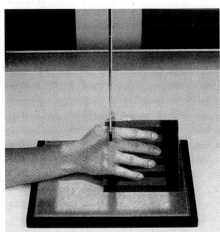

Fig. 4-55 PA oblique hand for demonstration of joint spaces.

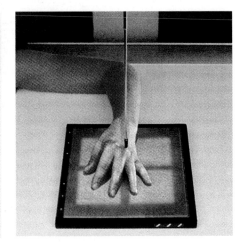

Fig. 4-56 PA oblique hand for demonstration of metacarpals.

Central ray

- Perpendicular to the third MCP joint

Structures shown

The resulting image shows a PA oblique projection of the bones and soft tissues of the hand (Figs. 4-57 and 4-58). This supplemental position is used for investigating fractures and pathologic conditions.

EVALUATION CRITERIA

The following should be clearly demonstrated:

- Minimal overlap of the third-fourth and fourth-fifth metacarpal shafts
- Slight overlap of the metacarpal bases and heads
- Separation of the second and third metacarpals
- Open interphalangeal and MCP joints
- Digits separated slightly with no overlap of their soft tissues
- All anatomy distal to the distal radius and ulna
- Soft tissue and bony trabeculation

NOTE: Lane, Kennedy, and Kuschner[1] recommend the inclusion of a reverse oblique projection to better demonstrate severe metacarpal deformities or fractures. This projection is accomplished by having the patient rotate the hand 45 degrees medially (internally) from the palm-down position.

Kallen[2] recommended using a tangential oblique projection to demonstrate metacarpal head fractures. From the PA hand position, the MCP joints are flexed 75 to 80 degrees with the dorsum of the digits resting on the cassette. The hand is rotated 40 to 45 degrees toward the ulnar surface. Then the hand is rotated 40 to 45 degrees forward until the affected MCP joint is projected beyond its proximal phalanx. The perpendicular central ray is directed tangentially to enter the MCP joint of interest. Variations of rotation are described to demonstrate the second metacarpal head free of superimposition.

---

[1]Lane CS, Kennedy JF, Kuschner SH: The reverse oblique x-ray film: metacarpal fractures revealed, *J Hand Surg* 17A(3):504, 1992.
[2]Kallen MJ: Kallen projection reveals metacarpal head fractures, *Radiol Technol* 65:229, 1994.

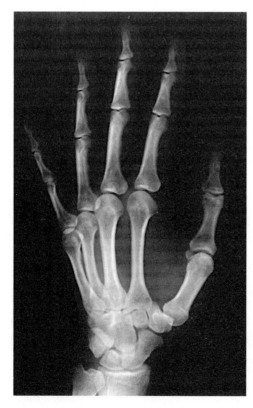

Fig. 4-57 PA oblique hand with digits on sponge to demonstrate open joints.

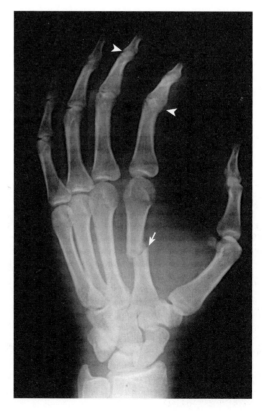

Fig. 4-58 PA oblique hand without support sponge, showing the fracture *(arrow)*. Note that the interphalangeal joints *(arrows)* are not entirely open, and phalanges are foreshortened.

⚜ LATERAL PROJECTION
Mediolateral or lateromedial
Extension and fan lateral

Image receptor: 8 × 10 inch (18 × 24 cm) for hand of average size or 24 × 30 cm (10 × 12 inch) crosswise for two images

Position of patient
- Seat the patient at the end of the radiographic table with the forearm in contact with the table and the hand in the lateral position with the ulnar aspect down (Fig. 4-59).
- Alternatively, place the radial side of the wrist against the cassette (Fig. 4-60). However, this position is more difficult for the patient to assume.
- If the elbow is elevated, support it with sandbags.

Position of part
- Extend the patient's digits and adjust the first digit at a right angle to the palm.
- Place the palmar surface perpendicular to the cassette.
- Center the cassette to the MCP joints, and adjust the midline to be parallel with the long axis of the hand and forearm. If the hand is resting on the ulnar surface, immobilization of the thumb may be necessary.
- The two extended digit positions result in superimposition of the phalanges. A modification of the lateral hand is the *fan lateral position,* which eliminates superimposition of all but the proximal phalanges. For the fan lateral position, place the digits on a sponge wedge. Abduct the thumb and place it on the radiolucent sponge for support (Fig. 4-61).
- *Shield gonads.*

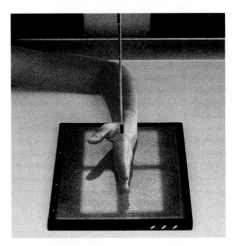

Fig. 4-59 Lateral hand with ulnar surface to cassette: lateromedial.

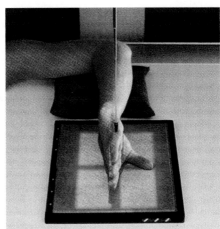

Fig. 4-60 Lateral hand with radial surface to cassette: mediolateral.

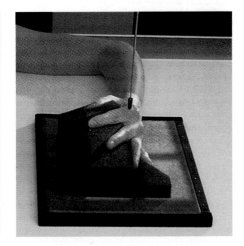

Fig. 4-61 Fan lateral hand.

Hand

Central ray

- Perpendicular to the *second digit* MCP joint

Structures shown

This image, which shows a lateral projection of the hand in extension (Fig. 4-62), is the customary position for localizing of foreign bodies and metacarpal fracture displacement. The exposure technique depends on the foreign body.

The fan lateral superimposes the metacarpals but demonstrates almost all of the individual phalanges. The most proximal portions of the proximal phalanges remain superimposed (Fig. 4-63).

EVALUATION CRITERIA

The following should be clearly demonstrated:

- Hand in a true lateral position if the following are seen:
  - Superimposed phalanges (individually demonstrated on fan lateral)
  - Superimposed metacarpals
  - Superimposed distal radius and ulna
- Extended digits
- Thumb free of motion and superimposition
- Each bone outlined through the superimposed shadows of the other metacarpals

NOTE: To better demonstrate fractures of the fifth metacarpal, Lewis[1] recommended rotating the hand 5 degrees posteriorly from the true lateral position. This positioning removes the superimposition of the second through fourth metacarpals. The thumb is extended as much as possible, and the hand is allowed to become hollow by relaxation. The central ray is angled so that it passes parallel to the extended thumb and enters the midshaft of the fifth metacarpal.

[1]Lewis S: New angles on the radiographic examination of the hand—II, *Radiogr Today* 54:29, 1988.

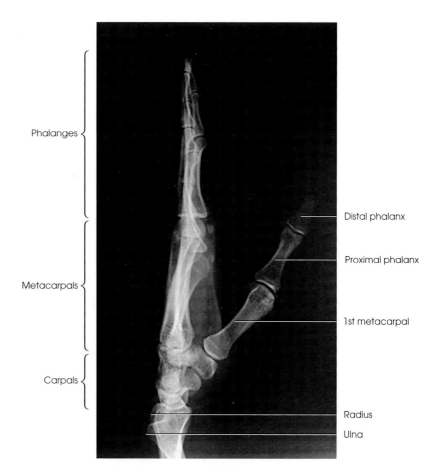

Phalanges

Metacarpals

Carpals

Distal phalanx

Proximal phalanx

1st metacarpal

Radius

Ulna

Fig. 4-62 Lateral hand.

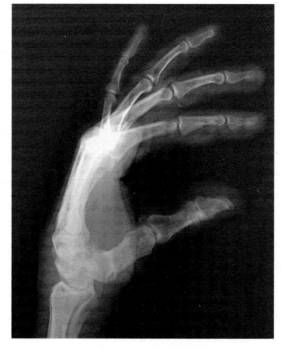

Fig. 4-63 Fan lateral hand.

LATERAL PROJECTION
Lateromedial in flexion

Image receptor: 8 × 10 inch (18 × 24 cm) lengthwise

Position of patient
- Seat the patient at the end of the radiographic table.
- Ask the patient to rest the forearm on the table, and place the hand on the cassette with the ulnar aspect down.

Position of part
- Center the cassette to the MCP joints, and adjust it so that its midline is parallel with the long axis of the hand and forearm.
- With the patient relaxing the digits to maintain the natural arch of the hand, arrange the digits so that they are perfectly superimposed (Fig. 4-64).
- Have the patient hold the thumb parallel with the cassette, or if necessary immobilize the thumb with tape or a sponge.
- *Shield gonads.*

Central ray
- Perpendicular to the MCP joints, entering MCP joint of the second digit

Structures shown
This projection produces a lateral image of the bony structures and soft tissues of the hand in their normally flexed position (Fig. 4-65). It also demonstrates anterior or posterior displacement in fractures of the metacarpals.

EVALUATION CRITERIA
The following should be clearly demonstrated:
- Superimposed phalanges and metacarpals
- Superimposed distal radius and ulna
- Flexed digits
- No motion or superimposition of the first digit
- Radiographic density similar to frontal and oblique hand images, which requires increased exposure factors to compensate for greater hand thickness
- Clear outline of each bone through the superimposed shadows of the other metacarpals

AP OBLIQUE PROJECTION
NORGAARD METHOD[1-3]
Medial rotation

The Norgaard method,[1-3] sometimes referred to as the *ball-catcher's position,* assists in detecting early radiologic changes needed to diagnose rheumatoid arthritis. Norgaard reported that it is often possible to make an early diagnosis of rheumatoid arthritis by using this position before laboratory tests are positive.[3] He also stated that extremely fine-grain intensifying screens should be used to demonstrate high resolution. Low kilovoltage peak (60 to 65) is recommended to obtain necessary contrast.

In a more recent article, Stapczynski[3] recommended this projection for the demonstration of fractures of the base of the fifth metacarpal.

Image receptor: 24 × 30 cm (10 × 12 inch) crosswise

Position of patient
- Seat the patient at the end of the radiographic table. Norgaard recommended that both hands be radiographed in the half-supinate position for comparison.

Position of part
- Have the patient place the palms of both hands together. Center the MCP joints on the medial aspect of both hands to the cassette. Both hands should be in the lateral position.
- Place two 45-degree radiolucent sponges against the posterior aspect of each hand.
- Rotate the patient's hands to a half-supinate position until the dorsal surface of each hand rests against each 45-degree sponge support (Fig. 4-66).
- Extend the patient's fingers, and abduct the thumbs slightly to avoid superimposition over the fingers.

[1]Norgaard F: Earliest roentgenological changes in polyarthritis of the rheumatoid type: rheumatoid arthritis, *Radiology* 85:325, 1965.
[2]Norgaard F: Early roentgen changes in polyarthritis of the rheumatoid type, *Radiology* 92:299, 1969.
[3]Stapczynski JS: Fracture of the base of the little finger metacarpal: importance of the "ball-catcher" radiographic view, *J Emerg Med* 9:145, 1991.

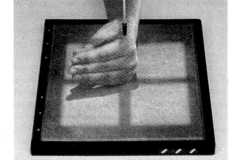

Fig. 4-64 Lateral hand in flexion.

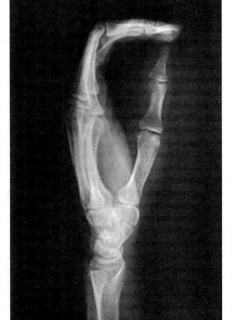

Fig. 4-65 Lateral hand in flexion.

- The original method of positioning the hands is often modified. The patient is positioned similar to the method described except that the fingers are not extended. Instead the fingers are cupped as if the patient were going to catch a ball (Fig. 4-67). Comparable diagnostic information is demonstrated using either position.
- *Shield gonads.*

Central ray

- Perpendicular to the point midway between both hands at the level of the MCP joints for either of the two patient positions

Structures shown

The resulting image shows an AP 45-degree oblique projection of both hands (Fig. 4-68). The early radiologic change significant in making the diagnosis of rheumatoid arthritis is a symmetric, very slight, indistinct outline of the bone corresponding to the insertion of the joint capsule dorsoradial on the proximal end of the first phalanx of the four fingers. In addition, associated demineralization of the bone structure is always present in the area directly below the contour defect.

EVALUATION CRITERIA

The following should be clearly demonstrated:
- Both hands from the carpal area to the tips of the digits
- Metacarpal heads free of superimposition
- Useful level of density over the heads of the metacarpals

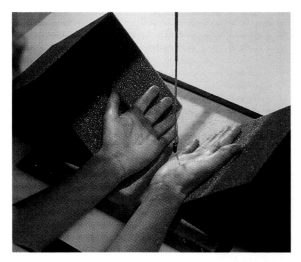

Fig. 4-66 AP oblique hands, semi-supinated position.

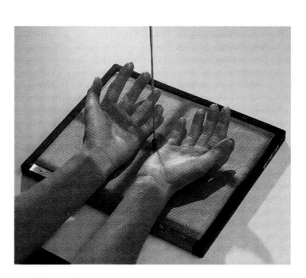

Fig. 4-67 Ball-catcher's position.

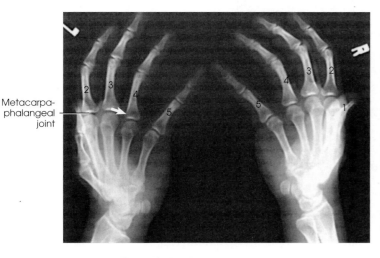

Metacarpa-phalangeal joint

A

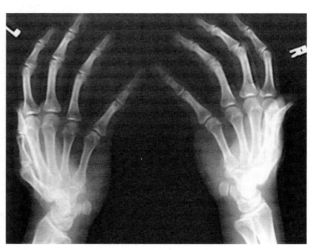

B

Fig. 4-68 A, AP oblique hands, ball-catcher's position, showing where indistinct area occurs *(arrow).* **B,** Ball-catcher's position.

Upper limb

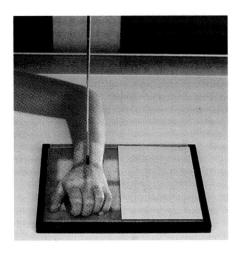

Fig. 4-69 PA wrist.

⚡ PA PROJECTION

Image receptor: 8 × 10 inch (18 × 24 cm) crosswise for two or more images on one cassette

Position of patient

- Seat the patient low enough to place the axilla in contact with the table, or elevate the limb to shoulder level on a suitable support. This position places the shoulder, elbow, and wrist joints in the same plane to permit right-angle rotation of the ulna and radius for the lateral position.

Position of part

- Have the patient rest the forearm on the table, and center the wrist to the cassette area.
- When it is difficult to determine the exact location of the carpals because of a swollen wrist, ask the patient to flex the wrist slightly and center the cassette to the point of flexion. When the wrist is in a cast or splint, the exact point of centering can be determined by comparison with the opposite side.
- Adjust the hand and forearm to lie parallel with the long axis of the cassette.
- Slightly arch the hand at the MCP joints by flexing the digits to place the wrist in close contact with the cassette (Fig. 4-69).
- When necessary, place a support under the digits to immobilize them.
- *Shield gonads.*

Central ray

- Perpendicular to the midcarpal area

Structures shown

A PA projection of the carpals, distal radius and ulna, and proximal metacarpals is shown (Fig. 4-70). The projection gives a slightly oblique rotation to the ulna. When the ulna is under examination, an AP projection should be taken.

EVALUATION CRITERIA

The following should be clearly demonstrated:

- Distal radius and ulna, carpals, and proximal half of metacarpals
- No rotation in carpals, metacarpals, or radius
- Soft tissue and bony trabeculation
- No excessive flexion to overlap and obscure metacarpals with digits

NOTE: To better demonstrate the scaphoid and capitate, Daffner, Emmerling, and Buterbaugh[1] recommended angling the central ray when the patient is positioned for a PA radiograph. A central ray angle of 30 degrees toward the elbow elongates the scaphoid and capitate, whereas an angle of 30 degrees toward the fingertips only elongates the capitate

[1]Daffner RH, Emmerling EW, Buterbaugh GA: Proximal and distal oblique radiography of the wrist: value in occult injuries, *J Hand Surg Am* 17:499, 1992.

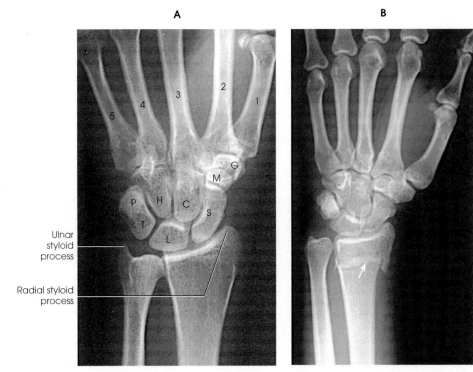

Ulnar styloid process

Radial styloid process

Fig. 4-70 A, PA wrist. (*S,* scaphoid; *L,* lunate; *T,* triquetrum; *P,* pisiform; *G,* trapezium; *M,* trapezoid; *C,* capitate; and *H,* hamate.) **B,** PA wrist showing fracture of the distal radius (*arrow*).

AP PROJECTION

Image receptor: 8 × 10 inch (18 × 24 cm) crosswise for two or more images on one cassette

Position of patient
- Seat the patient at the end of the radiographic table.

Position of part
- Have the patient rest the forearm on the table, with the arm and hand supinated.
- Place the cassette under the wrist, and center it to the carpals.
- Elevate the digits on a suitable support to place the wrist in close contact with the cassette.
- Have the patient lean laterally to prevent rotation of the wrist (Fig. 4-71).
- *Shield gonads.*

Central ray
- Perpendicular to the midcarpal area

Structures shown

The *carpal interspaces* are better demonstrated in the AP image than the PA image. Because of the oblique direction of the interspaces, they are more closely parallel with the divergence of the x-ray beam (Fig. 4-72).

EVALUATION CRITERIA

The following should be clearly demonstrated:
- Distal radius and ulna, carpals, and proximal half of the metacarpals
- No rotation of the carpals, metacarpals, radius, and ulna
- Well-demonstrated soft tissue and bony trabeculation
- No overlapping or obscuring of the metacarpals as a result of excessive flexion

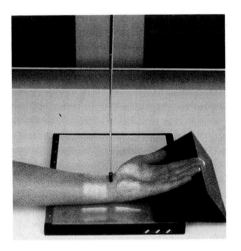

Fig. 4-71 AP wrist.

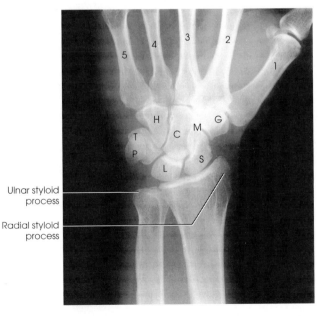

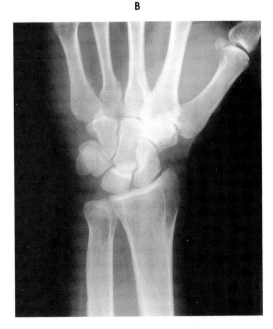

Fig. 4-72 A, AP wrist. (*S,* scaphoid; *L,* lunate; *T,* triquetrum; *P,* pisiform; *G,* trapezium; *M,* trapezoid; *C,* capitate; and *H,* hamate.) **B,** AP wrist.

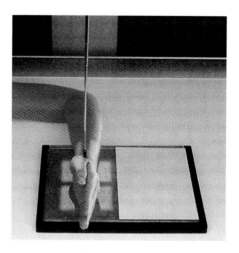

Fig. 4-73 Lateral wrist with ulnar surface to cassette.

🦅 LATERAL PROJECTION
Lateromedial

Image receptor: 8 × 10 inch (18 × 24 cm) for two images

Position of patient
- Seat the patient at the end of the radiographic table.
- Have the patient rest the arm and forearm on the table to ensure that the wrist is in a lateral position.

Position of part
- Have the patient flex the elbow 90 degrees to rotate the ulna to the lateral position.
- Center the cassette to the carpals, and adjust the forearm and hand so that the wrist is in a true lateral position (Fig. 4-73).
- *Shield gonads.*

Central ray
- Perpendicular to the wrist joint

Structures shown
This image shows a lateral projection of the proximal metacarpals, carpals, and distal radius and ulna (Fig. 4-74). An image obtained with the radial surface against the cassette (Fig. 4-75) is shown for comparison. This position can also be used to demonstrate anterior or posterior displacement in fractures.

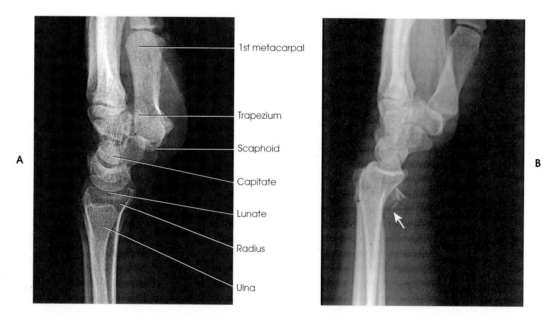

1st metacarpal

Trapezium

Scaphoid

Capitate

Lunate

Radius

Ulna

A

B

Fig. 4-74 A, Lateral wrist with ulnar surface to cassette.**B,** Lateral with fracture *(arrow)*. This is the same patient as in Fig. 4-70, *B.*

EVALUATION CRITERIA

The following should be clearly demonstrated:

- Distal radius and ulna, carpals, and proximal half of metacarpals
- Superimposed distal radius and ulna
- Superimposed metacarpals
- Radiographic density similar to PA or AP and oblique radiographs, which requires increased exposure factors to compensate for greater part thickness

NOTE: Burman et al[1] suggested that the lateral position of the scaphoid should be obtained with the wrist in palmar flexion because this action rotates the bone anteriorly into a dorsovolar position (Fig. 4-76, *A*). This position, however, is valuable only when sufficient flexion is permitted.

Fiolle[2,3] was the first to describe a small bony growth occurring on the dorsal surface of the third CMC joint. He termed the condition *carpe bossu (carpal boss)* and found that it is demonstrated best in a lateral position with the wrist in palmar flexion (Fig. 4-76, *B*).

[1]Burman MS et al: Fractures of the radial and ulnar axes, *AJR* 51:455, 1944.
[2]Fiolle J: Le "carpe bossu," *Bull Soc Chir Paris* 57:1687, 1931.
[3]Fiolle J et al: Nouvelle observation de "carpe bossu," *Bull Soc Chir Paris* 58:187, 1932.

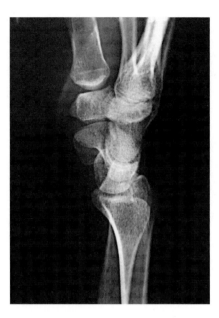

Fig. 4-75 Lateral wrist with radial surface to cassette.

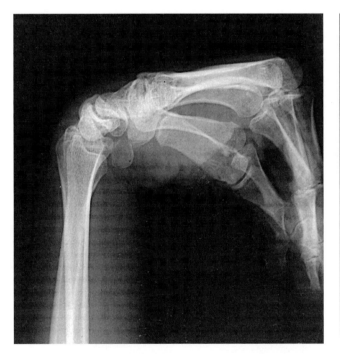
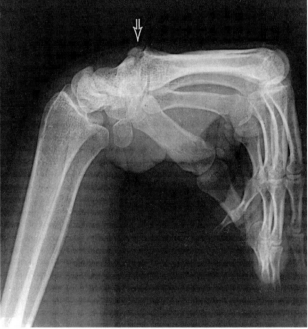

Fig. 4-76 A, Lateral wrist with palmar flexion of normal wrist. **B,** Lateral wrist with palmar flexion of wrist, showing carpal boss *(arrow)*.

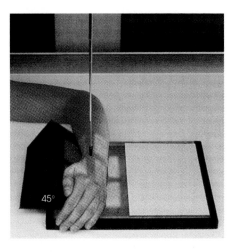

Fig. 4-77 PA oblique wrist: lateral rotation.

⚓ PA OBLIQUE PROJECTION
Lateral rotation

Image receptor: 8 × 10 inch (18 × 24 cm) crosswise for two images on one cassette

Position of patient
- Seat the patient at the end of the radiographic table, placing the axilla in contact with the table.

Position of part
- Rest the palmar surface of the wrist on the cassette.
- Adjust the cassette so that its center point is under the scaphoid when the wrist is rotated from the pronated position.
- From the pronated position, rotate the wrist laterally (externally) until it forms an angle of approximately 45 degrees with the plane of the cassette. For exact positioning and to ensure duplication in follow-up examinations, place a 45-degree foam wedge under the elevated side of the wrist.
- Extend the wrist slightly, and if the digits do not touch the table, support them in place (Fig. 4-77).
- When the scaphoid is under examination, adjust the wrist in ulnar deviation. Place a sandbag across the forearm.
- *Shield gonads.*

Central ray
- Perpendicular to the midcarpal area. It enters just distal to the radius.

Structures shown
This projection demonstrates the carpals on the lateral side of the wrist, particularly the trapezium and the scaphoid. The scaphoid is superimposed on itself in the direct PA projection (Figs. 4-78 and 4-79).

EVALUATION CRITERIA
The following should be clearly demonstrated:
- A well-demonstrated scaphoid and trapezium
- Distal radius and ulna, carpals and proximal half of metacarpals
- Usually, adequate amount of obliquity in the following circumstances:
  - ☐ Slight interosseus space between the third-fourth and fourth-fifth metacarpal shafts
  - ☐ Slight overlap of the distal radius and ulna
- Soft tissue and bony trabeculation

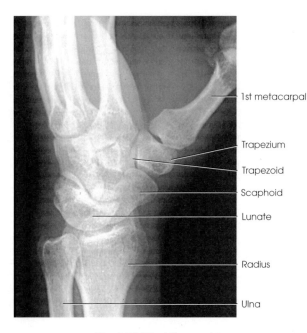

1st metacarpal

Trapezium

Trapezoid

Scaphoid

Lunate

Radius

Ulna

Fig. 4-78 PA oblique wrist.

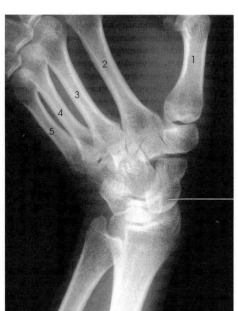

Scaphoid

Fig. 4-79 PA oblique wrist with ulnar deviation.

Wrist

AP OBLIQUE PROJECTION[1]
Medial rotation

Image receptor: 8 × 10 inch (18 × 24 cm) crosswise for two images on one cassette

Position of patient
- Seat the patient at the end of the radiographic table.
- Have the patient rest the forearm on the table in the supine position.

Position of part
- Place the cassette under the wrist and center it at the dorsal surface of the wrist.
- Rotate the wrist medially (internally) until it forms a semisupinated position of approximately 45 degrees to the cassette (Fig. 4-80).
- *Shield gonads.*

Central ray
- Perpendicular to the midcarpal area. It enters the anterior surface of the wrist midway between its medial and lateral borders.

Structures shown
This position separates the pisiform from the adjacent carpal bones. It also gives a more distinct radiograph of the triquetrum and hamate (unciform) (compare Figs. 4-81 and 4-82).

EVALUATION CRITERIA

The following should be clearly demonstrated:
- Carpals on medial side of wrist
- Triquetrum, hamate, and pisiform free of superimposition and in profile
- Distal radius and ulna, carpals and proximal half of metacarpals
- Radiographic quality soft tissue and bony trabeculation

---

[1]McBride E: Wrist joint injuries, a plea for greater accuracy in treatment, *J Okla Med Assoc* 19:67, 1926.

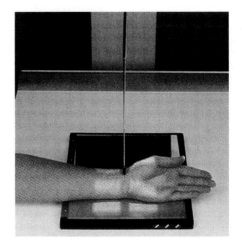

Fig. 4-80 AP oblique wrist: medial rotation.

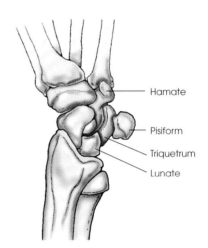

Hamate

Pisiform

Triquetrum

Lunate

Fig. 4-81 AP oblique wrist.

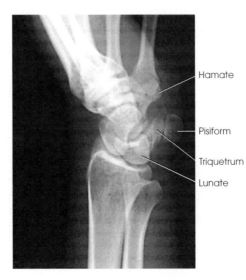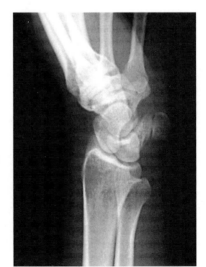

Hamate

Pisiform

Triquetrum

Lunate

Fig. 4-82 AP oblique wrist.

Upper limb

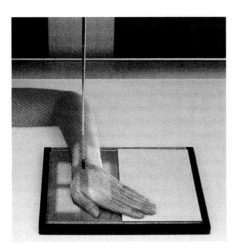

Fig. 4-83 PA wrist in ulnar deviation.

♠ PA PROJECTION
Ulnar deviation (flexion)

This position has historically been called *ulnar flexion* in radiography textbooks.[1] However, the orthopedic community consistently uses the term *ulnar deviation*. The term *ulnar deviation* is used in this text to prevent confusion in the clinical setting and to be consistent.

Image receptor: 8 × 10 inch (18 × 24 cm) for two images

Position of patient

- Seat the patient at the end of the radiographic table with the arm and forearm resting on the table.

Position of part

- Position the wrist on the cassette for a PA projection.
- With one hand cupped over the joint to hold it in position, move the elbow away from the patient's body and then turn the hand outward until the wrist is in extreme ulnar deviation (Fig. 4-83).
- *Shield gonads.*

---

[1]Frank, ED et al: Two terms, one meaning, *Radiol Technol* 69:517, 1998.

Central ray

- Perpendicular to the scaphoid.
- Clear delineation sometimes requires a central ray angulation of 10 to 15 degrees proximally or distally.

Structures shown

This position corrects foreshortening of the scaphoid, which occurs with a perpendicular central ray. It also opens the spaces between the adjacent carpals (Fig. 4-84).

EVALUATION CRITERIA

The following should be clearly demonstrated:

- Scaphoid with adjacent articulations open
- No rotation of wrist
- Extreme ulnar deviation, as revealed by the angle formed between longitudinal axes of the forearm compared with the longitudinal axes of the metacarpals
- Soft tissue and bony trabeculation

A **B**

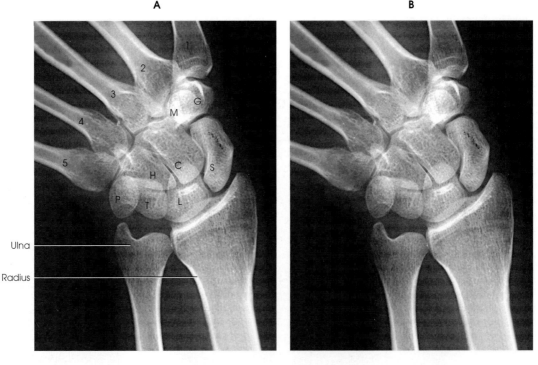

Fig. 4-84 A, PA wrist in ulnar deviation. (*S,* scaphoid; *L,* lunate; *T,* triquetrum; *P,* pisiform; *G,* trapezium; *M,* trapezoid; *C,* capitate; and *H,* hamate.) **B,** Wrist in ulnar flexion.

PA PROJECTION
Radial deviation (flexion)

This position has historically been called *radial flexion* in radiography textbooks.[1] However, the orthopedic community consistently uses the term *radial deviation*. The term *radial deviation* is used in this text to prevent confusion in the clinical setting and to be consistent.

Image receptor: 8 × 10 inch (18 × 24 cm) for two images

Position of patient
• Seat the patient at the end of the radiographic table.

Position of part
• Position the wrist on the cassette for a PA projection.
• Cup one hand over the wrist joint to hold it in position. Then move the elbow toward the patient's body and turn the hand medially until the wrist is in extreme radial deviation (Fig. 4-85).
• *Shield gonads.*

---

[1]Frank ED et al. Two terms, one meaning, *Radiol Technol* 69:517, 1998.

Central ray
• Perpendicular to the midcarpal area

Structures shown
Radial deviation opens the interspaces between the carpals on the medial side of the wrist (Fig. 4-86).

EVALUATION CRITERIA

The following should be clearly demonstrated:
■ Carpals and their articulations on the medial side of the wrist
■ No rotation of wrist
■ Extreme radial deviation, as revealed by the angle formed between longitudinal axes of forearm compared to the longitudinal axes of the metacarpals
■ Soft tissue and bony trabeculation

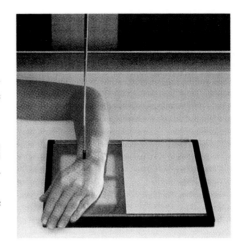

Fig. 4-85 PA wrist in radial deviation.

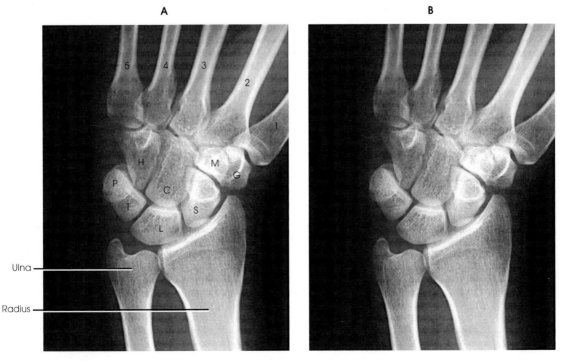

Fig. 4-86 A, PA wrist in radial deviation. (*S,* scaphoid; *L,* lunate; *T,* triquetrum; *P,* pisiform; *G,* trapezium; *M,* trapezoid; *C,* capitate; and *H,* hamate.) **B,** Wrist in radial flexion.

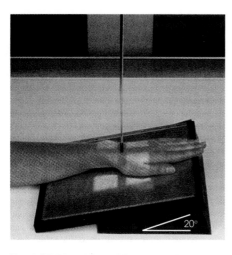

Fig. 4-87 PA axial wrist for scaphoid: Stecher method.

Scaphoid

⚛ PA AXIAL PROJECTION
STECHER METHOD[1]

Image receptor: 8 × 10 inch (18 × 24 cm)

Position of patient
- Seat the patient at the end of the radiographic table with the arm and axilla in contact with the table.
- Rest the forearm on the table.

Position of part
- Place one end of the cassette on a support and adjust the cassette so that the finger end of the cassette is elevated 20 degrees (Fig. 4-87).
- Adjust the wrist on the cassette for a PA projection, and center the wrist to the cassette.
- Bridgman[2] suggested positioning the wrist in ulnar deviation for this radiograph.
- *Shield gonads.*

---

[1]Stecher WR: Roentgenography of the carpal navicular bone, *AJR* 37:704, 1937.
[2]Bridgman CF: Radiography of the carpal navicular bone, *Med Radiogr Photogr* 25:104, 1949.

Central ray
- Perpendicular to the table and directed to enter the scaphoid

Structures shown
The 20-degree angulation of the wrist places the scaphoid at right angles to the central ray so that it is projected without self-superimposition (Figs. 4-88 and 4-89).

EVALUATION CRITERIA
The following should be clearly demonstrated:
- Scaphoid
- No rotation of carpals, metacarpals, radius, or ulna
- Distal radius and ulna, carpals, and proximal half of the metacarpals
- Soft tissue and bony trabeculation

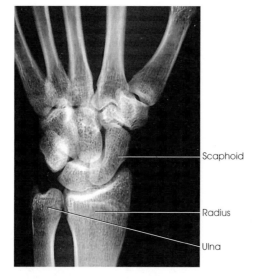

Scaphoid

Radius

Ulna

Fig. 4-88 PA axial wrist for scaphoid: Stecher method.

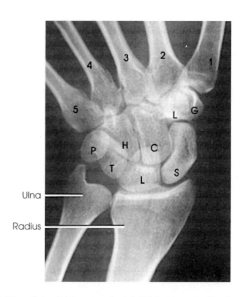

Ulna

Radius

Fig. 4-89 PA axial wrist for scaphoid: Bridgman method, ulnar flexion. (*S*, scaphoid; *L*, lunate; *T*, triquetrum; *P* pisiform; *G*, trapezium; *M*, trapezoid; *C*, capitate; and *H*, hamate.)

VARIATIONS

Stecher recommended the previous method as preferable; however, a similar position can be obtained by placing the cassette and wrist horizontally and directing the central ray 20 degrees toward the elbow (Fig. 4-90).

To demonstrate a fracture line that angles superoinferiorly, these positions may be reversed. In other words, the wrist may be angled inferiorly, or from the horizontal position the central ray may be angled toward the digits.

A third method recommended by Stecher is to have the patient clench the fist. This elevates the distal end of the scaphoid so that it lies parallel with the cassette; it also widens the fracture line. The wrist is positioned as for the PA projection, and no central ray angulation is used.

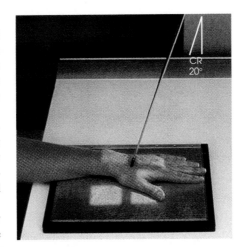

Fig. 4-90 PA axial wrist for scaphoid: Stecher method, angulation of central ray.

Scaphoid Series
PA AND PA AXIAL PROJECTIONS
RAFERT-LONG METHOD[1]
Ulnar deviation (flexion)
Scaphoid fractures account for 60% of all carpal bone injuries. In 1991, Rafert and Long[1] described this method of diagnosing scaphoid fractures using a four-image, multiple-angle central ray series. The series is performed after routine wrist radiographs do not identify a fracture.

Image receptor: 8 × 10 inch (18 × 24 cm) crosswise for two images

[1]Rafert JA, Long BW: Technique for diagnosis of scaphoid fractures, *Radiol Technol* 63:16, 1991.

Position of patient
- Seat the patient at the end of the radiographic table with the arm and forearm resting on the table.

Position of part
- Position the wrist on the cassette for a PA projection.
- Without moving the forearm, turn the hand outward until the wrist is in extreme ulnar deviation (Fig. 4-91).
- *Shield gonads.*

Central ray
- Perpendicular and with multiple cephalad angles. With the hand and wrist in the same position for each projection, four separate exposures are made at 0, 10, 20, and 30 degrees cephalad.
- The central ray should directly enter the scaphoid bone.
- Collimation should be close to improve image quality.

Structures shown
The scaphoid is demonstrated with minimal superimposition (Fig. 4-92).

EVALUATION CRITERIA
The following should be clearly demonstrated:
- No rotation of the wrist
- Scaphoid with adjacent articular areas open
- Extreme ulnar deviation

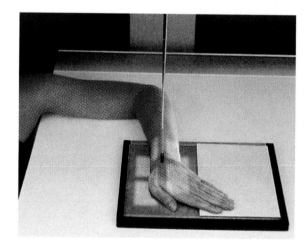

Fig. 4-91 PA wrist in ulnar deviation.

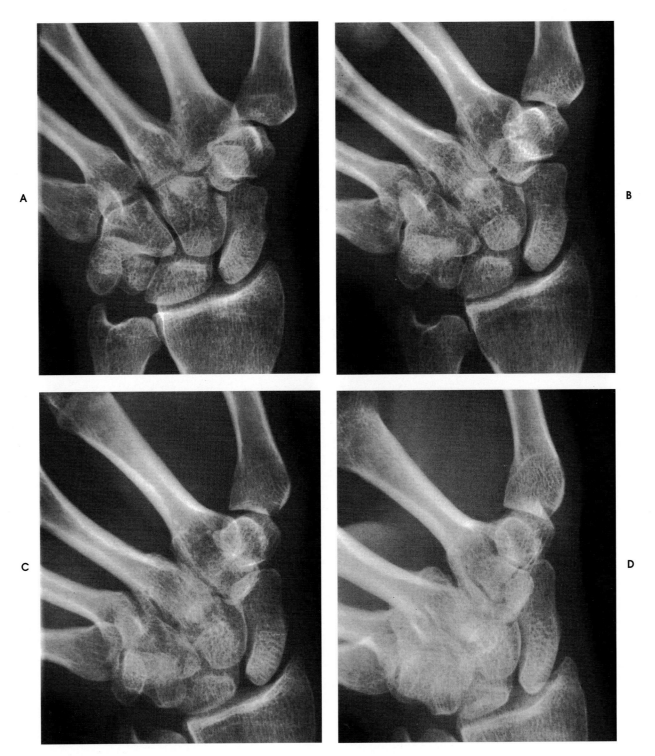

Fig. 4-92 PA and PA axial wrist in ulnar deviation for Rafert-Long method scaphoid series. Radiographs are all from the same patient. **A,** PA wrist with 0-degree central ray angle. **B,** PA axial wrist with 10-degree cephalad angle. **C,** PA axial wrist with 20-degree cephalad angle. **D,** PA axial wrist with 30-degree cephalad angle (From Rafert JA, Long BW: Technique for diagnosis of scaphoid fractures, *Radiol Technol,* 63:16, 1991.)

Trapezium
PA AXIAL OBLIQUE PROJECTION
CLEMENTS-NAKAYAMA METHOD[1]

Fractures of the trapezium are rare; however, if undiagnosed, these fractures can lead to functional difficulties. In certain cases the articular surfaces of the trapezium should be evaluated to treat the osteoarthritic patient.

Image receptor: 8 × 10 inch (18 × 24 cm)

Position of patient

- With the patient seated at the end of the radiographic table, place the hand on the cassette in the lateral position.

[1]Clements R, Nakayama H: Radiography of the polyarthritic hands and wrists, *Radiol Technol* 53:203, 1981.

Position of part

- Place the wrist in the lateral position, resting on the ulnar surface over the center of the cassette.
- Place a 45-degree sponge wedge against the anterior surface, and rotate the hand to come in contact with the sponge.
- If the patient is able to achieve ulnar deviation, adjust the cassette so that the long axis of the cassette and the forearm align with the central ray (Fig. 4-93).
- If the patient is unable to comfortably achieve ulnar deviation, align the straight wrist to the cassette and rotate the elbow end of the cassette and arm 20 degrees away from the central ray (Fig. 4-94).
- *Shield gonads.*

Central ray

- Angled 45 degrees distally to enter the anatomic snuffbox of the wrist and pass through the trapezium

Structures shown

The image clearly demonstrates the trapezium and its articulations with the adjacent carpal bones (Fig. 4-95). The articulation of the trapezium and scaphoid is not demonstrated on this image.

EVALUATION CRITERIA

The following should be clearly demonstrated:

- ■ Trapezium projected free of the other carpal bones with the exception of the articulation with the scaphoid

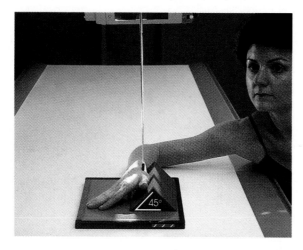

Fig. 4-93 PA axial oblique wrist for trapezium: Clements-Nakayama method; alignment with ulnar deviation.

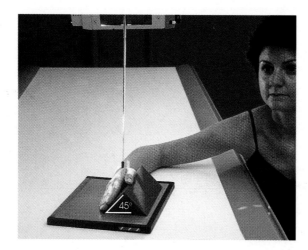

Fig. 4-94 PA axial oblique wrist for trapezium: Clements-Nakayama method; alignment without ulnar deviation.

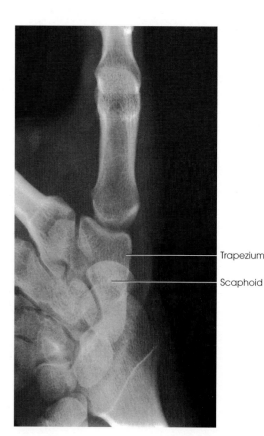

Trapezium

Scaphoid

Fig. 4-95 PA axial oblique wrist for trapezium: Clements-Nakayama method.

TANGENTIAL PROJECTION

Image receptor: 8 × 10 inch (18 × 24 cm) lengthwise

Position of patient
- Seat or stand the patient at the side of the radiographic table to permit the required manipulation of the arm or x-ray tube.

Position of part
- The originators[1] of this projection recommended that the hand lie palm upward on the cassette with the hand at right angle to the forearm (Fig. 4-96).

---

[1]Lentino W et al: The carpal bridge view, *J Bone Joint Surg* 39A:88, 1957.

- When the wrist is too painful to be adjusted in the position just described, a similar image can be obtained by elevating the forearm on sandbags or other suitable support. Then with the wrist flexed in right-angle position, place the cassette in the vertical position (Fig. 4-97).
- *Shield gonads.*

Central ray
- Directed to a point about 1½ inches (3.8 cm) proximal to the wrist joint at a caudal angle of 45 degrees

Structures shown
The carpal bridge is demonstrated on the image in Figs. 4-98 and 4-99. The originators recommended this procedure for demonstration of fractures of the scaphoid, lunate dislocations, calcifications and foreign bodies in the dorsum of the wrist, and chip fractures of the dorsal aspect of the carpal bones.

EVALUATION CRITERIA

The following should be clearly demonstrated:
- Dorsal aspect of the wrist
- Carpals
- Dorsal surface of the carpals free of superimposition by the metacarpal bases

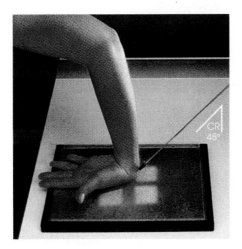

Fig. 4-96 Tangential carpal bridge, original method.

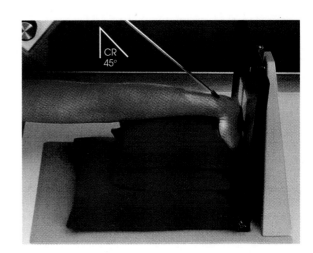

Fig. 4-97 Tangential carpal bridge, modified method.

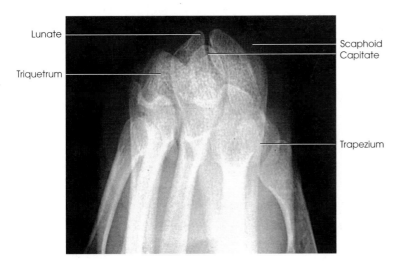

Lunate
Triquetrum
Scaphoid
Capitate
Trapezium

Fig. 4-98 Tangential carpal bridge, original method.

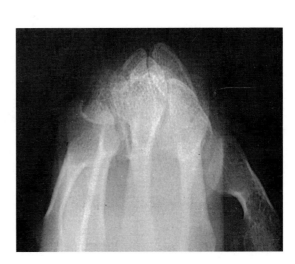

Fig. 4-99 Tangential carpal bridge, modified method.

Carpal Canal

⚡ TANGENTIAL PROJECTIONS
GAYNOR-HART METHOD[1]

The carpal canal contains the tendons of the flexors of the fingers and the median nerve. Compression of the median nerve results in pain. Radiography is performed to identify abnormality of the bones or soft tissue of the canal.

Fractures of the hook of hamate, pisiform, and trapezium are increasingly seen in athletes. The tangential projection is helpful in identifying fractures of these carpal bones. This projection was added as an essential projection based on the 1997 survey performed by Bontrager.[2]

Image receptor: 8 × 10 inch (18 × 24 cm)

Inferosuperior
Position of patient
- Seat the patient at the end of the radiographic table so that the forearm can be adjusted to lie parallel with the long axis of the table.

---

[1]Hart VL, Gaynor V: Roentgenographic study of the carpal canal, *J Bone Joint Surg* 23:382, 1941.
[2]Bontrager KL: *Textbook of radiographic positioning and related anatomy,* 4 ed, 1997, Mosby.

Position of part
- Hyperextend the wrist, and center the cassette to the joint at the level of the radial styloid process.
- For support, place a radiolucent pad approximately ¾ inch (1.9 cm) thick under the lower forearm.
- Adjust the position of the hand to make its long axis as vertical as possible.
- To prevent superimposition of the shadows of the hamate and pisiform bones, rotate the hand slightly toward the radial side.
- Have the patient grasp the digits with the opposite hand, or use a suitable device to hold the wrist in the extended position (Fig. 4-100).
- *Shield gonads.*

Central ray
- Directed to the palm of the hand at a point approximately 1 inch (2.5 cm) distal to the base of the third metacarpal and at an angle of 25 to 30 degrees to the long axis of the hand

Structures shown
This image of the carpal canal (carpal tunnel) shows the palmar aspect of the trapezium, the tubercle of the trapezium, and the scaphoid, capitate, hook of hamate, triquetrum, and entire pisiform (Fig. 4-101).

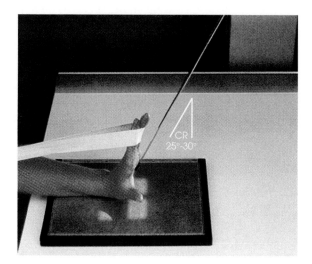

Fig. 4-100 Tangential (inferosuperior) carpal canal: Gaynor-Hart method.

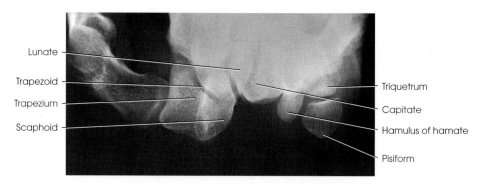

Fig. 4-101 Tangential (inferosuperior) carpal canal: Gaynor-Hart method.

Superoinferior
Position of patient

- When the patient cannot assume or maintain the previously described wrist position, a similar image may be obtained.
- Have the patient dorsiflex the wrist as much as is tolerable and lean forward to place the carpal canal tangent to the cassette (Fig. 4-102). The canal is easily palpable on the palmar aspect of the wrist as the concavity between the trapezium laterally and hook of hamate and pisiform medially.

Position of part

- When dorsiflexion of the wrist is limited, Marshall[1] suggested placing a 45-degree angle sponge under the palmar surface of the hand. This slightly elevates the wrist to place the carpal canal tangent to the central ray. A slight degree of magnification exists because of the increased object-to-image receptor distance (OID) (Fig. 4-103).

[1]Marshall J: Imaging the carpal tunnel, *Radiogr Today* 56:11, 1990.

Central ray

- Tangential to the carpal canal at the level of the midpoint of the wrist
- Angled toward the hand approximately 20 to 35 degrees from the long axis of the forearm

EVALUATION CRITERIA

With either approach, the following should be clearly demonstrated:

- Carpals in an arch arrangement
- Pisiform in profile and free of superimposition
- Hamulus of hamate
- All carpals

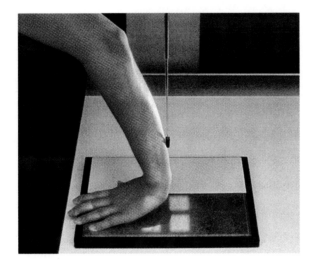

Fig. 4-102 Tangential (inferosuperior) carpal canal.

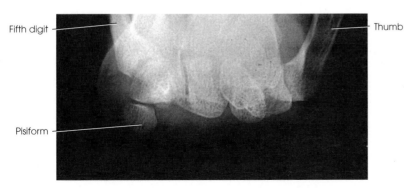

Fifth digit

Thumb

Pisiform

Fig. 4-103 Tangential (inferosuperior) carpal canal.

Forearm

⚘ AP PROJECTION

The cassette should be long enough to include the entire forearm from the olecranon process of the ulna to the styloid process of the radius. Both images of the forearm may be taken on one cassette by alternately covering one half of the cassette with a lead mask. Space should be allowed for the patient identification marker so that no part of the radiographic image is cut off.

Image receptor: Lengthwise—30 × 35 cm (11 × 14 inch) divided; 18 × 43 cm (7 × 17 inch) single; 35 × 43 cm (14 × 17 inch) divided

Position of patient

- Seat the patient close to the radiographic table and low enough to place the entire limb in the same plane.

Position of part

- Supinate the hand, extend the elbow, and center the unmasked half of the cassette to the forearm. Ensure that the joint of interest is included.
- Adjust the cassette so that the long axis is parallel with the forearm.
- Have the patient lean laterally until the forearm is in a true supinated position (Fig. 4-104).

- Because the proximal forearm is commonly rotated in this position, palpate and adjust the humeral epicondyles to be equidistant from the cassette.
- Ensure that the hand is supinated (Fig. 4-105). Pronation of the hand crosses the radius over the ulna at its proximal third and rotates the humerus medially, resulting in an oblique projection of the forearm (Fig. 4-106).
- *Shield gonads.*

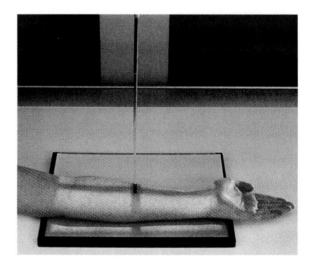

Fig. 4-104 AP forearm.

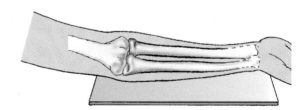

Fig. 4-105 AP forearm with hand supinated.

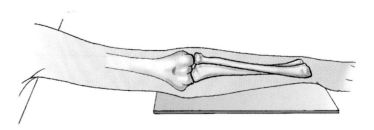

Fig. 4-106 AP forearm with hand pronated—incorrect.

Central ray

- Perpendicular to the midpoint of the forearm

Structures shown

An AP projection of the forearm demonstrates the elbow joint, the radius and ulna, and the proximal row of slightly distorted carpal bones (Fig. 4-107).

EVALUATION CRITERIA

The following should be clearly demonstrated:

- Wrist and distal humerus
- Slight superimposition of the radial head, neck, tuberosity over the proximal ulna
- No elongation or foreshortening of the humeral epicondyles
- Partially open elbow joint if the shoulder was placed in the same plane as the forearm
- Similar radiographic densities of the proximal and distal forearm

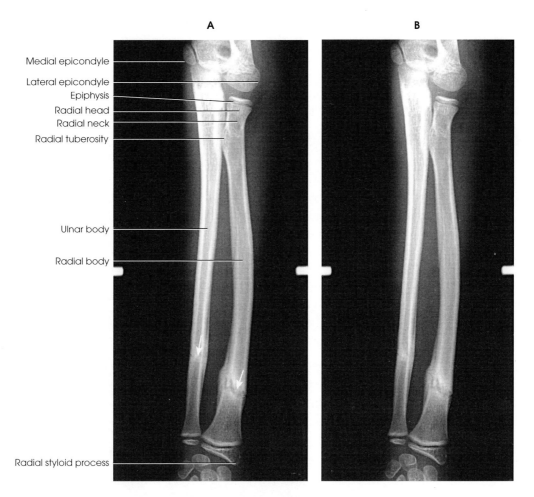

Medial epicondyle
Lateral epicondyle
Epiphysis
Radial head
Radial neck
Radial tuberosity

Ulnar body

Radial body

Radial styloid process

Fig. 4-107 A, AP forearm with fractured radius and ulna *(arrows)*. **B,** AP forearm. The elbow could not be exactly perpendicular because of the patient's condition.

Forearm

LATERAL PROJECTION
Lateromedial

Image receptor: Lengthwise—30 × 35 cm (11 × 14 inch) divided; 18 × 43 cm (7 × 17 inch) single; 35 × 43 cm (14 × 17 inch) divided

Position of patient
- Seat the patient close to the radiographic table and low enough that the humerus, shoulder joint, and elbow lie in the same plane.

Position of part
- Flex the elbow 90 degrees, and center the forearm over the unmasked half of the cassette and parallel with the long axis of the forearm.
- Make sure that the entire joint of interest is included.
- Adjust the limb in a true lateral position. The thumb side of the hand must be up (Fig. 4-108).
- *Shield gonads.*

Central ray
- Perpendicular to the midpoint of the forearm

Structures shown
The lateral projection demonstrates the bones of the forearm, the elbow joint, and the proximal row of carpal bones (Fig. 4-109).

EVALUATION CRITERIA
The following should be clearly demonstrated:
- Wrist and distal humerus
- Superimposition of the radius and ulna at their distal end
- Superimposition by the radial head over the coronoid process
- Radial tuberosity facing anteriorly
- Superimposed humeral epicondyles
- Elbow flexed 90 degrees
- Soft tissue and bony trabeculation along the entire length of the radial and ulnar shafts

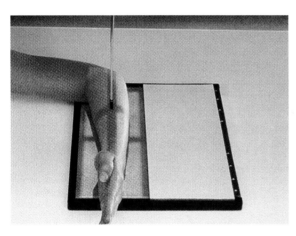

Fig. 4-108 Lateral forearm.

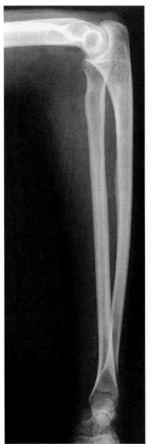

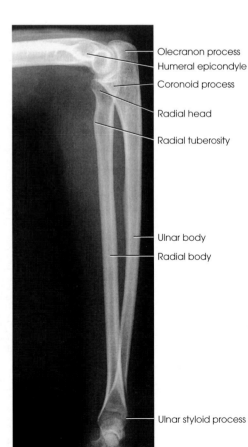

Olecranon process
Humeral epicondyle
Coronoid process

Radial head

Radial tuberosity

Ulnar body
Radial body

Ulnar styloid process

Fig. 4-109 Lateral forearm.

⚕ AP PROJECTION

Image receptor: 8 × 10 inch (18 × 24 cm) single or 24 × 30 cm (10 × 12 inch) divided

Position of patient

- Seat the patient near the radiographic table and low enough to place the shoulder joint, humerus, and elbow joint in the same plane.

Position of part

- Extend the elbow, supinate the hand, and center the cassette to the elbow joint.
- Adjust the cassette to make it parallel with the long axis of the part (Fig. 4-110).
- Have the patient lean laterally until the humeral epicondyles and anterior surface of the elbow are parallel with the plane of the cassette.
- Supinate the hand to prevent rotation of the bones of the forearm.
- *Shield gonads.*

Central ray

- Perpendicular to the elbow joint

Structures shown

An AP projection of the elbow joint, distal arm, and proximal forearm is presented (Fig. 4-111).

EVALUATION CRITERIA

The following should be clearly demonstrated:

- Radial head, neck, and tuberosity slightly superimposed over the proximal ulna
- Elbow joint open and centered to the central ray
- No rotation of humeral epicondyles
- Soft tissue and bony trabeculation

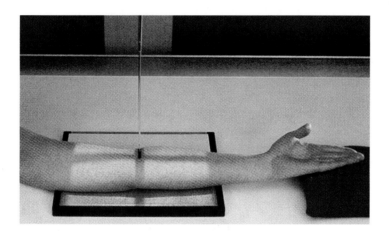

Fig. 4-110 AP elbow.

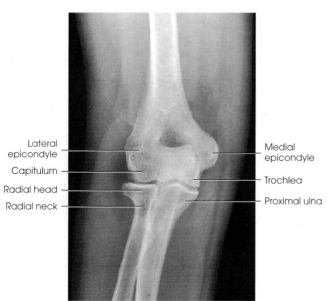
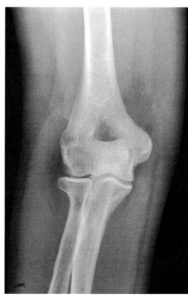

Lateral epicondyle
Capitulum
Radial head
Radial neck

Medial epicondyle
Trochlea
Proximal ulna

Fig. 4-111 AP elbow.

☀ LATERAL PROJECTION
Lateromedial

Griswold[1] gave two reasons for the importance of flexing the elbow 90 degrees: (1) the olecranon process can be seen in profile, and (2) the elbow fat pads are the least compressed. It must be realized that in partial or complete extension the olecranon process elevates the posterior elbow fat pad and simulates joint pathology.

Image receptor: 8 × 10 inch (18 × 24 cm) single or 24 × 30 cm (10 × 12 inch) divided

Position of patient
- Seat the patient at the end of the radiographic table low enough to place the humerus and elbow joint in the same plane.

---

[1]Griswold R: Elbow fat pads: a radiography perspective, *Radiol Technol* 53:303, 1982.

Position of part
- From the supine position, flex the elbow 90 degrees and place the humerus and forearm in contact with the table.
- Center the cassette to the elbow joint. Adjust the elbow joint so that its long axis is parallel with the long axis of the forearm (Figs. 4-112 and 4-113). On patients with muscular forearms, elevate the wrist to place the forearm parallel with the cassette.
- Adjust the cassette diagonally to include more of the arm and forearm (Fig. 4-114).
- To obtain a lateral projection of the elbow, adjust the hand in the lateral position and ensure that the humeral epicondyles are perpendicular to the plane of the cassette.
- *Shield gonads.*

Central ray
- Perpendicular to the elbow joint, regardless of its location on the cassette

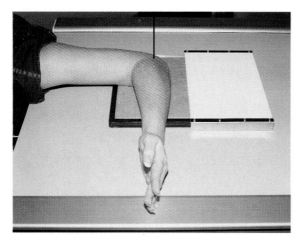

Fig. 4-112 Lateral elbow.

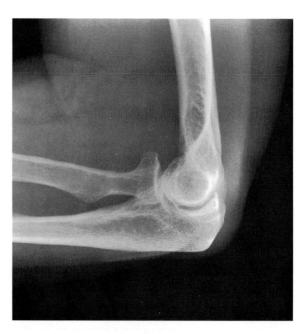

Fig. 4-113 Lateral elbow.

Structures shown

The lateral projection demonstrates the elbow joint, distal arm, and proximal forearm (see Figs. 4-113 and 4-114).

EVALUATION CRITERIA

The following should be clearly demonstrated:

- Open elbow joint centered to the central ray
- Elbow flexed 90 degrees
- Superimposed humeral epicondyles
- Radial tuberosity facing anteriorly
- Radial head partially superimposing the coronoid process
- Olecranon process seen in profile
- Bony trabeculation and any elevated fat pads in the soft tissue at the anterior and posterior distal humerus and the anterior proximal forearm

NOTE: When injury to the soft tissue around the elbow is suspected, the joint should be flexed only 30 or 35 degrees (Fig. 4-115). This partial flexion does not compress or stretch the soft structures as does the full 90-degree lateral flexion.

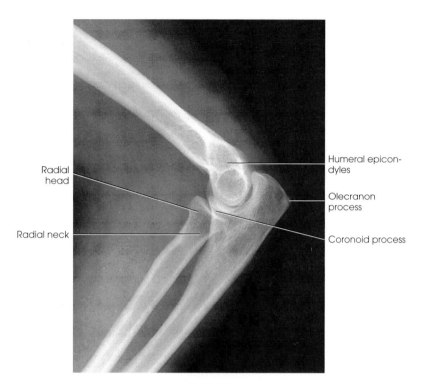

Radial head

Radial neck

Humeral epicondyles

Olecranon process

Coronoid process

Fig. 4-114 Lateral elbow.

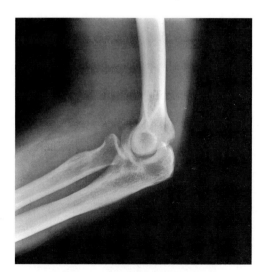

Fig. 4-115 Lateral elbow in partial flexion position for soft tissue image.

▲ AP OBLIQUE PROJECTION
Medial rotation

Image receptor: 8 × 10 inch (18 × 24 cm) single or 24 × 30 cm (10 × 12 inch) divided

Position of patient

- Seat the patient at the end of the radiographic table with the arm extended and in contact with the table.

Position of part

- Extend the limb in position for an AP projection, and center the midpoint of the cassette to the elbow joint (Fig. 4-116).
- Medially (internally) rotate or pronate the hand, and adjust the elbow to place its anterior surface at an angle of 45 degrees. This degree of obliquity usually clears the coronoid process of the radial head.
- *Shield gonads.*

Central ray

- Perpendicular to the elbow joint

Structures shown

The image shows an oblique projection of the elbow with the coronoid process projected free of superimposition (Fig. 4-117).

EVALUATION CRITERIA

The following should be clearly demonstrated:

- Coronoid process in profile
- Elongated medial humeral epicondyle
- Ulna superimposed by the radial head and neck
- Olecranon process within the olecranon fossa
- Soft tissue and bony trabeculation

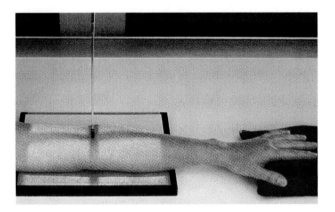

Fig. 4-116 AP oblique elbow: medial rotation.

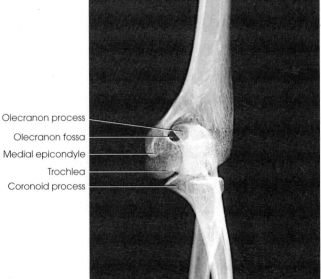
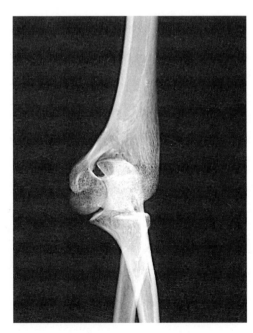

Olecranon process
Olecranon fossa
Medial epicondyle
Trochlea
Coronoid process

Fig. 4-117 AP oblique elbow.

✳ AP OBLIQUE PROJECTION
Lateral rotation

Image receptor: 8 × 10 inch (18 × 24 cm) single or 24 × 30 cm (10 × 12 inch) divided

Position of patient
• Seat the patient at the end of the radiographic table with the arm extended and in contact with the table.

Position of part
• Extend the patient's arm in position for an AP projection and center the midpoint of the cassette to the elbow joint.
• Rotate the hand laterally (externally) to place the posterior surface of the elbow at a 45-degree angle (Fig. 4-118). When proper lateral rotation is achieved, the patient's first and second digits should touch the table.
• *Shield gonads.*

Central ray
• Perpendicular to the elbow joint

Structures shown
The image shows an oblique projection of the elbow with the radial head and neck projected free of superimposition of the ulna (Fig. 4-119).

EVALUATION CRITERIA
The following should be clearly demonstrated:
■ Radial head, neck, and tuberosity projected free of the ulna
■ Open elbow joint
■ Soft tissue and bony trabeculation

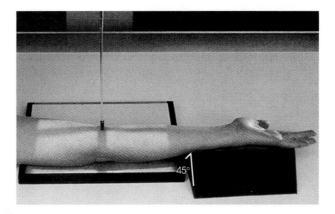

Fig. 4-118 AP oblique elbow: lateral rotation.

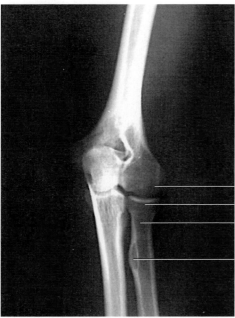
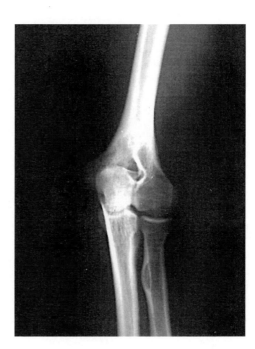

Capitulum
Radial head
Radial neck

Radial tuberosity

Fig. 4-119 AP oblique elbow.

Distal Humerus

☀ AP PROJECTION
Partial flexion

When the patient cannot completely extend the elbow, the lateral position is easily performed; however, two AP projections must be obtained to avoid distortion. A separate AP projection of the distal humerus and proximal forearm is required.

Image receptor: Both exposures can be made on one 8 × 10 inch (18 × 24 cm) cassette or on one cassette placed crosswise by alternately covering one half of the cassette with a lead mask.

Position of patient

- Seat the patient low enough to place the entire humerus in the same plane. Support the elevated forearm.

Position of part

- If possible, supinate the hand. Place the cassette under the elbow, and center it to the condyloid area of the humerus (Fig. 4-120).
- *Shield gonads.*

Central ray

- Perpendicular to the humerus, traversing the elbow joint.
- Depending on the degree of flexion, angle the central ray distally into the joint.

Structures shown

This projection shows the distal humerus when the elbow cannot be fully extended (Figs. 4-121 and 4-122).

EVALUATION CRITERIA

The following should be clearly demonstrated:

- Distal humerus without rotation or distortion
- Proximal radius superimposed over the ulna
- Closed elbow joint
- Greatly foreshortened proximal forearm
- Trabecular detail on the distal humerus

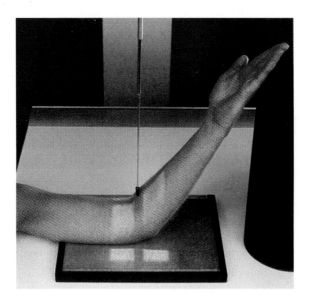

Fig. 4-120 AP elbow, partially flexed.

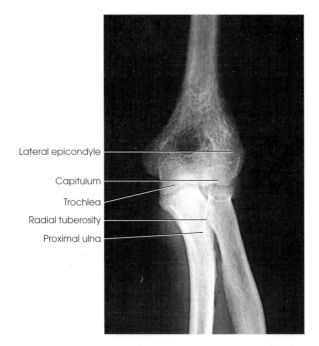

Lateral epicondyle
Capitulum
Trochlea
Radial tuberosity
Proximal ulna

Fig. 4-121 AP elbow, partially flexed, demonstrating distal humerus.

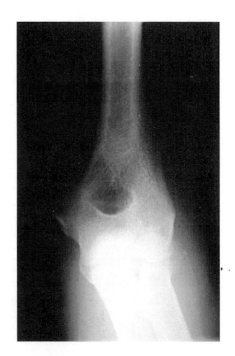

Fig. 4-122 AP elbow, partially flexed, demonstrating distal humerus.

Proximal Forearm

▲ AP PROJECTION
Partial flexion

Image receptor: 8 × 10 inch (18 × 24 cm)

Position of patient
Seat the patient at the end of the radiographic table with the hand supinated.

Position of part
- Seat the patient high enough to permit the dorsal surface of the forearm to rest on the table (Fig. 4-123). If this position is not possible, elevate the limb on a support, adjust the limb in the lateral position, place the cassette in the vertical position behind the upper end of the forearm, and direct the central ray horizontally.
- *Shield gonads.*

Central ray
- Perpendicular to the elbow joint and long axis of the forearm.
- Adjust the cassette so that the central ray passes to its midpoint.

Structures shown
This projection demonstrates the proximal forearm when the elbow cannot be fully extended (Figs. 4-124 and 4-125).

EVALUATION CRITERIA
The following should be clearly demonstrated:
- Proximal radius and ulna without rotation or distortion
- Radial head, neck, and tuberosity slightly superimposed over the proximal ulna
- Partially open elbow joint
- Foreshortened distal humerus
- Trabecular detail on the proximal forearm

NOTE: Holly[1] described a method of obtaining the AP projection of the radial head. The patient is positioned as described for the distal humerus. The elbow is extended as much as possible, and the forearm is supported. The forearm should be supinated enough to place the horizontal plane of the wrist at an angle of 30 degrees from horizontal.

[1]Holly EW: Radiography of the radial head, *Med Radiogr Photogr* 32:13, 1956.

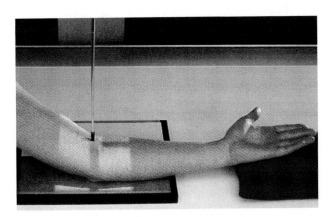

Fig. 4-123 AP elbow, partially flexed.

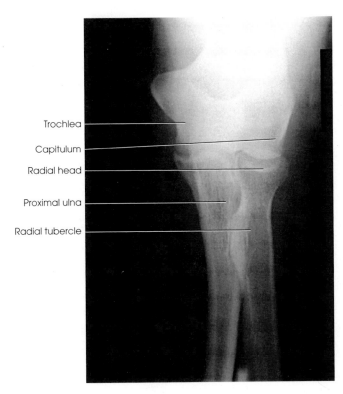

Trochlea
Capitulum
Radial head
Proximal ulna
Radial tubercle

Fig. 4-124 AP elbow, partially flexed, demonstrating proximal forearm. This is a view of the dislocated elbow of the patient shown in Fig. 4-125.

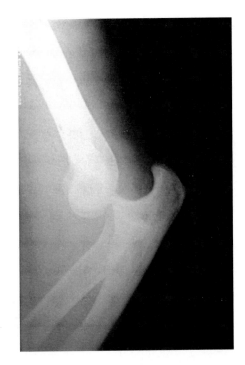

Fig. 4-125 Lateral elbow showing dislocation on same patient as shown in Figs. 4-122 and 4-124.

Distal Humerus
AP PROJECTION
Acute flexion

When fractures around the elbow are being treated using the Jones orthopedic technique (complete flexion), the lateral position offers little difficulty, but the frontal projection must be made through the superimposed bones of the AP arm and PA forearm.

Image receptor: 8 × 10 inch (18 × 24 cm); may be divided for two images on one cassette

Position of patient
• Seat the patient at the end of the radiographic table with the elbow fully flexed (unless contraindicated).

Position of part
• Center the cassette proximal to the epicondylar area of the humerus. The long axis of the arm and forearm should be parallel with the long axis of the cassette (Figs. 4-126 and 4-127).
• Adjust the arm or the radiographic tube and cassette to prevent rotation.
• *Shield gonads.*

Central ray
• Perpendicular to the humerus approximately 2 inches (5 cm) superior to the olecranon process

Structures shown
This position superimposes the bones of the forearm and arm. The olecranon process should be clearly demonstrated (Fig. 4-128).

EVALUATION CRITERIA

The following should be clearly demonstrated:
■ Forearm and humerus superimposed
■ No rotation
■ Olecranon process and distal humerus
■ Soft tissue outside the olecranon process

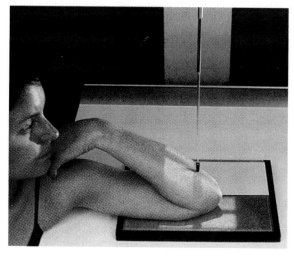

Fig. 4-126 AP distal humerus: acute flexion of elbow.

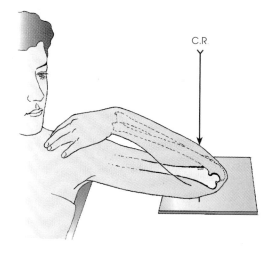

Fig. 4-127 AP distal humerus: acute flexion of elbow.

C.R.

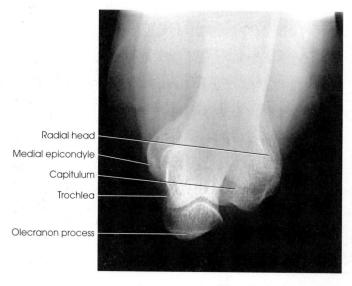

Radial head
Medial epicondyle
Capitulum
Trochlea
Olecranon process

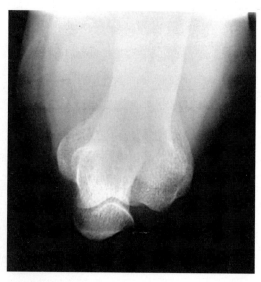

Fig. 4-128 AP distal humerus: acute flexion of elbow.

Proximal Forearm
PA PROJECTION
Acute flexion

Image receptor: 8 ×10 inch (18 × 24 cm)

Position of patient
- Seat the patient at the end of the radiographic table with the elbow fully flexed.

Position of part
- Center the flexed elbow joint to the center of the cassette. The long axis of the superimposed forearm and arm should be parallel with the long axis of the cassette (Figs. 4-129 and 4-130).
- Move the cassette toward the shoulder so that the central ray will pass to the midpoint.
- *Shield gonads.*

Central ray
- Perpendicular to the flexed forearm, entering approximately 2 inches (5 cm) distal to the olecranon process

Structures shown
The superimposed bones of the arm and forearm are outlined (Fig. 4-131). The elbow joint should be more open than for projections of the distal humerus.

EVALUATION CRITERIA

The following should be clearly demonstrated:
- Forearm and humerus superimposed
- No rotation
- Proximal radius and ulna

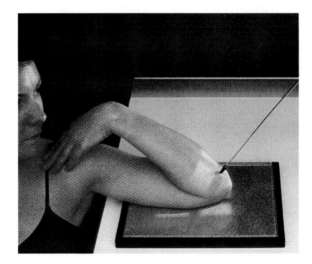

Fig. 4-129 PA proximal forearm: full flexion of elbow.

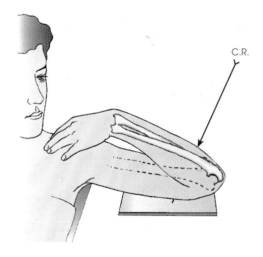

Fig. 4-130 PA proximal forearm: full flexion of elbow.

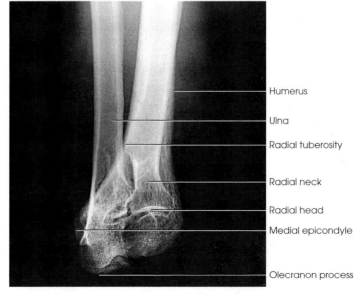

Humerus

Ulna

Radial tuberosity

Radial neck

Radial head

Medial epicondyle

Olecranon process

Fig. 4-131 PA proximal forearm: full flexion of elbow.

Radial Head
LATERAL PROJECTION
Lateromedial
Four-position series

Place the cassette in position, and cover the unused section with a sheet of lead. For demonstration of the entire circumference of the radial head free of superimposition, four projections with varying positions of the hand are performed.

Image receptor: 8 × 10 inch (18 × 24 cm) single or 24 × 30 cm (10 × 12 inch) divided

Position of patient
• Seat the patient low enough to place the entire arm in the same horizontal plane.

Position of part
• Flex the elbow 90 degrees, center the joint to the unmasked cassette, and place the joint in the lateral position.
• Make the first exposure with the hand supinated as much as is possible (Fig. 4-132).
• Shift the cassette and make the second exposure with the hand in the lateral position, that is, with the thumb surface up (Fig. 4-133).

• Shift the cassette, and make the third exposure with the hand pronated (Fig. 4-134).
• Shift the cassette, and make the fourth exposure with the hand in extreme internal rotation, that is, resting on the thumb surface (Fig. 4-135).
• *Shield gonads.*

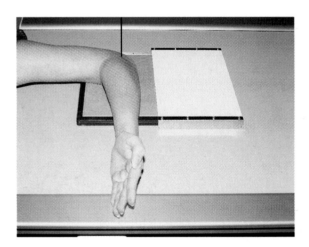

Fig. 4-132 Lateral elbow, radius with hand supinated as much as possible.

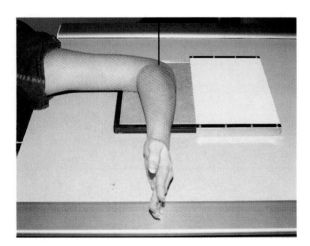

Fig. 4-133 Lateral elbow, radius with hand lateral.

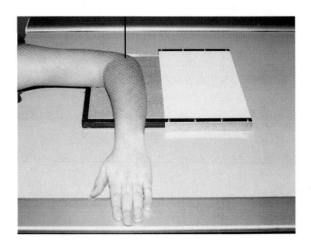

Fig. 4-134 Lateral elbow, radius with hand pronated.

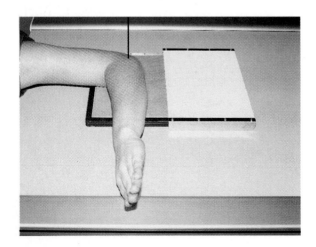

Fig. 4-135 Lateral elbow, radius with hand internally rotated.

Central ray
- Perpendicular to the elbow joint

Structures shown
The radial head is projected in varying degrees of rotation (Figs. 4-136 to 4-139).

EVALUATION CRITERIA
The following should be clearly demonstrated:
- Radial tuberosity facing anteriorly for the first and second images and posteriorly for the third and fourth images (see Figs. 4-136 to 4-139)
- Elbow flexed 90 degrees
- Radial head partially superimposing the coronoid process but seen in all images

NOTE: Greenspan and Norman[1] reported that the radial head can be projected more clearly with reduced superimposition by directing the central ray 45 degrees medially (toward the shoulder) when the structure is positioned as in Figs. 4-132 to 4-135. The resulting radiograph is shown in Fig. 4-140.

---

[1]Greenspan A, Norman A: The radial head, capitellum view: useful technique in elbow trauma, *AJR* 138:1186, 1982.

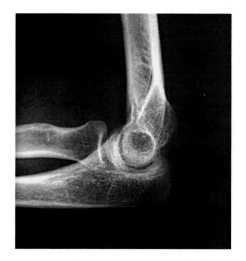

Fig. 4-136 Lateral elbow, radius with hand supinated.

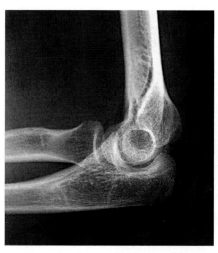

Fig. 4-137 Lateral elbow, radius with hand lateral.

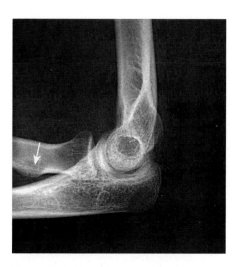

Fig. 4-138 Lateral elbow, radius with hand pronated (radial tuberosity, *arrow*).

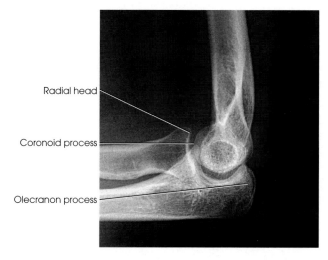

Radial head
Coronoid process
Olecranon process

Fig. 4-139 Lateral elbow, radius with hand internally rotated.

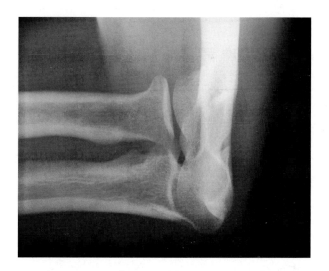

Fig. 4-140 Lateral elbow, radial head with central ray angled 45 degrees medially as described by Greenspan and Norman.

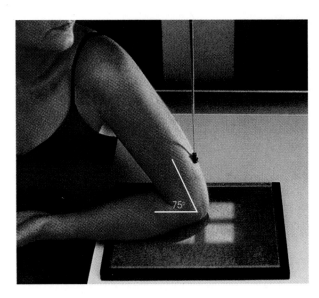

Fig. 4-141 PA axial distal humerus.

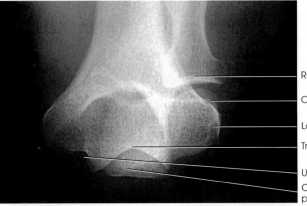

Radial head

Capitulum

Lateral epicondyle

Trochlea

Ulnar sulcus

Olecranon process

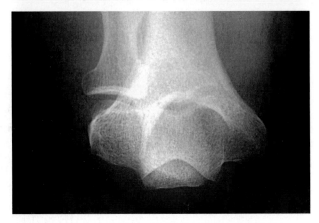

Fig. 4-142 PA axial distal humerus.

PA AXIAL PROJECTION

Image receptor: 8 × 10 inch (18 × 24 cm) for one or two images on one cassette

Position of patient
- Seat the patient high enough to enable the forearm to rest on the radiographic table with the arm in the vertical position. The patient must be seated so that the forearm can be adjusted parallel with the long axis of the table.

Position of part
- Ask the patient to rest the forearm on the table, and then adjust the forearm so that its long axis is parallel with the table.
- Center a point midway between the epicondyles and the center of the cassette.
- Flex the patient's elbow to place the arm in a nearly vertical position so that the humerus forms an angle of approximately 75 degrees from the forearm (approximately 15 degrees between the central ray and the long axis of the humerus).
- Confirm that the patient is not leaning anteriorly or posteriorly.
- Supinate the hand to prevent rotation of the humerus and ulna, and have the patient immobilize it with the opposite hand (Fig. 4-141).
- *Shield gonads.*

Central ray
- Perpendicular to the ulnar sulcus, entering at a point just medial to the olecranon process

Structures shown
This projection demonstrates the epicondyles, trochlea, ulnar sulcus (groove between the medial epicondyle and the trochlea), and olecranon fossa (Fig. 4-142). The projection is used in radiohumeral bursitis (tennis elbow) to detect otherwise obscured calcifications located in the ulnar sulcus.

EVALUATION CRITERIA
The following should be clearly demonstrated:
- Outline of the ulnar sulcus (groove)
- Soft tissue outside the distal humerus
- Forearm and humerus superimposed
- No rotation

Olecranon Process

PA AXIAL PROJECTION

Image receptor: 8 × 10 inch (18 × 24 cm)

Position of patient
- Seat the patient at the end of the radiographic table, high enough that the forearm can rest flat on the cassette.

Position of part
- Adjust the arm at an angle of 45 to 50 degrees from the vertical position and ensure that the patient is not leaning anteriorly or posteriorly.
- Supinate the hand and have the patient immobilize it with the opposite hand.
- Center a point midway between the epicondyles and the center of the cassette.
- *Shield gonads.*

Central ray
- Perpendicular to the olecranon process to demonstrate the dorsum of the olecranon process and at a 20-degree angle toward the wrist to demonstrate the curved extremity and articular margin of the olecranon process (Fig. 4-143)

Structures shown
The projection demonstrates the olecranon process and the articular margin of the olecranon and humerus (Figs. 4-144 to 4-146).

EVALUATION CRITERIA
The following should be clearly demonstrated:
- Olecranon process in profile
- Soft tissue outside the olecranon process
- Forearm and humerus superimposed
- No rotation

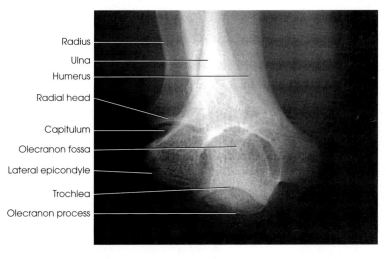

Fig. 4-143 PA axial olecranon process with central ray angled 20 degrees.

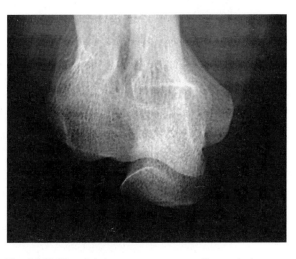

Fig. 4-144 PA axial olecranon process.

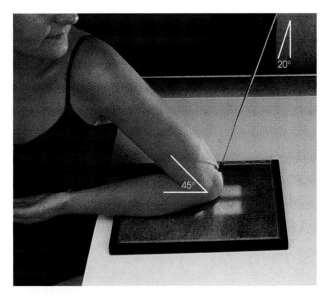

Radius
Ulna
Humerus
Radial head
Capitulum
Olecranon fossa
Lateral epicondyle
Trochlea
Olecranon process

Fig. 4-145 PA axial olecranon process with central ray angulation of 0 degrees.

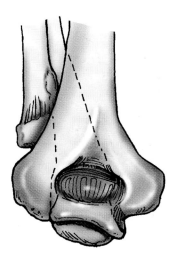

Fig. 4-146 PA axial olecranon process with central ray angulation of 20 degrees.

AP PROJECTION
Upright

Shoulder and arm abnormalities, whether traumatic or pathologic in origin, are extremely painful. For this reason an upright position, either standing or seated, should be used whenever possible. With rotation of the patient's body as required, the arm can be positioned quickly and accurately with minimal discomfort to the patient and, in the presence of fracture, with no danger of fragment displacement. The cassette selected should be long enough to include the humerus.

Image receptor: Lengthwise—30 × 35 cm (11 × 14 inch); 18 × 43 cm (7 × 17 inch); 35 × 43 cm (14 × 17 inch)

Position of patient

• Place the patient in a seated-upright or standing position facing the x-ray tube.
• Fig. 4-147 illustrates the body position used for an AP projection of the freely movable arm. The body position, whether oblique or facing toward or away from the cassette, is unimportant as long as a true frontal radiograph of the arm is obtained.

Position of part

• Adjust the height of the cassette to place its upper margin about 1½ inches (3.8 cm) above the head of the humerus.
• Abduct the arm slightly, and supinate the hand.
• A coronal plane passing through the epicondyles should be parallel with the cassette plane for the AP (or PA) projection (see Fig. 4-147).
• *Shield gonads.*
• *Respiration:* Suspend.

Central ray

• Perpendicular to the midportion of the humerus and the center of the cassette

Structures shown

The AP projection demonstrates the entire length of the humerus. The accuracy of the position is shown by the epicondyles (Fig. 4-148).

EVALUATION CRITERIA

The following should be clearly demonstrated:

■ Elbow and shoulder joints
■ Maximal visibility of epicondyles without rotation
■ Humeral head and greater tubercle in profile
■ Outline of the lesser tubercle, located between the humeral head and the greater tubercle
■ Beam divergence possibly partially closing the elbow joint
■ No great variation in radiographic densities of the proximal and distal humerus

NOTE: Radiographs of the humerus and shoulder may be taken with or without a grid. The size of the patient and the preferences of the radiographer and physician are often considered in reaching a decision. Most medical facilities establish a policy for the initial procedures. Whether the policy is to use a grid or not, the positioning of the body part remains the same.

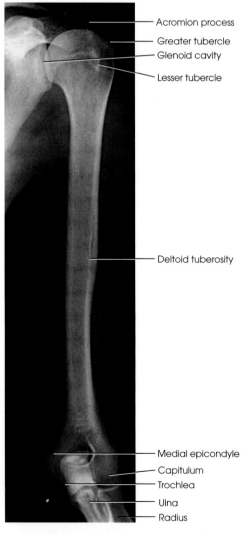

— Acromion process
— Greater tubercle
— Glenoid cavity
— Lesser tubercle

— Deltoid tuberosity

— Medial epicondyle
— Capitulum
— Trochlea
— Ulna
— Radius

Fig. 4-148 Upright AP humerus.

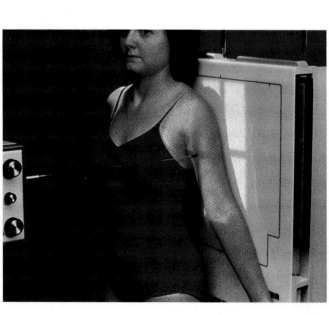

Fig. 4-147 Upright position for AP humerus.

Humerus

⚜ LATERAL PROJECTION
Lateromedial
Upright

Image receptor: 30 × 35 cm (11 × 14 inch); 18 × 43 cm (7 × 17 inch); 35 × 43 cm (14 × 17 inch)

Position of patient

- Place the patient in a seated-upright or standing position facing the x-ray tube. The body position, whether oblique or facing toward or away from the cassette, is not critical as long as a true projection of the lateral arm is obtained.

Position of part

- Place the top margin of the cassette approximately 1½ inches (3.8 cm) above the level of the head of the humerus.
- Unless contraindicated by possible fracture, internally rotate the arm, flex the elbow approximately 90 degrees, and place the patient's hand on the patient's hip. A coronal plane passing through the epicondyles should be perpendicular with the cassette plane (Fig. 4-149).
- *Shield gonads.*
- *Respiration:* Suspend.

Central ray

- Perpendicular to the midportion of the humerus and the center of the cassette

Structures shown

The lateral projection demonstrates the entire length of the humerus. A true lateral image is confirmed by superimposed epicondyles (Fig. 4-150).

EVALUATION CRITERIA

The following should be clearly demonstrated:

- Elbow and shoulder joints
- Superimposed epicondyles
- Lesser tubercle in profile
- Greater tubercle superimposed over the humeral head
- Beam divergence possibly partially closing the elbow joint
- No great variation in radiographic densities of the proximal and distal humerus

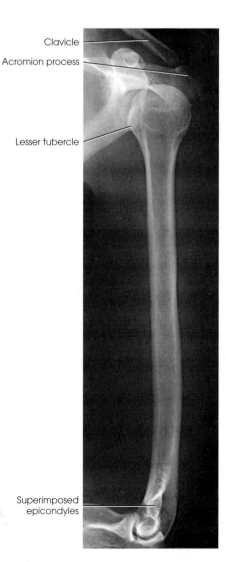

Clavicle

Acromion process

Lesser tubercle

Superimposed epicondyles

Fig. 4-150 Upright lateral humerus.

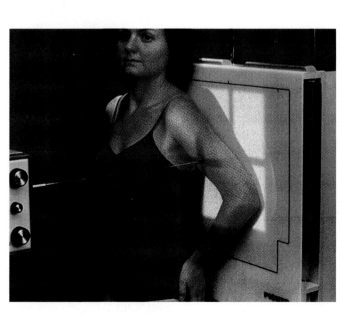

Fig. 4-149 Upright position for lateral humerus. Note the hand placement on the hip.

♣ AP PROJECTION
Recumbent

The cassette size selected should be long enough to include the entire humerus.

Image receptor: Lengthwise—30 × 35 cm (11 × 14 inch); 18 × 43 cm (7 × 17 inch); 35 × 43 cm (14 × 17 inch)

Position of patient

• With the patient in the supine position, adjust the cassette to include the entire length of the humerus.

Position of part

• Place the upper margin of the cassette approximately 1½ inches (3.8 cm) above the humeral head.
• Elevate the opposite shoulder on a sandbag to place the affected arm in contact with the cassette or elevate the arm and cassette on sandbags.
• Unless contraindicated, supinate the hand and adjust the limb to place the epicondyles parallel with the plane of the cassette (Fig. 4-151).
• *Shield gonads.*
• *Respiration:* Suspend.

Central ray

• Perpendicular to the midportion of the humerus and the center of the cassette

Structures shown

An AP projection of the entire humerus is presented (Fig. 4-152).

EVALUATION CRITERIA

The following should be clearly demonstrated:

■ Elbow and shoulder joints
■ Maximum visibility and no rotation of the epicondyles
■ Humeral head and greater tubercle in profile
■ Outline of the lesser tubercle located between the humeral head and the greater tubercle
■ No great variation in radiographic densities of the proximal and distal humerus
■ Possible partial closure of the elbow joint (by beam divergence)

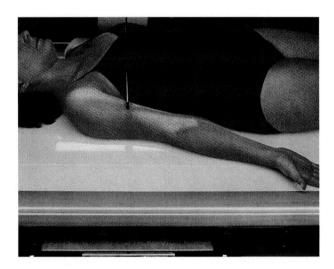

Fig. 4-151 Recumbent position for AP humerus. Note that the hand is supinated.

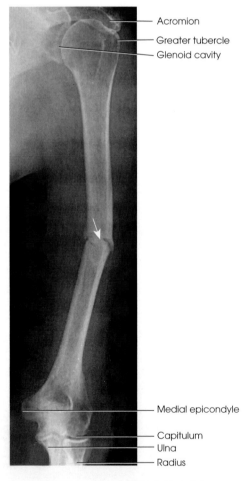

— Acromion
— Greater tubercle
— Glenoid cavity

— Medial epicondyle

— Capitulum
— Ulna
— Radius

Fig. 4-152 Recumbent AP humerus, showing healing fracture midshaft *(arrow).*

✱ LATERAL PROJECTION
Lateromedial
Recumbent

Image receptor: Lengthwise—30 × 35 cm (11 × 14 inch); 18 × 43 cm (7 × 17 inch); 35 × 43 cm (14 × 17 inch)

Position of patient
Place the patient in the supine position with the humerus centered to the cassette, or use a Bucky tray.

Position of part
- Adjust the top of the cassette to be approximately 1½ inches (3.8 cm) above the level of the head of the humerus.
- Unless contraindicated by possible fracture, abduct the arm somewhat and center the cassette under it.
- Rotate the forearm medially to place the epicondyles perpendicular to the plane of the cassette, and rest the *posterior aspect* of the hand against the patient's side. The elbow may be flexed for comfort.
- Adjust the position of the cassette to include the entire length of the humerus (Fig. 4-153).

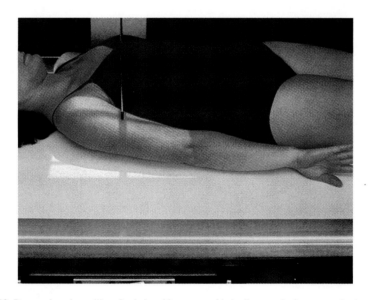

Fig. 4-153 Recumbent position for lateral humerus. Note the posterior aspect of patient's hand against thigh.

✺ LATERAL PROJECTION
Lateromedial
Lateral recumbent

- When a known or suspected fracture exists, position the patient in the lateral recumbent position, place the cassette close to the axilla, and center the humerus to the cassette's midline.
- Unless contraindicated, flex the elbow, turn the thumb surface of the hand up, and rest the humerus on a suitable support (Fig. 4-154).
- Adjust the position of the body to place the lateral surface of the humerus perpendicular to the central ray.
- *Shield gonads.*
- *Respiration:* Suspend.

Central ray
Recumbent
- Perpendicular to the midportion of the humerus and the center of the cassette (se Fig. 4-153)

Lateral recumbent
- Directed to the center of the cassette, which exposes only the distal humerus (see Fig. 4-154)

Structures shown
The lateral projection demonstrates either the entire humerus or the distal humerus depending on the condition of the patient (Fig. 4-155).

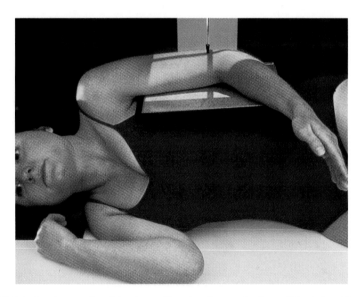

Fig. 4-154 Lateral recumbent body position for demonstration of the lateral humerus.

EVALUATION CRITERIA

The following should be clearly demonstrated:

■ Elbow and shoulder joints (recumbent)
■ Superimposed epicondyles

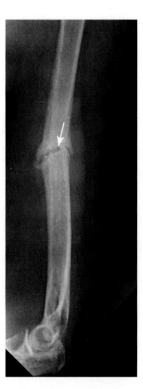

Fig. 4-155 Recumbent lateral humerus,
showing healing fracture *(arrow)*.

Upper limb

TRANSTHORACIC LATERAL PROJECTION
LAWRENCE METHOD[1]
R or L position

The Lawrence method[1] is used when trauma has occurred and the arm cannot be abducted or rotated for the AP or lateral projection. In most instances the arm cannot be moved and the projection is performed with the arm as is.

Image receptor: 24 × 30 cm (10 × 12 inch) lengthwise

---

[1]Lawrence WS: A method of obtaining an accurate lateral roentgenogram of the shoulder joint, *AJR* 5:193, 1918.

Position of patient
- Although the projection can be performed with the patient in the supine or upright position, the upright position is much easier on the trauma patient. The upright position also facilitates accurate adjustment of the shoulder.
- Seat or stand the patient in the lateral position before a vertical grid device.

Position of part
- Have the patient raise the uninjured arm, rest the forearm on the head, and elevate the shoulder as much as possible. Elevation of the uninjured shoulder will drop the injured side, thus separating the shoulders to prevent superimposition.
- Ensure that the midcoronal plane of the body is perpendicular to the cassette.

- Center the cassette to the region of the surgical neck of the affected humerus (Fig. 4-156).
- For nontrauma only, the epicondyles should be perpendicular to the plane of the cassette. On trauma patients the arm is not moved.
- *Shield gonads.*
- *Respiration:* Full inspiration. Having the lungs full of air increases the radiographic contrast and decreases the exposure necessary to penetrate the body. If the patient can be sufficiently immobilized to prevent voluntary motion, a breathing technique can be used. In this case, the patient should practice slow, deep breathing. A minimum exposure time of 3 seconds (4 to 5 seconds is desirable) provides excellent results when using a low milliamperage.

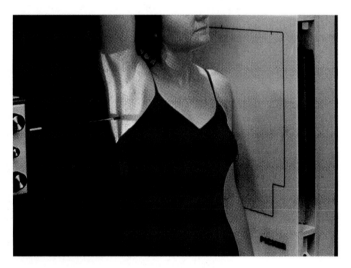

Fig. 4-156 Transthoracic lateral projection for demonstration of the proximal humerus.

Proximal Humerus

Central ray
- Perpendicular to the cassette at the level of the surgical neck.
- If the patient cannot elevate the unaffected shoulder, the central ray may be angled 10 to 15 degrees cephalad to obtain a comparable radiograph.

Structures shown
The resultant image shows a lateral projection of the proximal half or two thirds of the humerus, projected through the thorax. Although recorded detail may be poor, the outline of the humerus is clearly shown (Fig. 4-157).

The following should be clearly demonstrated:
- Proximal portion of the humerus
- Greater tubercle in profile on the anterior surface of the humeral head
- Outline of the proximal humerus clearly demonstrated through the ribs and lung fields
- No overlap of the area of interest by the unaffected humerus and shoulder
- No superimposition of the upper thoracic vertebrae by the humerus

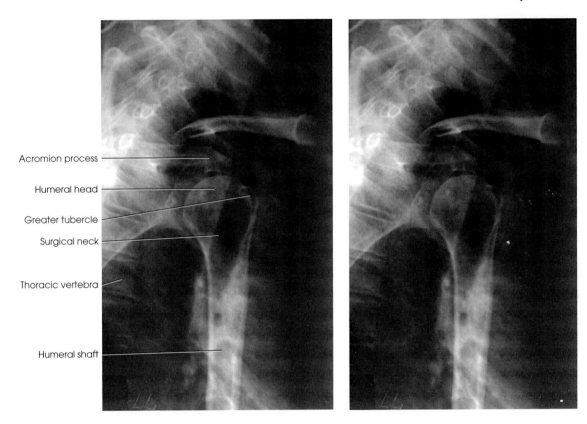

Acromion process
Humeral head
Greater tubercle
Surgical neck
Thoracic vertebra
Humeral shaft

Fig. 4-157 Transthoracic lateral proximal humerus: Lawrence method. The humerus was medially rotated in this image.

5

SHOULDER GIRDLE

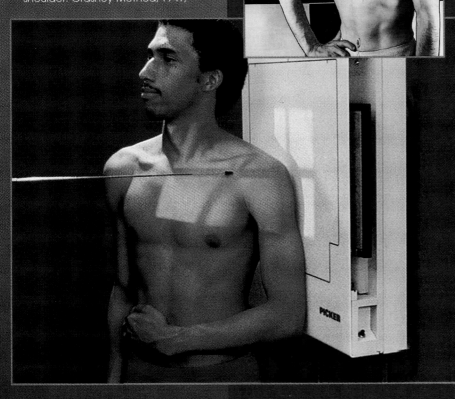

RIGHT: Positioning for AP oblique shoulder: Grashey Method, 1949,

LEFT: Positioning for AP oblique shoulder: Grashey method, 1999

SUMMARY OF PROJECTIONS

PROJECTIONS, POSITIONS & METHODS

Page	Essential	Anatomy	Projection	Position	Method
160	✦	Shoulder	AP	External rotation humerus	
163	✦	Shoulder	AP	Neutral rotation humerus	
164	✦	Shoulder	AP	Internal rotation humerus	
166	✦	Shoulder	Transthoracic lateral	R or L	LAWRENCE
168	✦	Shoulder joint	Inferosuperior axial		LAWRENCE
168		Shoulder joint	Inferosuperior axial		RAFERT
170		Shoulder joint	Inferosuperior axial		WEST POINT
172		Shoulder joint	Inferosuperior axial		CLEMENTS
174		Shoulder joint	Superoinferior axial		
176		Shoulder joint	Axial rolled film		CLEAVES
178		Shoulder joint	AP axial		
179	✦	Shoulder joint: *scapular Y*	PA oblique	RAO or LAO	
182		Shoulder joint: *glenoid cavity*	AP oblique	RPO or LPO	GRASHEY
184		Shoulder joint: *supraspinatus "outlet"*	Tangential	RAO or LAO	NEER
185		Shoulder joint: *proximal humerus*	AP axial		STRYKER "NOTCH"
186		Proximal humerus: *interubercular groove*	Tangential		FISK
188		Proximal humerus: *teres minor insertion*	PA		BLACKETT-HEALY
189		Proximal humerus: *subscapular insertion*	AP		BLACKETT-HEALY
190		Proximal humerus: *infraspinatus insertion*	AP axial		
190	✦	Acromioclavicular articulations	AP		PEARSON
192		Acromioclavicular articulations	AP axial		ALEXANDER
194		Acromioclavicular articulations	PA axial oblique	RAO OR LAO	ALEXANDER
195	✦	Clavicle	AP		
196	✦	Clavicle	PA		
197		Clavicle	AP axial	Lordotic	
198		Clavicle	PA axial		
198		Clavicle	Tangential		
200		Clavicle	Tangential		TARRANT
202	✦	Scapula	AP		
204	✦	Scapula	Lateral	RAO or LAO	
206		Scapula	PA oblique	RAO or LAO	LORENZ, LILIENFIELD
208		Scapula	AP oblique	RPO or LPO	
210		Scapula: *coracoid process*	AP axial		
212		Scapular spine	Tangential		LAQUERRIÈRE-PIERQUIN
214		Scapular spine	Tangential		

The icons in the Essential column indicate projections frequently performed in the United States and Canada. Students should become competent in these projections.

Shoulder Girdle

The *shoulder girdle* is formed by two bones, the *clavicle* and *scapula.* Their function is to connect the upper limb to the trunk. Although the alignment of these two bones is considered a girdle, it is incomplete both in front and in back. The girdle is completed in front by the sternum, which articulates with the medial end of the clavicle. The scapulae are widely separated in the back. The proximal portion of the humerus is part of the upper limb and not the shoulder girdle proper; however, because the proximal humerus is included in the shoulder joint, its anatomy is considered with that of the shoulder girdle (Fig. 5-1).

Clavicle

The *clavicle,* classified as a long bone, has a *body* and two articular extremities (Fig. 5-2). The clavicle lies in a horizontal oblique plane just above the first rib and forms the anterior part of the shoulder girdle. The lateral aspect is termed the *acromial extremity,* and it articulates with the acromion process of the scapula. The *medial* aspect, termed the *sternal extremity,* articulates with the manubrium of the sternum and the first costal cartilage. The clavicle, which serves as a fulcrum for the movements of the arm, is doubly curved for strength. The curvature is more acute in males than in females.

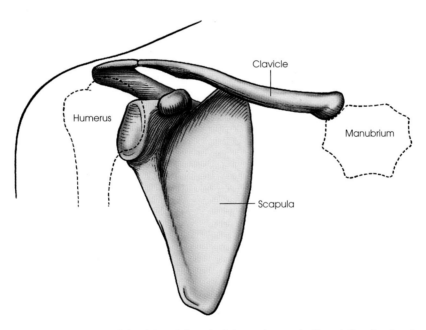

Fig. 5-1 Anterior aspect of shoulder girdle: clavicle and scapula. The girdle attaches to the humerus and manubrium of the sternum.

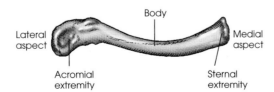

Fig. 5-2 Superior aspect of right clavicle.

Scapula

The *scapula*, classified as a flat bone, forms the posterior part of the shoulder girdle (Figs. 5-3 and 5-4). Triangular in shape, the scapula has two surfaces, three borders, and three angles. Lying on the superoposterior thorax between the second and seventh ribs, the scapula's *medial border* runs parallel with the vertebral column. The *body* of the bone is arched from top to bottom for greater strength, and its surfaces serve as the attachment sites of numerous muscles.

The *costal (anterior) surface* of the scapula is slightly concave and contains the *subscapular fossa.* It is filled almost entirely by the attachment of the subscapularis muscle. The anterior serratus muscle attaches to the medial border of the costal surface from the *superior angle* to the *inferior angle.*

The *dorsal (posterior) surface* is divided into two portions by a prominent spinous process. The *crest of spine* arises at the superior third of the medial border from a smooth, triangular area and runs obliquely superior to end in a flattened, ovoid projection called the *acromion.* The area above the spine is called the *supraspinous fossa* and gives origin to the supraspinatus muscle. The infraspinatus muscle arises from the portion below the spine, which is called the *infraspinous fossa.* The teres minor muscle arises from the superior two thirds of the lateral border of the dorsal surface and the teres major from the distal third and the inferior angle. The dorsal surface of the medial border affords attachment of the levator muscles of the scapulae, greater rhomboid muscle, and lesser rhomboid muscle.

The *superior border* extends from the superior angle to the *coracoid process* and at its lateral end has a deep depression, the *scapular notch.* The *medial border* extends from the superior to the inferior angles. The *lateral border* extends from the *glenoid cavity* to the inferior angle.

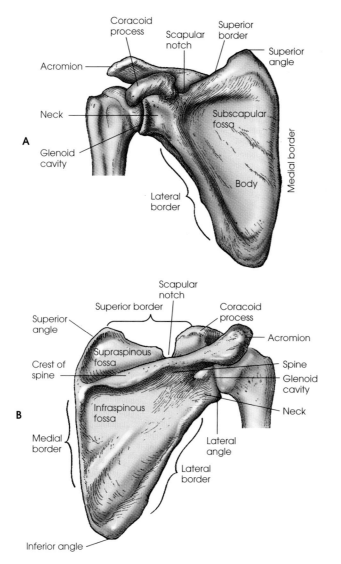

Fig. 5-3 Scapula. **A,** Costal surface (anterior aspect.). **B,** Dorsal surface (posterior aspect).

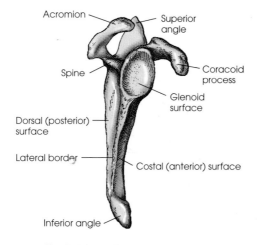

Fig. 5-4 Lateral aspect of scapula.

The *superior angle* is formed by the junction of the superior and medial borders. The *inferior angle* is formed by the junction of the medial (vertebral) and lateral borders and lies over the seventh rib. The *lateral angle,* the thickest part of the body of the scapula, ends in a shallow, oval depression called the *glenoid cavity.* The constricted region around the glenoid cavity is called the *neck* of the scapula. The coracoid process arises from a thick base that extends from the scapular notch to the superior portion of the neck of the scapula. This process projects first anteriorly and medially and then curves on itself to project laterally. The coracoid process can be palpated just distal and slightly medial to the acromioclavicular articulation.

Humerus

The proximal end of the *humerus* consists of a head, an anatomic neck, two prominent processes called the *greater* and *lesser tubercles,* and the surgical neck (Fig. 5-5). The *head* is large, smooth, and rounded, and it lies in an oblique plane on the superomedial side of the humerus. Just below the head, lying in the same oblique plane, is the narrow, constricted *anatomic neck.* The constriction of the body just below the tubercles is called the *surgical neck,* which is the site of many fractures.

The *lesser tubercle* is situated on the anterior surface of the bone, immediately below the anatomic neck (see Figs. 5-5 and 5-6). The tendon of the subscapular muscle inserts at the lesser tubercle. The *greater tubercle* is located on the lateral surface of the bone, just below the anatomic neck, and is separated from the lesser tubercle by a deep depression called the *intertubercular* (bicipital) *groove.* The superior surface of the greater tubercle slopes posteriorly at an angle of approximately 25 degrees and has three flattened impressions for muscle insertions. The anterior impression is the highest of the three and affords attachment to the tendon of the supraspinatus muscle. The middle impression is the point of insertion of the infraspinatus muscle. The tendon of the upper fibers of the teres minor muscle inserts at the posterior impression (the lower fibers insert into the *body* of the bone immediately below this point).

Bursae are small synovial fluid-filled sacs that relieve pressure and reduce friction in tissue. They are often found between the bones and the skin, and they allow the skin to move easily when the joint is moved. Bursae are found also between bones and ligaments, muscles, or tendons. One of the largest bursae of the shoulder is the *subacromial bursa* (Fig. 5-7). It is located under the acromion process and lies between the deltoid muscle and the shoulder joint capsule. It does not normally communicate with the joint. Other bursae of the shoulder are found superior to the acromion, between the coracoid process and the joint capsule, and between the capsule and the tendon of the subscapular muscle. Bursae become important radiographically when injury or age causes the deposition of calcium.

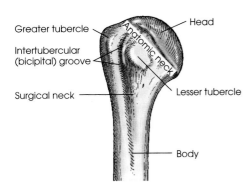

Fig. 5-5 Anterior aspect of right proximal humerus.

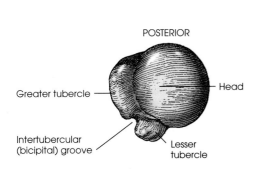

Fig. 5-6 Superior aspect of humerus.

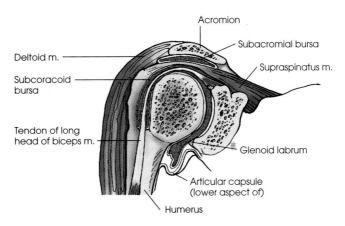

Fig. 5-7 Right shoulder bursae and muscles.

Shoulder Girdle Articulations

A summary of the three joints of the shoulder girdle is contained in Table 5-1, and a detailed description follows.

SCAPULOHUMERAL ARTICULATION

The *scapulohumeral* articulation between the glenoid cavity and the head of the humerus forms a *synovial ball-and-socket* joint, allowing movement in all directions (Fig. 5-8). Although many muscles connect with, support, and enter into the function of the shoulder joint, radiographers are chiefly concerned with the insertion points of the short rotator cuff muscles (Figs. 5-9 and 5-10). The insertion points of these muscles—the subscapular, supraspinatus, infraspinatus, and teres minor—have already been described.

TABLE 5-1

Joints of the shoulder girdle

| Joint | Structural classification | | Movement |
	Tissue	Type	
Scapulohumeral	Synovial	Ball and socket	Freely movable
Acromioclavicular	Synovial	Gliding	Freely movable
Sternoclavicular	Synovial	Double gliding	Freely movable

An articular capsule completely encloses the shoulder joint. The tendon of the long head of the biceps brachii muscle, which arises from the superior margin of the glenoid cavity, passes through the capsule of the shoulder joint, between its fibrous and synovial layers, arches over the head of the humerus, and descends through the intertubercular (bicipital) groove. The short head of the biceps arises from the coracoid process and, with the long head of the muscle, inserts in the radial tuberosity. Because it crosses with both the shoulder and elbow joints, the biceps help synchronize their action.

The interaction of movement between the wrist, elbow, and shoulder joints makes the position of the hand important in radiography of the upper limb. Any rotation of the hand also rotates the joints. The best approach to the study of the mechanics of joint and muscle action is to perform all movements ascribed to each joint and carefully note the reaction in remote parts.

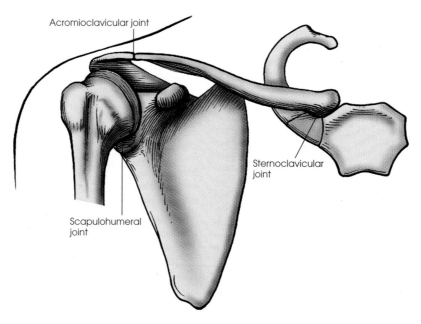

Fig. 5-8 Articulations of the scapula and humerus.

ACROMIOCLAVICULAR ARTICULATION

The *acromioclavicular* articulation between the *acromion* process of the scapula and the acromial extremity of the *clavicle* forms a *synovial gliding* joint (see Fig. 5-8). It permits both gliding and rotary (elevation, depression, protraction, and retraction) movement. Because the end of the clavicle rides higher than the adjacent surface of the acromion, the slope of the surfaces tends to favor displacement of the acromion downward and under the clavicle.

STERNOCLAVICULAR ARTICULATION

The *sternoclavicular* articulation is formed by the sternal extremity of the clavicle with two bones: the manubrium and the first rib cartilage (see Fig. 5-8).

The union of the clavicle with the manubrium of the sternum is the only bony union between the upper limb and trunk. This articulation is a *synovial double-gliding* joint. However, the joint is adapted by a fibrocartilaginous disk to provide movements similar to a ball-and-socket joint: circumduction, elevation, depression, and forward and backward movements. The clavicle carries the scapula with it through any movement.

SUMMARY OF ANATOMY

Shoulder girdle
clavicle
scapula

Clavicle
body
acromial extremity
sternal extremity

Scapula
medial border
body
costal surface
subscapular fossa

superior angle
inferior angle
dorsal surface
crest of spine
acromion
supraspinous fossa
infraspinous fossa
superior border
coracoid process
scapular notch
lateral border
glenoid cavity
lateral angle
neck

Humerus (proximal aspect)
head
anatomic neck
surgical neck
intertubercular groove
greater tubercles
lesser tubercles
body
bursae
subacromial bursa

Shoulder articulations
scapulohumeral
acromioclavicular
sternoclavicular

*See *Addendum* at the end of the volume for a summary of the changes in the anatomic terms used in this edition.

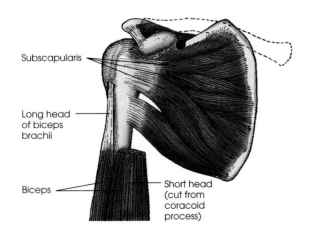

Fig. 5-9 Muscles on costal (anterior) surface of scapula and proximal humerus.

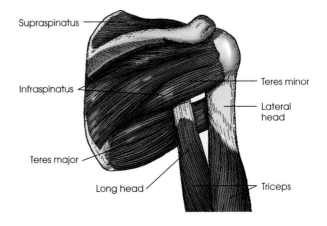

Fig. 5-10 Muscles on dorsal (posterior) surface of scapula and proximal humerus.

Shoulder girdle

Radiation Protection

Protection of the patient from unnecessary radiation is a professional responsibility of the radiographer (see Chapters 1 and 2 for specific guidelines). In this chapter, the *Shield gonads* statement at the end of the *Position of part* section indicates that the patient is to be protected from unnecessary radiation by using proper collimation *and* placing lead shielding between the gonads and the radiation source to restrict the radiation beam.

Shoulder

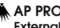 AP PROJECTION
External rotation humerus

NOTE: Do not have the patient rotate the arm if fracture or dislocation is suspected.

Image receptor: 24 × 30 cm (10 × 12 inch) crosswise

Position of patient

- Examine the patient in the upright or the supine position. Shoulder and arm lesions, whether traumatic or pathologic in origin, are extremely sensitive to movement and pressure. For this reason the upright position should be used whenever possible.

Position of part

- Center the shoulder joint to the midline of the grid.
- Adjust the position of the cassette so that its center is 1 inch (2.5 cm) inferior to the coracoid process.
- If necessary to overcome the curve of the back and the resultant obliquity of the shoulder structures, slightly rotate the patient enough to place the body of the scapula parallel with the plane of the cassette.
- If the patient is in the supine position, support the elevated (nonradiographed) shoulder and hip on sandbags.
- Ask the patient to supinate the hand, unless contraindicated (Table 5-2).
- Abduct the arm slightly, and rotate it so that the epicondyles are parallel with the plane of the cassette.

Text continued on p. 162

TABLE 5-2
The hand position and its effect on the proximal humerus

Description	Hand position	Proximal humerus position
Supinating the hand will position the humerus in *external rotation*.		AP shoulder. External rotation humerus. Greater tubercle *(arrow)*
The palm of the hand placed against the hip will position the humerus in *neutral rotation*.		AP shoulder. Neutral rotation humerus. Greater tubercle *(arrow)*
The posterior aspect of the hand placed against the hip will position the humerus in *internal rotation*.		AP shoulder. Internal rotation humerus. Greater tubercle *(arrow)*; lesser tubercle in profile

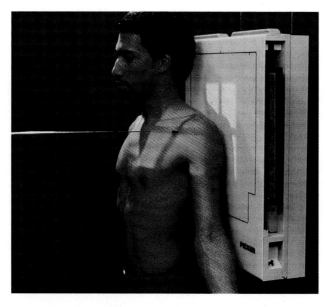

Fig. 5-11 AP shoulder, external rotation humerus.

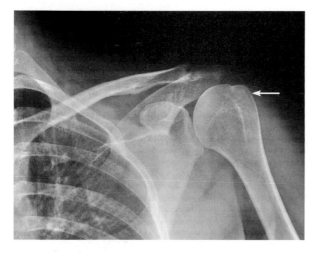

Fig. 5-12 AP shoulder, external rotation humerus: greater tubercle *(arrow)*.

- When the patient is upright, immobilize the arm by resting the hand against an IV pole or the back of a chair. Externally rotating the entire arm from the neutral position places the shoulder and entire humerus in the true anatomic position (Fig. 5-11).
- *Shield gonads.*
- *Respiration:* Suspend.

Central ray

- Perpendicular to a point 1 inch (2.5 cm) inferior to the coracoid process

COMPUTED RADIOGRAPHY

Both dense and nondense body areas will be exposed. The kilovolt (peak) kVp must be sufficient to penetrate the dense area. Collimation must be very close to keep unnecessary radiation from reaching the cassette phosphor.

Structures shown

External rotation of the humerus demonstrates the bony and soft structures of the shoulder and proximal humerus in the anatomic position (Fig. 5-12). The scapulohumeral joint relationship and the region of the subacromial bursa are seen. The greater tubercle of the humerus and the site of insertion of the supraspinatus tendon are visualized.

EVALUATION CRITERIA

The following should be clearly demonstrated:

- Superior scapula, lateral half of the clavicle, and proximal humerus
- Soft tissue around the shoulder, along with bony trabecular detail
- Humeral head in profile
- Greater tubercle in profile on the lateral aspect of the humerus
- Scapulohumeral joint visualized with slight overlap of humeral head on glenoid cavity
- Outline of lesser tubercle between the humeral head and greater tubercle

▲ AP PROJECTION
Neutral rotation humerus

Image receptor: 24 × 30 cm (10 × 12 inch) crosswise

Position of patient
- Examine the patient in the upright or the supine position. Shoulder and arm lesions, whether traumatic or pathologic in origin, are extremely sensitive to movement and pressure. For this reason the upright position should be used whenever possible.

Position of part
- Center the shoulder joint to the midline of the grid.
- Adjust the position of the cassette so that its center is 1 inch (2.5 cm) inferior to the coracoid process.
- If necessary to overcome the curve of the back and the resultant obliquity of the shoulder structures, slightly rotate the patient enough to place the body of the scapula parallel with the plane of the cassette.
- If the patient is in the supine position, support the elevated shoulder and hip on sandbags.

- Ask the patient to rest the palm of the hand against the thigh (see Table 5-2). This position of the arm rolls the humerus slightly internal into a neutral position, placing the epicondyles at an angle of about 45 degrees with the plane of the cassette (Fig. 5-13).
- *Shield gonads.*
- *Respiration:* Suspend.

Central ray
- Perpendicular to a point 1 inch (2.5 cm) inferior to the coracoid process

COMPUTED RADIOGRAPHY

Both dense and nondense body areas will be exposed. The kVp must be sufficient to penetrate the dense area. Collimation must be very close to keep unnecessary radiation from reaching the cassette phosphor.

Structures shown
Fig. 5-14 demonstrates the bony and soft tissue structures of the shoulder. Also seen is the posterior part of the supraspinatus insertion, which sometimes profiles small calcific deposits not otherwise visualized.

EVALUATION CRITERIA
The following should be clearly demonstrated:
- Superior scapula, lateral half of the clavicle, and proximal humerus
- Soft tissue around the shoulder, along with bony trabecular detail
- Greater tubercle partially superimposing the humeral head
- Humeral head in partial profile
- Slight overlap of the humeral head on the glenoid cavity

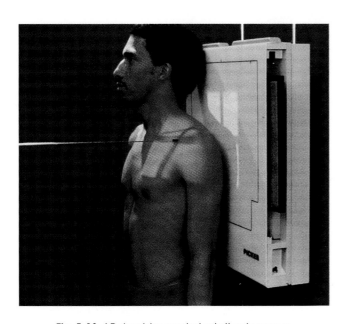

Fig. 5-13 AP shoulder, neutral rotation humerus.

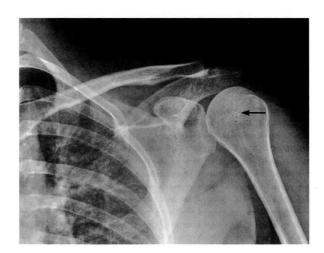

Fig. 5-14 AP shoulder, neutral rotation humerus: greater tubercle *(arrow)*.

▲ AP PROJECTION
Internal rotated humerus

Image receptor: 24 × 30 cm (10 × 12 inch) crosswise

Position of patient
- Examine the patient in the upright or the supine position. Shoulder and arm lesions, whether traumatic or pathologic in origin, are extremely sensitive to movement and pressure. For this reason the upright position should be used whenever possible.

Position of part
- Center the shoulder joint to the midline of the grid.
- Adjust the position of the cassette so that its center is 1 inch (2.5 cm) inferior to the coracoid process.
- If necessary to overcome the curve of the back and the resultant obliquity of the shoulder structures, slightly rotate the patient enough to place the body of the scapula parallel with the plane of the cassette.
- If the patient is in the supine position, support the elevated shoulder and hip on sandbags.

- Ask the patient to flex the elbow somewhat, rotate the arm internally, and rest the *back of the hand* on the hip (see Table 5-2).
- Adjust the arm to place the epicondyles perpendicular to the plane of the cassette (Fig. 5-15). When the shoulder is too painful for adequate internal rotation of the arm, turn the patient somewhat away from the cassette.
- *Shield gonads.*
- *Respiration:* Suspend.

Central ray
- Perpendicular to a point 1 inch (2.5 cm) inferior to the coracoid process

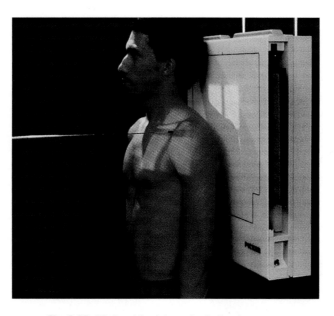

Fig. 5-15 AP shoulder, internal rotation humerus.

COMPUTED RADIOGRAPHY

Both dense and nondense body areas are exposed. The kVp must be sufficient to penetrate the dense area. Collimation must be very close to keep unnecessary radiation from reaching the cassette phosphor.

Structures shown

With the arm in internal rotation, the bony and soft tissue structures of the shoulder are seen. The proximal humerus is seen in a true lateral position. The region of the subacromial bursa is also demonstrated. When the arm can be abducted enough to clear the lesser tubercle of the head of the scapula, a profile image of the site of the insertion of the subscapular tendon is seen (Fig 5-16).

EVALUATION CRITERIA

The following should be clearly demonstrated:

- Superior scapula, lateral half of the clavicle, and proximal humerus
- Soft tissue around the shoulder, along with bony trabecular detail
- Lesser tubercle in profile and pointing medially
- Outline of the greater tubercle superimposing the humeral head
- Greater amount of humeral overlap of the glenoid cavity than in the external and neutral positions

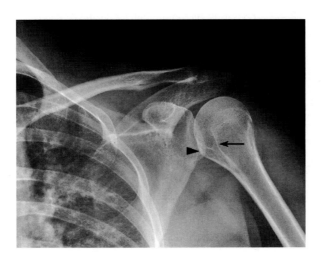

Fig. 5-16 AP shoulder, internal rotation humerus: greater tubercle *(arrow);* lesser tubercle in profile *(arrowhead).*

TRANSTHORACIC LATERAL PROJECTION
LAWENCE METHOD[1]
R or L position

The Lawrence method is used when trauma exists and the arm cannot be rotated or abducted because of an injury.

Image receptor: 24 × 30 cm (10 × 12 inch) lengthwise

Position of patient

- Although this position can be carried out with the patient in the upright or the supine position, the upright position is much easier on the trauma patient. It also facilitates accurate adjustment of the shoulder.
- For upright positioning, seat or stand the patient in the lateral position before a vertical grid device (Fig. 5-17).
- If an upright position is not possible, place the patient in a recumbent position on the table with radiolucent pads elevating the head and shoulders (Fig. 5-18).

---

[1] Lawrence WS: A method of obtaining an accurate lateral roentgenogram of the shoulder joint, *AJR* 5:193, 1918.

Position of part

- Have the patient raise the uninjured arm, rest the forearm on the head, and elevate the shoulder as much as possible (see Fig. 5-17). Elevation of the uninjured shoulder drops the injured side, separating the shoulders to prevent superimposition. Ensure that the midcoronal plane is perpendicular to the cassette.
- No attempt should be made to rotate or otherwise move the injured arm.
- Center the cassette to the surgical neck area of the affected humerus.
- *Shield gonads.*
- *Respiration:* Full inspiration. Having the lungs full of air improves the contrast and decreases the exposure necessary to penetrate the body.
- If the patient can be sufficiently immobilized to prevent voluntary motion, a breathing technique can be utilized. In this case, instruct the patient to practice slow, deep breathing. A minimum exposure time of 3 seconds (4 to 5 seconds is desirable) will give excellent results when a low milliamperage is used.

Central ray

- Perpendicular to the cassette, entering the midcoronal plane at the level of the surgical neck.
- If the patient cannot elevate the unaffected shoulder, angle the central ray 10 to 15 degrees cephalad to obtain a comparable radiograph.

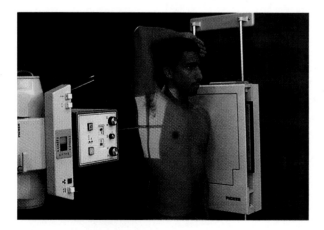

Fig. 5-17 Upright transthoracic lateral shoulder: Lawrence method.

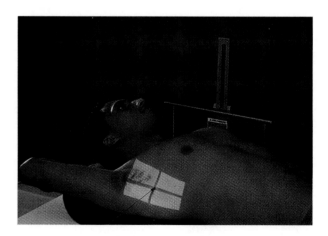

Fig. 5-18 Recumbent transthoracic lateral shoulder: Lawrence method.

Structures shown

A lateral image of the shoulder and proximal humerus is projected through the thorax (Figs. 5-19 and 5-20).

EVALUATION CRITERIA

The following should be clearly demonstrated:

- Proximal humerus
- Scapula, clavicle, and humerus seen through the lung field
- Scapula superimposed over the thoracic spine
- Unaffected clavicle and humerus projected above the shoulder closest to the cassette

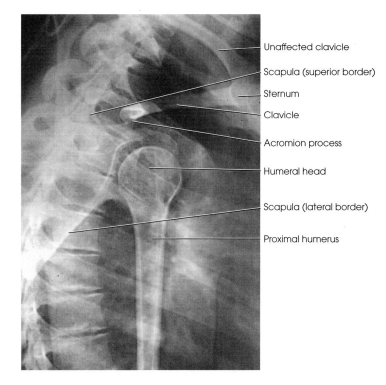

Unaffected clavicle
Scapula (superior border)
Sternum
Clavicle
Acromion process
Humeral head
Scapula (lateral border)
Proximal humerus

Fig. 5-19 Transthoracic lateral shoulder: Lawrence method.

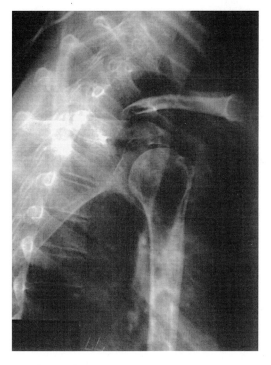

Fig. 5-20 Transthoracic lateral shoulder (patient breathing): Lawrence method.

INFEROSUPERIOR AXIAL PROJECTION
LAWRENCE METHOD[1]
INFEROSUPERIOR AXIAL PROJECTION
RAFERT ET AL[2] MODIFICATION

Image receptor: 8 × 10 inch (18 × 24 cm) crosswise, placed in the vertical position in contact with the superior surface of the shoulder

Position of patient
- With the patient in the supine position, elevate the head, shoulders, and elbow about 3 inches (7.6 cm).

---

[1]Lawrence WS: New position in radiographing the shoulder joint, *AJR* (2)728, 1915.
[2]Rafert JA et al: Axillary shoulder with exaggerated rotation: the Hill-Sachs defect, *Radiol Technol* 62(1):18, 1990.

Position of part
Lawrence method
- As much as possible, abduct the arm of the affected side at right angles to the long axis of the body.
- Keep the humerus in *external rotation,* and adjust the forearm and hand in a comfortable position, grasping a vertical support or extended on sandbags or a firm pillow. Support may be needed under the forearm and hand. Provide patient with an extension board for the arm.
- Have the patient turn the head away from the side being examined so that the cassette can be placed against the neck.
- Place the cassette on edge against the shoulder and as close as possible to the neck.
- Support the cassette in position with sandbags, or use a vertical cassette holder (Fig. 5-21).

Rafert modification
- Anterior dislocation of the humeral head can result in a wedge-shaped compression fracture of the articular surface of the humeral head, called the *Hill-Sachs defect.*[1] The fracture will be located on the posterolateral humeral head. An *exaggerated external rotation* of the arm may be required to see the defect.
- With the patient in position exactly as for the Lawrence method, externally rotate the extended arm until the hand forms a 45-degree oblique. The thumb will be pointing downward (Fig. 5-22).
- Assist the patient in rotating the arm to avoid overstressing the shoulder joint.
- *Shield gonads.*
- *Respiration:* Suspend.

---

[1]Hill H, Sachs M: The grooved defect of the humeral head. A frequently underrecognized complication of dislocations of the shoulder joint, *Radiology* 35:690, 1940.

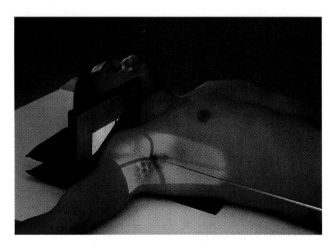

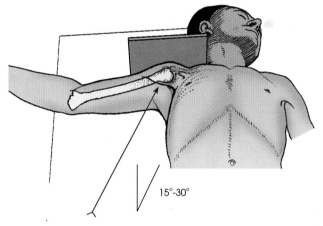

15°-30°

Fig. 5-21 Inferosuperior axial shoulder joint: Lawrence method.

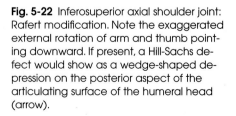

Fig. 5-22 Inferosuperior axial shoulder joint: Rafert modification. Note the exaggerated external rotation of arm and thumb pointing downward. If present, a Hill-Sachs defect would show as a wedge-shaped depression on the posterior aspect of the articulating surface of the humeral head (arrow).

(From Rafert JA et al: Axillary shoulder with exaggerated rotation: the Hill-Sachs defect, *Radiol Technol* 62:18, 1990.)

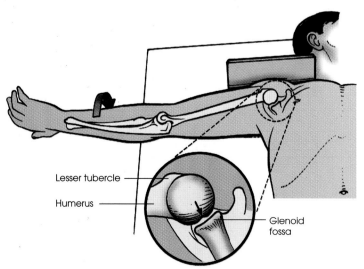

Lesser tubercle

Humerus

Glenoid fossa

Central ray

Lawrence method

- Horizontally through the axilla to the region of the acromioclavicular articulation. The degree of medial angulation of the central ray depends on the degree of abduction of the arm. The degree of medial angulation is often between 15 and 30 degrees. The greater the abduction, the greater the angle.

Rafert modification

- Horizontal and angled approximately 15 degrees medially, entering the axilla and passing through the acromioclavicular joint.

Structures shown

An inferosuperior axial image shows the proximal humerus, the scapulohumeral joint, the lateral portion of the coracoid process, and the acromioclavicular articulation. The insertion site of the subscapular tendon on the lesser tubercle of the humerus and the point of insertion of the teres minor tendon on the greater tubercle of the humerus are also shown. A Hill-Sachs compression fracture on the posterolateral humeral head may be seen using the Rafert modification (Figs. 5-23 and 5-24).

EVALUATION CRITERIA

The following should be clearly demonstrated:

- Scapulohumeral joint with slight overlap
- Coracoid process, pointing anteriorly
- Lesser tubercle in profile and directed anteriorly
- Acromioclavicular joint, acromion, and acromial end of clavicle projected through the humeral head
- Soft tissue in the axilla with bony trabecular detail
- Axillary structures

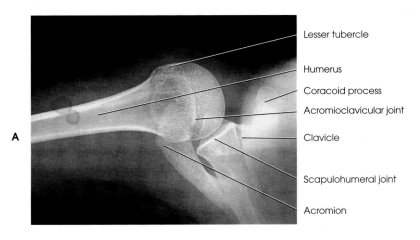
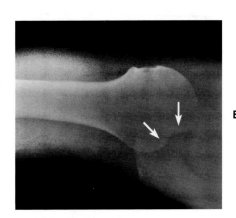

Lesser tubercle

Humerus

Coracoid process

Acromioclavicular joint

Clavicle

Scapulohumeral joint

Acromion

Fig. 5-23 A, Inferosuperior axial shoulder joint: Lawrence method. **B,** Inferosuperior axial shoulder joint: Rafert modification showing a Hill-Sachs defect *(arrows).*

(From Rafert JAet al: Axillary shoulder with exaggerated rotation: the Hill-Sachs defect, *Radiol Technol* 62:18, 1990.)

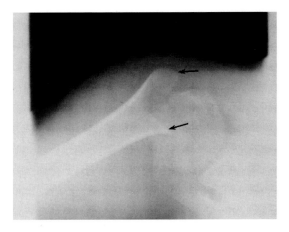

Fig. 5-24 Inferosuperior axial shoulder joint: Lawrence method with little arm abduction because of fracture of the surgical neck *(arrows).*

Shoulder girdle

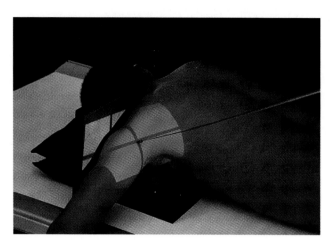

Fig. 5-25 Inferosuperior axial shoulder joint: West Point method.

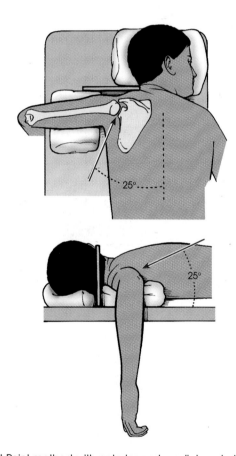

Fig. 5-26 West Point method with anterior and medial central ray angulation.

INFEROSUPERIOR AXIAL PROJECTION
WEST POINT METHOD[1]

Image receptor: 8 × 10 inch (18 × 24 cm) crosswise placed in the vertical position in contact with the superior surface of the shoulder

Position of patient
- Adjust the patient in the prone position with approximately a 3-inch (7.6-cm) pad under the shoulder being examined.
- Turn the patient's head away from the side being examined.

Position of part
- Abduct the arm of the affected side *90 degrees*, and rotate so that the forearm rests over the edge of the table or a Bucky tray, which may be used for support. (Figs. 5-25 and 5-26).
- Place a vertically supported cassette against the superior aspect of the shoulder with the edge of the cassette in contact with the neck.
- Support the cassette with sandbags or a vertical cassette holder.
- *Shield gonads.*
- *Respiration:* Suspend.

[1]Rokous JR, Feagin JA, Abbott HG: Modified axillary roentgenogram, *Clin Orthop* 82:84, 1972.

Central ray

- Directed at a dual angle of 25 degrees *anteriorly* from the horizontal and 25 degrees *medially.* The central ray enters approximately 5 inches (13 cm) inferior and 1½ inch (3.8 cm) medial to the acromial edge and exits the glenoid cavity.

Structures shown

The resulting image shows bony abnormalities of the anterior inferior rim of the glenoid in patients with instability of the shoulder (Fig. 5-27).

EVALUATION CRITERIA

The following should be clearly demonstrated:

- Humeral head projected free of the coracoid process
- Articulation between the head of the humerus and the glenoid cavity
- Acromion superimposed over the posterior portion of the humeral head
- Shoulder joint

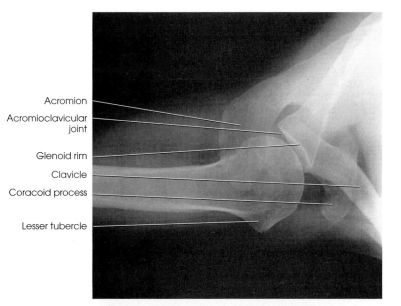

Acromion
Acromioclavicular joint
Glenoid rim
Clavicle
Coracoid process
Lesser tubercle

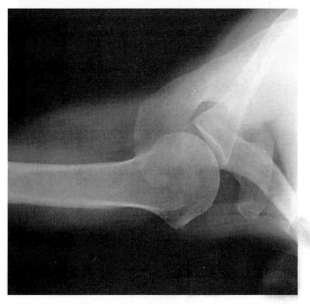

Fig. 5-27 Inferosuperior axial shoulder joint: West Point method.

INFEROSUPERIOR AXIAL PROJECTION
CLEMENTS MODIFICATION[1]

Image receptor: 8 × 10 inch (18 × 24 cm) placed in the vertical position in contact with the superior surface of the shoulder

Position of patient
- When the prone or supine position is not possible, Clements[1] suggested that the patient be radiographed in the lateral recumbent position lying, on the unaffected side.
- Flex the patient's hips and knees.

Position of part
- Abduct the affected arm 90 degrees, and point it toward the ceiling.
- Place the cassette against the superior aspect of the patient's shoulder, holding it in place with the unaffected arm or by securing it appropriately (Fig. 5-28, *A*).
- *Shield gonads.*
- *Respiration:* Suspend respiration.

Central ray
- Horizontal to the midcoronal plane, passing through the midaxillary region of the shoulder.
- Angled 5 to 15 degrees medially when the patient cannot abduct the arm a full 90 degrees (Fig. 5-28, *B*). The resulting radiograph is seen in Fig. 5-29.

---

[1]Clements RW: Adaptation of the technique for radiography of the glenohumeral joint in the lateral position, *Radiol Technol* 51:305, 1979.

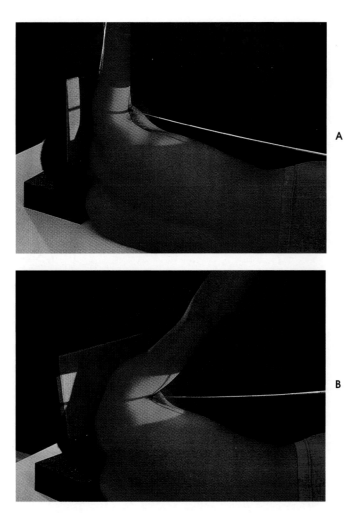

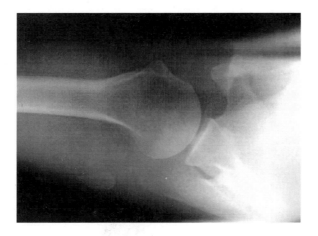

Fig. 5-28 Inferosuperior axial shoulder joint: Clements modification. **A,** Arm abducted 90 degrees. **B,** Arm partially abducted.

Fig. 5-29 Inferosuperior axial shoulder joint: Clements modification

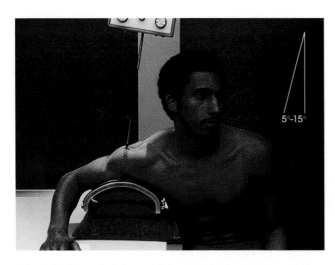

Fig. 5-30 Superoinferior axial shoulder joint: curved cassette.

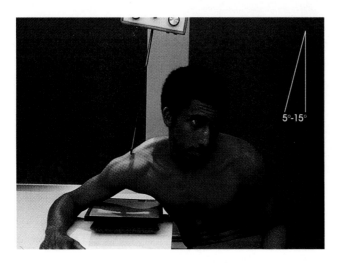

Fig. 5-31 Superoinferior axial shoulder joint: standard cassette.

SUPEROINFERIOR AXIAL PROJECTION

Before undertaking this position, verify the patient's ability to abduct the arm to a nearly right angle to the long axis of the body and the advisability of doing so.

Image receptor: 8 × 10 inch (18 × 24 cm) placed lengthwise for accurate centering to the shoulder joint. A curved cassette may be used for this position to reduce the object-to-image receptor distance.

Position of patient

- Seat the patient at the end of the table on a stool or chair high enough to enable extension of the shoulder under examination well over the cassette.
- Center the shoulder to the midline of the cassette.

Position of part

- Place the cassette near the end of the table and parallel with its long axis.
- Ask the patient to hold the hand of the affected side and raise the arm to a position as near as possible at right angles to the long axis of the body. Then have the patient lean laterally over the cassette until the shoulder joint is over the midpoint of the cassette.
- Bring the elbow to rest on the table.
- Flex the patient's elbow 90 degrees, and place the hand in the prone position (Figs. 5-30 and 5-31).
- Have the patient tilt the head toward the unaffected shoulder.
- To obtain direct lateral positioning of the head of the humerus, adjust any anterior or posterior leaning of the body to place the humeral epicondyles in the vertical position.
- *Shield gonads.*
- *Respiration:* Suspend.

Central ray

- Angled 5 to 15 degrees through the shoulder joint and toward the elbow

Structures shown

A superoinferior axial image shows the joint relationship of the proximal end of the humerus and the glenoid cavity (Figs. 5-32 and 5-33). The acromioclavicular articulation, the outer portion of the coracoid process, and the points of insertion of the subscapularis muscle (at body of scapula) and teres minor muscle (at inferior axillary border) are demonstrated. Depending on the flexibility of the patient, a greater or lesser portion of the medial structures is shown.

EVALUATION CRITERIA

The following should be clearly demonstrated:

- Open scapulohumeral joint (not open on patients with limited flexibility)
- Coracoid process projected above the clavicle
- Lesser tubercle in profile
- Acromioclavicular joint through the humeral head
- Soft tissue in the axilla with bony trabecular detail

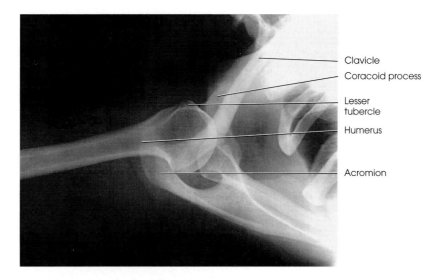

Clavicle
Coracoid process
Lesser tubercle
Humerus
Acromion

Fig. 5-32 Superoinferior axial shoulder joint.

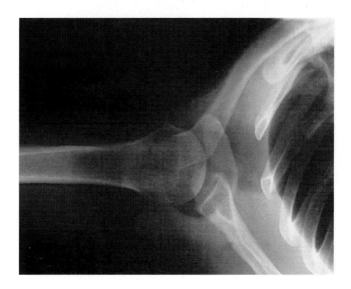

Fig. 5-33 Superoinferior axial shoulder joint.

Shoulder Joint

AXIAL PROJECTION
CLEAVES METHOD WITH ROLLED FILM

Cleaves[1] devised a method of obtaining an axial projection of the shoulder joint for use with patients who cannot or should not abduct the arm enough for one of the preliminary axial radiographs.

Image receptor: 8 × 10 inch (18 × 24 cm)

This position requires that an 8 × 10 inch film be enclosed in a lightproof envelope and gently curved around a small tube approximately 2 inches (5 cm) in diameter. A tube smaller than 2 inches (5 cm) will cause too much distortion on the radiograph, and a tube that is too large will be difficult to place high in the axilla.

The envelope used to enclose the film may include flexible intensifying screens to reduce radiation exposure to the patient. The loaded envelope is curved around the tube and secured at each end. If screens are used, extreme care must be taken to keep from damaging them when loading and unloading film.

---

[1]Cleaves EN: A new film holder for roentgen examination of the shoulder, *AJR* 45:288, 1941.

Position of patient
- Seat the patient laterally at the end of the table. When necessary, adapt this position for the supine patient.

Position of part
- Place the film roll as high in the axilla as possible and adjust it so that it is horizontal (Fig. 5-34). Ensure that the forearm is resting on the tabletop if the sitting position is used.
- *Shield gonads.*
- *Respiration:* Suspend.

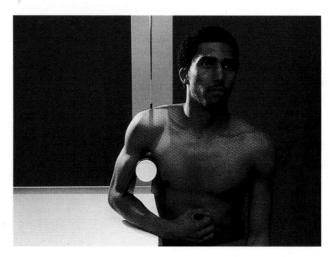

Fig. 5-34 Axial shoulder joint: Cleaves method, rolled film.

Central ray
- Perpendicular to the shoulder, entering ⅜ inch (1 cm) posterior to the acromioclavicular joint (Fig. 5-35).

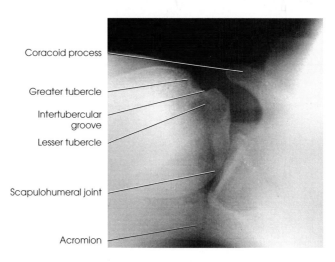

Coracoid process

Greater tubercle

Intertubercular groove

Lesser tubercle

Scapulohumeral joint

Acromion

Fig. 5-35 Axial shoulder joint: Cleaves method, angulation of 0 degrees.

Variations

- Directed to the acromioclavicular articulation at a 5-degree medial angulation to demonstrate the lesser tubercle and intertubercular (bicipital) groove (Fig. 5-36) and at a 5-degree lateral angulation to demonstrate the coracoid process (Fig. 5-37)

Structures shown

An axial image demonstrates the scapulohumeral joint, greater and lesser tubercles, intertubercular (bicipital) groove, and coracoid process (see Figs. 5-35 to 5-37).

EVALUATION CRITERIA

The following should be clearly demonstrated:

- Scapulohumeral joint open and visualized
- Coracoid, intertubercular (bicipital) groove, and humeral tubercles

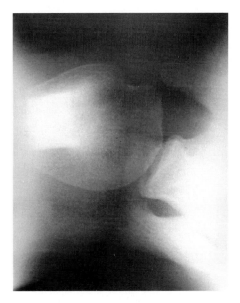 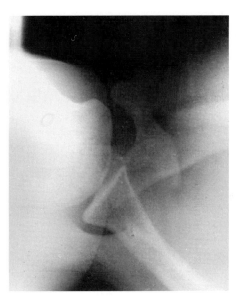

Fig. 5-36 Axial shoulder joint: Cleaves method, medial angulation of 5 degrees.

Fig. 5-37 Axial shoulder joint: Cleaves method, lateral angulation of 5 degrees.

Shoulder Joint

AP AXIAL PROJECTION

Image receptor: 8 × 10 inch (18 × 24 cm) crosswise

Position of patient
• Position the patient in the upright or supine body position.

Position of part
• Center the scapulohumeral joint of the shoulder being examined to the midline of the grid (Fig. 5-38).
• *Shield gonads.*
• *Respiration:* Suspend.

Central ray
• Directed through the scapulohumeral joint at a cephalic angle of 35 degrees

Structures shown
The axial image shows the relationship of the head of the humerus to the glenoid cavity. This is useful in diagnosing cases of posterior dislocation (Fig. 5-39).

EVALUATION CRITERIA

The following should be clearly demonstrated:
■ Scapulohumeral joint
■ Proximal humerus
■ Clavicle projected above superior angle of scapula

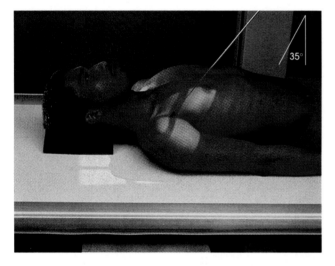

Fig. 5-38 AP axial shoulder joint.

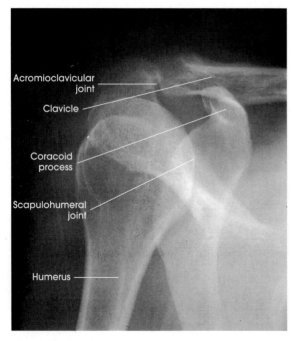
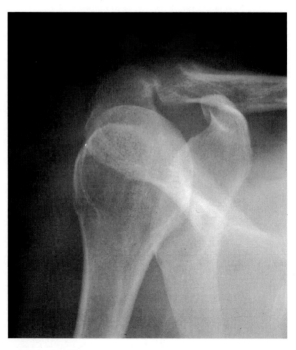

Acromioclavicular joint
Clavicle
Coracoid process
Scapulohumeral joint
Humerus

Fig. 5-39 AP axial shoulder joint.

Scapular Y

✹ PA OBLIQUE PROJECTION
RAO or LAO position

This projection, described by Rubin, Gray, and Green,[1] obtained its name as a result of the appearance of the scapula. The body of the scapula forms the vertical component of the Y, and the acromion and coracoid processes form the upper limbs. The projection is useful in the evaluation of suspected shoulder dislocations.

Image receptor: 24 × 30 cm (10 × 12 inch)

Position of patient

- Radiograph the patient in the upright or recumbent body position; the upright position is preferred.
- When the patient is severely injured, modify the anterior oblique position by placing the patient in the posterior oblique position.

[1]Rubin SA, Gray RL, Green WR: The scapular Y: a diagnostic aid in shoulder trauma, *Radiology* 110:725, 1974.

Position of part

- Position the anterior surface of the shoulder being examined against the upright table.
- Rotate the patient so that the midcoronal plane forms an angle of 45 to 60 degrees to the cassette. The position of the arm is not critical because it does not alter the relationship of the humeral head to the glenoid cavity (Fig. 5-40). Palpate the scapula, and place its flat surface perpendicular to the cassette.
- Position the center of the cassette at the level of the scapulohumeral joint.
- *Shield gonads.*
- *Respiration:* Suspend.

COMPUTED RADIOGRAPHY

Collimation must be very close to prevent unnecessary radiation from reaching the cassette phosphor.

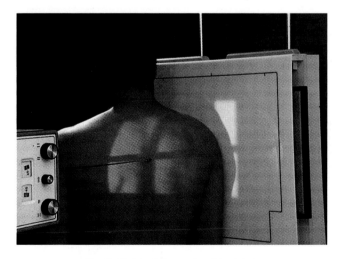

Fig. 5-40 PA oblique shoulder joint.

Shoulder Joint

Central ray
- Perpendicular to the scapulohumeral joint (Table 5-3)

Structures shown

The scapular Y is demonstrated on an oblique image of the shoulder. In the normal shoulder the humeral head is directly superimposed over the junction of the Y (Fig. 5-41). In anterior (subcoracoid) dislocations, the humeral head is beneath the coracoid process (Fig. 5-42); in posterior (subacromial) dislocations, it is projected beneath the acromion process. An AP shoulder projection is shown for comparison (Fig. 5-43).

EVALUATION CRITERIA

The following should be clearly demonstrated:
- No superimposition of the scapular body over the bony thorax
- Acromion projected laterally and free of superimposition
- Coracoid possibly superimposed or projected below the clavicle
- Scapula in lateral profile

TABLE 5-3
Similar shoulder projections

Name	Body rotation	Scapula relationship to cassette	Central ray angle*	Central ray entrance point*	Arm position*
Acromioclavicular articulation: Alexander method	45 to 60 degrees	Perpendicular	15 degrees caudad	Acromioclavicular joint	Across chest
Shoulder joint: Neer method	45 to 60 degrees	Perpendicular	10 to 15 degrees	Superior humeral border caudad	At side
Shoulder joint: scapular Y	45 to 60 degrees	Perpendicular	0 degrees	Scapulohumeral joint	At side
Scapula lateral	45 to 60 degrees	Perpendicular	0 degrees	Center of medial border of scapula	Variable

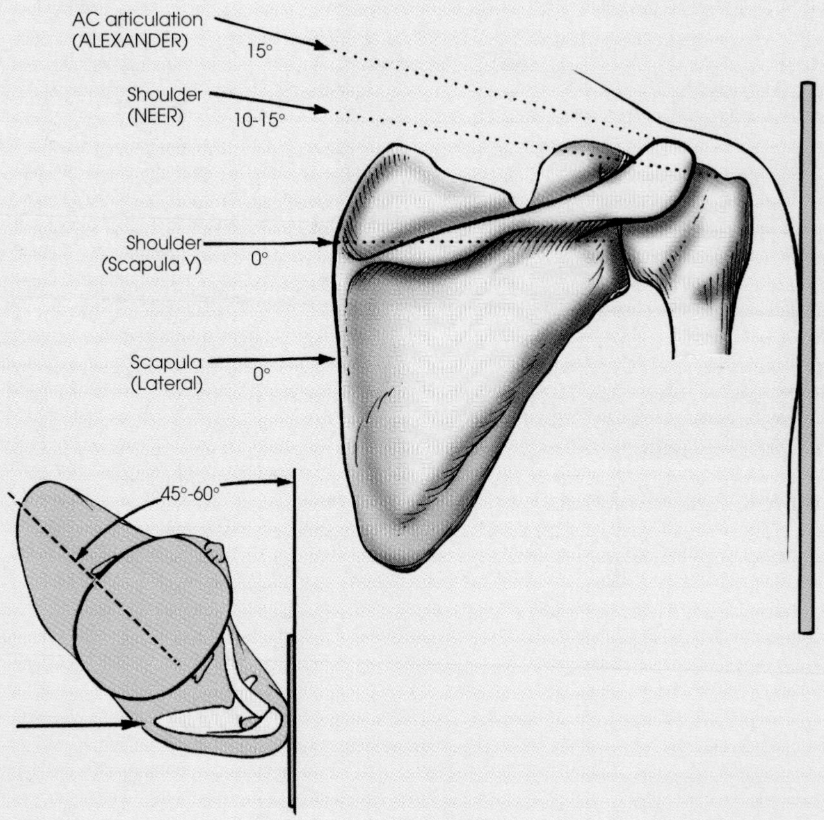

AC articulation (ALEXANDER) 15°
Shoulder (NEER) 10-15°
Shoulder (Scapula Y) 0°
Scapula (Lateral) 0°
45°-60°

*The central ray angles and entrance points and the arm positions are the only differences among these four projections.

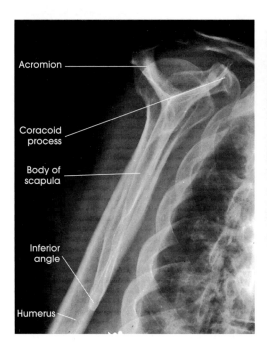

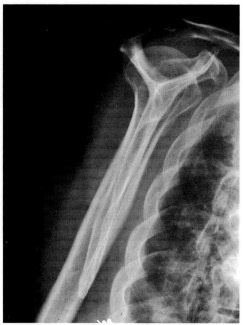

Fig. 5-41 PA oblique shoulder joint. Note the scapular Y components-body, acromion, and coracoid.

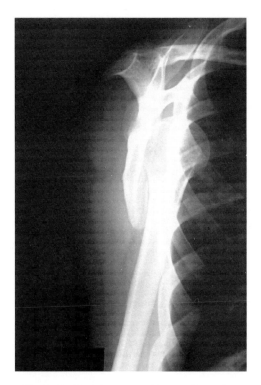

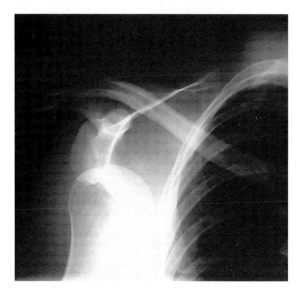

Fig. 5-42 PA oblique shoulder joint showing anterior dislocation (humeral head projected beneath coracoid process).

Fig. 5-43 AP shoulder (same patient as in Fig. 5-42).

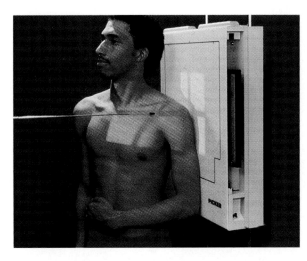

Fig. 5-44 Upright AP oblique glenoid cavity: Grashey method.

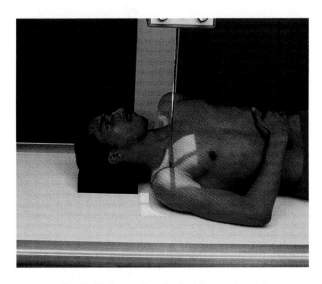

Fig. 5-45 Recumbent AP oblique glenoid cavity: Grashey method.

Glenoid Cavity
AP OBLIQUE PROJECTION
GRASHEY METHOD
RPO or LPO position

Image receptor: 8 × 10 inch (18 × 24 cm) crosswise

Position of patient
- Achieve this position with the patient in the supine or upright position. The upright position is more comfortable for the patient and facilitates accurate adjustment of the part.

Position of part
- Center the cassette to the scapulohumeral joint.
- Rotate the body approximately 35 to 45 degrees toward the affected side (Fig. 5-44).
- Adjust the degree of rotation to place the scapula parallel with the plane of the cassette. This allows the head of the humerus to be in contact with the cassette.
- If the patient is in the supine position, the body may need to be rotated more than 45 degrees to place the scapula parallel to the cassette.
- In addition, support the elevated shoulder and hip on sandbags (Fig. 5-45).
- Abduct the arm slightly in internal rotation, and place palm of the hand on the abdomen.
- *Shield gonads.*
- *Respiration:* Suspend.

Central ray

• Perpendicular to the glenoid cavity at a point 2 inches (5 cm) medial and 2 inches (5 cm) inferior to the superolateral border of the shoulder

Structures shown

The joint space between the humeral head and the glenoid cavity (scapulohumeral joint) is shown (Fig. 5-46).

EVALUATION CRITERIA

The following should be clearly demonstrated:

■ Open joint space between the humeral head and glenoid cavity
■ Glenoid cavity in profile
■ Soft tissue at the scapulohumeral joint along with trabecular detail on the glenoid and humeral head

NOTE: Kornguth and Salazar[1] reported a projection similar to the 45-degree AP oblique shoulder just described. For the apical oblique projection, the central ray enters the coracoid process with a caudal angulation of 45 degrees. The patient remains in a 45-degree oblique position with the affected shoulder against the cassette.

[1]Kornguth PJ, Salazar AM: The apical oblique view of the shoulder: its usefulness in acute trauma, *AJR* 149:113, 1987.

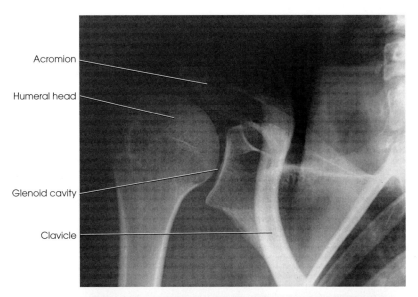

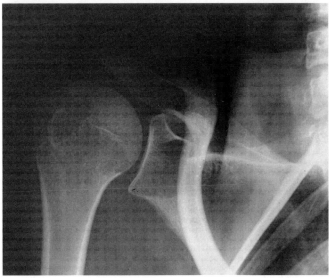

Acromion

Humeral head

Glenoid cavity

Clavicle

Fig. 5-46 AP oblique glenoid cavity: Grashey method.

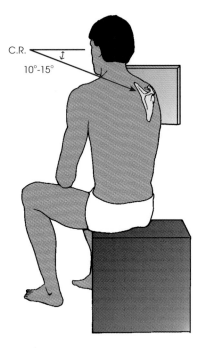

Fig. 5-47 Tangential supraspinatus "outlet" projection.

Supraspinatus "Outlet"

TANGENTIAL PROJECTION

NEER METHOD[1,2]

RAO or LAO position

This radiographic projection is useful to demonstrate tangentially the coracoacromial arch or outlet to diagnose shoulder impingement. The tangential image is obtained by projecting the x-ray beam under the acromion and acromioclavicular joint, which defines the superior border of the coracoacromial outlet.

Image receptor: 8 × 10 inch (18 × 24 cm) lengthwise

Position of patient

- Place the patient in a seated or standing position facing the vertical grid device.

---

[1]Neer CS II: Supraspinatus outlet, *Orthop Trans* 11:234, 1987.
[2]Neer CS II: *Shoulder reconstruction,* Philadelphia, 1990, WB Saunders, pp. 14-24.

Position of part

- With the patient's affected shoulder centered and in contact with the cassette, rotate the patient's unaffected side away from the cassette. Palpate the flat aspect of the affected scapula and place it perpendicular to the cassette. The degree of patient obliquity varies from patient to patient. The average degree of patient rotation varies from 45 to 60 degrees from the plane of the cassette (Fig. 5-47).
- Place the patient's arm at the patient's side.
- *Shield gonads.*
- *Respiration:* Suspend.

Central ray

- Angled 10 to 15 degrees caudad, entering the superior aspect of the humeral head (see Table 5-3)

Structures shown

The tangential outlet image demonstrates the posterior surface of the acromion and the acromioclavicular joint identified as the superior border of the coracoacromial outlet (Figs. 5-48 and 5-49).

EVALUATION CRITERIA

The following should be clearly demonstrated:

- Humeral head projected below the acromioclavicular joint
- Humeral head and acromioclavicular joint with bony detail
- Humerus and scapular body, generally parallel

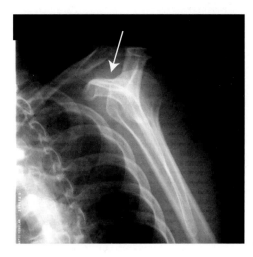

Fig. 5-48 Shoulder joint: Neer method. Supraspinatus outlet *(arrow).*

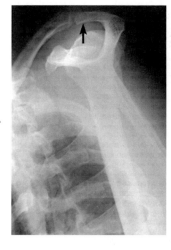

A

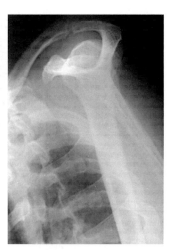

B

Fig. 5-49 A, Tangential supraspinatus outlet projection showing impingement of the shoulder outlet *(arrow).* **B,** Radiograph of same patient as in Fig. 5-48 after surgical removal of posterolateral surface of clavicle.

Proximal Humerus
AP AXIAL PROJECTION
STRYKER "NOTCH" METHOD[1]

Dislocations of the shoulder are frequently caused by posterior defects involving the posterolateral head of the humerus. Such defects, called *Hill-Sachs defects,*[2] are often not demonstrated using conventional radiographic positions. Hall, Isaac, and Booth[1] described the notch projection, from ideas expressed by W. S. Stryker, as being useful in identifying the cause of shoulder dislocation.

Image receptor: 24 × 30 cm (10 × 12 inch)

Position of patient
• Place the patient on the radiographic table in the supine position.

---

[1]Hall RH, Isaac F, Booth CR: Dislocations of the shoulder with special reference to accompanying small fractures, *J Bone Joint Surg* 41A:489, 1959.
[2]Hill H, Sachs M: The grooved defect of the humeral head: a frequently unrecognized complication of dislocations of the shoulder joint, *Radiology* 35:690, 1940.

Position of part
• With the coracoid process of the affected shoulder centered to the table, ask the patient to flex the arm slightly beyond 90 degrees and place the palm of the hand on top of the head with fingertips resting on the head. (This hand position places the humerus in a slight internal rotation position.) The body of the humerus is adjusted to be vertical so that it is parallel to the midsagittal plane of the body (Fig. 5-50).
• *Shield gonads.*
• *Respiration:* Suspend.

Central ray
• Angled 10 degrees cephalad, entering the coracoid process

Structures shown
The resulting image will show the posterosuperior and posterolateral areas of the humeral head (Fig. 5-51).

EVALUATION CRITERIA
The following should be clearly demonstrated:
■ Overlapping of coracoid process and clavicle
■ Long axis of the humerus aligned with the long axis of the patient's body
■ Bony trabeculation of the head of the humerus

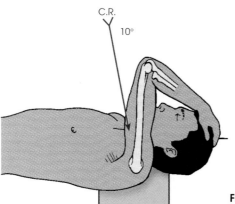

Fig. 5-50 AP axial humeral notch: Stryker notch method.

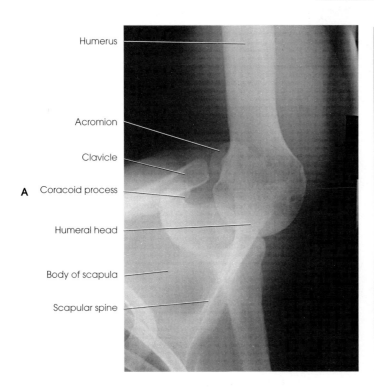

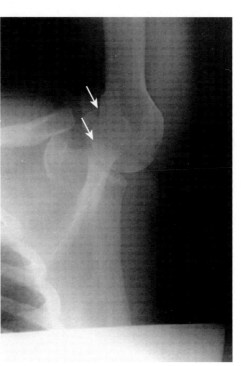

Humerus
Acromion
Clavicle
A Coracoid process
Humeral head
Body of scapula
Scapular spine

B

Fig. 5-51 A, AP axial humeral notch: Stryker notch method. **B,** Same projection in a patient with a small Hill-Sachs defect *(arrows).*

Intertubercular Groove

TANGENTIAL PROJECTION

FISK MODIFICATION[1]

In recent years, various modifications of the intertubercular groove image have been devised. In all cases the central ray is aligned to be tangential to the intertubercular groove, which lies on the anterior surface of the humerus.

A regular or flexible cassette (the type used for panoramic examinations containing intensifying screens) may be used. The flexible cassette allows the film to be placed closer to the shoulder than a rigid cassette does.

[1]Fisk C: Adaptation of the technique for radiography of the bicipital groove, *Radiol Technol* 34:47, 1965.

The x-ray tube head assembly may limit the performance of this examination. Some radiographic units have large collimators and/or handles that limit flexibility in positioning. A mobile radiographic unit may be used to reduce this difficulty.

Image receptor: 8 × 10 inch (24 × 30 cm)

Position of patient

- Place the patient in the supine, seated, or standing position.
- To improve centering, extend the chin or rotate the head away from the affected side.

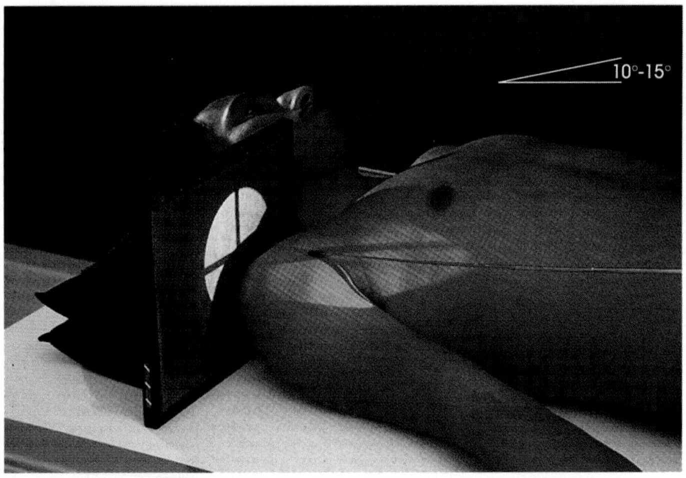

Fig. 5-52 Supine tangential intertubercular groove.

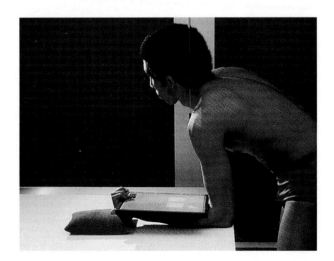

Fig. 5-53 Standing tangential intertubercular groove: Fisk modification.

Position of part

- With the patient supine, palpate the anterior surface of the shoulder to locate the intertubercular groove.
- With the patient's hand in the supinated position, place the cassette against the superior surface of the shoulder and immobilize the cassette as shown in Fig. 5-52.
- *Shield gonads.*
- *Respiration:* Suspend.

Fisk Modification

Fisk[1] first described this position with the patient standing at the end of the radiographic table. This employs a greater OID. The following steps are then taken with Fisk's technique:

- Instruct the patient to flex the elbow and lean forward far enough to place the posterior surface of the forearm on the table. The patient supports and grasps the cassette as depicted in Fig. 5-53.
- For radiation protection and to reduce backscatter to the film from the forearm, place a lead shielding between the cassette back and the forearm.
- Place a sandbag under the hand to place the cassette horizontal.
- Have the patient lean forward or backward as required to place the vertical humerus at an angle of 10 to 15 degrees.

[1]Fisk C: Adaptation of the technique for radiography of the bicipital groove, *Radiol Technol* 34:47, 1965.

Central ray

- Angled 10 to 15 degrees posterior (downward from horizontal) to the long axis of the humerus for the supine position (see Fig. 5-52)

Fisk Modification

- Perpendicular to the cassette when the patient is leaning forward and the vertical humerus is 10 to 15 degrees (see Fig. 5-53)

Structures shown

The tangential image profiles the intertubercular groove free from superimposition of the surrounding shoulder structures (Figs. 5-54 and 5-55).

EVALUATION CRITERIA

The following should be clearly demonstrated:

- Intertubercular groove in profile
- Soft tissue along with enhanced visibility of the intertubercular groove

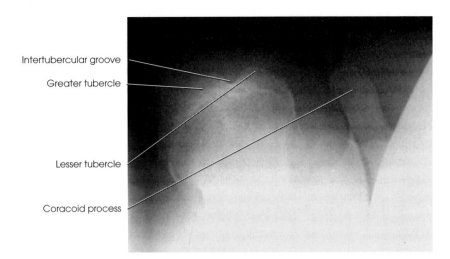

Intertubercular groove
Greater tubercle
Lesser tubercle
Coracoid process

Fig. 5-54 Supine tangential intertubercular groove.

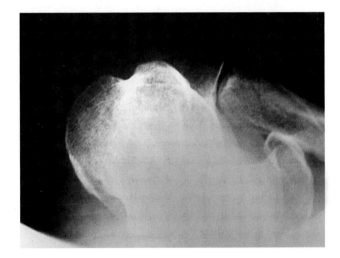

Fig. 5-55 Standing tangential intertubercular groove: Fisk modification.

Proximal Humerus

Teres Minor Insertion

PA PROJECTION
BLACKETT-HEALY METHOD

Image receptor: 8 × 10 inch (18 × 24 cm) crosswise

Position of patient
- Adjust the patient in the prone position, with the arms along the sides of the body and the head resting on the cheek of the affected side.
- Place support under the ankles for the patient's comfort.

Position of part
- Place the cassette under the shoulder, and center it to a point about 1 inch (2.5 cm) below the coracoid process.
- Turn the arm to a position of extreme internal rotation. If possible, flex the elbow and place the hand on the patient's back (Figs. 5-56 and 5-57).
- *Shield gonads.*
- *Respiration:* Suspend at the end of exhalation for a more uniform density.

Central ray
- Perpendicular to the head of the humerus

Structures shown
This position rotates the head of the humerus so that the greater tubercle is brought anteriorly, giving a tangential image of the insertion of the teres minor at the outer edge of the bone just below the articular surface of the head (Fig. 5-58).

EVALUATION CRITERIA

The following should be clearly demonstrated:
- Outline of the greater tubercle superimposing the humeral head
- Lesser tubercle in profile and pointing medially
- Soft tissue around the humerus along with trabecular detail on the humeral head

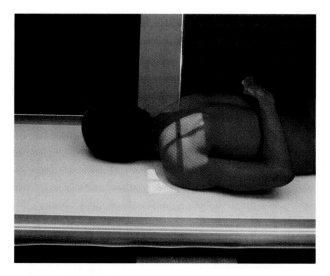

Fig. 5-56 PA proximal humerus for teres minor insertion.

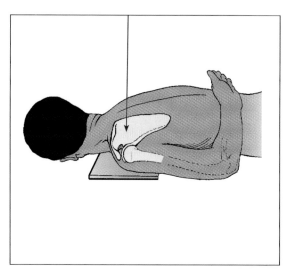

Fig. 5-57 PA proximal humerus for teres minor insertion.

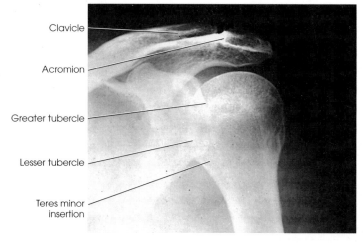

Clavicle

Acromion

Greater tubercle

Lesser tubercle

Teres minor insertion

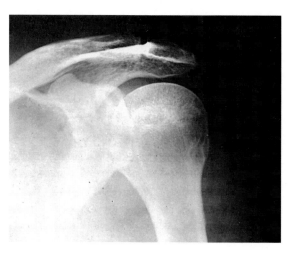

Fig. 5-58 PA proximal humerus for teres minor insertion.

Subscapular Insertion
AP PROJECTION
BLACKETT-HEALY METHOD

Image receptor: 8 × 10 inch (18 × 24 cm)

Position of patient
- Place the patient in the supine position, with the arms resting along the sides of the body.

Position of part
- Align the patient's body so that the affected shoulder joint is centered to the midline of the table.
- The opposite shoulder may be elevated approximately 15 degrees and supported with a sandbag.
- Abduct the affected arm to the long axis of the body, flex the elbow, and rotate the arm internally by pronating the hand (Figs. 5-59 and 5-60).
- Place one sandbag under the hand and another on top, if necessary, for immobilization.
- *Shield gonads.*
- *Respiration:* Suspend.

Central ray
- Perpendicular to the shoulder joint, entering the coracoid process

Structures shown
This method provides an image of the insertion of the subscapularis at the lesser tubercle (Fig. 5-61).

EVALUATION CRITERIA
The following should be clearly demonstrated:
- Lesser tubercle in profile and pointing inferiorly
- Outline of the greater tubercle superimposing the humeral head
- Soft tissue around the humerus along with trabecular detail on the humeral head

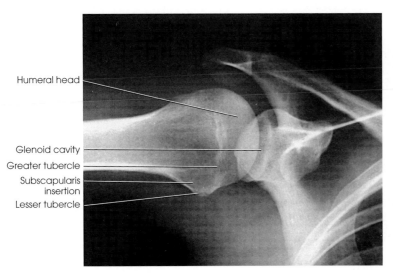

Fig. 5-59 AP proximal humerus for subscapularis insertion.

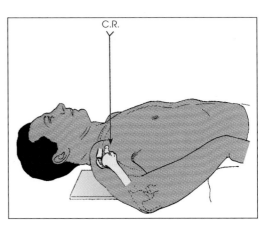

Fig. 5-60 AP proximal humerus for subscapularis insertion.

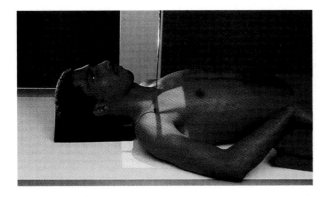
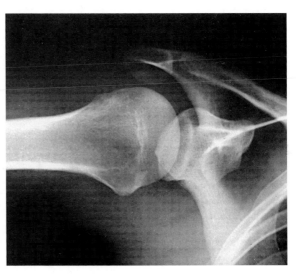

Humeral head
Glenoid cavity
Greater tubercle
Subscapularis insertion
Lesser tubercle

Fig. 5-61 AP proximal humerus for subscapularis insertion.

Shoulder girdle

Infraspinatus Insertion
AP AXIAL PROJECTION

Place the patient in the supine position with the affected arm by the patient's side. Turn the arm in external rotation to open the subacromial space (Fig. 5-62, *A*). Rotate the arm to the neutral position (Fig. 5-62, *B*) and then in complete internal rotation (Fig. 5-62, *C*) to allow full evaluation of the humeral head. Direct the central ray to enter the coracoid process at an angle of 25 degrees caudad. The image profiles the greater tubercle, the site of insertion of the infraspinatus tendon, and opens the subacromial space.

Acromioclavicular Articulations

AP PROJECTION
Bilateral
PEARSON METHOD

Image receptor: 18 × 43 cm (7 × 17 inch) or two 8 × 10 inch (18 × 24 cm), as needed to fit the patient

SID: 72 inches (183 cm). A longer SID reduces magnification, which enables both joints to be included on one image. It also reduces the distortion of the joint space resulting from central ray divergence.

Position of patient
- Place patient in an upright body position, either seated or standing, because dislocation of the acromioclavicular joint tends to reduce itself in the recumbent position. The positioning is easily modified to obtain a PA projection.

Position of part
- Place the patient in the upright position before a vertical grid device, and adjust the height of the cassette so that the midpoint of the cassette lies at the same level as the acromioclavicular joints (Fig. 5-63).
- Center the midline of the body to the midline of the grid.
- Ensure that the weight of the body is equally distributed on the feet to avoid rotation.
- With the patient's arms hanging by the sides, adjust the shoulders to lie in the same horizontal plane. It is important that the arms hang unsupported.
- Make two exposures: one in which the patient is standing upright *without* weights attached, and a second in which the patient has *equal weights* (5 to 8 lb) affixed to each wrist. [1,2]
- After the first exposure, slowly affix the weights to the patient's wrist using a band or strap.
- Instruct the patient not to favor (tense up) the injured shoulder.
- *Avoid having the patient hold weights in each hand;* this tends to make the shoulder muscles contract, thus reducing the possibility of demonstrating a small acromioclavicular separation.
- *Shield gonads.* Also use a thyroid collar, because the thyroid gland is exposed to the primary beam.
- *Respiration:* Suspend.

[1]Allman FL. Fractures and ligamentous injuries of the clavicle and its articulations, *J Bone Joint Surg* 49A:774, 1967.
[2]Rockwood CA, Green DP: *Fractures in adults,* ed 3, Philadelphia, 1991, Lippincott.

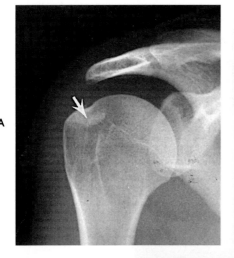
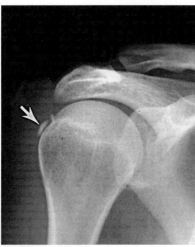
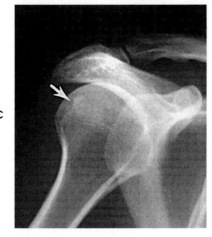

Fig. 5-62 AP axial, 25-degree caudal angulation, demonstrating calcareous peritendinitis *(arrows).* **A,** External rotation. **B,** Neutral position. **C,** Internal rotation.

Acromioclavicular Articulations

Central ray

- Perpendicular to the midline of the body at the level of the acromioclavicular joints for a single projection; directed at each respective acromioclavicular joint when two separate exposures are needed for each shoulder in broad-shouldered patients

COMPUTED RADIOGRAPHY

Collimation must be very close to keep unnecessary radiation from reaching the cassette phosphor.

Structures shown

Bilateral images of the acromioclavicular joints are demonstrated (Figs. 5-64 and 5-65). This projection is used to demonstrate dislocation, separation, and function of the joints.

EVALUATION CRITERIA

The following should be clearly demonstrated:

- Acromioclavicular joints visualized with some soft tissue and without excessive density
- Both acromioclavicular joints, with and without weights, entirely included on one or two single radiographs
- No rotation or leaning by the patient
- Right or left and weight or nonweight markers
- Separation, if done, clearly seen on the images with weights

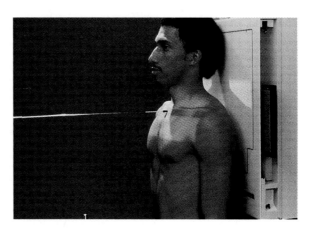

Fig. 5-63 Bilateral AP acromioclavicular articulations.

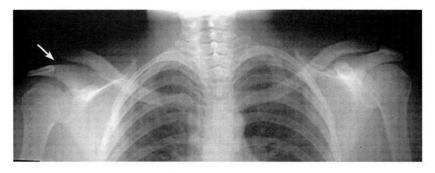

Fig. 5-64 Bilateral AP acromioclavicular joints demonstrating normal left joint and separation of right joint (arrow).

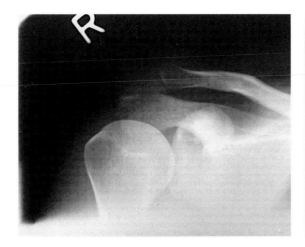
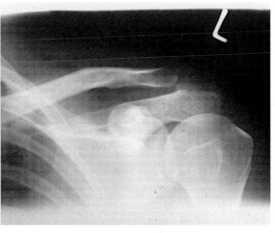

Fig. 5-65 Normal acromioclavicular joints requiring two separate radiographs.

AP AXIAL PROJECTION
ALEXANDER METHOD[1]

Alexander[1] suggested that both AP and PA axial oblique projections be used in cases of suspected acromioclavicular subluxation or dislocation. Each side is examined separately.

Image receptor: 8 × 10 inch (18 × 24 cm) lengthwise

Position of patient
- Place the patient in the upright position, either standing or seated.

[1]Alexander OM: Radiography of the acromioclavicular articulation, *Med Radiogr Photogr* 30:34, 1954.

Position of part
- Have the patient place the back against the vertical grid device and sit or stand upright.
- Center the affected shoulder under examination to the grid.
- Adjust the height of the cassette so that the midpoint of the film is at the level of the acromioclavicular joint.
- Adjust the patient's position to center the coracoid process to the cassette (Fig. 5-66).
- *Shield gonads.*
- *Respiration:* Suspend.

Central ray
- Directed to the coracoid process at a cephalic angle of 15 degrees (Fig. 5-67). This angulation projects the acromioclavicular joint above the acromion.

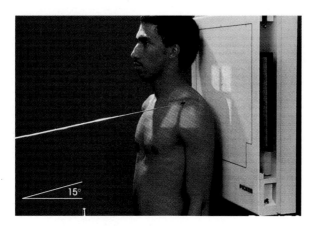

Fig. 5-66 Unilateral AP axial acromioclavicular articulation: Alexander method.

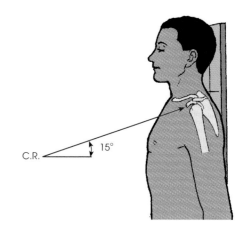

Fig. 5-67 AP axial acromioclavicular articulation: Alexander method.

Acromioclavicular Articulations

Structures shown

The resulting image will show the acromioclavicular joint projected slightly superiorly compared with an AP projection (Fig. 5-68).

The following should be clearly demonstrated:
- Acromioclavicular joint and clavicle projected above the acromion
- Acromioclavicular joint visualized with some soft tissue and without excessive density

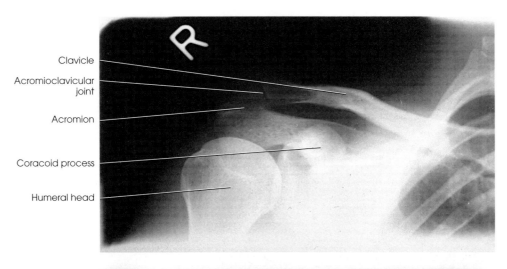

Clavicle
Acromioclavicular joint
Acromion
Coracoid process
Humeral head

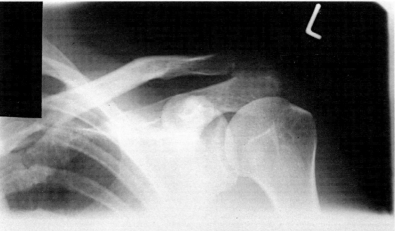

Fig. 5-68 AP axial acromioclavicular articulation: Alexander method.

PA AXIAL OBLIQUE PROJECTION
ALEXANDER METHOD[1]
RAO or LAO position

Image receptor: 8 × 10 inch (18 × 24 cm) lengthwise

[1]Alexander OM: Radiography of the acromioclavicular articulation, *Med Radiogr Photogr* 30:34, 1954.

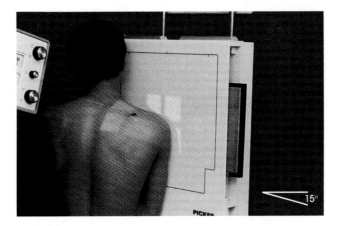

Fig. 5-69 PA axial oblique acromioclavicular articulation.

Position of part
- Stand or sit the patient facing the cassette, and place the hand of the affected side under the opposite axilla.
- Rotate the patient so the midcoronal plane forms an angle of 45 to 60 degrees from the cassette to place the scapula perpendicular to the cassette.
- Adjust the patient's position to center the acromioclavicular joint to the midline of the grid (Fig. 5-69).

- Just before making the exposure, have the patient lean the shoulder being examined against the cassette stand with the arm pulled firmly across the chest. Placing the arm across the chest draws the scapula laterally and forward. Although the projection can be done with the arm at the side, pulling the arm across the chest places the joint as close as possible to the cassette. The scapula and acromioclavicular joint are thus placed in the lateral position.
- *Shield gonads.*
- *Respiration:* Suspend.

Central ray
- Directed through the acromioclavicular joint at an angle of 15 degrees caudad (see Table 5-3)

Structures shown
The PA axial oblique image demonstrates the acromioclavicular joint and the relationship of the bones of the shoulder (Fig. 5-70).

EVALUATION CRITERIA
The following should be clearly demonstrated:
- Acromioclavicular articulation in profile
- Acromioclavicular joint visualized with some soft tissue without excessive density

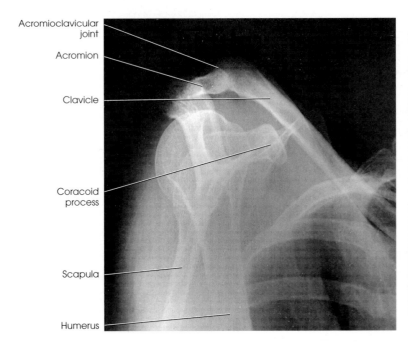

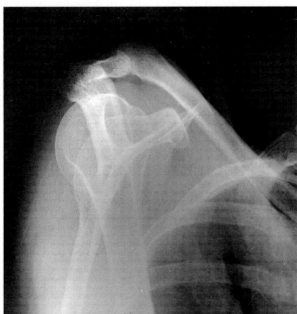

Acromioclavicular joint

Acromion

Clavicle

Coracoid process

Scapula

Humerus

Fig. 5-70 PA axial oblique acromioclavicular articulation.

Clavicle

☀ AP PROJECTION

Image receptor: 24 × 30 cm (10 × 12 inch) crosswise

Position of patient
- Place the patient in the supine or upright position.
- If the clavicle is being examined for a fracture or a destructive disease or if the patient cannot be placed in the upright position, use the supine position to reduce the possibility of fragment displacement or additional injury.

Position of part
- Adjust the body to center the clavicle to the midline of the table or vertical grid device.
- Place the arms along the sides of the body, and adjust the shoulders to lie in the same horizontal plane.
- Center the clavicle to the cassette (Fig. 5-71).
- *Shield gonads.*
- *Respiration:* Suspend at the end of exhalation to obtain a more uniform density image.

Central ray
- Perpendicular to the midshaft of the clavicle

COMPUTED RADIOGRAPHY

Collimation must be very close to keep unnecessary radiation from reaching the cassette phosphor.

Structures shown
This projection demonstrates a frontal image of the clavicle (Fig. 5-72).

EVALUATION CRITERIA
The following should be clearly demonstrated:
- Entire clavicle centered on the image
- Uniform density
- Lateral half of the clavicle above the scapula, with the medial half superimposing the thorax

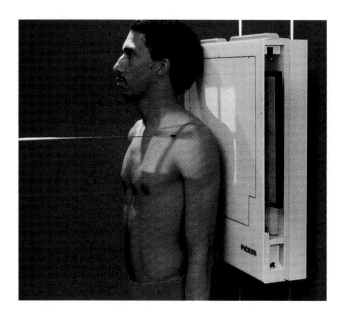

Fig. 5-71 AP clavicle.

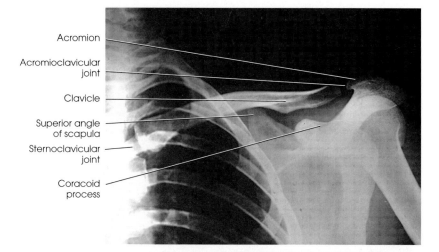

Acromion
Acromioclavicular joint
Clavicle
Superior angle of scapula
Sternoclavicular joint
Coracoid process

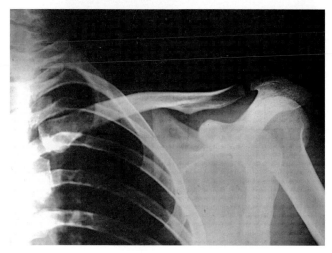

Fig. 5-72 AP clavicle.

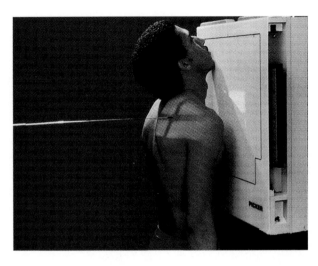

Fig. 5-73 PA clavicle.

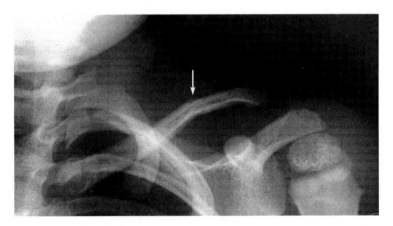

Fig. 5-74 PA clavicle in 3-year-old child showing fracture *(arrow)*. (See Fig. 5-77 for AP axial projection in the same patient.)

🔆 PA PROJECTION

The PA projection is generally well accepted by the patient who is able to stand, and it is most useful when improved recorded detail is desired. The advantage of the PA projection is that the clavicle is closer to the image receptor, thus reducing the OID. Positioning is similar to that of the AP projection. The differences are as follows:

- The patient is standing upright (back toward the x-ray tube) or prone (Fig. 5-73).
- The perpendicular central ray exits midshaft of the clavicle (Fig. 5-74).

Structures shown and evaluation criteria are the same as for the AP projection.

COMPUTED RADIOGRAPHY

Collimation must be very close to keep unnecessary radiation from reaching the cassette phosphor.

✹ AP AXIAL PROJECTION
Lordotic position

NOTE: If the patient is injured or unable to assume the lordotic position, a slightly distorted image results when the tube is angled. An optional approach for improved recorded detail is the PA axial projection.

Image receptor: 24 × 30 cm (10 × 12 inch) crosswise

Position of patient
- Stand or seat the patient 1 foot in front of the vertical cassette device, with the patient facing the x-ray tube.
- Alternatively, if the patient is unable to stand and assume the lordotic position, place the patient supine on the table.

Position of part
Standing lordotic position
- Temporarily support the patient in the lordotic position to estimate the required central ray angulation, and have the patient reassume the upright position while the equipment is adjusted.

- Have the patient lean backward in a position of extreme lordosis, and rest the neck and shoulder against the vertical grid device. The neck will be in extreme flexion (Figs. 5-75 and 5-76).
- Center the clavicle to the center of the cassette (see Fig. 5-76).
Supine position
- Center the cassette to the clavicle.
- *Shield gonads.*
- *Respiration:* Suspend at the end of full inspiration to further elevate and angle the clavicle.

Central ray
- Directed to enter the midshaft of the clavicle.
- Cephalic central ray angulation can vary from the long axis of the torso. Thinner patients require more angulation to project the clavicle off the scapula and ribs.

- For the *standing lordotic position,* 0 to 15 degrees is recommended (see Fig. 5-75).
- For the *supine position,* 15 to 30 degrees is recommended (see Fig. 5-76).

COMPUTED RADIOGRAPHY

Collimation must be very close to keep unnecessary radiation from reaching the cassette phosphor.

Structures shown
An axial image of the clavicle is projected above the ribs (Fig. 5-77).

EVALUATION CRITERIA
The following should be clearly demonstrated:
- Most of the clavicle projected above the ribs and scapula with the medial end overlapping the first or second rib
- Clavicle in a horizontal placement
- Entire clavicle along with the acromioclavicular and sternoclavicular joints

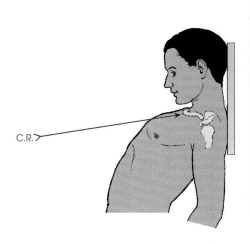
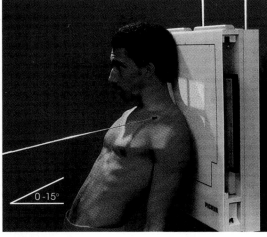

Fig. 5-75 AP axial clavicle, lordotic position.

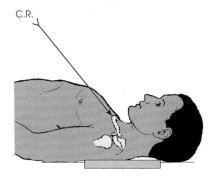

Fig. 5-76 AP axial clavicle.

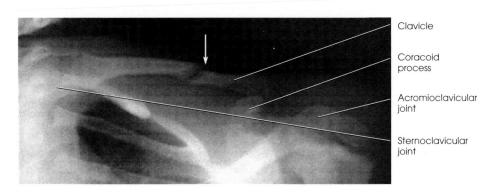

Fig. 5-77 AP axial clavicle of 3-year-old child, showing fracture *(arrow).* This is the same patient as Fig. 5-74.

197

🔻 PA AXIAL PROJECTION

Positioning of the PA axial clavicle is similar to the AP axial projection just described. The differences are as follows:
- The patient is prone or standing, facing the vertical grid device.
- The central ray is angled 15 to 30 degrees caudad. (Fig. 5-78).

Structures shown and evaluation criteria are the same as for the AP axial projection described previously.

COMPUTED RADIOGRAPHY

Collimation must be very close to keep unnecessary radiation from reaching the cassette phosphor.

TANGENTIAL PROJECTION

The tangential projection is similar to the AP axial projection described previously. However, the increased angulation of the central ray required for this approach places the central ray nearly parallel with the rib cage. The clavicle is thus projected free of the chest wall.

Image receptor: 8 × 10 inch (18 × 24 cm) crosswise

Position of patient
- With the patient in the supine position, place the arms along the sides of the body.

Position of part
- If possible, depress the shoulder to place the clavicle in a horizontal plane
- Have the patient turn the head away from the side being examined.
- Place the cassette on edge at the top of the shoulder and support it in position. The cassette should be as close to the neck as possible (Figs. 5-79 and 5-80).
- *Shield gonads.*
- *Respiration:* Suspend.

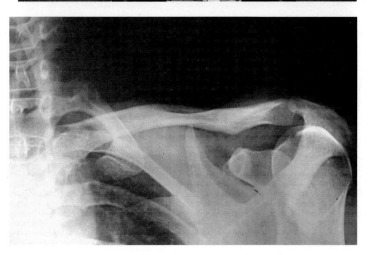

Fig. 5-78 PA axial clavicle.

Central ray

- Angled so that the central ray will pass between the clavicle and the chest wall, perpendicular to the plane of the cassette. The angulation will be about 25 to 40 degrees from the *horizontal.*
- If the medial third of the clavicle is in question, it is also necessary to angle the central ray laterally; 15 to 25 degrees is usually sufficient.

Structures shown

An inferosuperior image of the clavicle is demonstrated, projected free of superimposition (Fig. 5-81).

EVALUATION CRITERIA

The following should be clearly demonstrated:

- Midclavicle without superimposition
- Acromial and sternal ends superimposed
- Entire clavicle along with the acromioclavicular and sternoclavicular joints

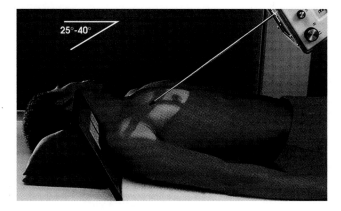

Fig. 5-79 Tangential clavicle.

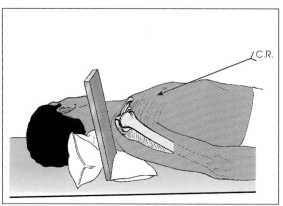

Fig. 5-80 Tangential alignment for clavicle.

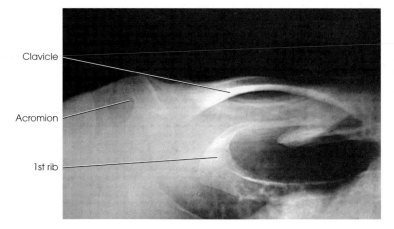
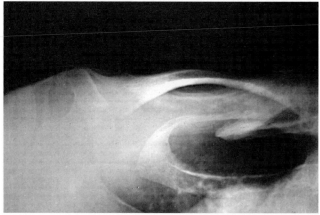

Clavicle

Acromion

1st rib

Fig. 5-81 Tangential clavicle.

TANGENTIAL PROJECTION
TARRANT METHOD[1]

The Tarrant method is particularly useful with patients who have multiple injuries or who cannot assume the lordotic or recumbent position.

Image receptor: 24 × 30 cm (10 × 12 inch) crosswise

Position of patient
- Place the patient in a seated position.

[1]Tarrant RM: The axial view of the clavicle, *Xray Techn* 21:358, 1950.

Position of part
- Adjust a sheet of leaded rubber over the gonad area. A folded pillow or blankets may be placed on the patient's lap to support the horizontally placed cassette if needed.
- Using the collimator light as the indicator, center the cassette to the projected clavicle area, and have the patient hold the cassette in position.
- Ask the patient to lean slightly forward (Fig. 5-82).
- *Shield gonads.*
- *Respiration:* Suspend.

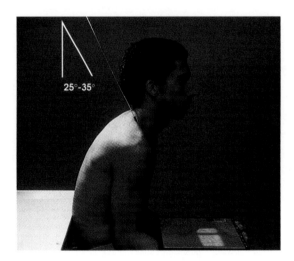

Fig. 5-82 Tangential clavicle: Tarrant method.

Central ray

- Directed anterior and inferior to the midshaft of the clavicle at a 25- to 35-degree angle. It should pass perpendicular to the longitudinal axis of the clavicle.
- Because of the considerable OID, an increased SID is recommended to reduce magnification.

Structures shown

The clavicle above the thoracic cage is demonstrated (Fig. 5-83).

EVALUATION CRITERIA

The following should be clearly demonstrated:

- Most of the clavicle above the ribs and scapula with the medial end overlapping the first or second ribs
- Clavicle in a horizontal orientation
- Entire clavicle along with the acromioclavicular and sternoclavicular joints

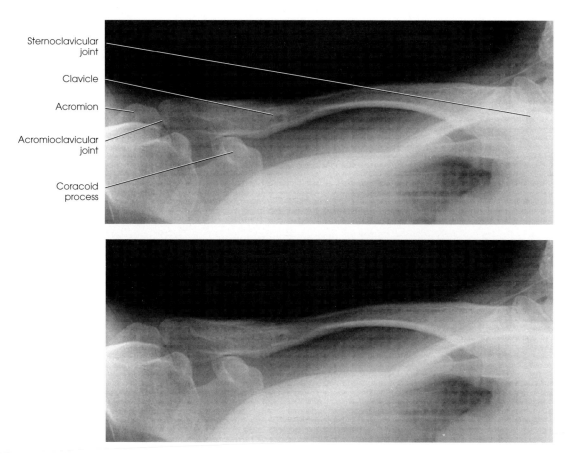

Sternoclavicular joint

Clavicle

Acromion

Acromioclavicular joint

Coracoid process

Fig. 5-83 Tangential clavicle: Tarrant method.

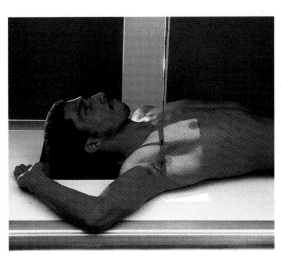

Fig. 5-84 AP scapula.

▲ AP PROJECTION

Image receptor: 24 × 30 cm (10 × 12 inch) lengthwise

Position of patient
- Place the patient in the upright or supine position. The upright position is preferred if the shoulder is tender.

Position of part
- Adjust the patient's body, and center the affected scapula to the midline of the grid.
- Abduct the arm to a right angle with the body to draw the scapula laterally. Then flex the elbow, and support the hand in a comfortable position.
- For this projection, do not rotate the body toward the affected side because the resultant obliquity would offset the effect of drawing the scapula laterally (Fig. 5-84).
- Position the top of the cassette 2 inches (5 cm) above the top of the shoulder.
- *Shield gonads.*
- *Respiration:* Make this exposure during slow breathing to obliterate lung detail.

Central ray

• Perpendicular to the midscapular area at a point approximately 2 inches (5 cm) inferior to the coracoid process

Structures shown

An AP projection of the scapula is demonstrated (Fig. 5-85).

EVALUATION CRITERIA

The following should be clearly demonstrated:

■ Lateral portion of the scapula free of superimposition from the ribs
■ Scapula horizontal and not obliqued
■ Scapular detail through the superimposed lung and ribs (Shallow breathing should help obliterate lung detail.)
■ Acromion process and inferior angle

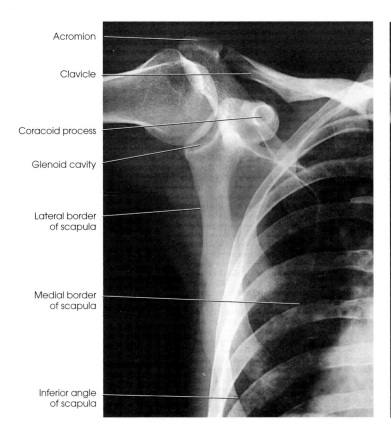
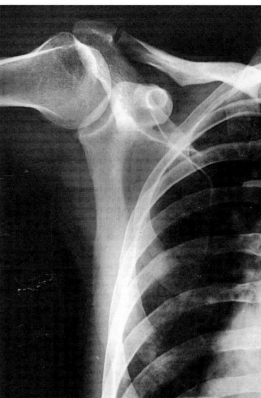

Acromion

Clavicle

Coracoid process

Glenoid cavity

Lateral border of scapula

Medial border of scapula

Inferior angle of scapula

Fig. 5-85 AP scapula.

⚡ LATERAL PROJECTION
RAO or LAO body position

Image receptor: 24 × 30 cm (10 × 12 inch) lengthwise

Position of patient
- Place the patient in the upright position, standing or seated, facing a vertical grid device.
- The prone position can be used, but the projection will be more difficult to perform. The supine position can also be used; however, the scapula will be magnified.

Position of part
- Adjust the patient in an RAO or LAO position, with the affected scapula centered to the grid. The average patient requires a 45- to 60-degree rotation from the plane of the cassette.
- Place the arm in one of two positions according to the area of the scapula to be demonstrated:
  - For delineation of the *acromion* and *coracoid processes* of the scapula, have the patient flex the elbow and place the hand on the posterior thorax at a level sufficient to prevent the humerus from overlapping the scapula (Figs. 5-86 and 5-87). Mazujian[1] suggested that the patient place the arm across the upper chest by grasping the opposite shoulder as shown in Fig. 5-88.
  - For demonstration of the *body* of the scapula, ask the patient to extend the arm upward and rest the forearm on the head or across the upper chest by grasping the opposite shoulder. (Figs. 5-88 and 5-89).

---

[1]Mazujian M: Lateral profile view of the scapula, *Xray Techn* 25:24, 1953.

- After placing the arm in any of the above positions, grasp the lateral and medial borders of the scapula between the thumb and index fingers of one hand. Make a final adjustment of the body rotation, placing the body of the scapula perpendicular to the plane of the cassette.
- *Shield gonads.*
- *Respiration:* Suspend.

Central ray
- Perpendicular to the midmedial border of the protruding scapula (see Table 5-3)

COMPUTED RADIOGRAPHY

Collimation must be very close to keep unnecessary radiation from reaching the cassette phosphor.

Structures shown
A lateral image of the scapula is demonstrated by this projection. The placement of the arm determines the portion of the superior scapula that is superimposed over the humerus.

EVALUATION CRITERIA
The following should be clearly demonstrated:
- Lateral and medial borders superimposed
- No superimposition of the scapular body on the ribs
- No superimposition of the humerus on the area of interest
- Inclusion of the acromion process and inferior angle
- Lateral thickness of scapula with proper density

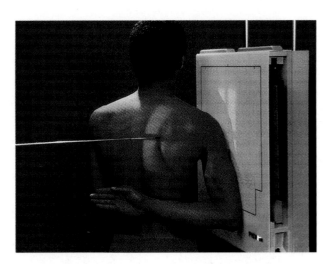

Fig. 5-86 Lateral scapula, RAO body position.

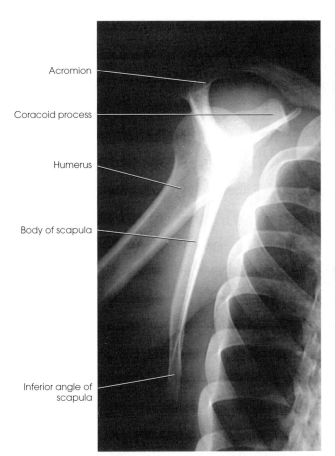

Acromion

Coracoid process

Humerus

Body of scapula

Inferior angle of scapula

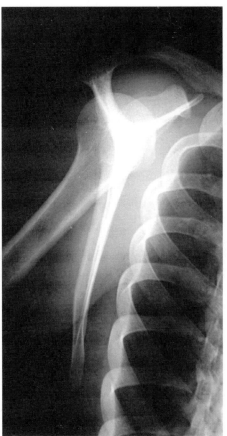

Fig. 5-87 Lateral scapula with arm on posterior chest.

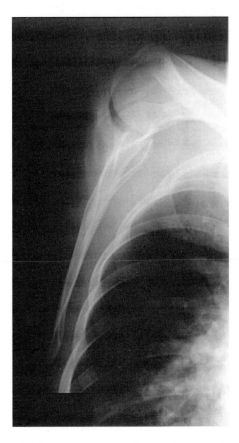

Fig. 5-88 Lateral scapula with arm across upper anterior thorax.

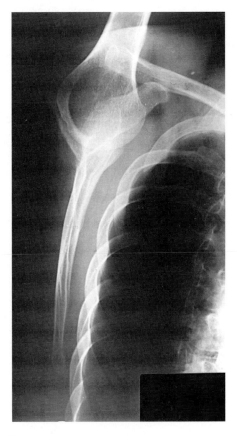

Fig. 5-89 Lateral scapula with arm extended above head.

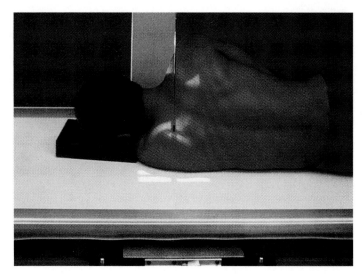

Fig. 5-90 PA oblique scapula: Lorenz method.

PA OBLIQUE PROJECTION
LORENZ AND LILIENFELD METHODS
RAO or LAO position

Image receptor: 24 × 30 cm (10 × 12 inch) lengthwise

Position of patient
- Place the patient in the upright or lateral recumbent position.
- When the shoulder is painful, use the upright position if possible.

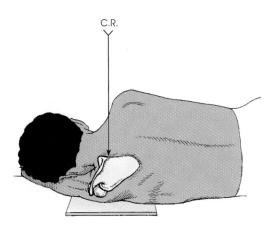

Fig. 5-91 PA oblique scapula: Lilienfeld method.

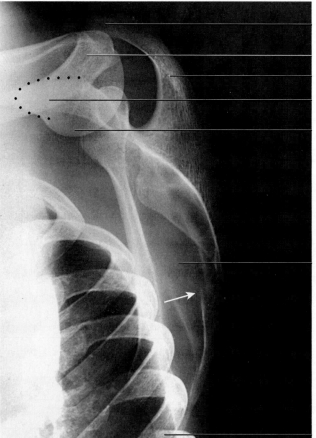

Acromioclavicular joint

Clavicle

Acromion

Coracoid process

Humeral head

Body of scapula

Inferior angle of scapula

Fig. 5-92 Lorenz method with scapula showing fracture *(arrow)*.

Position of part

- With the patient in the lateral position, upright or recumbent, align the body and center the scapula to the midline of the grid device.
- Adjust the arm according to the projection desired.

Lorenz method

- Adjust the arm of the affected side at a right angle to the long axis of the body, flex the elbow, and rest the hand against the patient's head.
- Rotate the body slightly forward, and have the patient grasp the side of the table or the stand for support (Fig. 5-90).

Lilienfeld method

- Extend the arm of the affected side obliquely upward, and have the patient rest the hand on his or her head.
- Rotate the body slightly forward, and have the patient grasp the side of the table or the stand for support (Fig. 5-91).

Both methods

- Grasp the lateral and medial borders of the scapula between the thumb and index fingers of one hand, and adjust the rotation of the body so that the scapula will be projected free of the rib cage.
- *Shield gonads.*
- *Respiration:* Suspend.

Central ray

- Perpendicular to the cassette, between the chest wall and the midarea of the protruding scapula

Structures shown

An oblique image of the scapula is shown. The degree of obliquity depends on the position of the arm. The delineation of the different parts of the bone in the two oblique projections are shown in Figs. 5-92 and 5-93.

EVALUATION CRITERIA

The following should be clearly demonstrated:

- Oblique scapula
- Medial border adjacent to the ribs
- Acromion process and inferior angle

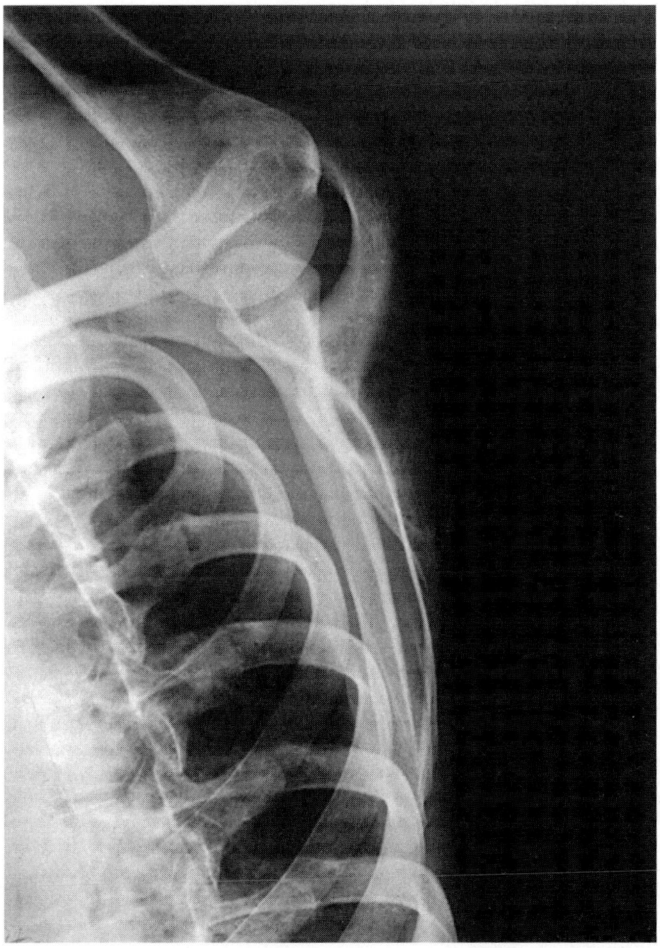

Fig. 5-93 PA oblique scapula: Lilienfeld method.

AP OBLIQUE PROJECTION
RPO or LPO position

Image receptor: 24 × 30 cm (10 × 12 inch) lengthwise

Position of patient
- Place the patient in the supine or upright position.
- Use the upright position when the shoulder is painful unless contraindicated.

Position of part
- Align the body and center the affected scapula to the midline of the grid.
- For moderate AP oblique projection, ask the patient to extend the arm superiorly, flex the elbow, and place the supinated hand under the head or have the patient extend the affected arm across the anterior chest.
- Have the patient turn away from the affected side enough to rotate the shoulder 15 to 25 degrees (Fig. 5-94).
- For a steeper oblique projection, ask the patient to extend the arm, rest the flexed elbow on the forehead, and rotate the body *away* from the affected side 25 to 35 degrees (Fig. 5-95).
- Grasp the lateral and medial borders of the scapula between the thumb and index fingers of one hand, and adjust the rotation of the body to project the scapula free of the rib cage.
- For a direct lateral projection of the scapula using this position, draw the arm across the chest, and adjust the body rotation to place the scapula perpendicular to the plane of the cassette as previously described and shown in Figs. 5-86 to 5-89.
- *Shield gonads.*
- *Respiration:* Suspend.

Central ray
- Perpendicular to the lateral border of the rib cage at the midscapular area

Structures shown
This projection shows oblique images of the scapula, projected free or nearly free of rib superimposition (Figs. 5-96 to 5-97).

EVALUATION CRITERIA
The following should be clearly demonstrated:
- Oblique scapula
- Lateral border adjacent to the ribs
- Acromion process and inferior angle

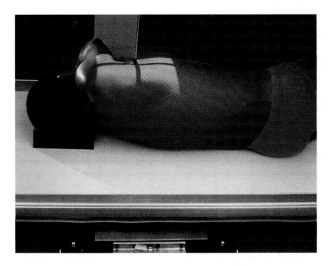

Fig. 5-94 AP oblique scapula, 20-degree body rotation.

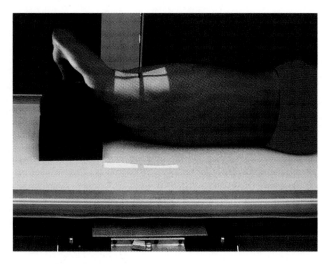

Fig. 5-95 AP oblique scapula, 35-degree body rotation.

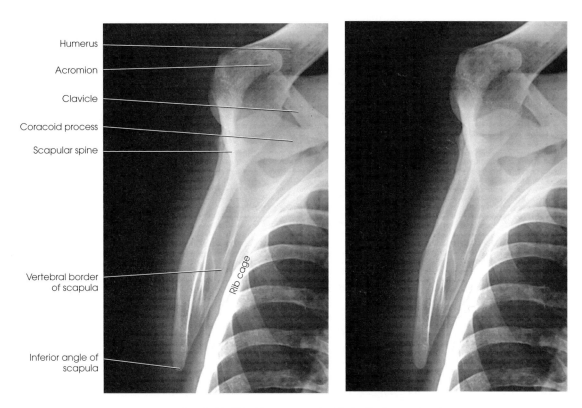

Humerus
Acromion
Clavicle
Coracoid process
Scapular spine
Vertebral border of scapula
Rib cage
Inferior angle of scapula

Fig. 5-96 AP oblique scapula, 15- to 25-degree body rotation.

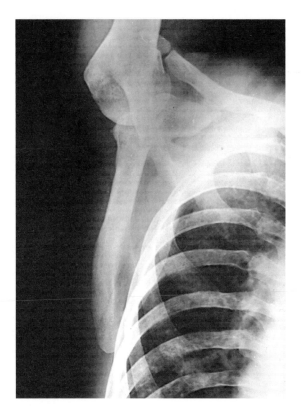

Fig. 5-97 AP oblique scapula, 25- to 30-degree body rotation.

Coracoid Process
AP AXIAL PROJECTION

Image receptor: 24 × 30 cm (10 × 12 inch) crosswise

Position of patient
• Place the patient in the supine position with the arms along the sides of the body.

Position of part
• Adjust the position of the body, and center the affected coracoid process to the midline of the grid.
• Position the cassette so that the midpoint of the cassette will coincide with the central ray.
• Adjust the shoulders to lie in the same horizontal plane.
• Abduct the arm of the affected side slightly, and supinate the hand, immobilizing it with a sandbag across the palm (Fig. 5-98).
• *Shield gonads.*
• *Respiration:* Suspend at the end of exhalation for a more uniform density.

Central ray
• Directed to enter the coracoid process at an angle of 15 to 45 degrees cephalad. Kwak, Espiniella, and Kattan[1] recommend 30 degrees. The degree of angulation depends on the shape of the patient's back. Round-shouldered patients require a greater angulation than those with a straight back (Fig. 5-99).

Structures shown
A slightly elongated inferosuperior image of the coracoid process is illustrated (Fig. 5-100). Because the coracoid is curved on itself, it casts a small, oval shadow in the direct AP projection of the shoulder.

EVALUATION CRITERIA
The following should be clearly demonstrated:
■ Coracoid process with minimal self-superimposition
■ Clavicle slightly superimposing the coracoid process

[1]Kwak DL, Espiniella JL, Kattan KR: Angled anteroposterior views of the shoulder, *Radiol Technol* 53:590, 1982.

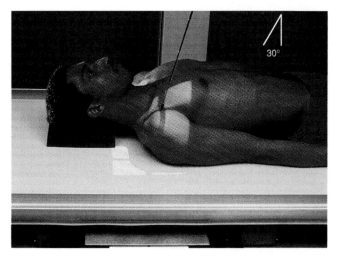

Fig. 5-98 AP axial coracoid process.

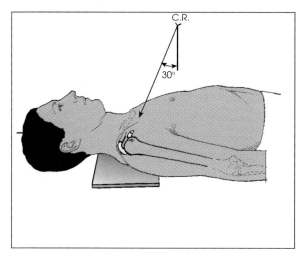

Fig. 5-99 AP axial coracoid process.

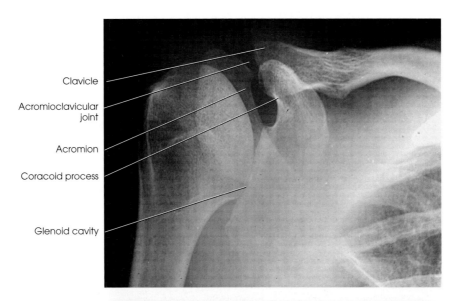

Clavicle

Acromioclavicular
joint

Acromion

Coracoid process

Glenoid cavity

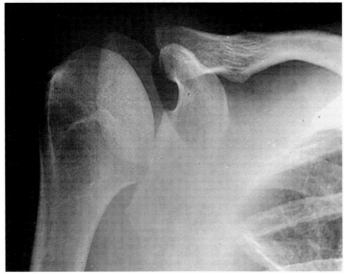

Fig. 5-100 AP axial coracoid process.

Shoulder girdle

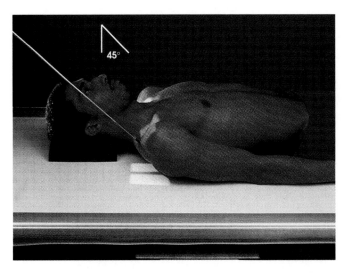

Fig. 5-101 Tangential scapular spine.

TANGENTIAL PROJECTION
LAQUERRIÈRE-PIERQUIN
METHOD[1]

Image receptor: 8 × 10 inch (18 × 24 cm) crosswise

Position of patient
• As described by Laquerrière and Pierquin,[1] place the patient in the supine position.

Position of part
• Center the shoulder to the midline of the grid.
• Adjust the patient's rotation to place the body of the scapula in a horizontal position. When this requires elevation of the opposite shoulder, support it on sandbags or radiolucent sponges.
• Turn the head away from the shoulder being examined enough to prevent superimposition (Fig. 5-101).
• Funke[2] found that in the examination of patients with small breasts, clavicular superimposition can be prevented by using a 15-degree radiolucent wedge to angle the shoulder caudally.
• *Shield gonads.*
• *Respiration:* Suspend.

[1]Laquerrière and Pierquin: De la nécessité d'employer une technique radiographique spéciale pour obtenir certains details squelettiques, *J Radiol Electr* 3:145, 1918.
[2]Funke T: Tangential view of the scapular spine, *Med Radiogr Photogr* 34:41, 1958.

Scapular Spine

Central ray

- Directed through the posterosuperior region of the shoulder at an angle of 45 degrees caudad. A 35-degree angulation suffices for obese and round-shouldered patients.
- After adjusting the x-ray tube, position the cassette so that it is centered to the central ray.

Structures shown

The spine of the scapula is shown in profile and is free of bony superimposition, except for the lateral end of the clavicle (Figs. 5-102 and 5-103).

EVALUATION CRITERIA

The following should be clearly demonstrated:

- Scapular spine superior to the scapular body
- Scapular spine with some soft tissue around it and without excessive density

NOTE: When the shoulder is too painful to tolerate the supine position, this projection can be obtained with the patient in the prone or upright position, as described on the following page.

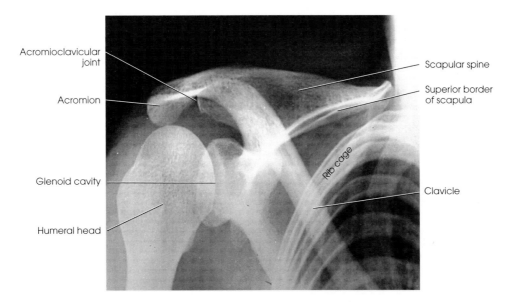

Fig. 5-102 Tangential scapular spine with 45-degree central ray angulation.

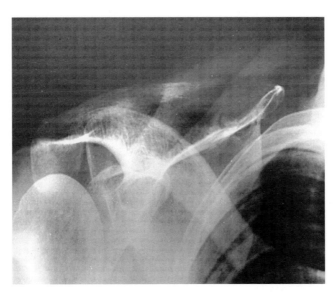

Fig. 5-103 Tangential scapular spine image with 30-degree central ray angulation.

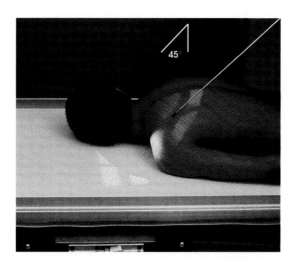

Fig. 5-104 Prone tangential scapular spine.

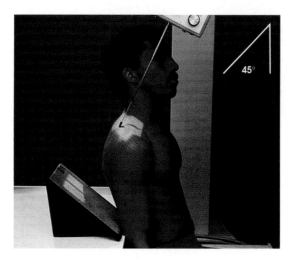

Fig. 5-105 Upright tangential scapular spine.

TANGENTIAL PROJECTION
Prone position

Image receptor: 8 × 10 inch (18 × 24 cm) crosswise

Position of part
- Place the patient in the prone position, and center the shoulder to the midline of the grid.
- Place the arms along the sides of the body, and adjust the shoulders to lie in the same horizontal plane.
- Take care to prevent lateral rotation of the scapula.
- Have the patient rest the head on the chin or the cheek of the affected side.
- Supinate the hand of the affected side (Fig. 5-104).
- Adjust a radiolucent wedge under the side of the shoulder and upper arm to place the scapula in the horizontal position.
- *Shield gonads.*
- *Respiration:* Suspend.

Central ray
- Direct through the scapular spine at an angle of 45 degrees cephalad. The central ray exits at the anterosuperior aspect of the shoulder.

Upright position
An increased SID is recommended because of the greater OID.

Position of part
- Seat the patient with his or her back toward and resting against the end of the table.
- Place the cassette on the table, center it in line with the shoulder, and adjust the cassette on a support to place it at an angle of 45 degrees (Fig. 5-105).
- *Shield gonads.*
- *Respiration:* Suspend.

Scapular Spine

Central ray

- Directed through the anterosuperior aspect of the shoulder at a posteroinferior angle of 45 degrees
- Perpendicular to the plane of the cassette

Structures shown

The tangential image shows the scapular spine in profile and free of superimposition of the scapular body (Figs. 5-106 and 5-107).

EVALUATION CRITERIA

The following should be clearly demonstrated:

- Scapular spine above the scapular wing
- Scapular spine with some soft tissue around it and without excessive density

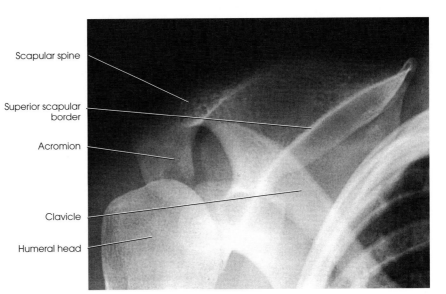

Scapular spine
Superior scapular border
Acromion
Clavicle
Humeral head

Fig. 5-106 Prone tangential scapular spine.

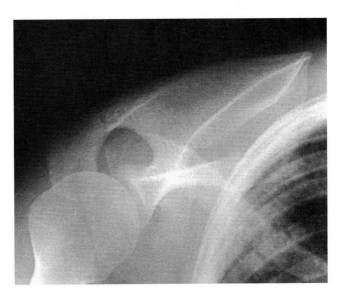

Fig. 5-107 Upright tangential scapular spine.

6

LOWER LIMB

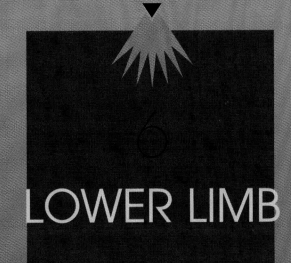

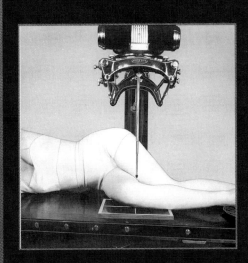

RIGHT Lateral knee showing 5-degree cephalic angulation, 1949.

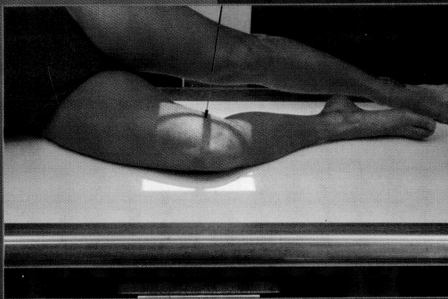

LEFT Lateral knee showing 5-degree cephalic angulation, 1999.

SUMMARY OF PROJECTIONS

PROJECTIONS, POSITIONS & METHODS

Page	Essential	Anatomy	Projection	Position	Method
230	▲	Toes	AP or AP axial		
232		Toes	PA		
233	▲	Toes	AP oblique	Medial rotation	
234		Toes	PA oblique	Medial rotation	
235	▲	Toes	Lateral (mediolateral or lateromedial)		
238		Sesamoids	Tangential		LEWIS and HOLLY
240		Sesamoids	Tangential		CAUSTON
242	▲	Foot	AP or AP axial		
244	▲	Foot	AP oblique	Medial rotation	
246		Foot	AP oblique	Lateral rotation	
248		Foot	PA oblique	Medial or lateral rotation	GRASHEY
250		Foot	PA oblique	Medial rotation	
251	▲	Foot	Lateral (mediolateral)		
252		Foot	Lateral (lateromedial)		
254		Foot: *longitudinal arch*	Lateral (lateromedial)	Standing	WEIGHT-BEARING
256		Feet	AP axial	Standing	WEIGHT-BEARING
257		Foot	AP axial	Standing	WEIGHT-BEARING COMPOSITE
259		Foot: *congenital clubfoot*	AP		KITE
260		Foot: *congenital clubfoot*	Lateral (mediolateral)		KITE
262		Foot: *congenital clubfoot*	Axial (dorsoplantar)		KANDEL
263	▲	Calcaneus	Axial (plantodorsal)		
264		Calcaneus	Axial (dorsoplantar)		
265		Calcaneus	Axial (dorsoplantar)	Standing	WEIGHT-BEARING
266	▲	Calcaneus	Lateral (mediolateral)		
267		Calcaneus	Lateromedial oblique		WEIGHT-BEARING
268		Subtalar joint	PA axial oblique	Lateral rotation	
269		Subtalar joint	AP axial oblique	Medial rotation	BRODEN
271		Subtalar joint	AP axial oblique	Lateral rotation	BRODEN
272		Subtalar joint	Lateromedial oblique	Medial rotation foot	ISHERWOOD
273		Subtalar joint	AP axial oblique	Medial rotation ankle	ISHERWOOD
274		Subtalar joint	AP axial oblique	Lateral rotation ankle	ISHERWOOD
275	▲	Ankle	AP		
276	▲	Ankle	Lateral (mediolateral)		
278		Ankle	Lateral (lateromedial)		

The icons in the Essential column indicate projections that are frequently performed in the United States and Canada. Students should be competent in these projections.

PROJECTIONS, POSITIONS & METHODS

Page	Essential	Anatomy	Projection	Position	Method
279	♠	Ankle	AP oblique	Medial rotation	
280	♠	Ankle: *mortise joint*	AP oblique	Medial rotation	
282		Ankle	AP oblique	Lateral rotation	
283	♠	Ankle	AP		STRESS
284	♠	Leg	AP		
286	♠	Leg	Lateral (mediolateral)		
288		Leg	AP oblique	Medial and lateral rotations	
290	♠	Knee	AP		
292		Knee	PA		
293	♠	Knee	Lateral (mediolateral)		
294	♠	Knees	AP	Standing	WEIGHT-BEARING
295		Knees	PA	Standing flexion	WEIGHT-BEARING
296	♠	Knee	AP oblique	Lateral rotation	
297	♠	Knee	AP oblique	Medial rotation	
298		Knee	PA oblique	Lateral rotation	
299		Knee	PA oblique	Medial rotation	
300	♠	Intercondylar fossa	PA axial		HOLMBLAD
302	♠	Intercondylar fossa	PA axial		CAMP-COVENTRY
304		Intercondylar fossa	AP axial		BÉCLÈRE
306	♠	Patella	PA		
307	♠	Patella	Lateral (mediolateral)		
308		Patella	PA oblique	Medial rotation	
309		Patella	PA oblique	Lateral rotation	
310		Patella	PA axial oblique	Lateral rotation	KUCHENDORF
311		Patella and patellofemoral joint	Tangential		HUGHSTON
312		Patella and patellofemoral joint	Tangential		MERCHANT
314	♠	Patella and patellofemoral joint	Tangential		SETTEGAST
316	♠	Femur	AP		
318	♠	Femur	Lateral (mediolateral)		
320		Lower limbs: *hips, knees, and ankles*	AP	Standing	WEIGHT-BEARING

The lower limb, or extremity, and its girdle (considered in Chapter 7) are studied in four parts: (1) foot, (2) leg, (3) thigh, and (4) hip. The bones are composed, shaped, and placed so that they can carry the body in the upright position and transmit its weight to the ground with a minimal amount of stress to the individual parts.

Foot

The *foot* consists of 26 bones (Figs. 6-1 and 6-2):
- 14 phalanges (bones of the toes)
- 5 metatarsals (bones of the instep)
- 7 tarsals (bones of the ankle)

The bones of the foot are similar to those in the hand. The structural differences, however, permit walking and support of the body's weight. For descriptive purposes the foot is sometimes divided into the forefoot, midfoot, and hindfoot. The forefoot includes the metatarsals and toes. The midfoot includes five tarsals— the cuneiforms, navicular, and cuboid bones. The hindfoot includes the talus and calcaneus. The bones of the foot are shaped and joined together to form a series of longitudinal and transverse arches. The longitudinal arch functions as a shock absorber to distribute the weight of the body in all directions, which permits smooth walking (see Fig. 6-2). The transverse arch runs from side to side and assists in supporting the longitudinal arch. The superior surface of the foot is termed the *dorsum* or *dorsal surface,* and the inferior, or posterior, aspect of the foot is termed the *plantar surface.*

PHALANGES

Each foot has 14 *phalanges*— two in the great toe and three in each of the other toes. The phalanges of the great toe are termed the *distal* and *proximal phalanges.* Those of the other toes are termed the *proximal, middle,* and *distal phalanges.* Each phalanx is composed of a *body* and two expanded articular ends— the proximal *base* and the distal *head.*

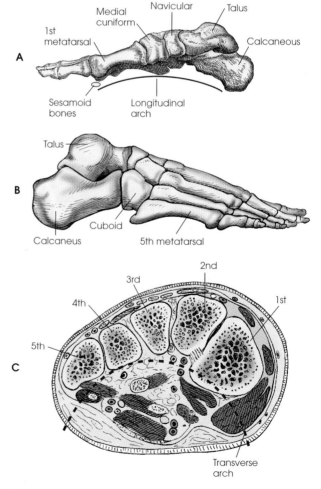

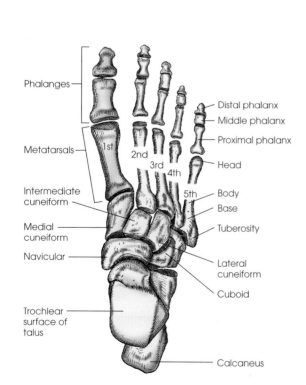

Fig. 6-1 Dorsal (superior) aspect of right foot.

Fig. 6-2 Right foot. **A**, Medial aspect. **B**, Lateral aspect. **C**, Coronal section near base of metatarsals. Transverse arch shown.

METATARSALS

The five *metatarsals* are numbered one to five beginning at the medial or great toe side of the foot. The metatarsals consist of a *body* and two articular ends. The expanded proximal end is called the *base,* and the small, rounded distal end is termed the *head.* The five heads form the "ball" of the foot. The first metatarsal is the shortest and thickest. The second metatarsal is the longest. The base of the fifth metatarsal contains a prominent *tuberosity,* which is a common site of fractures.

TARSALS

The ankle contains seven *tarsals* (see Fig. 6-1):
• Calcaneus
• Talus
• Navicular bone
• Cuboid
• Medial cuneiform
• Intermediate cuneiform
• Lateral cuneiform

Beginning at the medial side of the foot, the cuneiforms are described as *medial, intermediate,* and *lateral.*

The *calcaneus* is the largest and strongest tarsal bone (Fig. 6-3). It projects posteriorly and medially at the distal part of the foot. The long axis of the calcaneus is directed inferiorly and forms an angle of approximately 30 degrees. The posterior and inferior portions of the calcaneus contain the posterior *tuberosity* for attachment of the Achilles tendon. Superiorly, three articular facets join with the talus. They are called the *anterior, middle,* and *posterior facets.* Between the middle and posterior talar articular facets is a groove, the *calcaneal sulcus,* which corresponds to a similar groove on the inferior surface of the talus. Collectively these sulci comprise the *sinus tarsi.* The medial aspect of the calcaneus extends outward as a shelflike overhang and is termed the *sustentaculum tali.* The lateral surface of the calcaneus contains the *trochlea.*

The *talus,* irregular in form and occupying the most superior position of the foot, is the second largest of the tarsal bones (see Figs. 6-1 and 6-2). The talus articulates with four bones—the tibia, fibula, calcaneus, and navicular bone. The superior surface, the *trochlear surface,* articulates with the tibia. The head of the talus is directed anteriorly and has articular surfaces that join the navicular bone and calcaneus. On the inferior surface is a groove, the *sulcus tali,* that forms the roof of the sinus tarsi. Posterior to the sinus tali is the posterior articular surface for articulation with the calcaneus.

The *cuboid* bone lies on the lateral side of the foot between the calcaneus and the fourth and fifth metatarsals (see Fig. 6-1). The *navicular* bone lies on the medial side of the foot between the talus and the three cuneiforms. The *cuneiforms* lie at the central and medial aspect of the foot between the navicular bone and the first, second, and third metatarsals. The *medial* cuneiform is the largest of the three cuneiform bones, and the *intermediate* is the smallest.

The seven tarsals can be remembered using the following mnemonic:

Chubby	Calcaneus
Twisted,	Talus
Never	Navicular
Could	Cuboid
Cha	Cuneiform—medial
Cha	Cuneiform—intermediate
Cha	Cuneiform—lateral

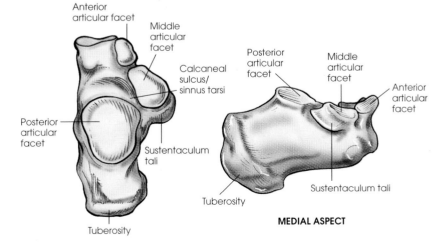

Fig. 6-3 Articular surfaces of right calcaneus.

SESAMOID BONES

Beneath the head of the first metatarsal are two small bones called *sesamoid* bones. They are detached from the foot and embedded within two tendons. These bones are seen on most adult foot radiographs. They are a common site of fractures and must be demonstrated radiographically (see Fig. 6-2).

Leg

The leg has two bones: the *tibia* and *fibula*. The tibia, the second largest bone in the body, is situated on the medial side of the leg. Slightly posterior to the tibia on the lateral side of the leg is the fibula.

TIBIA

The *tibia* (Fig. 6-4) is the larger of the two bones of the leg and consists of one *body* and two expanded extremities. The proximal end of the tibia has two prominent processes—the *medial* and *lateral condyles.* The superior surfaces of the condyles form smooth facets for articulation with the condyles of the femur. These two flatlike superior surfaces are called the *tibial plateaus,* and they slope posteriorly about 10 to 20 degrees. Between the two articular surfaces is a sharp projection, the *intercondylar eminence,* which terminates in two peaklike processes called the *medial* and *lateral intercondylar tubercles.* The lateral condyle has a facet at its distal posterior surface for articulation with the *head* of the fibula. On the anterior surface of the tibia, just below the condyles, is a prominent process called the *tibial tuberosity,* to which the ligamentum patellae attaches. Extending along the anterior surface of the tibial body, beginning at the tuberosity, is a sharp ridge called the *anterior crest.*

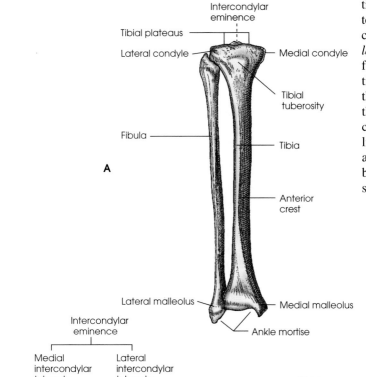

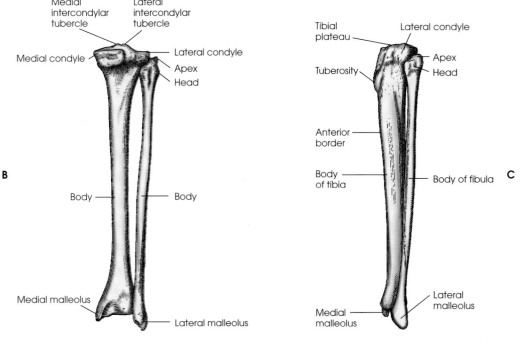

Fig. 6-4 Right tibia and fibula. **A,** Anterior aspect. **B,** Posterior aspect. **C,** Lateral aspect.

The distal end of the tibia (Fig. 6-5) is broad, and its medial surface is prolonged into a large process called the *medial malleolus*. Its anterolateral surface contains the *anterior tubercle*, which overlays the fibula. The lateral surface is flattened and contains the triangular *fibular notch* for articulation with the fibula. The surface under the distal tibia is smooth and shaped for articulation with the talus.

FIBULA

The *fibula* is slender in comparison to its length and consists of one *body* and two articular extremities. The proximal end of the fibula is expanded into a *head,* which articulates with the lateral condyle of the tibia. At the lateroposterior aspect of the head is a conical projection called the *apex.* The enlarged distal end of the fibula is the *lateral malleolus.* The lateral malleolus is pyramidal and marked by several depressions at its inferior and posterior surfaces.

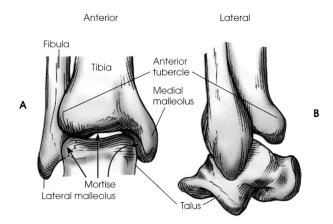

Fig. 6-5 Right distal tibia and fibula in true anatomic position. **A,** Mortise joint and surrounding anatomy. Note the slight overlap of the anterior tubercle of the tibia and the superolateral talus over the fibula. **B,** Lateral aspect showing fibula positioned slightly posterior to the tibia.

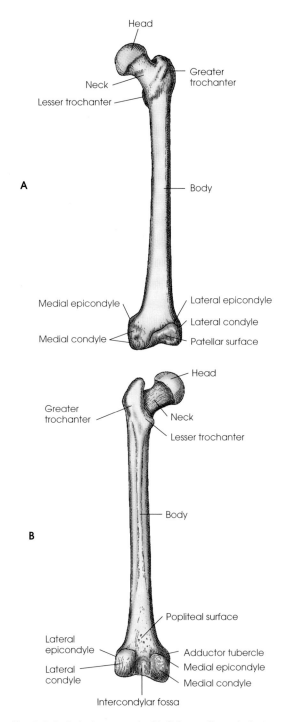

Fig. 6-6 **A**, Anterior aspect of left femur. **B**, posterior aspect.

Femur

The *femur* is the longest, strongest, and heaviest bone in the body (Figs. 6-6 and 6-7). This bone consists of one body and two articular extremities. The *body* is cylindrical, slightly convex anteriorly, and slants medially from 5 to 15 degrees. (The extent of medial inclination depends on the breadth of the pelvic girdle.) When the femur is vertical, the medial condyle is lower than the lateral condyle (Figs. 6-7 and 6-8). About a 5- to 7-degree difference exists between the two condyles. Because of this difference, on lateral radiographs of the knee the central ray is angled 5 to 7 degrees cephalad to "open" the joint space of the knee. The superior portion of the femur articulates with the acetabulum of the hip joint (considered with the pelvic girdle in Chapter 7.)

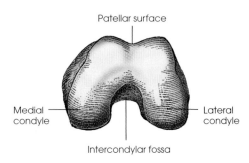

Fig. 6-7 Inferior aspect of left femur.

The distal end of the femur is broadened and has two large eminences: the larger *medial condyle* and the smaller *lateral condyle*. Anteriorly the condyles are separated by the *patellar surface,* a shallow, triangular depression. Posteriorly the condyles are separated by a deep depression called the *intercondylar fossa.* A slight prominence above and within the curve of each condyle forms the *medial* and *lateral epicondyles.* The medial condyle contains the *adductor tubercle,* which is located on the posterolateral aspect. The tubercle is a raised bony area that receives the tendon of the adductor muscle. This tubercle is important to identify on lateral knee radiographs because it assists in identifying overrotation or underrotation. The triangular area superior to the intercondylar fossa on the posterior femur is the *popliteal surface,* over which the popliteal blood vessels and nerves pass.

Patella

The *patella,* or knee cap (see Fig. 6-8), is the largest and most constant sesamoid bone in the body (see Chapter 3). The patella is a flat, triangular bone situated at the distal anterior surface of the femur. The patella develops in the tendon of the quadriceps femoris muscle between the ages of 3 and 5 years. The *apex,* or tip, is directed inferiorly, lies $\frac{1}{2}$ inch (1.3 cm) above the joint space of the knee, and is attached to the tuberosity of the tibia by the patellar ligament. Interestingly, the superior border of the patella is called the *base.*

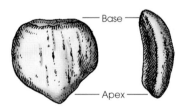

Base

Apex

Fig. 6-8 Anterior and lateral aspects of patella.

Knee Joint

The knee joint is one of the most complex joints in the human body. The femur, tibia, fibula, and patella are held together by a complex group of ligaments. These ligaments work together to provide stability for the knee joint. Although radiographers do not produce images of these ligaments, they need to have a basic understanding of their positions and interrelationship.

Many patients with knee injuries do not have fractures, but they may have torn one or more of these ligaments, which can cause great pain and may alter the position of the bones. Figs. 6-9 and 6-10 show the following important ligaments of the knee:
- Posterior cruciate ligament
- Anterior cruciate ligament
- Tibial collateral ligament
- Fibular collateral ligament

The knee joint contains two fibrocartilage disks called the *lateral* and *medial meniscus* (see Fig. 6-10). The circular menisci lie on the tibial plateaus. They are thick at the outer margin of the joint and taper off toward the center of the tibial plateau. The center of the tibial plateau contains cartilage that articulates directly with the condyles of the knee. The menisci provide stability for the knee and also act as a shock absorber. The menisci are commonly torn during injury. Either a knee arthrogram or a magnetic resonance imaging (MRI) scan must be performed to visualize a meninscular tear.

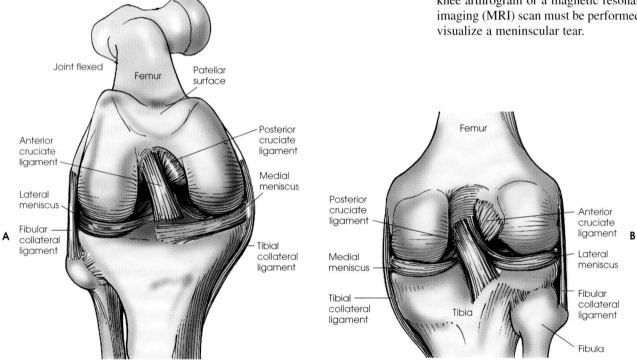

Fig. 6-9 Knee joint. **A**, Anterior aspect with femur flexed. **B** Posterior aspect.

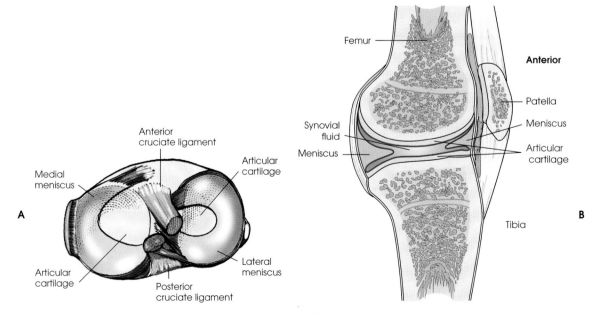

Fig. 6-10 Knee joint. **A**, Superior surface of tibia. **B**, Sagittal section.

Lower Limb Articulations

The joints of the lower limb are summarized in Table 6-1. Beginning with the most distal portion of the lower limb, the articulations are as follows.

The *interphalangeal articulations*, between the phalanges, are *synovial hinges* that allow only flexion and extension (Fig. 6-11, *A*). The joints between the distal and middle phalanges are the *distal interphalangeal (DIP)* joints. Articulations between the middle and proximal phalanges are the *proximal interphalangeal (PIP)* joints. With only two phalanges in the great toe, the joint is known simply as the *interphalangeal* joint.

TABLE 6-1

Joints of the lower limb

Joint	Structural classification		Movement
	Tissue	Type	
Interphalangeal	Synovial	Hinge	Freely movable
Metatarsophalangeal	Synovial	Ellipsoidal	Freely movable
Intermetatarsal	Synovial	Gliding	Freely movable
Tarsometatarsal	Synovial	Gliding	Freely movable
Intertarsal:			
Subtalar	Synovial	Gliding	Freely movable
Talocalcaneonavicular	Synovial	Ball and socket	Freely movable
Calcaneocuboid	Synovial	Gliding	Freely movable
Ankle mortise*	Synovial	Hinge	Freely movable
Tibiofibular:			
Proximal	Synovial	Gliding	Freely movable
Distal	Fibrous	Syndesmosis	Slightly movable
Knee:			
Patella femoral	Synovial	Gliding	Freely movable
Femorotibial	Synovial	Hinge modified	Freely movable

*The mortise joint can be divided specifically into the talofibular and talotibial joints (superior and medial aspects). The joint includes the medial malleolar, lateral malleolar, and superior aspects of the talus.

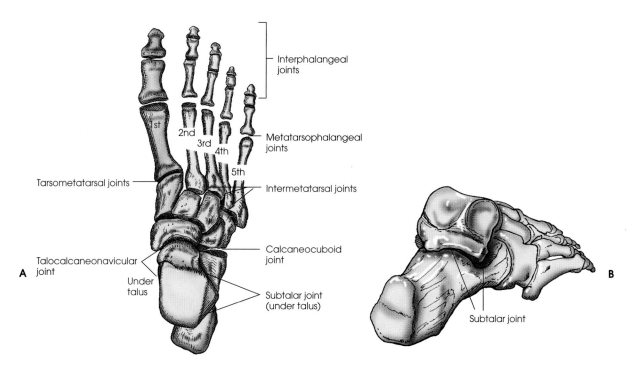

Fig. 6-11 A and **B**, Joints of the right foot.

The distal heads of the metatarsals articulate with the proximal ends of the phalanges at the *metatarsophalangeal* articulations to form *synovial ellipsoidal* joints, which have movements of flexion, extension, and slight adduction and abduction. The proximal bases of the metatarsals articulate with one another (*intermetatarsal* articulations) and with the tarsals (*tarsometatarsal* articulations) to form *synovial gliding* joints, which permit flexion, extension, adduction, and abduction movements.

The *intertarsal* articulations allow only slight gliding movements between the bones and are classified as *synovial gliding* or *synovial ball-and-socket* joints (see Table 6-1). The joint spaces are narrow and obliquely situated. Those lying in the horizontal plane slant inferiorly and posteriorly at a vertical angle of approximately 15 degrees. When the joint surfaces of these bones are in question, it is necessary to angle the x-ray tube or adjust the foot to place the joint spaces parallel with the central ray.

The calcaneus supports the talus and articulates with it by an irregularly shaped, three-faceted joint surface, forming the *subtalar joint.* This joint is classified as *synovial gliding.* Anteriorly the calcaneus articulates with the cuboid at the calcaneocuboid joint. This joint is a synovial gliding joint. The talus rests on top of the calcaneus (see Fig. 6-11). It articulates with the navicular bone anteriorly, supports the tibia above, and articulates with the malleoli of the tibia and fibula at its sides.

Each of the three parts of the subtalar joint is formed by reciprocally shaped facets on the inferior surface of the talus and the superior surface of the calcaneus. Study of the superior and medial aspects of the calcaneus (see Fig. 6-3) will help the radiographer to better understand the problems involved in radiography of this joint.

The *ankle joint* is commonly called the *ankle mortise,* or *mortise joint.* It is formed by the articulations between the lateral malleolus of the fibula and the inferior surface and medial malleolus of the tibia (Fig. 6-12). These form a socket type of structure that articulates with the superior portion of the talus. The talus fits inside the mortise. The articulation is a *synovial hinge* type of joint. The primary action of the ankle joint is dorsiflexion (flexion) and plantar flexion (extension); however, in full plantar flexion a small amount of rotation and abduction-adduction is permitted. Other movements at the ankle largely depend on the gliding movements of the intertarsal joints, particularly the one between the talus and calcaneus.

The fibula articulates with the tibia at both its distal and proximal ends. The *distal tibiofibular* joint is a *fibrous syndesmosis* joint allowing slight movement. The head of the fibula articulates with the posteroinferior surface of the lateral condyle of the tibia, which forms the *proximal tibiofibular joint,* which is a *synovial gliding* joint (Fig. 6-12).

The patella articulates with the patellar surface of the femur and protects the front of the knee joint. This articulation is called the *patellofemoral joint,* when the knee is extended and relaxed, the patella is freely movable over the patellar surface of the femur. When the knee is flexed, which is also a *synovial gliding* joint, the patella is locked in position in front of the patellar surface. The knee joint, or *femorotibial* joint, is the largest joint in the body. It is called a *synovial modified-hinge* joint. In addition to flexion and extension, the knee joint allows slight medial and lateral rotation in the flexed position. The joint is enclosed in an articular capsule and held together by numerous ligaments (Fig. 6-13).

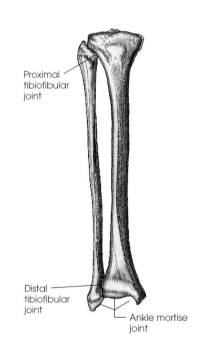

Proximal tibiofibular joint

Distal tibiofibular joint

Ankle mortise joint

Fig. 6-12 Joints of the right tibia and fibula.

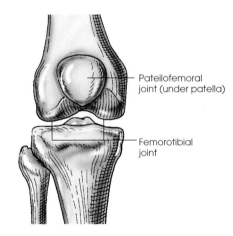

Patellofemoral joint (under patella)

Femorotibial joint

Fig. 6-13 Joints of the right knee.

SUMMARY OF ANATOMY*

Foot
phalanges
metatarsals
tarsals
dorsum (dorsal surface)
plantar surface

Phalanges (14)
proximal phalanx
middle phalanx
distal phalanx
body
base
head

Metatarsals (5)
First metatarsal
Second metatarsal
Third metatarsal
Fourth metatarsal
Fifth metatarsal
body
base
head
tuberosity (5th)

Tarsals (7)
calcaneus
   tuberosity
   anterior facet

middle facet
posterior facet
calcaneal sulcus
sinus tarsi
sustentaculum tali
trochlea
talus
   trochlear surface
   sulcus tali
   posterior articular
      surface
cuboid
navicular
medial cuneiform
intermediate cuneiform
lateral cuneiform

Others
sesamoid bones

Leg
tibia
fibula

Tibia
body
medial condyle
lateral condyle
tibial plateau
intercondylar eminence

medial intercondylar
   tubercle
lateral intercondylar
   tubercle
tibial tuberosity
anterior crest
medial malleolus
anterior tubercle
fibular notch

Fibula
body
head
apex
lateral malleolus

Thigh
femur
body
medial condyle
lateral condyle
patellar surface
intercondylar fossa
medial epicondyle
lateral epicondyle
adductor tubercle
popliteal surface

Patella
apex
base

Knee joint
posterior cruciate liga-
   ment
anterior cruciate liga-
   ment
tibial collateral ligament
fibular collateral liga-
   ment
lateral meniscus
medial meniscus

Articulations
interphalangeal
metatarsophalangeal
intermetatarsal
tarsometatarsal
intertarsal
   subtalar
   talocalcaneonavicular
   calcaneocuboid
ankle mortise
tibiofibular
   proximal
   distal
knee
   patellofemoral
   femorotibial

*See *Addendum* at the end of the volume for a summary of changes in the anatomic terms used in this edition.

Lower limb articulations

Lower limb

Radiation Protection

Protecting the patient from unnecessary radiation is a professional responsibility of the radiographer (see Chapter 1 for specific guidelines). In this chapter, the *Shield gonads* statement at the end of the *Position of part* sections indicates that the patient is to be protected from unnecessary radiation by restricting the radiation beam, using proper collimation, *and* placing lead shielding between the gonads and the radiation source.

Toes

☀ AP OR AP AXIAL PROJECTIONS

Because of the natural curve of the toes, the interphalangeal joint spaces are not best demonstrated on the AP projection. When demonstration of these joint spaces is not critical, an AP projection may be performed (Figs. 6-14 and 6-15). An AP axial projection is recommended to open the joint spaces and reduce foreshortening (Figs. 6-16 and 6-17).

Image receptor: 8×10 inch (18×24 cm) crosswise for two images on one cassette

Position of patient

- Have the patient seated or placed supine on the radiographic table.

Position of part

- With the patient in the supine or seated position, flex the knees, separate the feet about 6 inches (15 cm), and touch the knees together for immobilization.
- Center the toes directly over one half of the cassette (see Figs. 6-14 and 6-16), or place a 15-degree foam wedge well under the foot and rest the toes near the elevated base of the wedge (Fig. 6-18).
- Adjust the cassette half with its midline parallel to the long axis of the foot, and center it to the third metatarsophalangeal joint.
- *Shield gonads.*

NOTE: Some institutions may demonstrate the entire foot, whereas others radiograph only the toe(s) of interest.

Central ray

- Perpendicular through the third metatarsophalangeal joint (see Fig. 6-14) when demonstration of the joint spaces is not critical. To open the joint spaces, either direct the central ray 15 degrees posteriorly through the third metatarsophalangeal joint (see Fig. 6-16), or if the 15-degree foam wedge is used, direct the central ray perpendicularly (Fig. 6-18).

Structures shown

The images demonstrate the 14 phalanges of the toes; the distal portions of the metatarsals; and, on the axial projections, the interphalangeal joints.

EVALUATION CRITERIA

The following should be clearly demonstrated:
- No rotation of phalanges
- Open interphalangeal and metatarsophalangeal joint spaces on the axial projections
- Toes separated from each other
- Distal ends of the metatarsals
- Soft tissues and bony trabecular detail

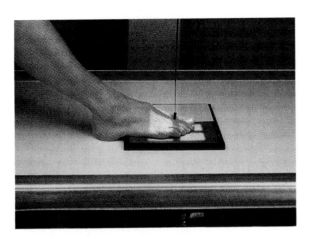

Fig. 6-14 AP toes, perpendicular central ray.

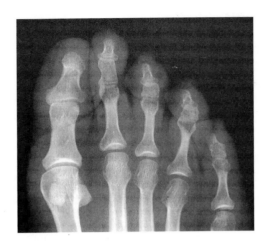

Fig. 6-15 AP toes, perpendicular central ray.

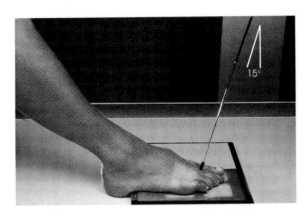

Fig. 6-16 AP axial toes, central ray angulation of 15 degrees.

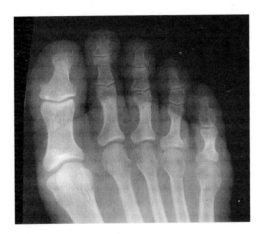

Fig. 6-17 AP axial toes, central ray angulation of 15 degrees.

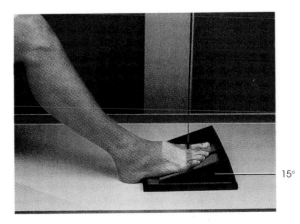

Fig. 6-18 AP axial, 15-degree foam wedge.

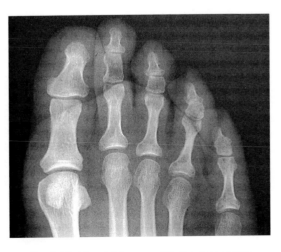

Fig. 6-19 AP axial, toes on 15-degree wedge.

PA PROJECTION

Image receptor: 8 × 10 inch (18 × 24 cm) crosswise for two images on one cassette

Position of patient

- Have patient lie prone on the radiographic table because this position naturally turns the foot over so that the dorsal aspect is in contact with the cassette.

Position of part

- Place the toes in the appropriate position by elevating them on one or two small sandbags and adjusting the support to place the toes horizontal.
- Place the cassette half under the toes with the midline of the side used parallel with the long axis of the foot, and center it to the third metatarsophalangeal joint (Fig. 6-20).
- *Shield gonads.*

NOTE: Some institutions may demonstrate the entire foot, whereas others radiograph only the toe(s) of interest.

Central ray

- Perpendicular to the midpoint of the cassette entering the third metatarsophalangeal joint (see Fig. 6-20). The interphalangeal joint spaces are shown well because the natural divergence of the x-ray beam coincides closely with the position of the toes (Fig. 6-21).

Structures shown

- This projection will demonstrate the 14 phalanges of the toes, the interphalangeal joints, and the distal portions of the metatarsals.

EVALUATION CRITERIA

The following should be clearly demonstrated:

- No rotation of phalanges
- Open interphalangeal and metatarsophalangeal joint spaces
- Toes separated from each other
- Distal ends of the metatarsals
- Soft tissues and bony trabecular detail

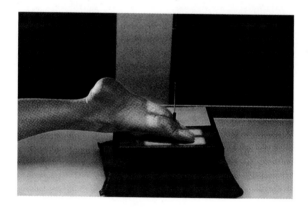

Fig. 6-20 PA toes.

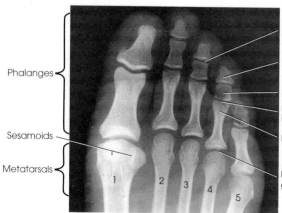

Fig. 6-21 PA toes.

⚕ AP OBLIQUE PROJECTION
Medial rotation

Image receptor: 8 × 10 inch (18 × 24 cm) crosswise for two images on one cassette

Position of patient
- Place the patient in the supine or seated position on the radiographic table.
- Flex the knee of the affected side enough to have the sole of the foot resting firmly on the table.

Position of part
- Position the cassette half under the toes.
- Medially rotate the lower leg and foot, and adjust the plantar surface of the foot to form a 30- to 45-degree angle from the plane of the cassette (Fig. 6-22).
- Center the proximal phalanx of the third toe to the cassette.
- *Shield gonads.*

Central ray
- Perpendicular and entering the third metatarsophalangeal joint

NOTE: Oblique projections of individual toes may be obtained by centering the affected toe to the portion of the cassette being used and collimating closely. The foot may be placed in a medial oblique position for the first and second toes and in a lateral oblique position for the fourth and fifth toes. Either oblique position is adequate for the third (middle) toe.

Structures shown
An AP oblique projection of the phalanges shows the toes and the distal portion of the metatarsals rotated medially (Fig. 6-23).

EVALUATION CRITERIA
The following should be clearly demonstrated:
- All phalanges
- Oblique toes
- Open interphalangeal and second through fifth metatarsophalangeal joint spaces
- First metatarsophalangeal joint (not always opened)
- Toes separated from each other
- Distal ends of the metatarsals
- Soft tissue and bony trabecular detail

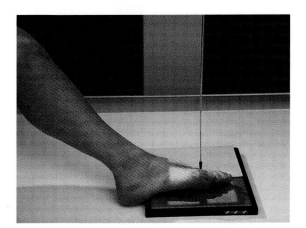

Fig. 6-22 AP oblique toes, medial rotation.

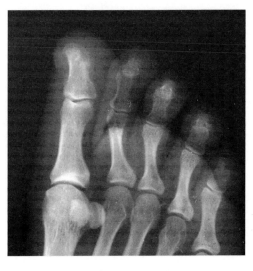

Fig. 6-23 AP oblique toes.

PA OBLIQUE PROJECTION
Medial rotation

Image receptor: 8 × 10 inch (18 × 24 cm) crosswise for two exposures on one cassette

Position of patient
- Have the patient lie in the lateral recumbent position on the affected side.

Position of part
- Adjust the affected limb in a partially extended position.
- Have the patient turn toward the prone position until the ball of the foot forms an angle of approximately 30 degrees to the horizontal, or have the patient rest the foot against a foam wedge or sandbag (Fig. 6-24).
- Center the cassette half to the third metatarsophalangeal joint, and adjust it so that its midline is parallel with the long axis of the foot.
- *Shield gonads.*

Central ray
- Perpendicular to the third metatarsophalangeal joint

Structures shown
A PA oblique projection of the phalanges shows the toes and the distal portion of the metatarsals rotated laterally (Fig. 6-25).

EVALUATION CRITERIA

The following should be clearly demonstrated:
- All phalanges
- Oblique toes
- Open interphalangeal and second through fifth metatarsophalangeal joint spaces
- First metatarsophalangeal joint (not always opened)
- Toes separated from each other
- Distal ends of the metatarsals
- Soft tissue and bony trabecular detail

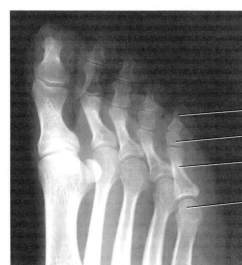

Distal phalanx

Middle phalanx

Proximal phalanx

Metatarsal head

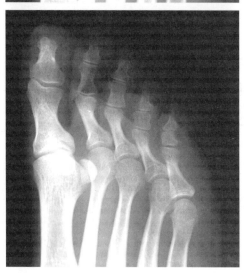

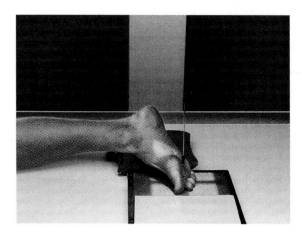

Fig. 6-24 PA oblique toes, medial rotation.

Fig. 6-25 PA oblique toes.

✹ LATERAL PROJECTIONS
Mediolateral or lateromedial

Image receptor: 8 × 10 inch (18 × 24 cm) crosswise for multiple exposures on one cassette

Position of patient
- Have the patient lie in the lateral recumbent position on the *unaffected* side.
- Support the affected limb on sandbags, and adjust it in a comfortable position.
- To prevent superimposition, tape the toes above the one being examined into a flexed position; a 4 × 4 inch gauze pad also may be used to separate the toes.

Position of part
Great toe, second toe
- Place an 8 × 10 inch (18 × 24 cm) cassette under the toe, and center it to the proximal phalanx.
- Grasp the patient's limb by the heel and knee, and adjust its position to place the toe in a true lateral position.
- Adjust the long axis of the cassette so that it is parallel with the long axis of the toe (Figs. 6-26, 6-27, and 6-28).

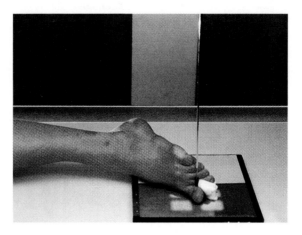

Fig. 6-26 Lateral great toe.

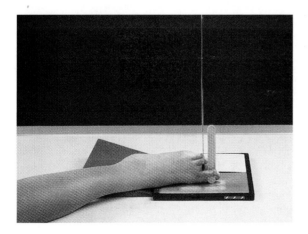

Fig. 6-27 Lateral second toe.

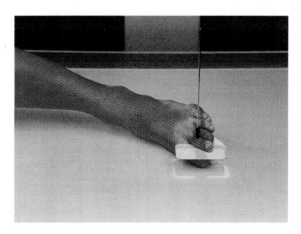

Fig. 6-28 Lateral second toe using occlusal film.

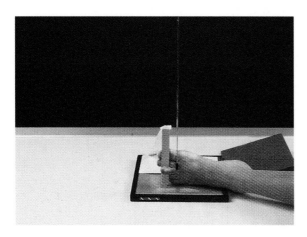

Fig. 6-29 Lateral third toe.

Third, fourth, fifth toes

- Place the patient on the *affected* side for these three toes.
- Select an 8 × 10 inch (18 × 24 cm) cassette or an occlusal film.
- If the occlusal film is used, place it with the pebbled surface up between the toe being examined and the subadjacent toe.
- Adjust the position of the limb to place the toe of interest and the cassette or film in a parallel position, placing the toe as close to the cassette or film as possible.
- Support the elevated heel on a sandbag or sponge for immobilization (Figs. 6-29, 6-30, and 6-31).
- *Shield gonads.*

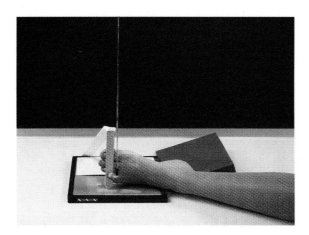

Fig. 6-30 Lateral fourth toe.

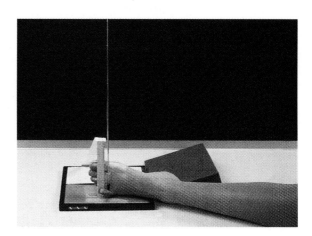

Fig. 6-31 Lateral fifth toe.

Central ray

- Perpendicular to the plane of the cassette or film, entering the metatarsophalangeal joint of the great toe or the proximal interphalangeal joint of the lesser toes

Structures shown

The resulting images show a lateral projection of the phalanges of the toe and the interphalangeal articulations projected free of the other toes (Figs. 6-32 through 6-36).

EVALUATION CRITERIA

The following should be clearly demonstrated:

- Phalanges in profile (toenail should appear lateral).
- Phalanx, without superimposition of adjacent toes. When superimposition cannot be avoided, the proximal phalanx must be demonstrated.
- Open interphalangeal and metatarsophalangeal joint spaces.
- Soft tissue and bony trabecular detail.

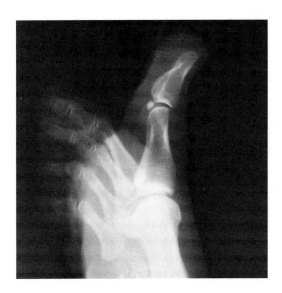

Fig. 6-32 Lateral great toe.

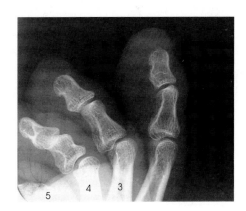

Fig. 6-33 Lateral second toe.

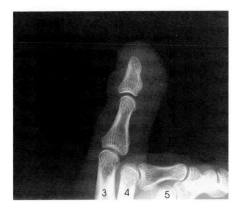

Fig. 6-34 Lateral third toe.

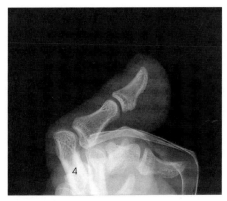

Fig. 6-35 Lateral fourth toe.

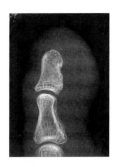

Fig. 6-36 Lateral fifth toe.

TANGENTIAL PROJECTION
LEWIS[1] AND HOLLY[2] METHODS

Image receptor: 8 × 10 inch (18 × 24 cm) crosswise for multiple exposures on one cassette

[1]Lewis RW: Non-routine views in roentgen examination of the extremities, *Surg Gynecol Obstet* 69:38, 1938.
[2]Holly EW: Radiography of the tarsal sesamoid bones, *Med Radiogr Photogr* 31:73, 1955.

Position of patient
• Place the patient in the prone position.
• Elevate the ankle of the affected side on sandbags for stability, if needed. A folded towel may be placed under the knee for comfort.

Position of part
• Rest the great toe on the table in a position of dorsiflexion, and adjust it to place the ball of the foot perpendicular to the horizontal plane.
• Center the cassette to the second metatarsal (Fig. 6-37).
• *Shield gonads.*

Central ray
• Perpendicular and tangential to the first metatarsophalangeal joint

Structures shown
The resulting image shows a tangential projection of the metatarsal head in profile and the sesamoids (Fig. 6-38).

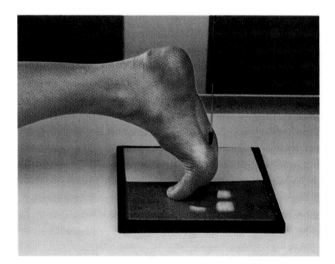

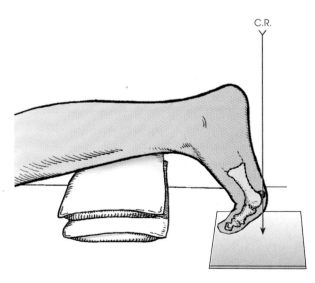

Fig. 6-37 Tangential sesamoids: Lewis method.

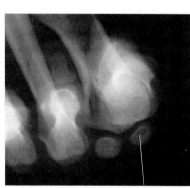

Sesamoid

Fig. 6-38 Tangential sesamoids: Lewis method with toes against cassette.

Sesamoids

EVALUATION CRITERIA

The following should be clearly demonstrated:

- Sesamoids free of any portion of the first metatarsal
- Metatarsal heads

NOTE: Holly[1] described a position that he believed was more comfortable for the patient. With the patient seated on the table, the foot is adjusted so that the medial border is vertical and the plantar surface is at an angle of 75 degrees with the plane of the cassette. The patient holds the toes in a flexed position with a strip of gauze bandage. The central ray is directed perpendicular to the head of the first metatarsal bone (Figs. 6-39 and 6-40).

[1]Holly EW: Radiography of the tarsal sesamoid bones, *Med Radiogr Photogr* 31:73, 1955.

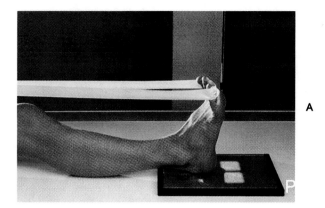

A

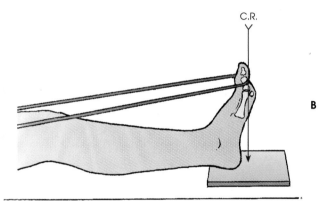

B

Fig. 6-39 Tangential sesamoids: Holly method.

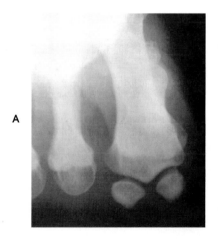

A

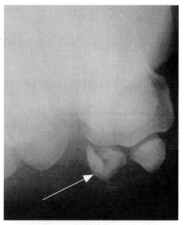

B

Fig. 6-40 A, Tangential sesamoids: Holly method with heel against cassette. **B,** Sesamoid with fracture (*arrow*).

TANGENTIAL PROJECTION
CAUSTON METHOD[1]

Image receptor: 8 × 10 inch (18 × 24 cm)

Position of patient
- Place the patient in the lateral recumbent position on the unaffected side, and flex the knees.

[1]Causton J: Projection of sesamoid bones in the region of the first metatarsophalangeal joint, *Radiology* 9:39, 1943.

Position of part
- Partially extend the limb being examined and put sandbags under the knee and foot.
- Adjust the height of a sandbag under the knee to place the foot in the *lateral position,* with the first metatarsophalangeal joint perpendicular to the horizontal plane of the cassette
- Place the cassette under the distal metatarsal region, and adjust it so that the midpoint will coincide with the central ray (Figs. 6-41 and 6-42).
- *Shield gonads.*

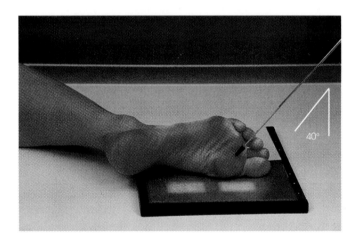

Fig. 6-41 Tangential sesamoids.

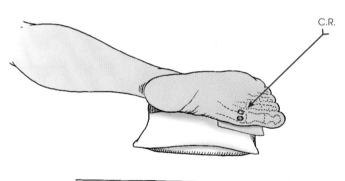

Fig. 6-42 Tangential sesamoids using occlusal film.

Central ray

• Directed to the prominence of the first metatarsophalangeal joint at an angle of 40 degrees toward the heel

Structures shown

The tangential image shows the sesamoid bones projected axiolaterally with a slight overlap (Fig 6-43).

The following should be clearly demonstrated:

■ First metatarsophalangeal sesamoids with little overlap

Occlusal film technique

For improved detail, a similar projection may be performed using an occlusal film. The film is placed on a sandbag as illustrated in Fig. 6-42 and then is appropriately processed.

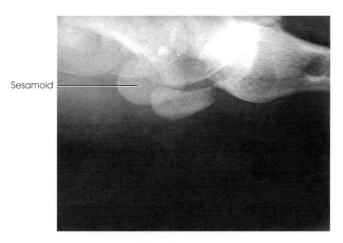

Sesamoid

Fig. 6-43 Tangential sesamoids.

🦅 AP OR AP AXIAL PROJECTION

Radiographs may be obtained by directing the central ray perpendicular to the plane of the cassette or by angling the central ray 10 degrees posteriorly. When a 10-degree posterior angle is used, the central ray is perpendicular to the metatarsals, therefore reducing foreshortening. The tarsometatarsal joint spaces of the midfoot are also demonstrated better (Figs. 6-44 and 6-45).

Image receptor: 8 × 10 inch (18 × 24 cm) or 24 × 30 cm (10 × 12 inch), depending on the length of the foot

Position of patient
- Place the patient in the supine position.
- Flex the knee of the affected side enough to rest the sole of the foot firmly on the radiographic table.

Position of part
- Position the cassette under the patient's foot, center it to the base of the third metatarsal, and adjust it so that its long axis is parallel with the long axis of the foot.
- Hold the leg in the vertical position by having the patient flex the opposite knee and lean it against the knee of the affected side.
- In this foot position the entire plantar surface rests on the cassette; thus it is necessary to take precautions against the cassette slipping.
- Ensure that no rotation of the foot occurs.
- *Shield gonads.*

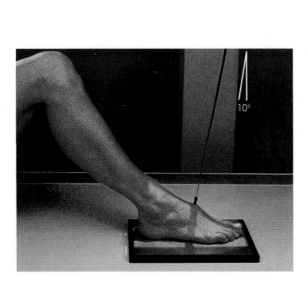

Fig. 6-44 AP axial foot with posterior angulation of 10 degrees.

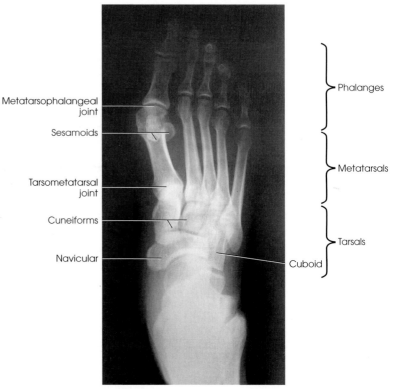

Fig. 6-45 AP axial foot with posterior angulation of 10 degrees.

Central ray

- Directed one of two ways: (1) 10 degrees toward the heel to the base of the third metatarsal (see Fig. 6-44) or (2) perpendicular to the cassette and toward the base of the third metatarsal (Fig. 6-46)

Structures shown

The resulting image shows an AP (dorsoplantar) projection of the tarsals anterior to the talus, metatarsals, and phalanges (Figs. 6-45, 6-47, and 6-48). This projection is used for localizing foreign bodies, determining the location of fragments in fractures of the metatarsals and anterior tarsals, and performing general surveys of the bones of the foot.

EVALUATION CRITERIA

The following should be clearly demonstrated:

- No rotation of the foot
- Equal amount of space between the adjacent midshafts of the second through fourth metatarsals
- Overlap of the second through fifth metatarsal bases
- Visualization of the phalanges and tarsals distal to the talus, as well as the metatarsals

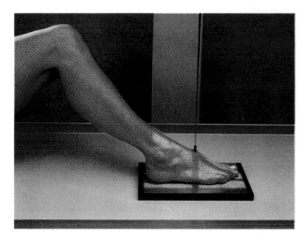

Fig. 6-46 AP foot with perpendicular central ray.

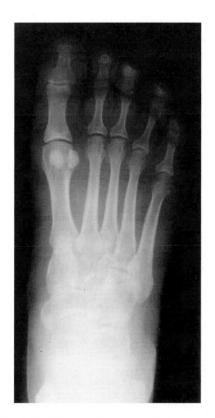

Fig. 6-47 AP foot with perpendicular central ray.

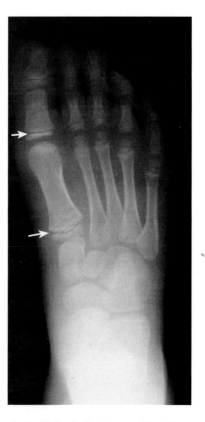

Fig. 6-48 AP foot of a 6-year-old patient. Note the epiphyseal centers of ossification (*arrows*).

AP OBLIQUE PROJECTION
Medial rotation

Image receptor: 8 × 10 inch (18 × 24 cm) or 24 × 30 cm (10 × 12 inch), depending on the length of the foot

Position of patient
- Place the patient in the supine position.
- Flex the knee of the affected side enough to have the plantar surface of the foot rest firmly on the radiographic table.

Position of part
- Place the cassette under the patient's foot, parallel with its long axis, and center it to the midline of the foot at the level of the base of the third metatarsal.
- Rotate the patient's leg medially until the plantar surface of the foot forms an angle of 30 degrees to the plane of the cassette (Fig. 6-49). If the angle of the foot is increased more than 30 degrees, the lateral cuneiform tends to be thrown over the other cuneiforms.[1]
- *Shield gonads.*

Central ray
- Perpendicular to the base of the third metatarsal

NOTE: A similar projection using a 45-degree medial rotation of the foot and a PA oblique projection is described on page 250. A greater rotation can be helpful in demonstrating the joint spaces of the foot.

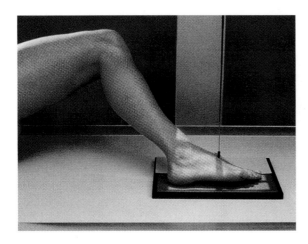

Fig. 6-49 AP oblique foot, medial rotation.

[1]Doub HP: A useful position for examining the foot, *Radiology* 16:764, 1931.

Foot

Structures shown

The resulting image shows the interspaces between the following: the cuboid and the calcaneus; the cuboid and the fourth and fifth metatarsals; the cuboid and the lateral cuneiform; and the talus and the navicular bone. The cuboid is shown in profile. The sinus tarsi is also well demonstrated (Fig. 6-50).

EVALUATION CRITERIA

The following should be clearly demonstrated:

- Third through fifth metatarsal bases free of superimposition
- Lateral tarsals with less superimposition than in the AP projection
- Lateral tarsometatarsal and intertarsal joints
- Sinus tarsi
- Tuberosity of the fifth metatarsal
- Bases of the first and second metatarsals
- Equal amount of space between the shafts of the second through fifth metatarsals
- Sufficient density to demonstrate the phalanges, metatarsals, and tarsals

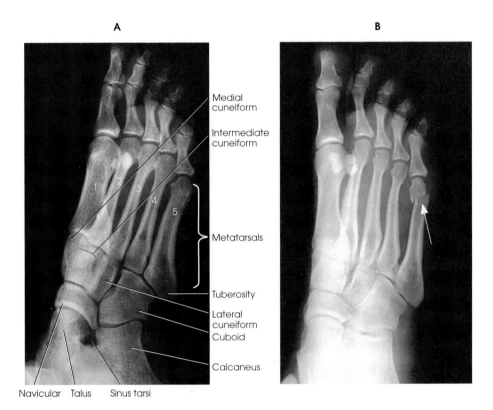

A

B

Medial cuneiform

Intermediate cuneiform

Metatarsals

Tuberosity

Lateral cuneiform

Cuboid

Calcaneus

Navicular   Talus   Sinus tarsi

Fig. 6-50 AP oblique projection foot; medial rotation. **B**, Fracture of the distal aspect of the fifth metatarsal (*arrow*).

AP OBLIQUE PROJECTION
Lateral rotation

Image receptor: 8 × 10 inch (18 × 24 cm) or 24 × 30 cm (10 × 12 inch), depending on the length of the foot

Position of patient
- Place the patient in the supine position.
- Flex the knee of the affected side enough for the plantar surface of the foot to rest firmly on the radiographic table.

Position of part
- Place the cassette under the patient's foot, parallel with its long axis, and center it to the midline of the foot at the level of the base of the third metatarsal.
- Rotate the leg laterally until the plantar surface of the foot forms an angle of 30 degrees to the cassette.
- Support the elevated side of the foot on a 30-degree foam wedge to ensure consistent results (Fig. 6-51).
- *Shield gonads.*

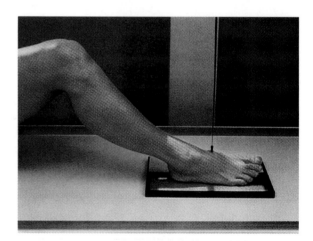

Fig. 6-51 AP oblique foot, lateral rotation.

Central ray

• Perpendicular to the base of the third metatarsal

Structures shown

The resulting image shows the interspaces between the first and second metatarsals and between the medial and intermediate cuneiforms (Fig. 6-52).

EVALUATION CRITERIA

The following should be clearly demonstrated:

■ Separate first and second metatarsal bases
■ No superimposition of the medial and intermediate cuneiforms
■ Navicular bone more clearly demonstrated than in the medial rotation
■ Sufficient density to demonstrate the phalanges, metatarsals, and tarsals

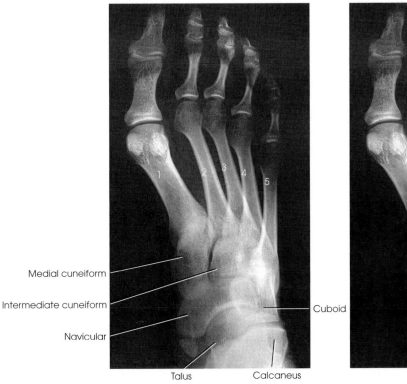

Fig. 6-52 AP oblique foot.

PA OBLIQUE PROJECTIONS
GRASHEY METHODS
Medial or lateral rotations

Image receptor: 8 × 10 inch (18 × 24 cm) or 24 × 30 cm (10 × 12 inch), depending on the length of the foot

Position of patient
- Place the patient in the prone position.
- Elevate the affected foot on sandbags. If desired, place a folded towel under the knee.

Position of part
- Adjust the elevation of the patient's foot to place its dorsal surface in contact with the cassette.
- Position the cassette under the foot, parallel with its long axis, and center it to the base of the third metatarsal.
- To demonstrate the interspace between the first and second metatarsals, rotate the *heel* medially approximately 30 degrees (Figs. 6-53 and 6-54).
- To demonstrate the interspaces between the second and third, the third and fourth, and the fourth and fifth metatarsals, adjust the foot so that the *heel* is rotated laterally approximately 20 degrees (see Fig. 6-54).
- *Shield gonads.*

Central ray
- Perpendicular to the base of the third metatarsal

Structures shown
The resulting image shows a PA oblique projection of the bones of the foot and the interspaces of the proximal ends of the metatarsals.

The following should be clearly demonstrated:

Heel medially rotated 30 degrees (Fig. 6-55)
- First and second metatarsal bases free of superimposition
- Medial cuneiform projected without superimposition
- Navicular bone seen in profile

Heel laterally rotated 20 degrees (Fig. 6-56)
- Third through fifth metatarsal bases free of superimposition
- Tuberosity of the fifth metatarsal and cuboid

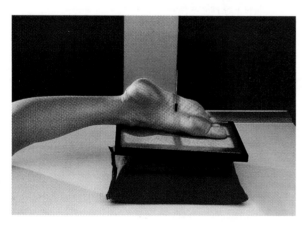

Fig. 6-53 PA oblique foot, heel medially rotated 30 degrees.

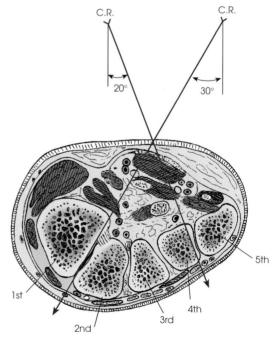

Fig. 6-54 Coronal section near base of metatarsals of right foot.

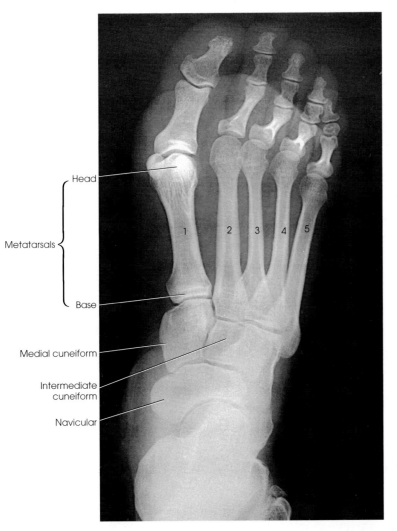
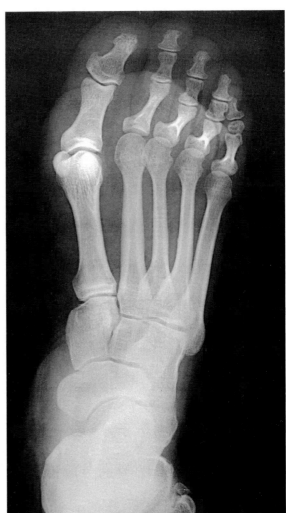

Head

Metatarsals

1 2 3 4 5

Base

Medial cuneiform

Intermediate
cuneiform

Navicular

Fig. 6-55 PA oblique foot, heel medially rotated 30 degrees.

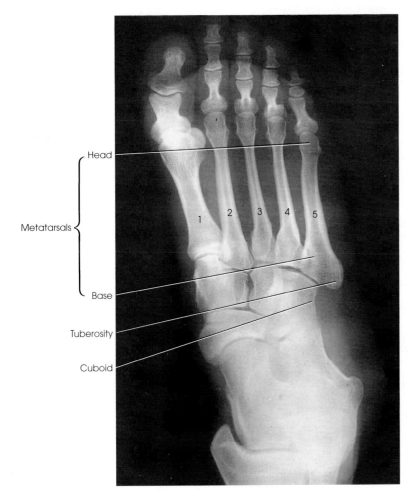
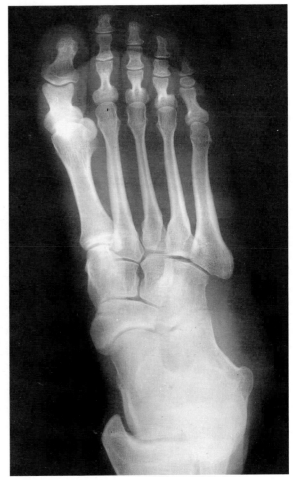

Head

Metatarsals

1 2 3 4 5

Base

Tuberosity

Cuboid

Fig. 6-56 PA oblique foot, heel laterally rotated 20 degrees.

PA OBLIQUE PROJECTION
Medial rotation

NOTE: This is essentially the same projection as the AP oblique foot projection described on page 244. Placing the lateral aspect of the foot closer to the cassette and using a 45-degree medial rotation can provide better visualization of the bones of the foot.

Image receptor: 8 × 10 inch (18 × 24 cm) or 24 × 30 cm (10 × 12 inch), depending on the length of the foot

Position of patient
• Place the patient in the lateral recumbent position on the affected side, and flex the knees.

Position of part
• Fully extend the leg of the side being examined.
• Have the patient turn toward the prone position until the plantar surface of the foot forms an angle of 45 degrees to the plane of the cassette.
• Center the cassette opposite the base of the fifth metatarsal, and adjust it so that its midline is parallel with the long axis of the foot.
• Rest the dorsum of the foot against a foam wedge. The general survey study is usually made with the foot at an angle of 45 degrees to obtain uniform results (Fig. 6-57).
• *Shield gonads.*

Central ray
• Perpendicular to the midline of the foot at the level of the base of the fifth metatarsal

Structures shown
The resulting image shows a PA oblique projection of the bones of the foot. The articulations between the cuboid and the adjacent bones (the calcaneus, lateral cuneiform, and fourth and fifth metatarsals) are clearly shown (Fig. 6-58). The articulations between the following bones are usually shown: talus and navicular bone; navicular bone and cuneiforms; and sustentaculum tali and talus. The cuboid is shown in profile.

EVALUATION CRITERIA
The following should be clearly demonstrated:
■ A more oblique projection than obtained with the Grashey method
■ Third through fifth metatarsal bases and the tarsals
■ Tarsometatarsal and intertarsal joints
■ Tuberosity of the fifth metatarsal
■ Some superimposition of the first and second metatarsals
■ Sufficient density to demonstrate the phalanges, metatarsals, and tarsals

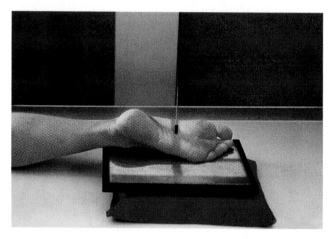

Fig. 6-57 PA oblique foot, medial rotation.

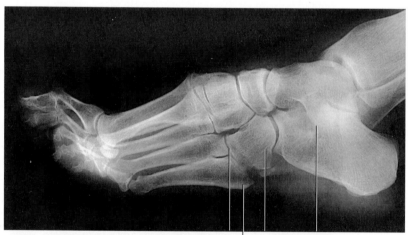

Tarsometatarsal joint   Cuboid   Calcaneus
Fifth metatarsal tuberosity

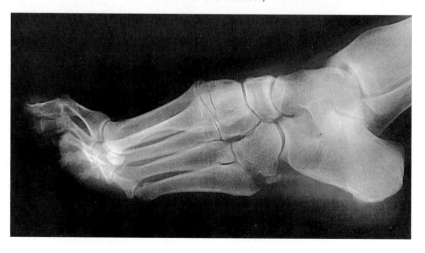

Fig. 6-58 PA oblique foot.

Foot

☀ LATERAL PROJECTION
Mediolateral

The lateral (mediolateral) projection is routinely used in most radiology departments because it is a comfortable position for the patient to assume. The *lateromedial* projection, however, is the recommended alternative when the patient's condition permits.

Image receptor: 8 × 10 inch (18 × 24 cm) or 24 × 30 cm (10 × 12 inch), depending on the size of the foot

Position of patient

- Have the patient lie on the radiographic table and turn toward the affected side until the leg and foot are lateral.
- Place the opposite leg behind the patient.

Position of part

- Elevate the patient's knee enough to place the patella perpendicular to the horizontal plane, and adjust a sandbag support under the knee (Fig. 6-59).
- Center the cassette to the midarea of the foot, and adjust it so that its long axis is parallel with the long axis of the foot.
- Dorsiflex the foot to form a 90-degree angle with the lower leg.
- *Shield gonads.*

Central ray

- Perpendicular to the base of the third metatarsal

Structures shown

- The resulting image shows the entire foot in profile, the ankle joint, and the distal ends of the tibia and fibula (Fig. 6-60).

EVALUATION CRITERIA

The following should be clearly demonstrated:

- Metatarsals nearly superimposed
- Distal leg
- Fibula overlapping the posterior portion of the tibia
- Tibiotalar joint
- Sufficient density to demonstrate the superimposed tarsals and metatarsals

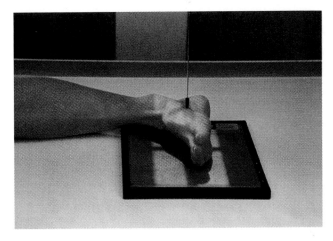

Fig. 6-59 Lateral foot.

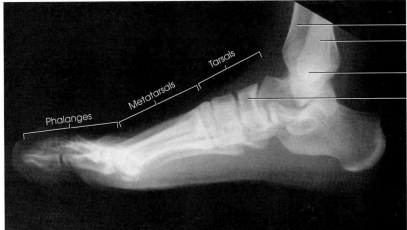

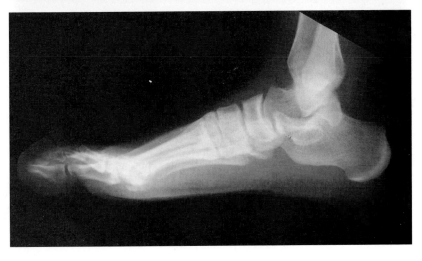

Fig. 6-60 Lateral foot.

LATERAL PROJECTION
Lateromedial

Whenever possible, lateral projections of the foot should be made with the medial side in contact with the cassette. In the absence of an unusually prominent medial malleolus, hallux valgus, or other deformity, the foot assumes an exact or nearly exact lateral position when resting on its medial side. Although the medial position may be more difficult for some patients to achieve, true lateral projections are more easily and consistently obtained with the foot in this position.

Image receptor: 8 × 10 inch (18 × 24 cm) or 24 × 30 cm (10 × 12 inch), depending on the length of the foot

Position of patient

- Place the patient in the supine position.
- Turn the patient onto the *unaffected* side until the affected leg and foot are laterally placed. The patient's body will be in an LPO or RPO position.

Position of part

- Elevate the patient's knee enough to place the patella perpendicular to the horizontal plane, and support the knee on a sandbag or sponge (Fig. 6-61).
- Center the cassette to the middle area of the foot, and adjust it so that its long axis is parallel with the long axis of the foot.
- Adjust the foot so that the plantar surface is perpendicular to the cassette.
- *Shield gonads.*

Central ray

- Perpendicular to the base of the third metatarsal

Structures shown

The resulting image shows a true lateromedial projection of the foot, ankle joint, and distal ends of the tibia and fibula (Fig. 6-62).

The following should be clearly demonstrated:

- Metatarsals usually more superimposed than in the mediolateral image, depending on the transverse arch of the foot
- Distal leg
- Fibula overlapping the posterior portion of the tibia
- Tibiotalar joint
- Sufficient density to demonstrate the superimposed tarsals and metatarsals

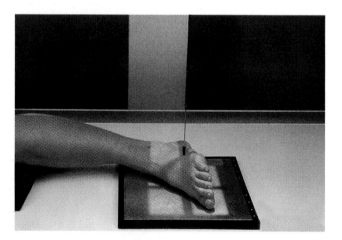

Fig. 6-61 Lateral foot.

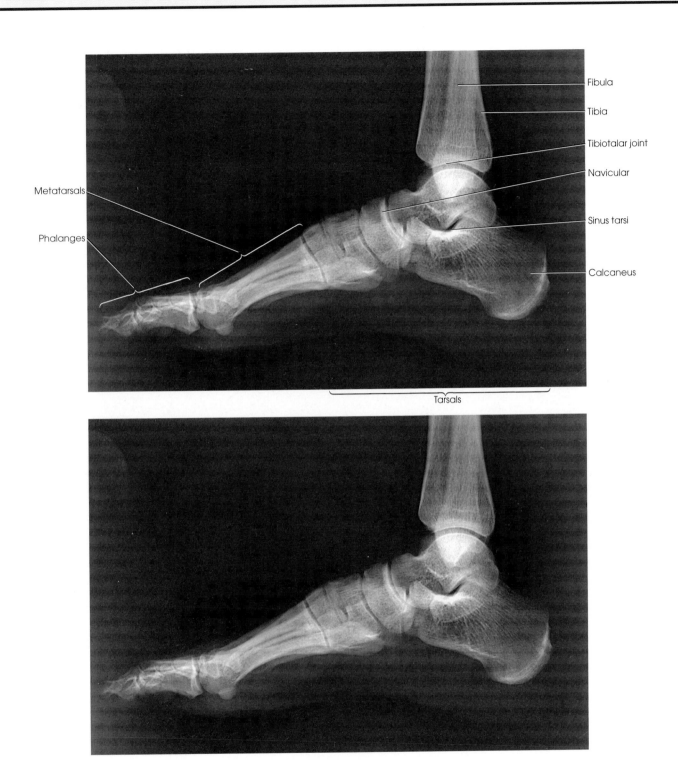

Fibula

Tibia

Tibiotalar joint

Navicular

Sinus tarsi

Calcaneus

Metatarsals

Phalanges

Tarsals

Fig. 6-62 Lateral foot.

Longitudinal Arch
LATERAL PROJECTION
Lateromedial
WEIGHT-BEARING METHOD
Standing

Image receptor: 8 × 10 inch (18 × 24 cm) or 24 × 30 cm (10 × 12 in), depending on the length of the foot and whether a unilateral or a bilateral examination is being performed

Position of patient
- Place the patient in the upright position, preferably on a low stool that has a cassette well. If such a stool is not available, use blocks to elevate the feet to the level of the x-ray tube (Figs. 6-63 and 6-64).
- If needed, use a mobile unit to allow the x-ray tube to reach the floor level.

Position of part
- Place the cassette in the cassette groove of the stool or between blocks with a sheet of leaded rubber to protect its lower half.
- Have the patient stand in a natural position, one foot on each side of the cassette, with the weight of the body equally distributed on the feet.
- Adjust the cassette so that it is centered to the base of the third metatarsal.
- After the first exposure has been made, remove the cassette, turn it over to face the opposite foot, and place it back into the cassette groove (if the same cassette is used), being careful to center to the same point.
- Rotate the tube 180 degrees to the opposite side, and make the second exposure.
- *Shield gonads.*

Central ray
- Perpendicular to a point just above the base of the third metatarsal

Structures shown
The resulting image shows a lateromedial projection of the bones of the foot with weight-bearing. The projection is used to demonstrate the structural status of the longitudinal arch. The right and left sides are examined for comparison (Fig. 6-65).

EVALUATION CRITERIA
- Superimposed plantar surfaces of the metatarsal heads
- Entire foot and distal leg
- Fibula overlapping the posterior portion of the tibia
- Sufficient density to visualize the superimposed tarsals and metatarsals

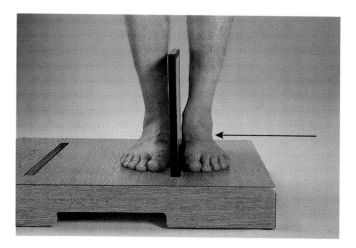

Fig. 6-63 Weight-bearing lateral foot.

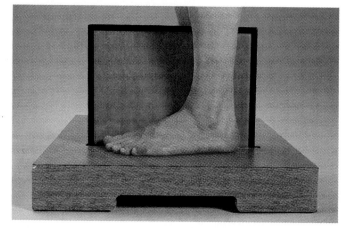

Fig. 6-64 Weight-bearing lateral foot.

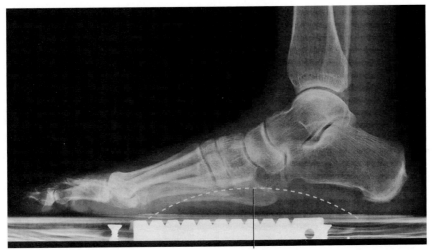

Longitudinal arch

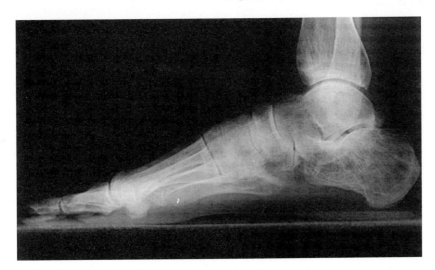

Fig. 6-65 Weight-bearing lateral foot.

AP AXIAL PROJECTION
WEIGHT-BEARING METHOD
Standing

Image receptor: 24 × 30 cm (10 × 12 inch) crosswise for both feet on one image

SID: 48 inches (122 cm). This SID is used to reduce magnification and improve recorded detail in the image.

Position of patient
• Place the patient in the standing-upright position.

Position of part
• Place the cassette on the floor, and have the patient stand on the cassette with the feet centered on each side.

• Pull the patient's pants up to the knee level, if necessary.
• Ensure that right and left markers and an upright marker are placed on the cassette.
• Ensure that the patient's weight is distributed equally on each foot (Fig. 6-66).
• The patient may hold the x-ray tube crane for stability.
• *Shield gonads.*

Central ray
• Angled 10 degrees toward the heel is optimal. A minimum of 15 degrees is usually necessary to have enough room to position the tube and allow the patient to stand. The central ray is positioned between the feet and at the level of the base of the third metatarsal.

Structures shown
The resulting image demonstrates a weight-bearing AP axial projection of both feet permitting an accurate evaluation and comparison of the tarsals and metatarsals (Fig. 6-67).

EVALUATION CRITERIA
The following should be clearly demonstrated:
■ Both feet centered on one image
■ Phalanges, metatarsals, and distal tarsals.
■ Correct right and left marker placement and a weight-bearing marker
■ Correct exposure technique to visualize all the components

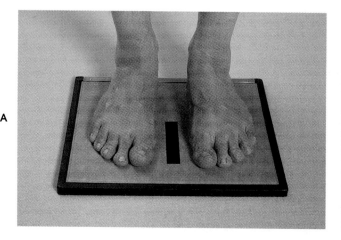
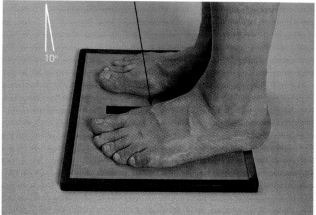

Fig. 6-66 Weight-bearing AP both feet, standing. **A,** Correct position of both feet on cassette. **B,** Lateral perspective of the same projection shows the position of the feet on cassette and the central ray.

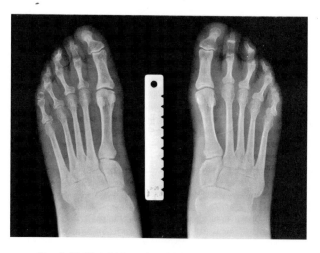

Fig. 6-67 Weight-bearing AP both feet, standing.

Foot

AP AXIAL PROJECTION
WEIGHT-BEARING COMPOSITE
METHOD
Standing

Image receptor: 8 × 10 inch (18 × 24 cm) or 24 × 30 cm (10 × 12 inch), depending on the length of the foot

Position of patient
- Place the patient in the standing-upright position. The patient should stand at a comfortable height on a low stool or on the floor.

Position of part
- With the patient standing upright, adjust the cassette under the foot and center its midline to the long axis of the foot.
- To prevent superimposition of the leg shadow on that of the ankle joint, have the patient place the opposite foot one step backward for the exposure of the forefoot and one step forward for the exposure of the hindfoot or calcaneus.
- *Shield gonads.*

Central ray
- To use the masking effect of the leg, direct the central ray along the plane of alignment of the foot in both exposures.
- With the tube in front of the patient and adjusted for a posterior angulation of 15 degrees, center the central ray to the base of the third metatarsal for the first exposure (Figs. 6-68 and 6-69).

- Caution the patient to carefully maintain the position of the affected foot and place the opposite foot one step forward in preparation for the second exposure.
- Move the tube behind the patient, adjust it for an anterior angulation of 25 degrees, and direct the central ray to the posterior surface of the ankle. The central ray emerges on the plantar surface at the level of the lateral malleolus (Figs. 6-70 and 6-71). An increase in technical factors is recommended for this exposure.

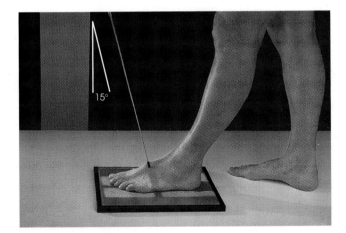

Fig. 6-68 Composite AP axial foot, posterior angulation of 15 degrees.

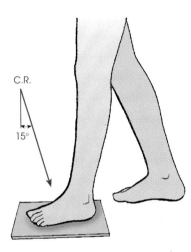

Fig. 6-69 Composite AP axial foot, posterior angulation of 15 degrees.

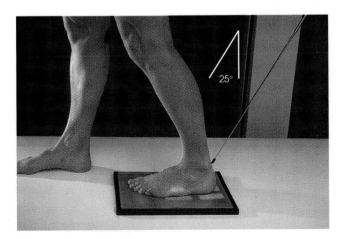

Fig. 6-70 Composite AP axial foot, anterior angulation of 25 degrees.

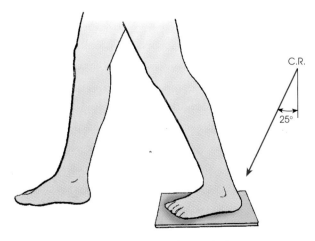

Fig. 6-71 Composite AP axial foot, anterior angulation of 25 degrees.

Structures shown

The resulting image shows a weight-bearing AP axial projection of all bones of the foot. The full outline of the foot is projected free of the leg (Fig. 6-72).

EVALUATION CRITERIA

The following should be clearly demonstrated:

- All tarsals
- Shadow of leg not overlapping the tarsals
- Foot not rotated
- Tarsals, metatarsals, and toes with similar densities

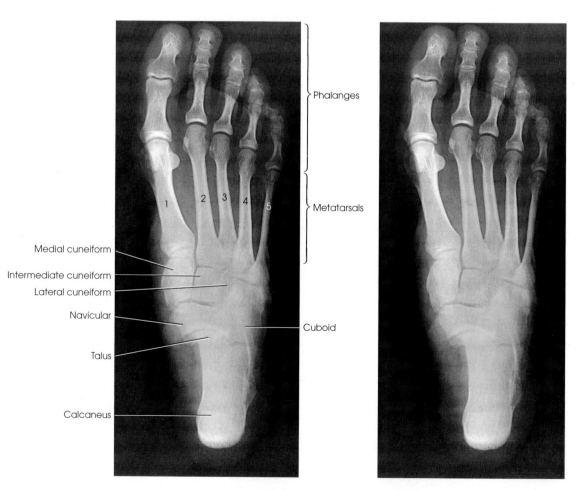

Phalanges

Metatarsals

Medial cuneiform

Intermediate cuneiform

Lateral cuneiform

Navicular

Cuboid

Talus

Calcaneus

Fig. 6-72 Composite AP axial foot.

Congenital Clubfoot
AP PROJECTION
KITE METHODS[1,2]

The typical clubfoot, called *talipes equinovarus*, shows three deviations from the normal alignment of the foot in relation to the weight-bearing axis of the leg. These deviations are plantar flexion and inversion of the calcaneus (equinus), medial displacement of the forefoot (adduction), and elevation of the medial border of the foot (supination). The typical clubfoot has numerous variations. Furthermore, each of the typical abnormalities just described has varying degrees of deformity.

The classic Kite methods—exactly placed AP and lateral projections—for radiography of the clubfoot are used to demonstrate the anatomy of the foot and the bones or ossification centers of the tarsals and their relation to one another. *A primary objective makes it essential that no attempt be made to change the abnormal alignment of the foot when placing it on the cassette.* Davis and Hatt[3] stated that even slight rotation of the foot can result in marked alteration in the radiographically projected relation of the ossification centers.

[1]Kite JH: Principles involved in the treatment of congenital clubfoot, *J Bone Joint Surg* 21:595, 1939.
[2]Kite JH: *The clubfoot,* New York, 1964, Grune & Stratton.
[3]Davis LA, Hatt WS: Congenital abnormalities of the feet, *Radiology* 64:818, 1955.

The AP projection demonstrates the degree of adduction of the forefoot and the degree of inversion of the calcaneus.

Image receptor: 8 × 10 inch (18 × 24 cm).

Position of patient
• Place the infant in the supine position, with the hips and knees flexed to permit the foot to rest flat on the cassette. Elevate the body on firm pillows to knee height to simplify both gonad shielding and leg adjustment.

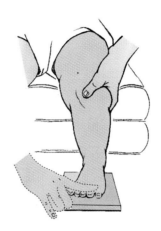

Fig. 6-73 AP foot for demonstration of clubfoot deformity.

Position of part
• Rest the feet flat on the cassette with the ankles extended slightly to prevent superimposition of the leg shadow.
• Hold the infant's knees together or in such a way that the legs are exactly vertical (i.e., so that they do not lean medially or laterally).
• Using a lead glove, hold the infant's toes. When the adduction deformity is too great to permit correct placement of the legs and feet for bilateral images without overlap of the feet, they must be examined separately (Figs. 6-73 and 6-74).
• *Shield gonads.*

Central ray
• Perpendicular to the tarsals, midway between the tarsal areas for a bilateral projection.
• An approximately 15-degree posterior angle is generally required for the central ray to be perpendicular to the tarsals.
• Kite[1,2] stressed the importance of directing the central ray vertically for the purpose of projecting the true relationship of the bones and ossification centers.

[1]Kite JH: Principles involved in the treatment of congenital clubfoot, *J Bone Joint Surg* 21:595, 1939.
[2]Kite JH: *The clubfoot,* New York, 1964, Grune & Stratton.

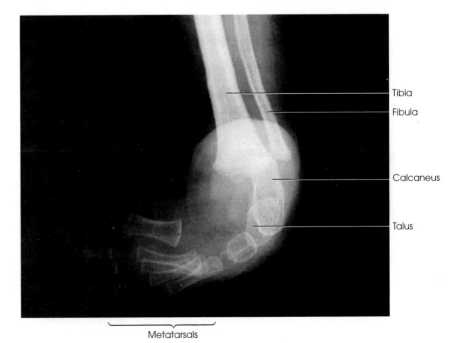

Metatarsals

Fig. 6-74 AP projection showing nearly 90-degree adduction of forefoot.

Congenital Clubfoot
LATERAL PROJECTION
Mediolateral
KITE METHOD

The Kite method lateral radiograph demonstrates the anterior talar subluxation and the degree of plantar flexion (equinus).

Position of patient
- Place the infant on his or her side in as near the lateral position as possible.
- Flex the uppermost limb, draw it forward, and hold it in place.

Position of part
- After adjusting the cassette under the foot, place a support that has the same thickness as the cassette under the infant's knee to prevent angulation of the foot and to ensure a lateral foot position.
- Hold the infant's toes in position with tape or a protected hand (Figs. 6-75 to 6-79).
- *Shield gonads.*

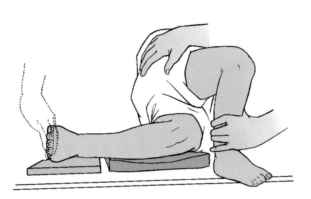

Fig. 6-75 Lateral foot.

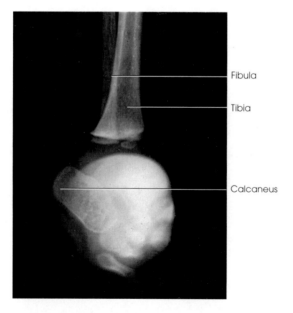

Fig. 6-76 Lateral foot projection showing pitch of calcaneus. Other tarsals are obscured by the adducted forefoot.

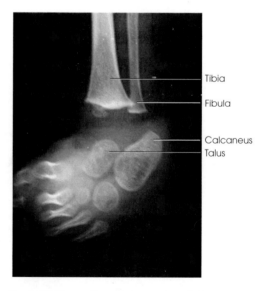

Fig. 6-77 Nonroutine 45-degree medial rotation showing extent of talipes equinovarus.

Central ray

• Perpendicular to the midtarsal area

EVALUATION CRITERIA

The following should be clearly demonstrated:

■ No medial or lateral angulation of the leg
■ Fibula in lateral projection overlapping the posterior half of the tibia
■ The need for a repeat examination if slight variations in rotation are seen in either image when compared with previous radiographs
■ Sufficient density of the talus, calcaneus, and metatarsals to allow assessment of alignment variations.

NOTE: Freiberger, Hersh, and Harrison[1] recommended that dorsiflexion of the infant foot could be obtained by pressing a small plywood board against the sole of the foot. The older child or adult is placed in the upright position for a horizontal projection. With the upright position the patient leans the leg forward to dorsiflex the foot.

NOTE: Conway and Cowell[2] recommended tomography for the demonstration of coalition at the middle facet and particularly for the hidden coalition involving the anterior facet.

[1]Freiberger RH, Hersh A, Harrison MO: Roentgen examination of the deformed foot, *Semin Roentgenol* 5:341, 1970.
[2]Conway JJ, Cowell HR: Tarsal coalition: clinical significance and roentgenographic demonstration, *Radiology* 92:799, 1969.

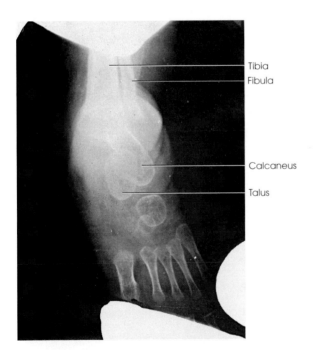

Fig. 6-78 AP projection after treatment (same patient as in Fig. 6-77).

Tibia
Fibula

Calcaneus

Talus

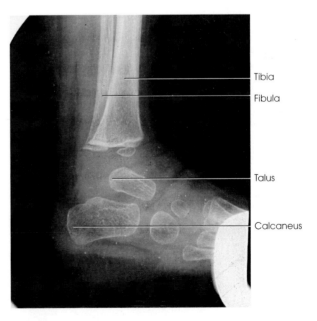

Fig. 6-79 Lateral projection after treatment (same patient as in Fig. 6-76).

Tibia
Fibula

Talus

Calcaneus

Congenital Clubfoot
AXIAL PROJECTION
Dorsoplantar
KANDEL METHOD[1]

Kandel[1] recommended the inclusion of a dorsoplantar axial projection in the examination of the patient with a clubfoot (Fig. 6-80).

For this method the infant is held in a vertical or a bending-forward position. The plantar surface of the foot should rest on the cassette, although a moderate elevation of the heel is acceptable when the equinus deformity is well marked. The central ray is directed 40 degrees anteriorly through the lower leg, as for the usual dorsoplantar projection of the calcaneus (Fig. 6-81).

[1]Kandel B: The suroplantar projection in the congenital clubfoot of the infant, *Acta Orthop Scand* 22:161, 1952.

Freiberger, Hersh, and Harrison[1] stated that sustentaculum talar joint fusion cannot be assumed on one projection, because the central ray may not have been parallel with the articular surfaces. They recommended that three radiographs be obtained with varying central ray angulations (35, 45, and 55 degrees).

[1]Freiberger RH, Hersh A, Harrison MO: Roentgen examination of the deformed foot, *Semin Roentgenol* 5:341, 1970.

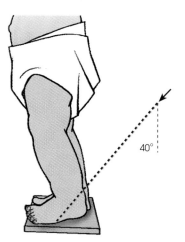

Fig. 6-80 Axial foot (dorsoplantar): Kandel method.

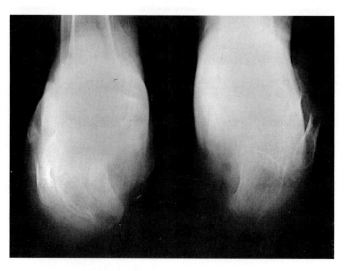

Fig. 6-81 Axial foot (dorsoplantar): Kandel method.

Calcaneus

AXIAL PROJECTION
Plantodorsal

Image receptor: 8 × 10 inch (18 × 24 cm)

Position of patient
- Place the patient in the supine or seated position with the legs fully extended.

Position of part
- Place the cassette under the patient's ankle, centered to the midline of the ankle (Figs. 6-82 and 6-83).
- Place a long strip of gauze around the ball of the foot. Have the patient grasp the gauze to hold the ankle in right-angle dorsiflexion.
- If the patient's ankles cannot be flexed enough to place the plantar surface of the foot perpendicular to the cassette, elevate the leg on sandbags to obtain the correct position.
- *Shield gonads.*

Central ray
- Directed to the midpoint of the cassette at a cephalic angle of 40 degrees to the long axis of the foot. The central ray enters the base of the third metatarsal.

Structures shown
The resulting image shows an axial projection of the calcaneus from the tuberosity to the sustentaculum tali and trochlear process (Fig. 6-84).

EVALUATION CRITERIA
The following should be clearly demonstrated:
- Calcaneus and subtalar joint.
- No rotation of the calcaneus—the first or fifth metatarsals not projected to the sides of the foot.
- Anterior portion of the calcaneus without excessive density over the posterior portion. Otherwise two images may be needed for the two regions of thickness.

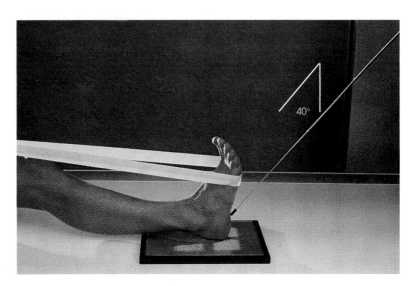

Fig. 6-82 Axial (plantodorsal) calcaneus.

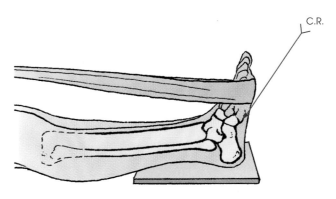

Fig. 6-83 Axial (plantodorsal) calcaneus.

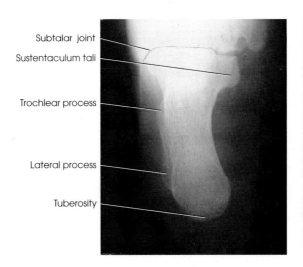
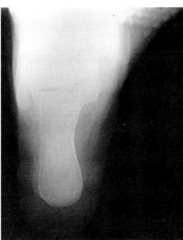

Subtalar joint
Sustentaculum tali
Trochlear process
Lateral process
Tuberosity

Fig. 6-84 Axial (plantodorsal) calcaneus.

263

AXIAL PROJECTION
Dorsoplantar

Image receptor: 8 × 10 inch (18 × 24 cm)

Position of patient
• Place the patient in the prone position.

Position of part
• Elevate the patient's ankle on sandbags.
• Adjust the height and position of the sandbags under the ankle in such a way that the patient can dorsiflex the ankle enough to place the long axis of the foot perpendicular to the tabletop.
• Place the cassette against the plantar surface of the foot, and support it in position with sandbags or a portable cassette holder (Figs. 6-85 and 6-86).
• *Shield gonads.*

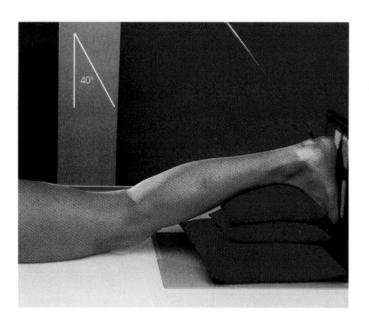

Fig. 6-85 Axial (dorsoplantar) calcaneus.

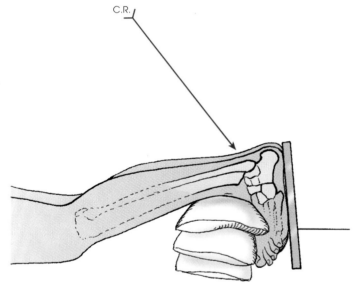

Fig. 6-86 Axial (dorsoplantar) calcaneus.

Central ray

- Directed to the midpoint of the cassette at a caudal angle of 40 degrees to the long axis of the foot. The central ray enters the dorsal surface of the ankle joint and emerges on the plantar surface parallel with the base of the third metatarsal.

Structures shown

The resulting image shows an axial projection of the calcaneus and the subtalar joint (Fig. 6-87).

EVALUATION CRITERIA

The following should be clearly demonstrated:

- Calcaneus and the subtalar joint.
- Sustentaculum tali.
- Calcaneus not rotated—the first or fifth metatarsals not projected to the sides of the foot.

- Anterior portion of the calcaneus without excessive density over posterior portion. Otherwise, two images may be needed for the two regions of thickness.

WEIGHT-BEARING "COALITION METHOD[1]"

This method, described by Lilienfeld[1] (cit. Holzknecht), has come into use for the demonstration of calcaneotalar coalition.[2-4] For this reason it has been called the "coalition position."

---

[1]Lilienfeld L: Anordnung der normalisierten Röntgenaufnahmen des menschlichen Körpers, ed 4, Berlin, 1927, Urban & Schwarzenberg.
[2]Harris RI, Beath T: Etiology of peroneal spastic flat foot, *J Bone Joint Surg* 30B:624, 1948.
[3]Coventry MB: Flatfoot with special consideration of tarsal coalition, *Minn Med* 33:1091, 1950.
[4]Vaughan WH, Segal G: Tarsal coalition, with special reference to roentgenographic interpretation, *Radiology* 60:855, 1953.

Position of patient

- Place the patient in the standing-upright position.

Position of part

- Center the cassette to the long axis of the calcaneus, with the posterior surface of the heel at the edge of the cassette.
- To prevent superimposition of the leg shadow, have the patient place the opposite foot one step forward (Fig. 6-88).

Central ray

- Angled exactly 45 degrees anteriorly and directed through the posterior surface of the flexed ankle to a point on the plantar surface at the level of the base of the fifth metatarsal

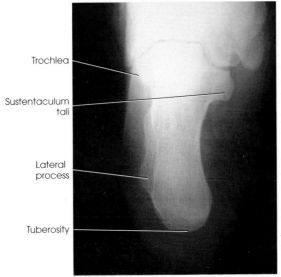
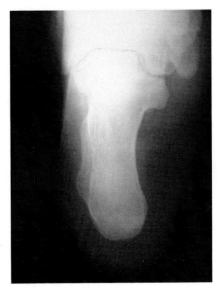

Trochlea

Sustentaculum tali

Lateral process

Tuberosity

Fig. 6-87 Axial (dorsoplantar) calcaneus.

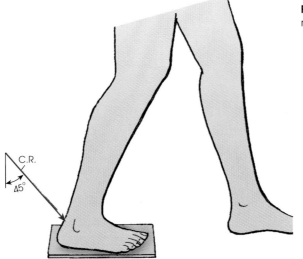

Fig. 6-88 Weight-bearing "coalition method."

C.R.

45°

Calcaneus

 LATERAL PROJECTION
Mediolateral

Image receptor: 8 × 10 inch (18 × 24 cm)

Position of patient
- Have the supine patient turn toward the affected side until the leg is approximately lateral. A support may be placed under the knee.

Position of part
- Adjust the calcaneus to the center of the cassette.
- Adjust the cassette so that the long axis is parallel with the plantar surface of the heel (Fig. 6-89).
- *Shield gonads.*

Central ray
- Perpendicular to the midportion of the calcaneus, which is about 1 inch (2.5 cm) distal to the medial malleolus

Structures shown
The resulting radiograph shows the ankle joint and the calcaneus in lateral profile (Fig. 6-90).

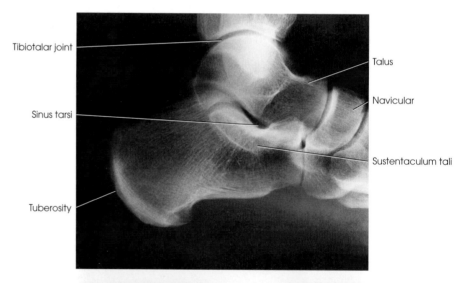

Tibiotalar joint — Talus — Navicular — Sinus tarsi — Sustentaculum tali — Tuberosity

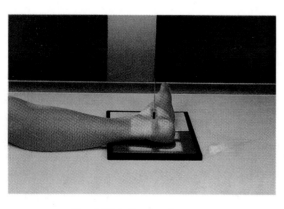

Fig. 6-89 Lateral calcaneus.

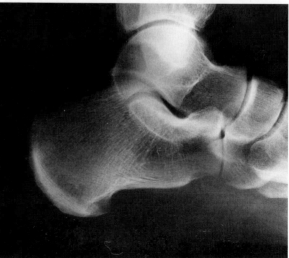

Fig. 6-90 Lateral calcaneus.

Lower limb

Calcaneus

LATEROMEDIAL OBLIQUE PROJECTION
WEIGHT-BEARING METHOD

Image receptor: 8 × 10 inch (18 × 24 cm)

Position of patient
- Have the patient stand with the affected heel centered toward the lateral border of the cassette (Fig. 6-91).
- A mobile radiographic unit may assist in this examination.

Position of part
- Adjust the patient's leg to ensure that it is exactly perpendicular.
- Center the calcaneus so that it will be projected to the center of the cassette.
- Center the lateral malleolus to the midline axis of the cassette.
- *Shield gonads.*

Central ray
- Directed medially at a caudal angle of 45 degrees to enter the lateral malleolus.

Structures shown
The resulting image shows the calcaneal tuberosity and is useful in diagnosing stress fractures of the calcaneus or tuberosity (Fig. 6-92).

EVALUATION CRITERIA

The following should be clearly demonstrated:
- Calcaneal tuberosity
- Sinus tarsi
- Cuboid

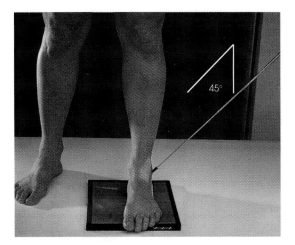

Fig. 6-91 Weight-bearing lateromedial oblique calcaneus.

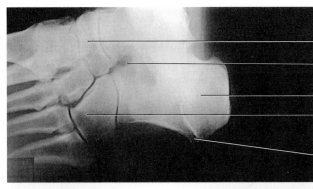

Navicular

Sinus tarsi

Calcaneus

Cuboid

Tuberosity

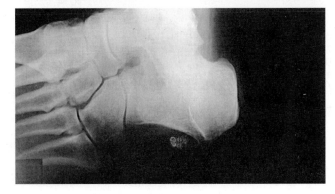

Fig. 6-92 Weight-bearing lateromedial oblique calcaneus.

PA AXIAL OBLIQUE PROJECTION
Lateral rotation

The calcaneus has three articular surfaces: anterior, middle, and posterior. These surfaces are located on the superior calcaneus and articulate with the inferior talus. The articulations form the subtalar (talocalcaneal) joint (see Fig. 6-11). This projection best demonstrates the anterior and posterior articulations.

Image receptor: 8 × 10 inch (18 × 24 cm)

Position of patient
- Have the patient lie on the affected side in the lateral position.
- Flex the uppermost knee to a comfortable position, and support it on sandbags to prevent too much forward rotation of the body (Fig. 6-93).

Position of part
- Ask the patient to extend the affected limb.
- Roll the limb slightly forward from the lateral position.
- Center the cassette 1 to 1½ inches (2.5 to 3.8 cm) distal to the ankle joint and adjust it so that its midline is parallel with the long axis of the leg.

- Adjust the obliquity of the foot so that the heel is elevated about 1½ inches (3.8 cm) from the exact lateral position. The ball of the foot (the metatarsophalangeal area) will be angled forward approximately 25 degrees.
- *Shield gonads.*

Central ray
- Directed to the ankle joint at a double angle of 5 degrees anterior and 23 degrees caudal

Structures shown
The resulting image shows the middle and posterior articulations of the subtalar joint and gives an "end-on" image of the sinus tarsi and an unobstructed projection of the lateral malleolus (Fig. 6-94).

EVALUATION CRITERIA

The following should be clearly demonstrated:

- Open subtalar (talocalcaneal) joint articulations
- Sinus tarsi
- Lateral malleolus seen in profile

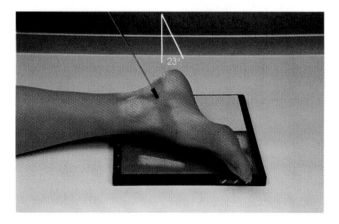

Fig. 6-93 PA axial oblique subtalar joint, lateral rotation.

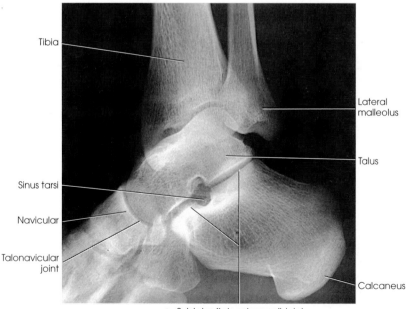
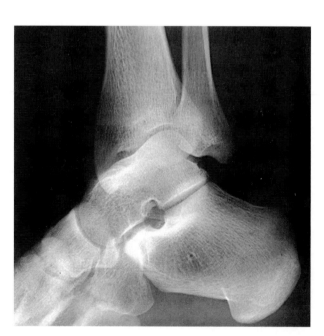

Fig. 6-94 PA axial oblique subtalar joint.

AP AXIAL OBLIQUE PROJECTION
BRODEN METHOD[1]
Medial Rotation

Broden[1] recommended the lateromedial and mediolateral right-angle oblique projections for demonstration of the *posterior articular* facet of the calcaneus to determine the presence of joint involvement in cases of comminuted fracture.

Image receptor: 8 × 10 inch (18 × 24 cm).

[1]Broden B: Roentgen examination of the subtaloid joint in fractures of the calcaneus, *Acta Radiol* 31:85, 1949.

Position of patient
- Place the patient in the supine position.
- Adjust a small sandbag under each knee.

Position of part
- Place the cassette under the patient's lower leg and heel with its midline parallel with and centered to the leg.
- Adjust the cassette so that the lower edge is about 1 inch (2.5 cm) distal to the plantar surface of the heel.

- Loop a strip of bandage around the ball of the foot. Have the patient grasp the ends of the bandage and dorsiflex the foot enough to obtain right-angle flexion at the ankle joint. Ask the patient to maintain the flexion for the exposure.
- With patient's ankle joint maintained in right-angle flexion, rotate the leg and foot 45 degrees medially, and rest the foot against a 45-degree foam wedge (Fig. 6-95).
- *Shield gonads.*

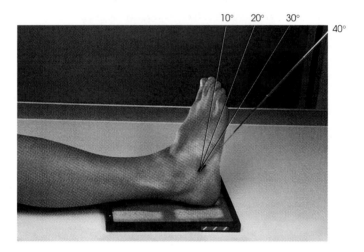

Fig. 6-95 AP axial oblique subtalar joint, medial rotation.

Subtalar Joint

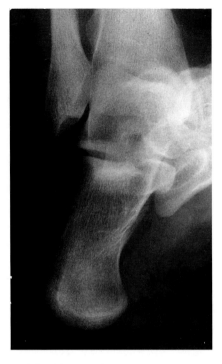

Fig. 6-96 AP axial oblique subtalar joint with angulation of 40 degrees.

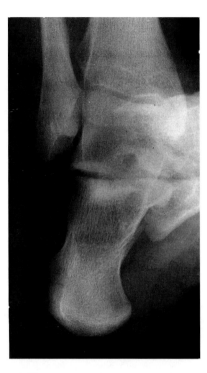

Fig. 6-97 AP axial oblique subtalar joint with angulation of 30 degrees.

Central ray

- Angled cephalad at 40, 30, 20, and 10 degrees, respectively. Four separate images are obtained
- For each image, direct the central ray to a point 2 or 3 cm caudoanteriorly to the lateral malleolus, to the midpoint of an imaginary line extending between the most prominent point of the lateral malleolus and the base of the fifth metatarsal (Figs. 6-96 to 6-99).

Structures shown

The anterior portion of the posterior facet is shown best in the 40-degree projection. The 10-degree projection shows the posterior portion. The articulation between the talus and sustentaculum tali (middle facet) is usually shown best in one of the intermediate projections.

EVALUATION CRITERIA

The following should be clearly demonstrated:

- Anterior and posterior portions of the posterior subtalar joint

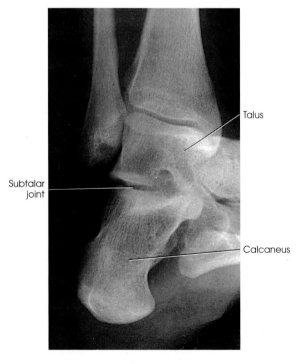

Fig. 6-98 AP axial oblique subtalar joint with angulation of 20 degrees.

Talus

Subtalar joint

Calcaneus

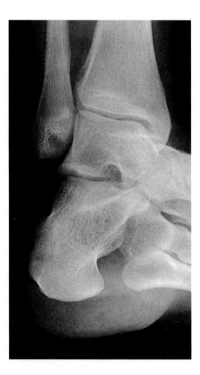

Fig. 6-99 AP axial oblique subtalar joint with angulation of 10 degrees.

AP AXIAL OBLIQUE PROJECTION
BRODEN METHOD
Lateral rotation

Image receptor: 8 × 10 inch (18 × 24 cm)

Position of patient
- Place the patient in the supine position.
- Adjust a small sandbag under each knee.

Position of part
- With the patient's ankle joint held in right-angle flexion, rotate the leg and foot 45 degrees laterally (Fig. 6-100).
- The foot may rest against a 45-degree foam wedge.
- *Shield gonads.*

Central ray
- Directed to a point 2 cm distal and 2 cm anterior to the medial malleolus, at a cephalic angle of 15 degrees for the first exposure (Fig. 6-101).
- Two or three images may be made with a 3- or 4-degree difference in central ray angulation (Fig. 6-102).

Structures shown
The posterior facet of the calcaneus is shown in profile. The articulation between the talus and sustentaculum tali is usually shown.

EVALUATION CRITERIA
The following should be clearly demonstrated:
- Posterior portion of the subtalar joint

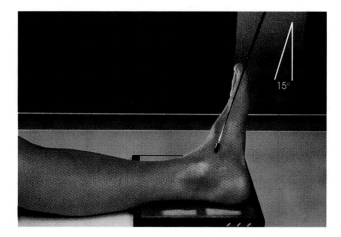

Fig. 6-100 AP axial oblique subtalar joint, lateral rotation.

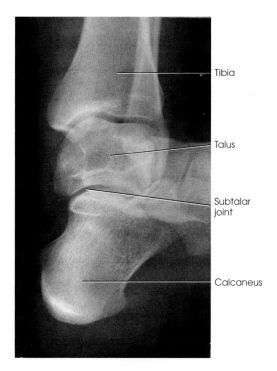

Tibia

Talus

Subtalar joint

Calcaneus

Fig. 6-101 AP axial oblique subtalar joint with angulation of 15 degrees.

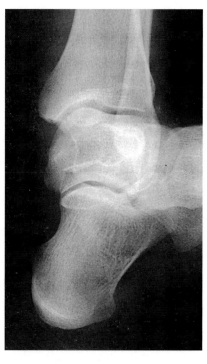

Fig. 6-102 AP axial oblique subtalar joint with angulation of 18 degrees.

LATEROMEDIAL OBLIQUE PROJECTION

ISHERWOOD METHOD[1]

Medial rotation foot

Isherwood[1] devised a method for each of the three separate articulations of the subtalar joint: (1) a *medial rotation foot* position for the demonstration of the anterior talar articular surface, (2) a *medial rotation ankle* position for the middle talar articular surface, and (3) a *lateral rotation ankle* position for the posterior talar articular surface. Feist[2] later described a similar position.

Image receptor: 8 × 10 inch (18 × 24 cm) for each position

Position of patient

- Place the patient in a semisupine or seated position, turned away from the side being examined
- Ask the patient to flex the knee enough to place the ankle joint in nearly right-angle flexion and then to lean the leg and foot medially.

---

[1]Isherwood I: A radiological approach to the subtalar joint, *J Bone Joint Surg* 43B:566, 1961.
[2]Feist JH, Mankin HJ: The tarsus: basic relationships and motions in the adult and definition of optimal recumbent oblique projection, *Radiology* 79:250, 1962.

Position of part

- With the medial border of the foot resting on the cassette, place a 45-degree foam wedge under the elevated leg.
- Adjust the leg so that its long axis is in the same plane as the central ray.
- Adjust the foot to be at a right angle.
- Place a support under the knee (Fig. 6-103).
- *Shield gonads.*

Central ray

- Perpendicular to a point 1 inch (2.5 cm) distal and 1 inch (2.5 cm) anterior to the lateral malleolus

Structures shown

The resulting image shows the anterior subtalar articular surface and an oblique projection of the tarsals (Fig. 6-104). The Feist-Mankin method produces a similar image representation.

EVALUATION CRITERIA

The following should be clearly demonstrated:

- Anterior talar articular surface

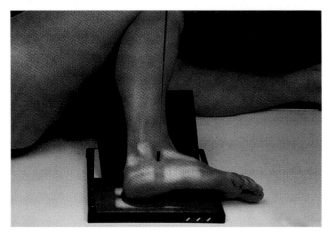

Fig. 6-103 Lateromedial oblique subtalar joint, medial rotation: Isherwood method.

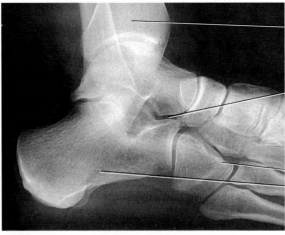
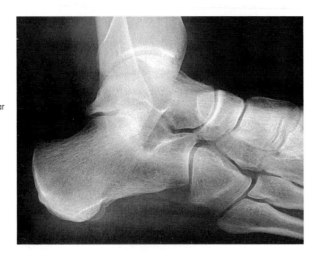

Tibia

Anterior talar articular surface

Cuboid
Calcaneus

Fig. 6-104 Lateromedial oblique subtalar joint demonstrating anterior articular surface: Isherwood method.

AP AXIAL OBLIQUE PROJECTION
ISHERWOOD METHOD
Medial rotation ankle

Image receptor: 8 × 10 in (18 × 24 cm)

Position of patient
- Have the patient assume a seated position on the radiographic table and turn with body weight resting on the flexed hip and thigh of the unaffected side.
- If a semilateral recumbent position is more comfortable, adjust the patient accordingly.

Position of part
- Ask the patient to rotate the leg and foot medially enough to rest the side of the foot and affected ankle on an optional 30-degree foam wedge (Fig. 6-105).
- Place a support under the knee. If the patient is recumbent, place another under the greater trochanter
- Dorsiflex the foot, then invert it if possible, and have the patient maintain the position by pulling on a strip of 2- or 3-inch (5- to 7.6-cm) bandage looped around the ball of the foot.
- *Shield gonads.*

Central ray
- Directed to a point 1 inch (2.5 cm) distal and 1 inch (2.5 cm) anterior to the lateral malleolus at an angle of 10 degrees cephalad.

Structures shown
The resulting image shows the middle articulation of the subtalar joint and an "end-on" projection of the sinus tarsi (Fig. 6-106).

EVALUATION CRITERIA
The following should be clearly demonstrated:
- Middle (subtalar) articulation
- Open sinus tarsi

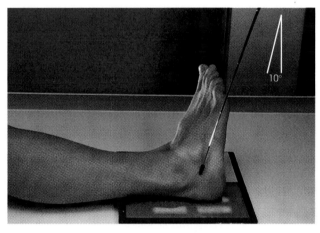

Fig. 6-105 AP axial oblique subtalar joint, medial rotation: Isherwood method.

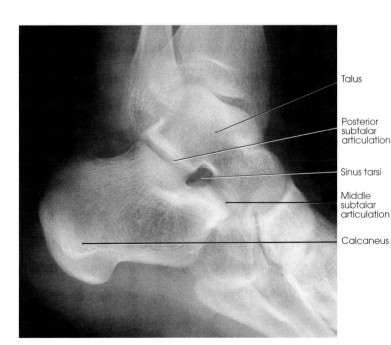
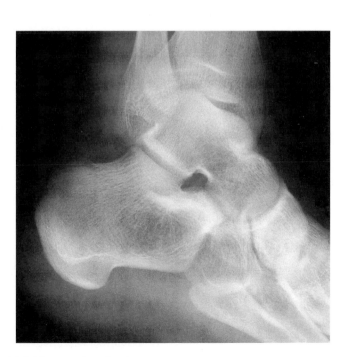

Talus

Posterior subtalar articulation

Sinus tarsi

Middle subtalar articulation

Calcaneus

Fig. 6-106 AP axial oblique subtalar joint: Isherwood method.

AP AXIAL OBLIQUE PROJECTION
ISHERWOOD METHOD
Lateral rotation ankle

Image receptor: 8 × 10 inch (18 × 24 cm)

Position of patient
- Place the patient in the supine or seated position.

Position of part
- Ask the patient to rotate the leg and foot laterally until the side of the foot and ankle rests against an optional 30-degree foam wedge.
- Dorsiflex the foot, evert it if possible, and have the patient maintain the position by pulling on a broad bandage looped around the ball of the foot (Fig. 6-107).
- *Shield gonads.*

Central ray
- Directed to a point 1 inch (2.5 cm) distal to the medial malleolus at an angle of 10 degrees cephalad

Structures shown
The resulting image shows the posterior articulation of the subtalar joint in profile (Fig. 6-108).

EVALUATION CRITERIA
The following should be clearly demonstrated:
- Posterior subtalar articulation

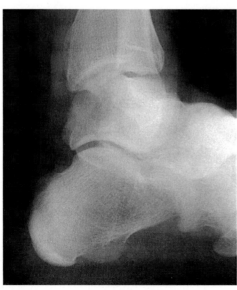

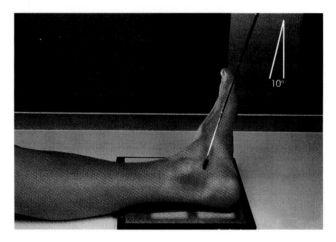

Fig. 6-107 AP axial oblique subtalar joint, lateral rotation: Isherwood method.

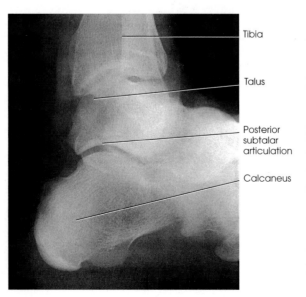

Tibia

Talus

Posterior subtalar articulation

Calcaneus

Fig. 6-108 AP oblique subtalar joint: Isherwood method.

☙ AP PROJECTION

Image receptor: 8 × 10 inch (18 × 24 cm) lengthwise or 24 × 30 cm (10 × 12 inch) crosswise for two images on one cassette

Position of patient

• Place the patient in the supine position with the affected limb fully extended.

Position of part

• Adjust the ankle joint in the anatomic position to obtain a true AP projection. Flex the ankle and foot enough to place the long axis of the foot in the vertical position. The leg should have no rotation (Fig. 6-109).
• Ball and Egbert[1] stated that the appearance of the ankle mortise is not appreciably altered by moderate plantar flexion or dorsiflexion as long as the leg is rotated neither laterally nor medially.
• *Shield gonads.*

Central ray

• Perpendicular to the ankle joint at a point midway between the malleoli.
• If an image of the larger area of the leg is desired, use a larger cassette and position the plantar surface of the heel to

[1]Ball RP, Egbert EW: Ruptured ligaments of the ankle, *AJR* 50:770, 1943.

the lower edge of the cassette. However, if the joint is involved, *always* direct the central ray to the joint.

Structures shown

The resulting image shows a true AP projection of the ankle joint, the distal ends of the tibia and fibula, and the proximal portion of the talus.

NOTE: The inferior tibiofibular articulation and the talofibular articulation will not be "open" nor shown in profile in the true AP projection. This is a positive sign for the radiologist because it indicates that the patient has no ruptured ligaments or other type of separations. For this reason it is important that the position of the ankle be anatomically "true" for the AP projection demonstrated (Fig. 6-110).

The following should be clearly demonstrated:

■ Tibiotalar joint space
■ Ankle joint centered to exposure area
■ Normal overlapping of the tibiofibular articulation with the anterior tubercle slightly superimposed over the fibula
■ Talus slightly overlapping the distal fibula
■ No overlapping of the medial talomalleolar articulation
■ Medial and lateral malleoli
■ Talus with proper density
■ Soft tissue

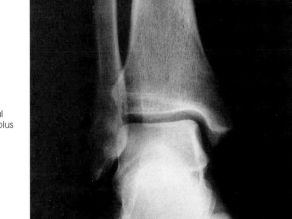

Fig. 6-109 AP ankle.

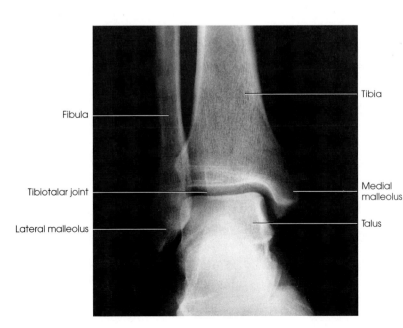
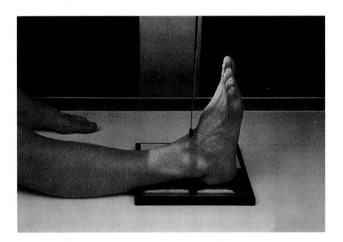

Fig. 6-110 AP ankle.

🔺 LATERAL PROJECTION
Mediolateral

Image receptor: 8 × 10 inch (18 × 24 cm)

Position of patient
- Have the supine patient turn toward the affected side until the ankle is lateral (Fig. 6-111).

Position of part
- Place the long axis of the cassette parallel with the long axis of the patient's leg and center it to the ankle joint.
- Have the patient turn anteriorly or posteriorly as required to place the patella perpendicular to the horizontal plane, and place a support under the knees.
- Dorsiflex the foot, and adjust it in the lateral position. Dorsiflexion is required to prevent lateral rotation of the ankle.
- *Shield gonads.*

Central ray
- Perpendicular to the ankle joint, entering the medial malleolus

Structures shown
The resulting image shows a true lateral projection of the lower third of the tibia and fibula, the ankle joint, and the tarsals (Fig. 6-112).

EVALUATION CRITERIA
The following should be clearly demonstrated:
- Ankle joint centered to exposure area
- Tibiotalar joint well visualized, with the medial and lateral talar domes superimposed
- Fibula over the posterior half of the tibia
- Distal tibia and fibula, talus, and adjacent tarsals
- Density of the ankle sufficient to see the outline of distal portion of the fibula

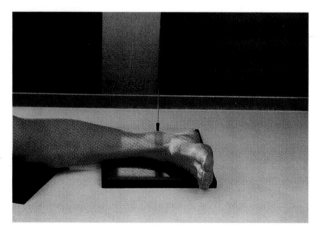

Fig. 6-111 Lateral ankle, mediolateral.

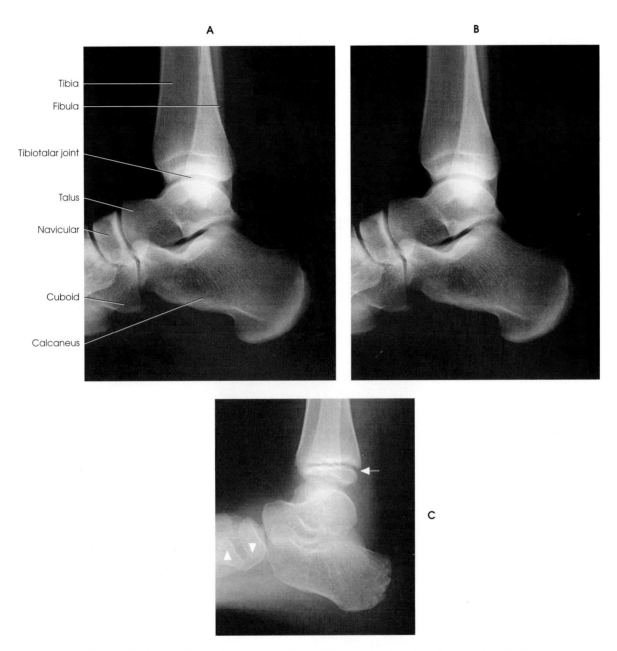

A

B

Tibia

Fibula

Tibiotalar joint

Talus

Navicular

Cuboid

Calcaneus

C

Fig. 6-112 A and **B**, Lateral ankle, mediolateral. **C**, Lateral ankle of an 8-year-old patient. Note the tibial epiphysis (*arrow*) and developing tarsals (*arrowhead*).

Lower limb

LATERAL PROJECTION
Lateromedial

It is often recommended that the lateral projection of the ankle joint be made with the medial side of the ankle in contact with the cassette. This position places the joint closer to the cassette and thus provides an improved image. A further advantage is that exact positioning of the ankle is more easily and more consistently obtained when the limb is rested on its comparatively flat medial surface.

Image receptor: 8 × 10 inch (18 × 24 cm)

Position of patient
- Have the supine patient turn away from the affected side until the extended leg is placed laterally.

Position of part
- Center the cassette to the ankle joint, and adjust the cassette so that its long axis is parallel with the long axis of the leg.
- Adjust the foot in the lateral position.
- Have the patient turn anteriorly or posteriorly as required to place the patella perpendicular to the horizontal plane (Fig. 6-113).
- If necessary, place a support under the patient's knee.
- *Shield gonads.*

Central ray
- Perpendicular through the ankle joint, entering $^1/_2$ inch (1.3 cm) superior to the lateral malleolus

Structures shown
The resulting image shows a lateral projection of the lower third of the tibia and fibula, the ankle joint, and the tarsals (Fig. 6-114).

The following should be clearly demonstrated:
- Ankle joint centered to exposure area
- Tibiotalar joint well visualized, with the medial and lateral talar domes superimposed
- Fibula over the posterior half of the tibia
- Distal tibia and fibula, talus, and adjacent tarsals
- Density of the ankle sufficient to see the outline of distal portion of the fibula

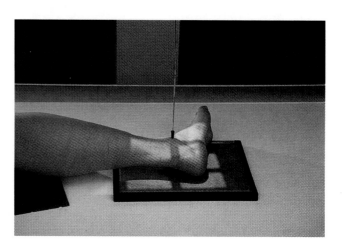

Fig. 6-113 Lateral ankle, lateromedial.

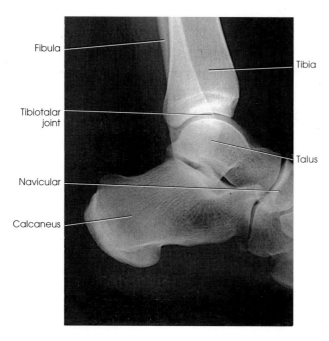
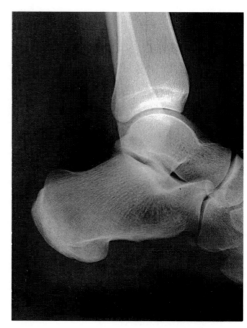

Fig. 6-114 Lateral ankle, lateromedial.

🦅 AP OBLIQUE PROJECTION
Medial rotation

Image receptor: 8 × 10 inch (18 × 24 cm) lengthwise or 24 × 30 cm (10 × 12) in crosswise for two images on one cassette

Position of patient
- Place the patient in the supine position with the affected limb fully extended.

Position of part
- Center the cassette to the ankle joint midway between the malleoli, and adjust the cassette so that its long axis is parallel with the long axis of the leg.
- Dorsiflex the foot enough to place the ankle at nearly right-angle flexion (Fig. 6-115). The ankle may be immobilized with sandbags placed against the sole of the foot or by having the patient hold the ends of a strip of bandage looped around the ball of the foot.
- Rotate the patient's *leg* primarily and the *foot* for all oblique projections of the ankle. Because the knee is a hinge joint, rotation of the leg can come only from the hip joint. Positioning the ankle for the oblique projection requires that the *leg* and *foot* be medially rotated 45 degrees.
- Grasp the lower femur area with one hand and the foot with the other. Internally rotate the entire leg and foot together until the 45-degree position is achieved.
- The foot can be placed against a foam wedge for support.
- *Shield gonads.*

Central ray
- Perpendicular to the ankle joint, entering midway between the malleoli

Structures shown
The 45-degree medial oblique projection demonstrates the distal ends of the tibia and fibula, parts of which are often superimposed over the talus. The tibiofibular articulation also should be demonstrated (Fig. 6-116).

The following should be clearly demonstrated:
- Distal tibia, fibula, and talus
- Distal tibia and fibula overlap some of the talus
- Talus and distal tibia and fibula adequately penetrated
- Tibiofibular articulation

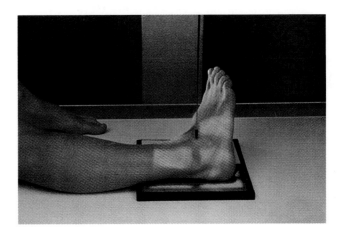

Fig. 6-115 AP oblique ankle, 45-degree medial rotation.

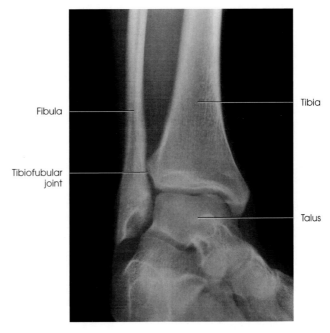

Fig. 6-116 AP oblique ankle, 45-degree medial rotation.

Mortise Joint[1]

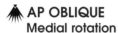 AP OBLIQUE
Medial rotation

Image receptor: 8 × 10 inch (18 × 24 cm) lengthwise or 24 × 30 cm (10 × 12 inch) crosswise for two images on one cassette

Position of patient
• Place the patient in the supine position.

[1]Frank ED et al: Radiography of the ankle mortise, *Radiol Technol* 62:354, 1991.

Position of part
• Center the patient's ankle joint to the cassette.
• Grasp the distal femur area with one hand and the foot with the other. Assist the patient by internally rotating the *entire leg* and *foot* together 15 to 20 degrees until the intermalleolar plane is parallel with the cassette (Fig. 6-117).

• The plantar surface of the foot should be placed at a right angle to the leg (Fig. 6-118).
• *Shield gonads.*

Central ray
• Perpendicular, entering the ankle joint midway between the malleoli

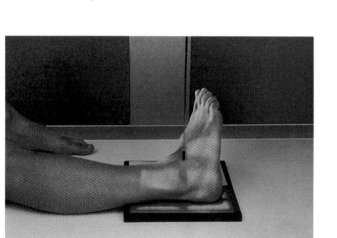

Fig. 6-117 AP oblique ankle, 15- to 20-degree medial rotation for demonstration of the ankle mortise joint.

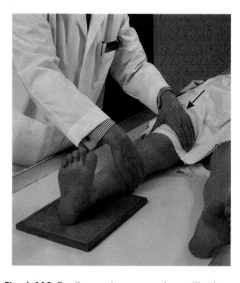

Fig. 6-118 Radiographer properly positioning the leg for demonstration of the ankle mortise joint. Note the action of the left hand *(arrow)* in turning the *leg medially.* Proper positioning requires turning the leg but not the foot.

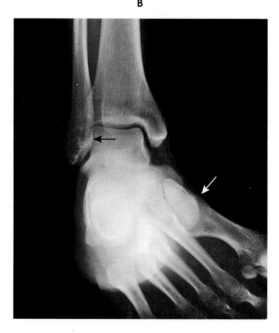

Fig. 6-119 AP oblique ankle, 15- to 20-degree medial rotation for demonstration of the ankle mortise joint. **A,** Properly positioned leg for demonstration of the mortise joint. **B,** Poorly positioned leg; radiograph had to be repeated. The foot was turned medially *(white arrow)* but not the leg. Note that the lateral mortise is closed *(black arrow)* because the "leg" was not medially rotated.

♠ AP PROJECTION

STRESS METHOD

Stress studies of the ankle joint usually are obtained after an inversion or eversion injury to verify the presence of a ligamentous tear. Rupture of a ligament is demonstrated by widening of the joint space on the side of the injury when, without moving or rotating the lower leg from the supine position, the foot is forcibly turned toward the opposite side.

When the injury is recent and the ankle is acutely sensitive to movement, the orthopedic surgeon may inject a local anesthetic into the sinus tarsi preceding the examination. The physician adjusts the foot when it must be turned into extreme stress and holds or straps it in position for the exposure. The patient usually can hold the foot in the stress position when the injury is not too painful or after he or she has received a local anesthestic by asymmetrically pulling on a strip of bandage looped around the ball of the foot (Figs. 6-123 to 6-126).

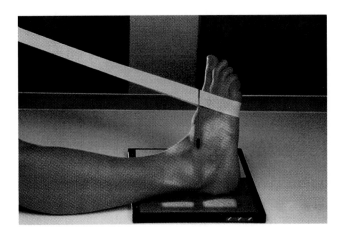

Fig. 6-123 AP ankle in neutral position. Use of lead glove and stress of the joint is required to obtain inversion and eversion radiographs (see Figs. 6-125 and 6-126).

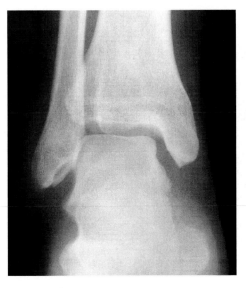

Fig. 6-124 AP ankle, neutral position.

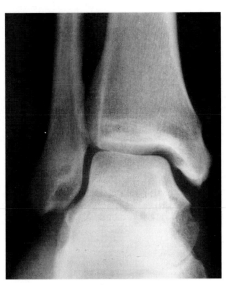

Fig. 6-125 Eversion stress. No damage to the medial ligament is indicated.

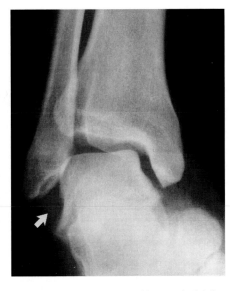

Fig. 6-126 Inversion stress. Change in joint and rupture of lateral ligament (*arrow*) are seen.

🔺 AP PROJECTION

For this projection, as well as the lateral and oblique projections described in the following sections, the long axis of the cassette is placed parallel with the long axis of the leg and centered to the midshaft. Unless the leg is unusually long, the cassette will extend beyond the knee and ankle joints enough to prevent their being projected off the cassette by the divergency of the x-ray beam. The cassette should extend from 1 to 1½ (2.5 to 3.8 cm) inches beyond the joints. When the leg is too long for these allowances and the site of the lesion is not known, two images should be made. The longer cassette is placed high enough to include the knee joint, and a small cassette is used for the distal end of the leg. If the site of the lesion has been localized, the cassette is adjusted to include the closest joint. Diagonal use of a 35 × 43 cm (14 × 17 inch) cassette is also an option if the leg is too long to fit lengthwise and if such use is permitted by the facility

Image receptor: 18 × 43 cm (7 × 17 inch) or 35 × 43 cm (14 × 17 inch) for two images on one cassette

Position of patient
- Place the patient in the supine position.

Position of part
- Adjust the patient's body so that the pelvis is not rotated.
- Adjust the leg so that the femoral condyles are parallel with the cassette and the foot is vertical.
- Flex the ankle until the foot is in the vertical position.
- If necessary, place a sandbag against the plantar surface of the foot to immobilize it in the correct position (Fig. 6-127).
- *Shield gonads.*

Central ray
- Perpendicular to the center of the leg

COMPUTED RADIOGRAPHY

If one cassette is used for two images, the unexposed side must be covered with lead. Scattered radiation reaching the cassette phosphor will produce an undiagnostic image or computer artifacts on both sides.

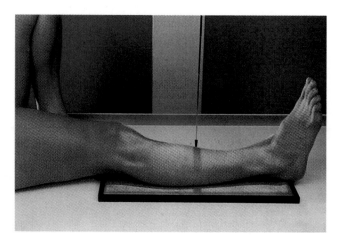

Fig. 6-127 AP tibia and fibula.

Structures shown

The resulting image shows the tibia, fibula, and adjacent joints (Fig. 6-128).

EVALUATION CRITERIA

The following should be clearly demonstrated:

- Ankle and knee joints on one or more AP projections
- Ankle and knee joints without rotation
- Proximal and distal articulations of the tibia and fibula moderately overlapped
- Trabecular detail and soft tissue for the entire leg

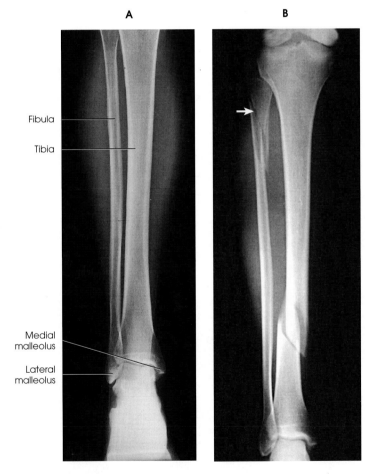

Fig. 6-128 A, AP tibia and fibula. Long leg length prevented demonstration of the entire leg. A separate knee projection had to be performed on this patient. **B,** Short leg length allowed the entire leg to be shown. A spiral fracture of the distal tibia with accompanying spiral fracture of the proximal fibula (*arrow*) is seen. This radiograph demonstrates the importance of including the entire length of a long bone in trauma cases.

🦅 LATERAL PROJECTION
Mediolateral

Image receptor: 18 × 43 cm (7 × 17 inch) or 35 × 43 centimeters (14 × 17 inch) for two images on one cassette

Position of patient
- Place the patient in the supine position.

Position of part
- Turn the patient toward the affected side with the leg on the cassette.
- Adjust the rotation of the body to place the patella perpendicular to the cassette, and ensure that a line drawn through the femoral condyles is also perpendicular.
- Place sandbag supports where needed for the patient's comfort and to stabilize the body position (Fig. 6-129).

Alternate method
- When the patient cannot be turned from the supine position, the lateral projection may be taken cross-table using a horizontal central ray.
- Lift the leg enough for an assistant to slide a rigid support under the patient's leg.
- The cassette may be placed between the legs and the central ray directed from the lateral side.
- *Shield gonads.*

Central ray
- Perpendicular to the midpoint of the leg

COMPUTED RADIOGRAPHY

Structures shown
The resulting image shows the tibia, fibula, and adjacent joints (Fig. 6-130).

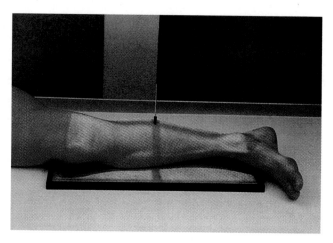

Fig. 6-129 Lateral tibia and fibula.

EVALUATION CRITERIA

The following should be clearly demonstrated:

- Ankle and knee joints on one or more images
- Distal fibula lying over the posterior half of the tibia
- Slight overlap of the tibia on the proximal fibular head
- Ankle and knee joints not rotated
- Possibly no superimposition of femoral condyles because of divergence of the beam
- Moderate separation of the tibial and fibular bodies, or shafts except at their articular ends
- Trabecular detail and soft tissue

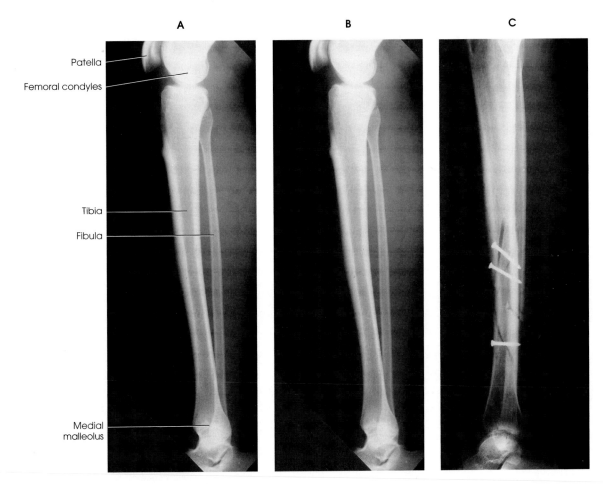

A   B   C

Patella
Femoral condyles

Tibia
Fibula

Medial
malleolus

Fig. 6-130 A and **B**, Lateral tibia and fibula. **C**, Lateral postreduction tibia and fibula, showing a fixation device.

AP OBLIQUE PROJECTIONS
Medial and lateral rotations

Image receptor: 18 × 43 cm (7 × 17 inch) or 35 × 43 cm (14 × 17 inch) for two exposures on one cassette

Position of patient
- Place the patient in the supine position on the radiographic table.

Position of part
- Take oblique projections of the leg by alternately rotating the limb 45 degrees medially (Fig. 6-131) or laterally (Fig. 6-132). Adjustment of the leg for the lateral oblique projection usually requires that the lateral side of the foot and ankle be rested against a 45-degree foam wedge.
- For the medial oblique projection, elevate the affected hip enough to rest the medial side of the foot and ankle against a 45-degree foam wedge, and place a support under the greater trochanter.
- *Shield gonads.*

Central ray
- Perpendicular to the midpoint of the cassette

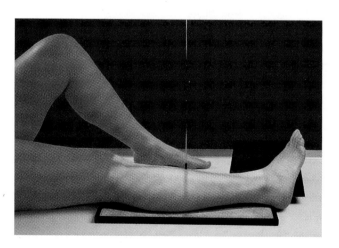

Fig. 6-131 AP oblique leg, medial rotation.

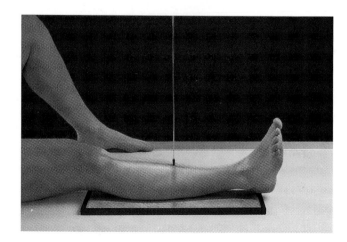

Fig. 6-132 AP oblique leg, lateral rotation.

COMPUTED RADIOGRAPHY

If one cassette is used for two images, ensure that the unexposed side is covered with lead. Scattered radiation reaching the cassette phosphor will produce an undiagnostic image or computer artifacts, on both sides.

Structures shown

The resulting image shows a 45-degree oblique projection of the bones and soft tissues of the leg and one or both of the adjacent joints (Figs. 6-133 and 6-134).

EVALUATION CRITERIA

The following should be clearly demonstrated:

Medial rotation
- Proximal and distal tibiofibular articulations
- Maximum interosseous space between the tibia and fibula
- Ankle and knee joints

Lateral rotation
- Fibula superimposed by lateral portion of tibia
- Ankle and knee joints

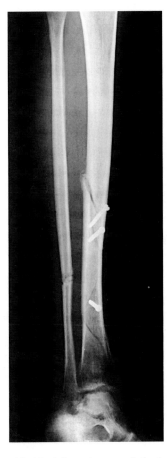

Fig. 6-133 AP oblique leg, medial rotation, showing a fixation device.

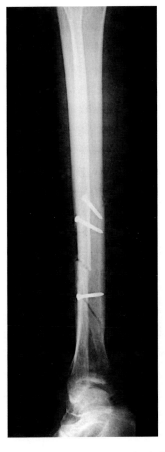

Fig. 6-134 AP oblique leg, lateral rotation, with a fixation device in place.

Lower limb

⚕ AP PROJECTION

Radiographs of the knee may be taken with or without use of a grid. The size of the patient's knee and the preference of the radiographer and physician are the factors considered in reaching a decision. Most medical facilities establish a policy for the routine knee procedure; whether the policy is to use a grid or nongrid technique, the positioning of the body part remains the same.

Attention is again called to the need for gonad shielding in examinations of the lower limbs. (Lead shielding is not shown on illustrations of the patient model because it would obstruct demonstration of the body position.)

Image receptor: 24 × 30 cm (10 × 12 inch) lengthwise.

Position of patient

- Place the patient in the supine position, and adjust the body so that the pelvis is not rotated.

Position of part

- With the cassette under the patient's knee, flex the joint slightly, locate the apex of the patella, and as the patient extends the knee, center the cassette about ½ inch (1.3 cm) below the patellar apex. This will center the cassette to the joint space.
- Adjust the patient's leg by placing the femoral epicondyles parallel with the cassette for a true AP projection (Fig. 6-135). The patella will lie slightly off center to the medial side. If the knee cannot be fully extended, a curved cassette may be used.
- *Shield gonads.*

Central ray

- Directed to a point ½ inch (1.3 cm) inferior to the patellar apex .
- Variable, depending on the measurement between the anterior superior iliac spine (ASIS) and the tabletop (Fig. 6-136), as follows[1]:

19 cm	3 to 5 degrees *caudad* (thin pelvis)
19 to 24 cm	0 degrees
24 cm	3 to 5 degrees *cephalad* (large pelvis)

[1]Martensen KM: Alternate AP knee method assures open joint space, *Radiol Technol* 64:19, 1992.

When radiographing the distal end of the femur or the proximal ends of the tibia and fibula, the central ray may be directed perpendicular to the joint.

Structures shown

The resulting image shows an AP projection of the knee structures (Fig. 6-137).

EVALUATION CRITERIA

The following should be clearly demonstrated:

- Open femorotibial joint space
- Knee fully extended if patient's condition permits
- Interspaces of equal width on both sides if the knee is normal
- Patella completely superimposed on the femur
- No rotation of the femur and tibia
- Slight superimposition of the fibular head if the tibia is normal
- Soft tissue around the knee joint
- Bony detail surrounding the patella on the distal femur

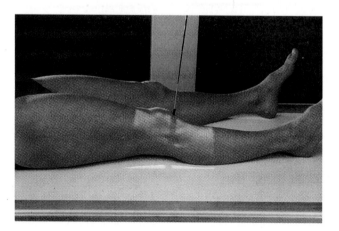

Fig. 6-135 AP knee.

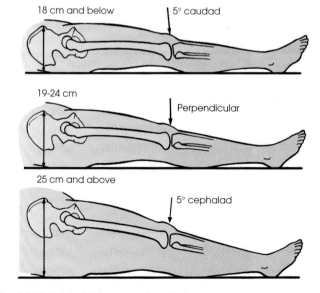

Fig. 6-136 Pelvic thickness and central ray angles for AP knee radiographs.

(Modified from Martensen KM: Alternate AP knee method assures open joint space, *Radiol Technol* 64:19, 1992.)

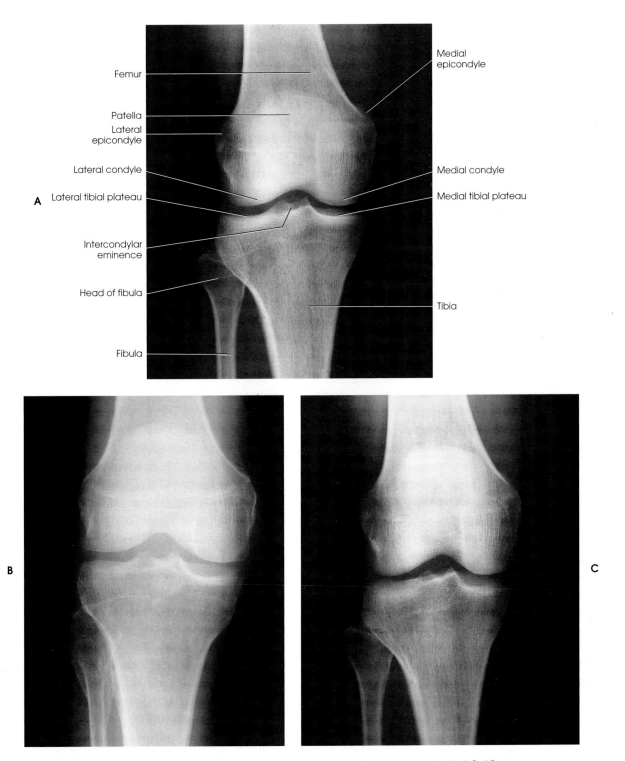

Femur

Patella

Lateral
epicondyle

Lateral condyle

A Lateral tibial plateau

Intercondylar
eminence

Head of fibula

Fibula

Medial
epicondyle

Medial condyle

Medial tibial plateau

Tibia

B

C

Fig. 6-137 A, AP knee. **B,** AP knee with central ray angled 5 degrees cephalad. **C,** AP knee with perpendicular central ray (same patient as in **A** and **B**).

Knee

PA PROJECTION

Image receptor: 24 × 30 cm (10 × 12 inch) lengthwise.

Position of patient

- Place the patient in the prone position with toes resting on the radiographic table, or place sandbags under the ankle for support.

Position of part

- Center a point ½ inch (1.3 cm) below the patellar apex to the center of the cassette, and adjust the patient's leg so that the femoral epicondyles are parallel with the tabletop. Because the knee is balanced on the medial side of the obliquely located patella, care must be used in adjusting the knee (Fig. 6-138).
- *Shield gonads.*

Central ray

- Perpendicular to exit a point ½ inch (1.3 cm) inferior to the patellar apex. Because the tibia and fibula are slightly inclined, the central ray will be parallel with the tibial plateau.

Structures shown

The resulting image shows a PA projection of the knee (Fig. 6-139).

EVALUATION CRITERIA

The following should be clearly demonstrated:

- Open femorotibial joint space
- Knee fully extended if the patient's condition permits
- Interspaces of equal width on both sides if the knee is normal
- No rotation of femur if tibia is normal
- Slight superimposition of the fibular head with the tibia
- Soft tissue around the knee joint
- Bony detail surrounding the patella

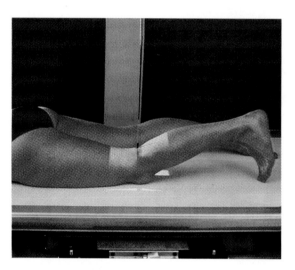

Fig. 6-138 PA knee.

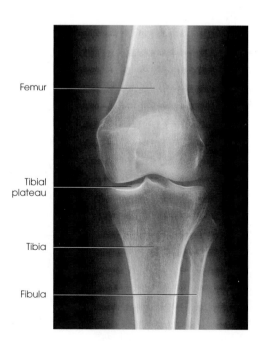

Femur

Tibial plateau

Tibia

Fibula

Fig. 6-139 PA knee.

▲ LATERAL PROJECTION
Mediolateral

Image receptor: 24 × 30 cm (10 × 12 inch) lengthwise

Position of patient
- Ask the patient to turn onto the affected side.
- For a standard lateral projection, have the patient bring the knee forward and extend the other limb behind it (Fig. 6-140). When the knee is examined in extension or partial flexion, the opposite limb may be brought forward and the flexed knee supported to prevent forward rotation of the pelvis.

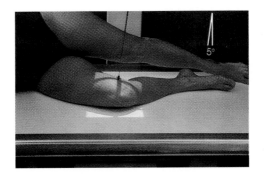

Fig. 6-140 Lateral knee showing 5-degree cephalad angulation of central ray.

Position of part
- A flexion of 20 to 30 degrees is usually preferred because this position relaxes the muscles and shows the maximum volume of the joint cavity.[1]
- To prevent fragment separation in new or unhealed patellar fractures, the knee should not be flexed more than 10 degrees.
- Flex the knee to the desired angle.
- Place a support under the ankle.
- Grasp the epicondyles and adjust them so that they are perpendicular to the cassette (condyles superimposed). The patella will be perpendicular to the plane of the cassette.
- *Shield gonads.*

Central ray
- Directed to the knee joint 1 inch (2.5 cm) distal to the medial epicondyle at an angle of 5 to 7 degrees cephalad. This slight angulation of the central ray will prevent the joint space from being obscured by the magnified image of the medial femoral condyle. In addition, in the lateral recumbent position, the medial condyle will be slightly inferior to the lateral condyle.
- Center the cassette to the central ray.

[1]Sheller S: Roentenographic studies on epiphyseal growth and ossification in the knee, *Acta Radiol* 195:12, 1960.

Structures shown
The resulting radiograph shows a lateral image of the distal end of the femur, patella, knee joint, proximal ends of the tibia and fibula, and adjacent soft tissue (Figs. 6-141 and 6-142).

EVALUATION CRITERIA
The following should be clearly demonstrated:
- Femoral condyles superimposed (Locate the adductor tubercle on the posterior surface of the medial condyle to identify the medial condyle to determine whether the knee is overrotated or underrotated.)
- Open joint space between femoral condyles and tibia
- Patella in a lateral profile
- Open patellofemoral joint space
- Fibular head and tibia slightly superimposed (Overrotation causes less superimposition, and underrotation causes more superimposition.)
- Knee flexed 20 to 30 degrees
- All soft tissue around the knee
- Femoral condyles with proper density

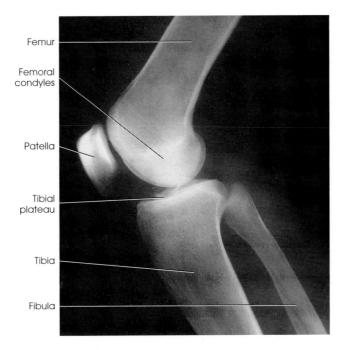

Fig. 6-141 Lateral knee.

Femur
Femoral condyles
Patella
Tibial plateau
Tibia
Fibula

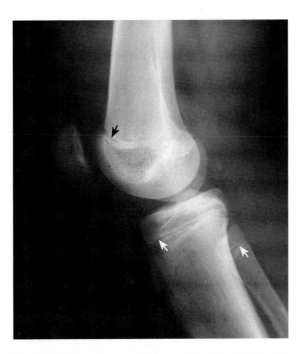

Fig. 6-142 Lateral knee of 15-year-old patient. Note epiphyses (*arrows*) of femur, tibia, and fibula.

Lower limb

☀ AP PROJECTION
WEIGHT-BEARING METHOD
Standing

Leach, Gregg, and Siber[1] recommended that a bilateral weight-bearing AP projection be routinely included in the radiographic examination of arthritic knees. They found that a weight-bearing study often reveals narrowing of a joint space that appears normal on the non–weight-bearing study.

Image receptor: 35 × 43 cm (14 × 17 inch) crosswise for bilateral image

[1]Leach RE, Gregg T, and Siber FJ: Weight-bearing radiography in osteoarthritis of the knee, *Radiology* 97:265, 1970.

Position of patient
- Place the patient in the upright position with back toward a vertical grid device.

Position of part
- Adjust the patient's position to center the knees to the cassette.
- Place the toes straight ahead, with the feet separated enough for good balance.
- Ask the patient to stand straight with knees fully extended and weight equally distributed on the feet
- Center the cassette ½ inch (1.3 cm) below the apices of the patellae (Fig. 6-143).
- *Shield gonads.*

Central ray
- Horizontal and perpendicular to the center of the cassette, entering at a point ½ inch (1.3 cm) below the apices of the patellae

Structures shown

The resulting image shows the joint spaces of the knees. Varus and valgus deformities can also be evaluated with this procedure (Fig. 6-144).

EVALUATION CRITERIA

The following should be clearly demonstrated:
- No rotation of the knees
- Both knees
- Knee joint space centered to the exposure area
- Adequate cassette size to demonstrate the longitudinal axis of the femoral and tibial bodies or shafts

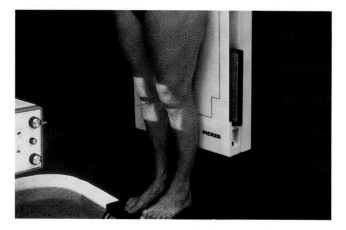

Fig. 6-143 AP bilateral weight-bearing knees.

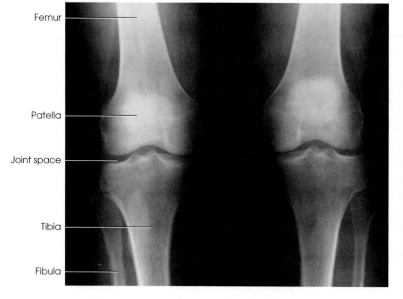

Femur

Patella

Joint space

Tibia

Fibula

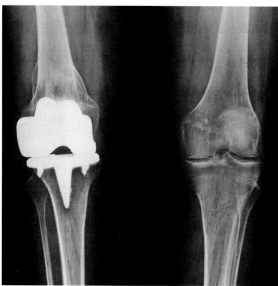

Fig. 6-144 AP bilateral weight-bearing knees.

PA PROJECTION
WEIGHT-BEARING METHOD[1]
Standing Flexion

Image receptor: 35 × 43 cm (14 × 17 inch) crosswise for bilateral knees.

Position of patient
- Place the patient in the standing position with the anterior aspect of the knees centered to the vertical grid device.

Position of part
- For a direct PA projection, have the patient stand upright with knees in contact with the vertical grid device.
- Center the cassette at a level ½ inch (1.3 cm) below the apices of the patellae.
- Have the patient grasp the edges of the grid device and flex knees to place the femurs at an angle of 45 degrees (Fig. 6-145).
- *Shield gonads.*

Central ray
- Horizontal and angled 10 degrees caudad through the tibiofibular joint spaces located ½ inch (1.3 cm) below the patellar apices

Structures shown
PA weight-bearing method is useful for evaluating joint space narrowing and demonstrating articular cartilage disease (Fig. 6-146). The image is similar to those obtained when radiographing the intercondylar fossa.

EVALUATION CRITERIA
The following should be clearly demonstrated:
- No rotation of the knees
- Both knees
- Knee joint centered to the exposure area

NOTE: For a weight-bearing study of a single knee, the patient puts full weight on the affected side. The patient may balance with slight pressure on the toes of the unaffected side.

[1]Rosenberg TD, et al: The forty-five degree posteroanterior flexion weight-bearing radiograph of the knee, *J Bone Joint Surg* 70A:1479, 1988.

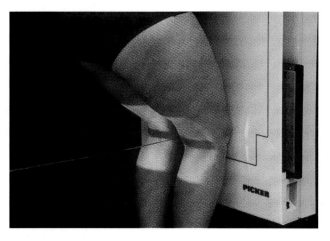

Fig. 6-145 PA projection with patient's knees flexed degrees using a perpendicular central ray.

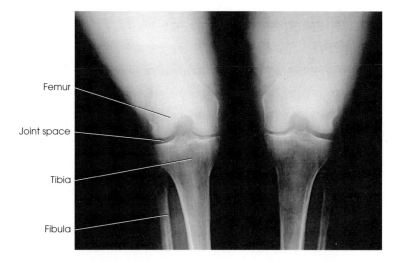

Femur

Joint space

Tibia

Fibula

Fig. 6-146 PA projection with knees flexed 45 degrees and central ray directed 10 degrees caudad.

🔥 AP OBLIQUE PROJECTION
Lateral rotation

Image receptor: 24 × 30 cm (10 × 12 inch) lengthwise

Position of patient
- Place the patient on the radiographic table in the supine position, and support the ankles.

Position of part
- If necessary, elevate the hip of the *unaffected* side enough to rotate the affected limb.
- Support the elevated hip and knee of the unaffected side (Fig. 6-147).
- Center the cassette ½ inch (1.3 cm) below the apex of the patella.
- Externally rotate the limb 45 degrees.
- *Shield gonads.*

Central ray
- Directed ½ inch (1.3 cm) inferior to the patellar apex. The angle is variable, depending on measurement between the ASIS and the tabletop, as follows:

19 cm	3 to 5 degrees *caudad*
19 to 24 cm	0 degrees
24 cm	3 to 5 degrees *cephalad*

Structures shown
The resulting image shows an AP oblique projection of the laterally rotated femoral condyles, patella, tibial condyles, and head of the fibula (Fig. 6-148).

EVALUATION CRITERIA
The following should be clearly demonstrated:
- Medial femoral and tibial condyles
- Tibial plateaus
- Open knee joint
- Fibula superimposed over the lateral half of the tibia
- Margin of the patella projected slightly beyond the edge of the lateral femoral condyle
- Soft tissue around the knee joint
- Bony detail on the distal femur and proximal tibia

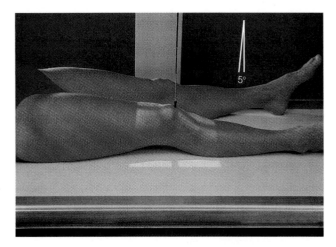

Fig. 6-147 AP oblique knee, lateral rotation.

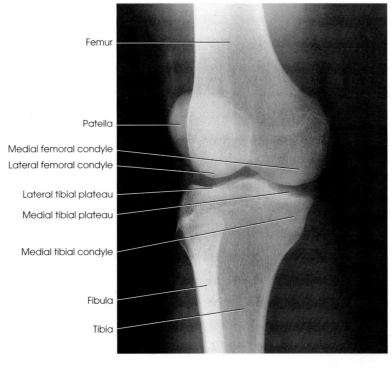

Femur

Patella

Medial femoral condyle
Lateral femoral condyle

Lateral tibial plateau
Medial tibial plateau

Medial tibial condyle

Fibula

Tibia

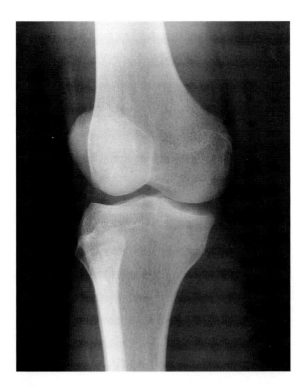

Fig. 6-148 AP oblique knee.

☀ AP OBLIQUE PROJECTION
Medial rotation

Image receptor: 24 × 30 cm (10 × 12 inches) lengthwise

Position of patient
- Place the patient on the table in the supine position, and support the ankles.

Position of part
- Medially rotate the limb, and elevate the hip of the *affected* side enough to rotate the limb 45 degrees.
- Place a support under the hip, if needed (Fig. 6-149).
- *Shield gonads.*

Central ray
- Directed ½ inch (1.3 cm) inferior to the patellar apex; the angle is variable, depending on the measurement between the ASIS and the tabletop, as follows:

19 cm	3 to 5 degrees *caudad*
19 to 24 cm	0 degrees
24 cm	3 to 5 degrees *cephalad*

Structures shown
The resulting image shows an AP oblique projection of the medially rotated femoral condyles, patella, tibial condyles, proximal tibiofibular joint, and head of the fibula (Fig. 6-150).

EVALUATION CRITERIA
The following should be clearly demonstrated:
- Tibia and fibula separated at their proximal articulation
- Posterior tibia
- Lateral condyles of the femur and tibia
- Both tibial plateaus
- Open knee joint
- Margin of the patella projecting slightly beyond the medial side of the femoral condyle
- Soft tissue around the knee joint
- Bony detail on the distal femur and proximal tibia

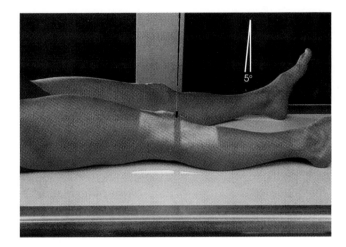

Fig. 6-149 AP oblique knee, medial rotation.

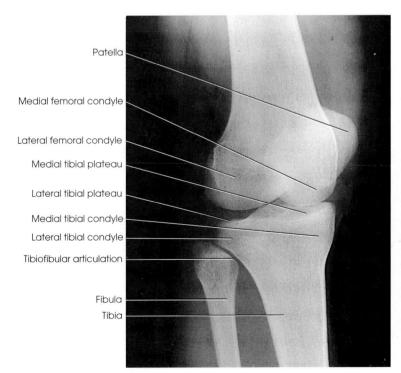
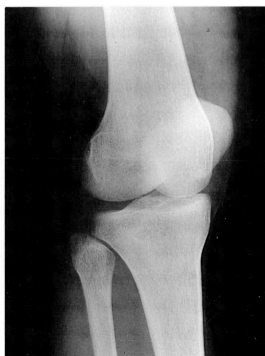

Patella
Medial femoral condyle
Lateral femoral condyle
Medial tibial plateau
Lateral tibial plateau
Medial tibial condyle
Lateral tibial condyle
Tibiofibular articulation
Fibula
Tibia

Fig. 6-150 AP oblique knee.

PA OBLIQUE PROJECTION
Lateral rotation

Image receptor: 24 × 30 cm (10 × 12 inch) lengthwise

Position of patient

- Place the patient on the radiographic table in the prone position.

Position of part

- Elevate the hip of the affected side, and laterally rotate the toes and knee to form a 45-degree angle.
- Support the hip (Fig. 6-151).
- *Shield gonads.*
- Holmblad[1] recommended that the knee be flexed about 10 degrees

---

[1]Holmblad EC: Improved x-ray technic in studying knee joints, *South Med* J 32:240, 1939.

Central ray

- Perpendicular through the knee joint at a level ½ inch (1.3 cm) below the patellar apex

Structures shown

The resulting image shows a PA oblique projection of the laterally rotated femoral condyles, patella, tibial condyles, and fibular head (Fig. 6-152).

The following should be clearly demonstrated:

- Medial femoral and tibial condyles
- Tibial plateaus
- Open knee joint
- Fibula superimposed over the lateral portion of the tibia
- Patellar margin projecting slightly beyond the side of the lateral femoral condyle
- Soft tissue around the knee joint
- Bony detail on the distal femur and proximal tibia

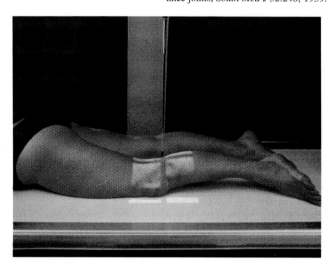

Fig. 6-151 PA oblique knee, lateral rotation.

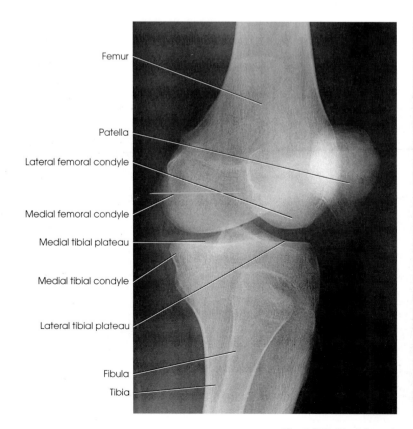
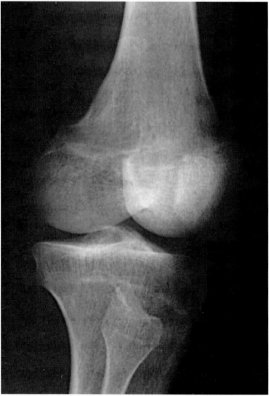

Femur

Patella

Lateral femoral condyle

Medial femoral condyle

Medial tibial plateau

Medial tibial condyle

Lateral tibial plateau

Fibula

Tibia

Fig. 6-152 PA oblique knee.

PA OBLIQUE PROJECTION
Medial rotation

Image receptor: 24 × 30 cm (10 × 12 inch) lengthwise

Position of patient
• Place the patient in the prone position.

Position of part
• Medially rotate the leg and foot, and elevate the hip of the unaffected side to rotate the limb 45 degrees medially.
• Place a support under the hip, if needed (Fig. 6-153).
• *Shield gonads.*

Central ray
• Perpendicular through the knee joint at the level $\frac{1}{2}$ inch (1.3 cm) below the apex of the patella

Structures shown
The resulting image shows a PA oblique projection of the medially rotated femoral condyles, patella, tibial condyles, proximal tibiofibular joint, and fibular head (Fig. 6-154).

EVALUATION CRITERIA
The following should be clearly demonstrated:
■ Tibia and fibula separated at their proximal articulation
■ Posterior tibia
■ Lateral condyles of the femur and tibia
■ Both tibial plateaus
■ Open knee joint
■ Margin of the patella projecting slightly beyond the side of the medial femoral condyle
■ Soft tissue around the knee joint
■ Bony detail on the distal femur and proximal tibia

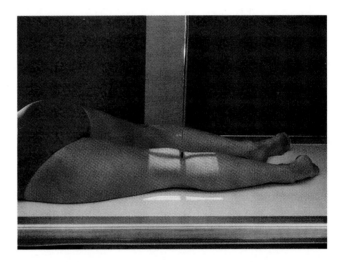

Fig. 6-153 PA oblique knee, medial rotation.

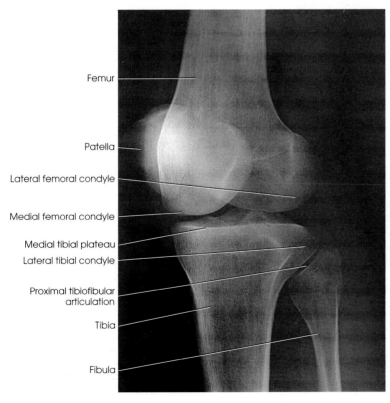
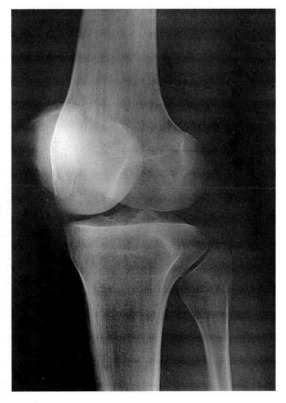

Femur

Patella

Lateral femoral condyle

Medial femoral condyle

Medial tibial plateau
Lateral tibial condyle

Proximal tibiofibular articulation

Tibia

Fibula

Fig. 6-154 PA oblique knee.

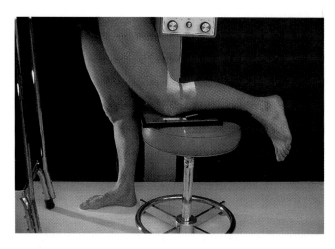

Fig. 6-155 PA axial intercondylar fossa, upright with knee on stool.

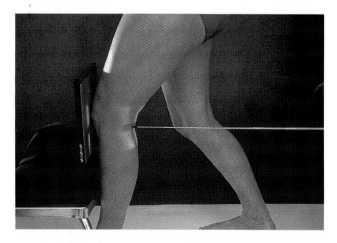

Fig. 6-156 PA axial intercondylar fossa, standing using horizontal central ray.

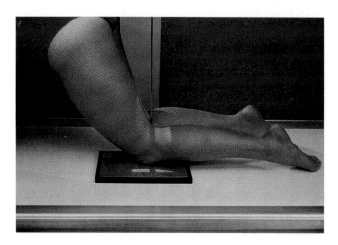

Fig. 6-157 PA axial intercondylar fossa, kneeling on radiographic table: original Holmblad method.

PA AXIAL PROJECTION
HOLMBLAD METHOD[1]

The PA axial, or "tunnel," projection, first described by Holmblad in 1937, required that the patient assume a kneeling position on the radiographic table. In 1983 the Holmblad method was modified so that if the patient's condition allowed, a standing position could be used.[2]

Image receptor: 8 × 10 inch (18 × 24 cm)

Position of patient

- After consideration of the patient's safety, place the patient in one of three positions: (1) standing with the knee of interest flexed and resting on a stool at the side of the radiographic table (Fig. 6-155), (2) standing at the side of the radiographic table with the affected knee flexed and placed in contact with the front of the cassette (Fig. 6-156), or (3) kneeling on the radiographic table as originally described by Holmblad, with the affected knee over the cassette (Fig. 6-157). In all three approaches, the patient leans on the radiographic table for support.

[1]Holmblad EC: Postero-anterior x-ray view of the knee in flexion, *JAMA* 109:1196, 1937.
[2]Turner GW, Burns CB, Previtte RG: Erect positions for "tunnel" views of the knee, *Radiol Technol* 55:640, 1983.

Intercondylar Fossa

Position of part
- For all positions, place the cassette against the anterior surface of the patient's knee, and center the cassette to the apex of the patella. Flex the knee 70 degrees from full extension (20-degree difference from the central ray, as shown in Fig. 6-158).
- *Shield gonads.*

Central ray
- Perpendicular to the lower leg, entering the midpoint of the cassette for all three positions

Structures shown
The resulting image shows the intercondylar fossa of the femur and the medial and lateral intercondylar tubercles of the intercondylar eminence in profile (Fig. 6-159). Holmblad[1] stated that the degree of flexion used in this position widens the joint space between the femur and tibia and gives an improved image of the joint and the surfaces of the tibia and femur.

---

[1]Holmblad EC: Postero-anterior x-ray view of the knee in flexion, *JAMA* 109:1196, 1937.

EVALUATION CRITERIA
The following should be clearly demonstrated:
- Open fossa
- Posteroinferior surface of the femoral condyles
- Intercondylar eminence and knee joint space
- Apex of the patella not superimposing the fossa
- No rotation, evident by slight tibiofibular overlap
- Soft tissue in the fossa and interspaces
- Bony detail on the intercondylar eminence, distal femur, and proximal tibia

NOTE: The bilateral examination is described on p. 295 (also see Figs. 6-145 and 6-146).

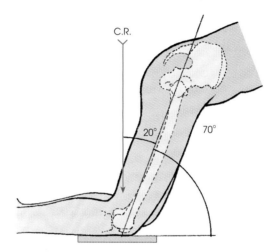

Fig. 6-158 Alignment relationship for any of three intercondylar fossa approaches: Holmblad method.

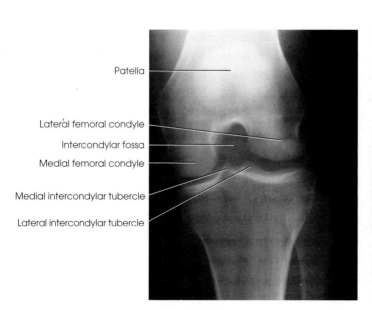
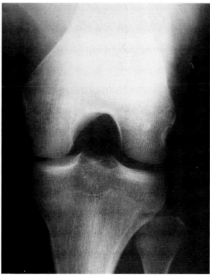

Patella

Lateral femoral condyle

Intercondylar fossa

Medial femoral condyle

Medial intercondylar tubercle

Lateral intercondylar tubercle

Fig. 6-159 PA axial ("tunnel") intercondylar fossa: Holmblad method.

♠ PA AXIAL PROJECTION
CAMP-COVENTRY METHOD[1]

Image receptor: 8 × 10 inch (18 × 24 cm) lengthwise

Position of patient
• Place the patient in the prone position, and adjust the body so that it is not rotated.

[1]Camp JD, Coventry MB: Use of special views in roentgenography of the knee joint, *US Naval Med Bull* 42:56, 1944.

Position of part
• Flex the patient's knee to either a 40- or 50-degree angle, and rest the foot on a suitable support.
• Center the upper half of the cassette to the knee joint; the central ray angulation projects the joint to the center of the cassette (Figs. 6-160 and 6-161).
• A protractor may be used beside the leg to determine the correct leg angle.
• Adjust the leg so that the knee has no medial or lateral rotation.
• *Shield gonads.*

Central ray
• Perpendicular to the long axis of the leg and centered to the knee joint (i.e., over the popliteal depression)
• Angled 40 degrees when the knee is flexed 40 degrees and 50 degrees when the knee is flexed 50 degrees

Structures shown
This axial image demonstrates an unobstructed projection of the intercondyloid fossa and the medial and lateral intercondylar tubercles of the intercondylar eminence (Figs. 6-162 and 6-163).

The following should be clearly demonstrated:
■ Open fossa
■ Posteroinferior surface of the femoral condyles
■ Intercondylar eminence and knee joint space
■ Apex of the patella not superimposing the fossa
■ No rotation, evident by slight tibiofibular overlap
■ Soft tissue in the fossa and interspaces
■ Bony detail on the intercondylar eminence, distal femur, and proximal tibia

NOTE: In routine examinations of the knee joint, an intercondylar fossa projection is usually included to detect loose bodies ("joint mice"). The projection is also used in evaluating split and displaced cartilage in osteochondritis dissecans and flattening, or underdevelopment, of the lateral femoral condyle in congenital slipped patella.

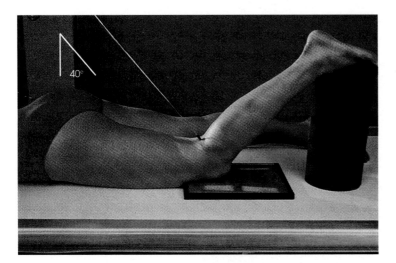

Fig. 6-160 PA axial ("tunnel") intercondylar fossa: Camp-Coventry method.

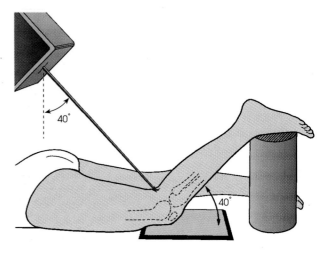

Fig. 6-161 PA axial ("tunnel") intercondylar fossa: Camp-Coventry method.

A

B

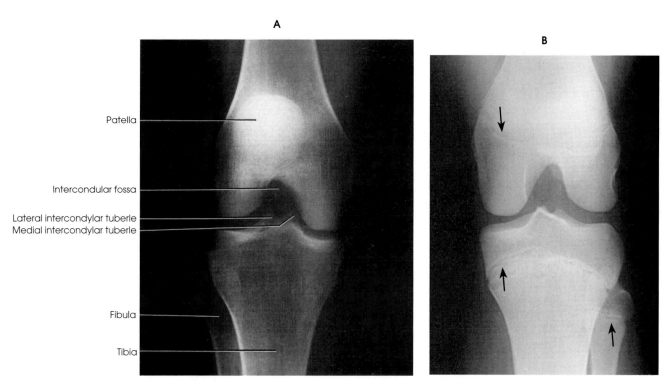

Patella

Intercondular fossa

Lateral intercondylar tuberle
Medial intercondylar tuberle

Fibula

Tibia

Fig. 6-162 Camp-Coventry method. **A**, Flexion of knee at 40 degrees (same patient as in Fig. 6-163). **B**, Flexion of knee at 40 degrees in a 13-year-old patient. Note epiphyses (*arrows*).

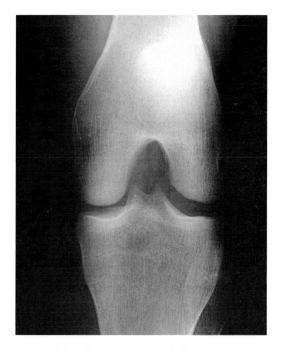

Fig. 6-163 Flexion of knee at 50 degrees (same patient as in Fig. 6-157): Camp-Coventry method.

AP AXIAL PROJECTION
BÉCLÈRE METHOD

Image receptor: 8 × 10 inch (18 × 24 cm)

A curved cassette is preferred to obtain a closer object-to-image receptor distance. An 8 × 10 inch (18 × 24 cm) transverse cassette supported on sandbags also may be used.

Position of patient
• Place the patient in the supine position, and adjust the body so that it is not rotated.

Position of part
• Flex the affected knee enough to place the long axis of the femur at an angle of 60 degrees to the long axis of the tibia.
• Support the knee on sandbags (Figs. 6-164 and 6-165).
• Place the cassette under the knee, and position the cassette so that the center point coincides with the central ray.
• Adjust the leg so that the femoral condyles are equidistant from the cassette. Immobilize the foot with sandbags.
• *Shield gonads.*

Central ray
• Perpendicular to the long axis of the tibia, entering the knee joint ½ inch (1.3 cm) below the patellar apex

Structures shown
The resulting image shows the intercondylar fossa, intercondylar eminence, and knee joint (Fig. 6-166).

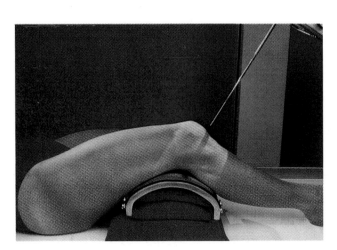

Fig. 6-164 AP axial intercondylar fossa with curved cassette: Béclère method.

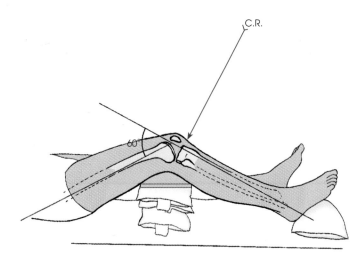

Fig. 6-165 AP axial intercondylar fossa with transverse cassette: Béclère method.

Intercondylar Fossa

EVALUATION CRITERIA

The following should be clearly demonstrated:

- Open intercondylar fossa
- Posteroinferior surface of the femoral condyles
- Intercondylar eminence and knee joint space
- No superimposition of the fossa by the apex of the patella
- No rotation, evident by slight tibiofibular overlap
- Soft tissue in the fossa and interspaces
- Bony detail on the intercondylar eminence, distal femur, and proximal tibia

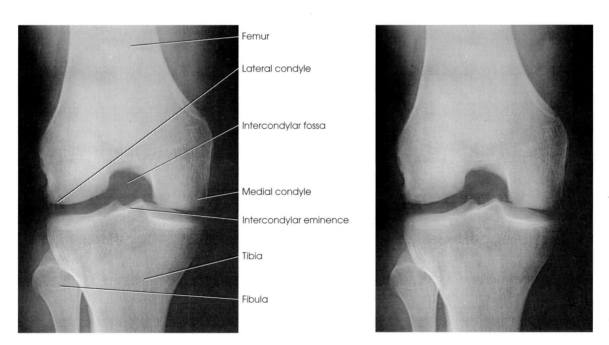

Femur

Lateral condyle

Intercondylar fossa

Medial condyle

Intercondylar eminence

Tibia

Fibula

Fig. 6-166 AP axial intercondylar fossa: Béclère method.

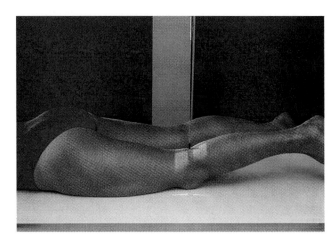

Fig. 6-167 PA patella.

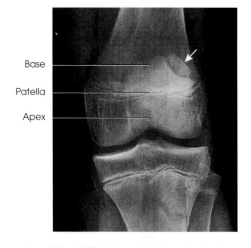

Base

Patella

Apex

Fig. 6-168 AP patella showing fracture (*arrow*).

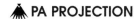

PA PROJECTION

Image receptor: 8 × 10 inch (18 × 24 cm) lengthwise

Position of patient
- Place the patient in the prone position.
- If the knee is painful, place one sand-bag under the thigh and another under the leg to relieve pressure on the patella.

Position of part
- Center the cassette to the patella.
- Adjust the position of the leg to place the patella parallel with the plane of the cassette. This usually requires that the heel be rotated 5 to 10 degrees laterally (Fig. 6-167).
- *Shield gonads.*

Central ray
- Perpendicular to the midpopliteal area exiting the patella.
- Collimate closely to the patellar area.

Structures shown
The PA projection of the patella provides sharper recorded detail than in the AP projection because of a closer object-to-image receptor distance (OID) (Figs. 6-168 and 6-169).

EVALUATION CRITERIA
The following should be clearly demonstrated:
- Patella completely superimposed by the femur
- Adequate penetration for visualization of the patella clearly through the superimposing femur
- No rotation

Fig. 6-169 A, Conventional PA projection of the patella shows a vertical radiolucent line (*arrow*) passing through the junction of the lateral and middle third of the patella.
B, On tomography this defect extends from the superior to the inferior margin of the patella. It is a bipartite patella and not a fracture.

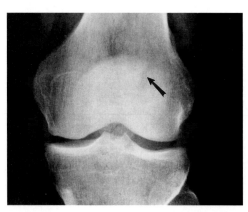

A

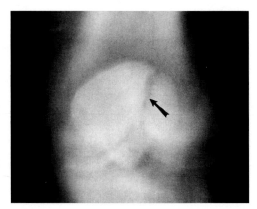

B

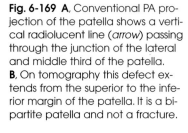

⚜ LATERAL PROJECTION
Mediolateral

Image receptor: 8 × 10 inch (18 × 24 cm) lengthwise

Position of patient
- Place the patient in the lateral recumbent position.

Position of part
- Ask the patient to turn onto the affected hip. A sandbag may be placed under the ankle for support.
- Have the patient flex the unaffected knee and hip, and place the unaffected foot in front of the affected limb for stability.
- Flex the affected knee approximately 5 to 10 degrees. Increasing the flexion reduces the patellofemoral joint space.
- Adjust the knee in the lateral position so that the femoral epicondyles are superimposed and the patella is perpendicular to the cassette (Fig. 6-170).
- *Shield gonads.*
- Center the cassette to the patella.

Central ray
- Perpendicular to the cassette, entering the knee at the midpatellofemoral joint.
- Collimate closely to the patellar area.

COMPUTED RADIOGRAPHY
Collimation must be close to keep unnecessary radiation from reaching the cassette phosphor.

Structures shown
The resulting image shows a lateral projection of the patella and patellofemoral joint space (Fig. 6-171).

EVALUATION CRITERIA
The following should be clearly demonstrated:
- Knee flexed 5 to 10 degrees
- Open patellofemoral joint space
- Patella in lateral profile
- Close collimation

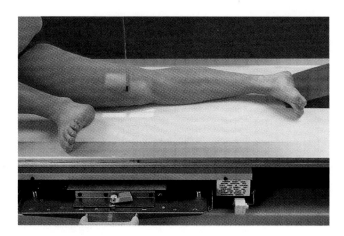

Fig. 6-170 Lateral patella, mediolaterial.

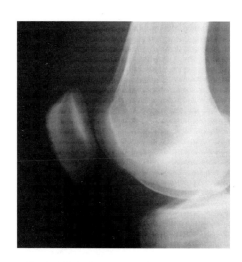

Fig. 6-171 Lateral patella, mediolaterial.

Patella

PA OBLIQUE PROJECTION
Medial rotation

Image receptor: 8 × 10 inch (18 × 24 cm) lengthwise

Position of patient
- Place the patient in the prone position.

Position of part
- Flex the patient's knee approximately 5 to 10 degrees.
- Medially rotate the knee 45 to 55 degrees from the prone position.
- Center the medial portion of the patella to the cassette (Fig. 6-172).
- *Shield gonads.*

Central ray
- Perpendicular to the cassette, exiting the palpated patella.
- Collimate closely to the patellar area.

Structures shown
A PA oblique image of the medial portion of the patella is demonstrated free of the femur (Fig. 6-173).

The following should be clearly demonstrated:
- Majority of the medial patella free of superimposition of the femur
- Lateral margin of patella superimposed over the femur
- Closely collimated image

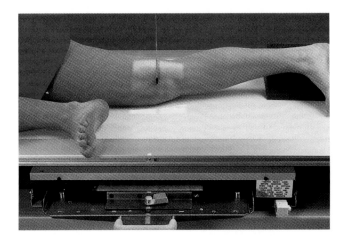

Fig. 6-172 PA oblique patella, medial rotation.

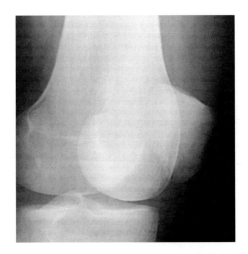

Fig. 6-173 PA oblique patella.

PA OBLIQUE PROJECTION
Lateral rotation

Image receptor: 8 × 10 inch (18 × 24 cm) lengthwise

Position of patient
- Place the patient in the prone position.

Position of part
- Flex the patient's knee 5 to 10 degrees, and externally (laterally) rotate the knee 45 to 55 degrees from the prone position.
- Center the lateral portion of the patella to the cassette (Fig. 6-174).
- *Shield gonads.*

Central ray
- Perpendicular to the cassette, exiting the palpated patella.
- Collimate closely to the patellar area.

Structures shown
The resulting image shows an oblique projection of the lateral aspect of the patella free of the femur (Fig. 6-175).

EVALUATION CRITERIA
The following should be clearly demonstrated:
- Majority of the patella free of superimposition of the femur
- Medial margin of patella superimposed over the femur
- Closely collimated image

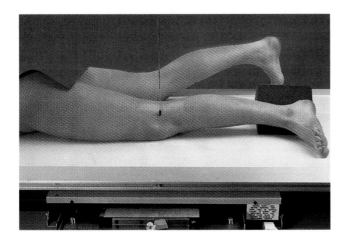

Fig. 6-174 PA oblique patella, lateral rotation.

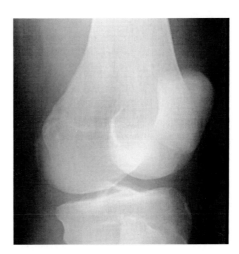

Fig. 6-175 PA oblique patella, lateral rotation.

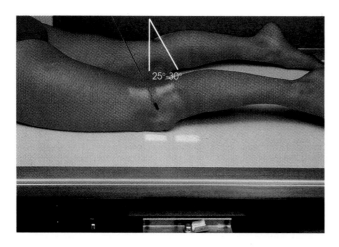

Fig. 6-176 PA axial oblique patella, lateral rotation.

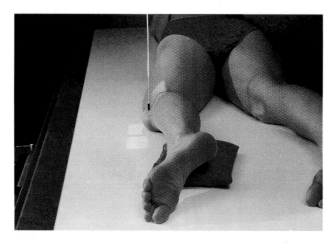

Fig. 6-177 PA axial oblique patella, lateral rotation.

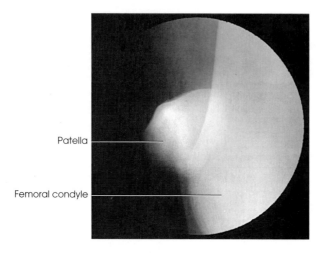

Patella

Femoral condyle

Fig. 6-178 PA axial oblique patella.

PA AXIAL OBLIQUE PROJECTION
KUCHENDORF METHOD
Lateral rotation

Image receptor: 8 × 10 inch (18 × 24 cm) lengthwise

Position of patient
- Place the patient in the prone position.
- Elevate the hip of the affected side 2 or 3 inches.
- Place a sandbag under the ankle and foot, and adjust it so that the knee is slightly flexed (approximately 10 degrees) to relax the muscles.

Position of part
- Center the cassette to the patella.
- Laterally rotate the knee approximately 35 to 40 degrees from the prone position (this position is more comfortable for the patient than the direct prone, because no pressure is placed on the injured patella. The patient rarely objects to the slight pressure required to displace the patella laterally).
- Place the index finger against the medial border of the patella, and press it laterally.
- Rest the knee on its anteromedial side to hold the patella in a position of lateral displacement (Figs. 6-176 and 6-177).
- *Shield gonads.*

Central ray
- Directed to the joint space between the patella and the femoral condyles at an angle of 25 to 30 degrees caudad. It enters the posterior surface of the patella.

Structures shown
The resulting image will show a slightly oblique PA projection of the patella, with most of the patella free of superimposed structures (Fig. 6-178).

EVALUATION CRITERIA

The following should be clearly demonstrated:
- Majority of the patella free of superimposition by the femur
- Patella and its outline where it is superimposed by the femur

TANGENTIAL PROJECTION
HUGHSTON METHOD[1,2]

Radiography of the patella has been the topic of hundreds of articles. For a tangential radiograph, the patient may be placed in any of the following body positions: prone, supine, lying on the side, seated on the table, seated on the radiographic table with the leg hanging over the edge, or standing.

Various authors have described the degree of flexion of the knee joint as being as little as 20 degrees to as much as 120 degrees. Laurin[3] reported that patellar subluxation is easier to demonstrate when the knee is flexed 20 degrees and noted a limitation of using this small angle. Modern radiographic equipment often will not permit such small angles because of the large size of the collimator.

Fodor, Malott, and Weinberg[4] and Merchant et al[5] recommended a 45-degree flexion of the knee, and Hughston[6] recommended an approximately 55-degree angle with the central ray angled 45 degrees.

Image receptor: 8 × 10 inch (18 × 24 cm) for unilateral examination; 24 × 30 cm (10 × 12 inch) crosswise for bilateral examination

Position of patient
- Place the patient in a prone position with the foot resting on the radiographic table.
- Adjust the body so that it is not rotated.

Position of part
- Place the cassette under the patient's knee, and slowly flex the affected knee so that the tibia and fibula form a 50- to 60-degree angle from the table.
- Rest the foot against the collimator, or support it in position (Fig. 6-179).

[1]Hughston JC: Subluxation of the patella, *J Bone Joint Surg* 50A:1003, 1968.
[2]Kimberlin GE: Radiological assessment of the patellofemoral articulation and subluxation of the patella, *Radiol Technol* 45:129, 1973.
[3]Laurin CA: The abnormal lateral patellofemoral angle, *J Bone Joint Surg* 60A:55, 1968.
[4]Fodor J, Malott JC, Weinberg S: Accurate radiography of the patellofemoral joint, *Radiol Technol* 53:570, 1982.
[5]Merchant AC et al: Roentgenographic analysis of patellofemoral congruence, *J Bone Joint Surg* 56A:1391, 1974.
[6]Hughston JC: Subluxation of the patella, *J Bone Joint Surg* 50A:1003, 1968.

- Ensure that the collimator surface is not hot because this could burn the patient.
- Adjust the patient's leg so that it is not rotated medially or laterally from the vertical plane.
- *Shield gonads.*

Central ray
- Angled 45 degrees cephalad and directed through the patellofemoral joint

Structures shown
The tangential image shows subluxation of the patella and patellar fractures and allows radiologic assessment of the femoral condyles. Hughston recommended that both knees be examined for comparison (Fig. 6-180).

EVALUATION CRITERIA
The following should be clearly demonstrated:
- Patella in profile
- Open patellofemoral articulation
- Surfaces of the femoral condyles
- Soft tissue of the femoropatellar articulation
- Bony recorded detail on the patella and femoral condyles

NOTE: Care must be taken to ensure that the foot does not come in contact with the hot collimator housing, which is heated by the light. In addition, the x-ray tube and support mechanism must be properly grounded.

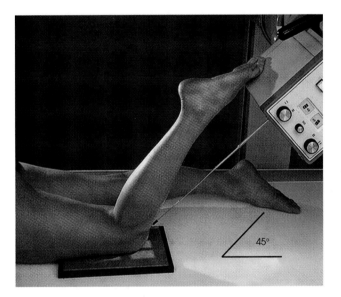

Fig. 6-179 Tangential patella and patellofemoral joint: Hughston method.

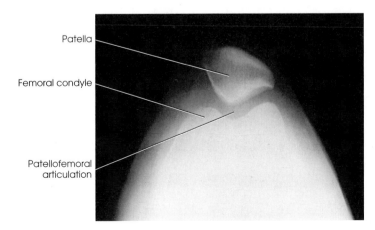

Patella

Femoral condyle

Patellofemoral articulation

Fig. 6-180 Tangential patellofemoral joint: Hughston method.

TANGENTIAL PROJECTION
MERCHANT METHOD[1]

Image receptor: 24 × 30 cm (10 × 12 inch) crosswise for bilateral examination

SID: A 6-foot (2-m) SID is recommended to reduce magnification.

Position of patient
- Place the patient supine with both knees at the end of the radiographic table.
- Support the knees and lower legs by an adjustable cassette-holding device.[2]
- To increase comfort and relaxation of the quadriceps femoris, place pillows or a foam wedge under the patient's head and back.

[1]Merchant AC et al: Roentgenographic analysis of patellofemoral congruence, *J Bone Joint Surg* 56A:1391, 1974.
[2]Merchant AC: "The Axial Viewer," Orthopedic Products, 2500 Hospital Dr., Bldg. 7, Mountain View, CA 94040.

Position of part
- Using the "axial viewer" device, elevate the patient's knees approximately 2 inches to place the femora parallel with the tabletop (Figs. 6-181 and 6-182).
- Adjust the angle of knee flexion to 40 degrees. (Merchant reported that the degree of angulation may be varied between 30 to 90 degrees to demonstrate various patellofemoral disorders.)
- Strap both legs together at the calf level to control leg rotation and allow patient relaxation.
- Place the cassette perpendicular to the central ray and resting on the patient's shins (a thin foam pad aids comfort) approximately 1 foot distal to the patellae.

- Ensure that the patient is able to relax. Relaxation of the quadriceps femoris is critical for an accurate diagnosis. If these muscles are not relaxed, a subluxed patella may be pulled back into the intercondylar sulcus, showing a false normal appearance.
- Record the angle of knee flexion for reproducibility during follow-up examinations, because the severity of patella subluxation commonly changes inversely with the angle of knee flexion.
- *Shield gonads.*

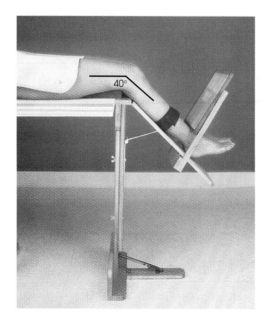

Fig. 6-181 Tangential patella and patellofemoral joint: Merchant method.

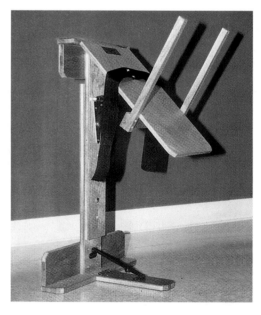

Fig. 6-182 "The axial viewer" device.

Patella and Patellofemoral Joint

Central ray

- Perpendicular to the cassette
- With 40-degree knee flexion, angle the central ray 30 degrees caudad from the horizontal plane (60 degrees from vertical) to achieve a 30-degree central ray-to-femur angle. The central ray enters midway between the patellae at the level of the patellofemoral joint.

Structures shown

The bilateral tangential image demonstrates an axial projection of the patellae and patellofemoral joints (Fig. 6-183). Because of the right-angle alignment of the cassette and central ray, the patellae are seen as nondistorted albeit slightly magnified images.

EVALUATION CRITERIA

The following should be clearly demonstrated:

- Patellae in profile
- Femoral condyles and intercondylar sulcus
- Open patellofemoral articulations

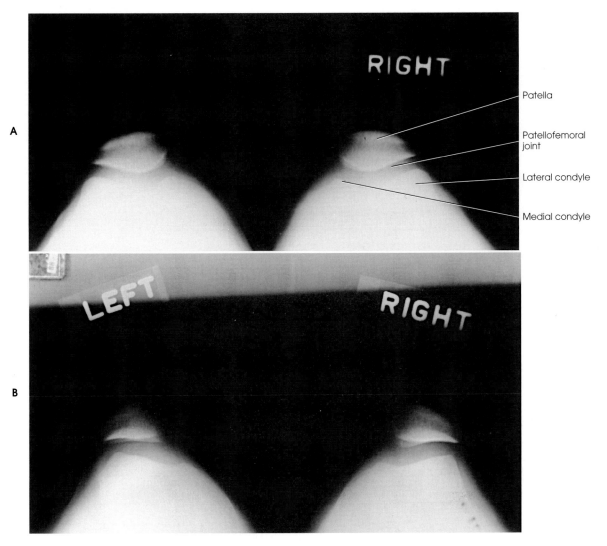

Fig. 6-183 A, Normal tangential radiograph of congruent patellofemoral joints, showing the patellae to be well centered with a normal trabecular pattern. **B,** Abnormal tangential radiograph showing abnormally shallow intercondylar sulci (*arrow*), misshapen and laterally subluxed patellae, and incongruent patellofemoral joints (left worse than right).

(Courtesy Alan J. Merchant.)

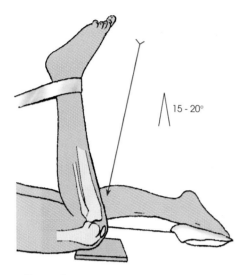

Fig. 6-184 Tangential patella and patellofemoral joint: Settegast method.

⚜ TANGENTIAL PROJECTION
SETTEGAST METHOD

Because of the danger of fragment displacement by the acute knee flexion required for this procedure, this projection should not be attempted until a transverse fracture of the patella has been ruled out with a lateral image.

Image receptor: 8 × 10 inch (18 × 24 cm)

Position of patient

- Place the patient in the supine or prone position. The latter is preferable because the knee can usually be flexed to a greater degree and immobilization is easier (Figs. 6-184 and 6-185).

- If the patient is seated on the radiographic table, hold the cassette securely in place (Fig. 6-186). Alternative positions are shown in Figs. 6-187 and 6-188.

Position of part

- Flex the patient's knee slowly as much as possible or until the patella is perpendicular to the cassette if the patient's condition permits. With *slow, even flexion,* the patient will be able to tolerate the position, whereas quick, uneven flexion may cause too much pain.

- If desired, loop a long strip of bandage around the patient's ankle or foot. Have the patient grasp the ends over the shoulder to hold the leg in position. Gently adjust the leg so that its long axis is vertical.

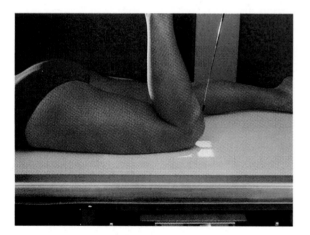

Fig. 6-185 Tangential patella and patellofemoral joint: Settegast method.

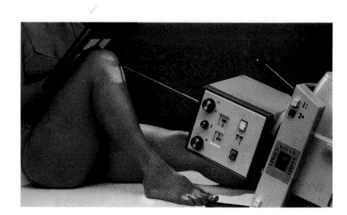

Fig. 6-186 Tangential patella and patellofemoral joint: Settegast method.

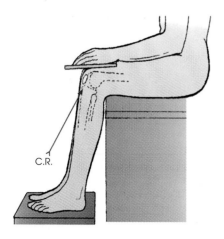

Fig. 6-187 Tangential patella and patellofemoral joint: patient seated.

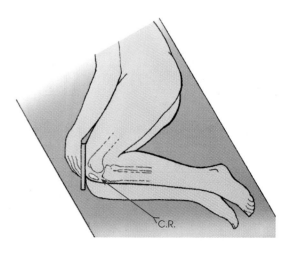

Fig. 6-188 Tangential patella and patellofemoral joint: patient lateral.

Patella and Patellofemoral Joint

- Place the cassette transversely under the knee, and center it to the joint space between the patella and the femoral condyles.
- *Shield gonads.*
- By maintaining the same OID and SID relationships, this position can be obtained with the patient in a lateral or seated position (see Figs. 6-187 and 6-188).

NOTE: When the central ray is directed toward the patient's upper body (see Figs. 6-186 and 6-187), the thorax and thyroid should be shielded. Gonad shielding (not shown) should be used in all patients.

Central ray

- Perpendicular to the joint space between the patella and the femoral condyles when the joint is perpendicular. When the joint is not, the degree of central ray angulation depends on the degree of flexion of the knee. The angulation typically will be 15 to 20 degrees.
- Close collimation is recommended.

COMPUTED RADIOGRAPHY

Collimation must be close to prevent unnecessary radiation from reaching the cassette phosphor.

Structures shown

The resulting image shows vertical fractures of bone and the articulating surfaces of the patellofemoral articulation (Figs. 6-189 and 6-190).

EVALUATION CRITERIA

The following should be clearly demonstrated:

- Patella in profile
- Open patellofemoral articulation
- Surfaces of the femoral condyles
- Soft tissue of the patellofemoral articulation
- Bony detail on the patella and femoral condyles

A   B

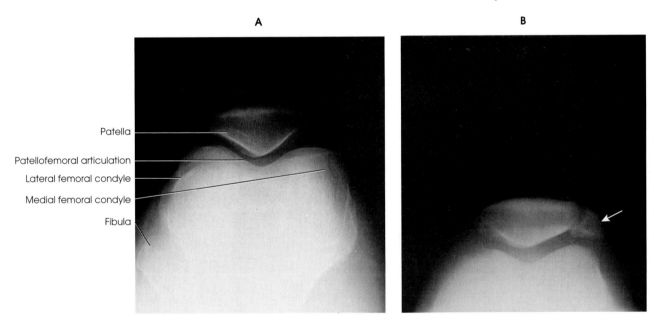

Patella
Patellofemoral articulation
Lateral femoral condyle
Medial femoral condyle
Fibula

Fig. 6-189 A, Tangential patella and patellofemoral joint: Settegast method. **B**, Fracture (*arrow*).

(Courtesy Dorothy Wilson.)

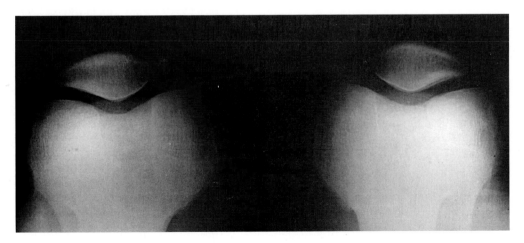

Fig. 6-190 Bilateral patella examination. For this examination, the legs should be strapped together at the level of the calf, using an appropriate binding to control femoral rotation.

🐦 AP PROJECTION

If the femoral heads are separated by an unusually broad pelvis, the bodies (shafts) will be more strongly angled toward the midline.

Image receptor: 18 × 43 cm (7 × 17 inch) or 35 × 43 cm (14 × 17 inch)

Position of patient

- Place the patient in the supine position.
- Check the pelvis to ensure it is not rotated.

Position of part

- Center the affected thigh to the midline of the cassette. When the patient is too tall to include the entire femur, include the joint closest to the area of interest on one image (Fig. 6-191).

With the knee included

- For projection of the *distal* femur, rotate the patient's limb internally to place it in true anatomic position. The limb will naturally be turned externally when laying on the table. Ensure that the epicondyles are parallel with the cassette.
- Place the bottom of the cassette 2 inches (5 cm) below the knee joint.

With the hip included

- For projection of the *proximal* femur, which must include the hip joint, place the top of the cassette at the level of the ASIS.
- Rotate the limb internally 10 to 15 degrees to place the femoral neck in profile.
- *Shield gonads.*

Central ray

- Perpendicular to the midfemur and the center of the cassette

Structures shown

The resulting image shows an AP projection of the femur, including the knee joint and/or hip (Figs. 6-192 and 6-193).

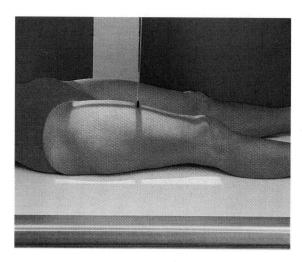

Fig. 6-191 AP distal femur.

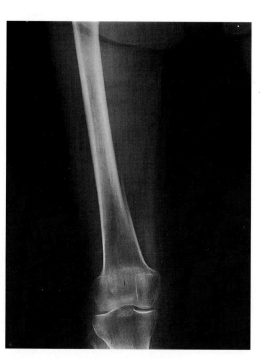

Fig. 6-192 AP distal femur.

EVALUATION CRITERIA

The following should be clearly demonstrated:

- Majority of the femur and the joint nearest to the pathologic condition or site of injury (A second projection of the other joint is recommended.)
- Femoral neck not foreshortened on the proximal femur
- Lesser trochanter not seen beyond the medial border of the femur or only a very small portion seen on the proximal femur
- No knee rotation on the distal femur
- Gonad shielding when indicated, but the shield not covering proximal femur
- Any orthopedic appliance in its entirety
- Trabecular recorded detail on the femoral shaft

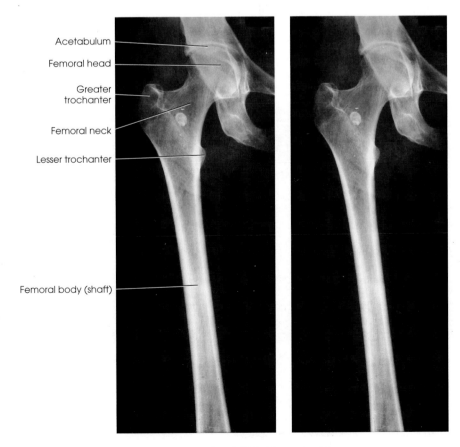

Acetabulum
Femoral head
Greater trochanter
Femoral neck
Lesser trochanter
Femoral body (shaft)

Fig. 6-193 AP proximal femur.

⬥ LATERAL PROJECTION
Mediolateral

Image receptor: 18 × 43 cm (7 × 17 inch) or 35 × 43 cm (14 × 17 inch) lengthwise

Position of patient

- Ask the patient to turn onto the affected side.
- Adjust the body position, and center the affected thigh to the midline of the grid.

Position of part
With the knee included

- For projection of the *distal* femur, draw the patient's uppermost limb forward and support it at hip level on sandbags.
- Adjust the pelvis in a true lateral position (Fig. 6-194).
- Flex the affected knee about 45 degrees, place a sandbag under the ankle, and adjust the body rotation to place the epicondyles perpendicular to the tabletop.
- Adjust the position of the Bucky tray so that the cassette projects approximately 2 inches (5 cm) beyond the knee to be included.

With the hip included

- For projection of the *proximal* femur, place the top of the cassette at the level of the ASIS.
- Draw the upper limb posteriorly, and support it.
- Adjust the pelvis so that it is rolled posteriorly just enough to prevent superimposition; 10 to 15 degrees from the lateral position is sufficient (Fig. 6-195).
- *Shield gonads.*

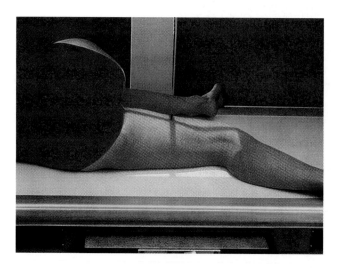

Fig. 6-194 Lateral distal femur

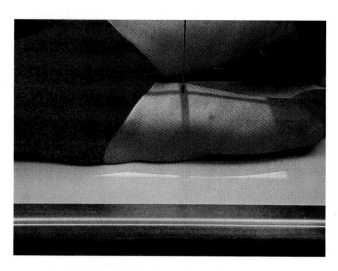

Fig. 6-195 Lateral proximal femur.

Central ray

• Perpendicular to the midfemur and the center of the cassette

Structures shown

The resulting image shows a lateral projection of about three fourths of the femur and the adjacent joint. If needed, use two cassettes for demonstration of the entire length of the adult femur (Figs. 6-196 and 6-197).

EVALUATION CRITERIA

The following should be clearly demonstrated:

■ Majority of the femur and the joint nearest to the pathologic condition or site of injury (A second radiograph of the other end of the femur is recommended.)
■ Any orthopedic appliance in its entirety
■ Trabecular detail on the femoral body

With the knee included

■ Superimposed anterior surface of the femoral condyles
■ Patella in profile
■ Open patellofemoral space
■ Inferior surface of the femoral condyles not superimposed because of divergent rays

With the hip included:

■ Opposite thigh not over area of interest
■ Greater and lesser trochanters not prominent

NOTE: Because of the danger of fragment displacement, the aforementioned position is not recommended for patients with fracture or patients who may have destructive disease. Patients with these conditions should be examined in the supine position by placing the cassette vertically along the medial or lateral aspect of the thigh and knee and then directing the central ray horizontally. A wafer grid or a grid-front cassette should be used to minimize secondary radiation.

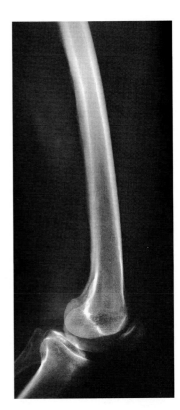

Fig. 6-196 Lateral distal femur.

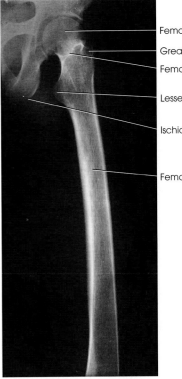

Femoral head
Greater trochanter
Femoral neck
Lesser trochanter
Ischial tuberosity
Femoral body (shaft)

Fig. 6-197 Lateral proximal femur.

Lower limb

Hips, Knees, and Ankles
AP PROJECTION
WEIGHT-BEARING METHOD[1,2]
Standing

NOTE: A specially built, long grid holder consisting of three grids, each 17 inches (43 cm) long, is required to hold the 51-inch cassette and its trifold film.

Image receptor: 14 × 51 inch (31 × 130 cm) lengthwise

SID: 8 feet (244 cm). This minimum-length SID is required to open the collimators wide enough to expose the entire 51-inch length of the cassette.

Position of patient
- Stand the patient with the back against the upright grid unit.

[1]Krushell R et al: A comparison of the mechanical and anatomical axes in arthritic knees. In *Proceedings of the Knee Society,* 1985-1986, Aspen, 1987
[2]Peterson TD, Rohr W: Improved assessment of lower extremity alignment using new roentgenographic techniques, *Clin Orthop Rel Res* 219, June 1987

Position of part
- Have the patient stand on a 2-inch (5 cm) riser so that the ankle joint is visible on the image. The bottom of the grid unit is positioned behind and below the riser.
- Measure both lateral malleoli, and position the legs so that they are exactly *20 cm* apart. If this distance cannot be achieved, measure the width of the malleoli and indicate this number on the request form. This image must be performed the same way for each return visit by the patient.
- Ensure that the patient's toes are positioned straight forward in the anatomic position (Fig 6-198).
- Ensure that the patient is distributing weight equally on both feet.
- Mark with a right or left side marker, and place a magnification marker in the area of the knee.
- Place a wedge filter (commercially available for this projection) in the appropriate position on the collimater (Fig. 6-199). This filter is necessary to compensate for the difference in thickness between the hip joint and ankle joint.
- *Shield gonads.*
- *Respiration:* Suspend.

Central ray
- Perpendicular to the cassette, entering midway between the knees at the level of the *knee joint.*
- Collimate appropriately, and ensure that the hip joints and ankle joints will be seen on the image.

Structures shown
This projection demonstrates the entire right and left limbs from the hip joint to the ankle joint (Fig. 6-200).

EVALUATION CRITERIA
The following should be clearly demonstrated:
- Appropriate density to visualize the hips to the ankles
- Both feet in anatomic position
- Hips, knees, and ankles
- Right or left marker and a magnification marker near the knee

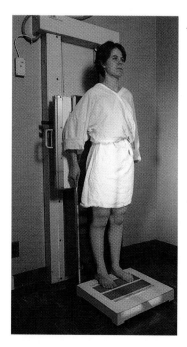

Fig. 6-198 Patient in position for radiograph of lower limbs: hips, knees, and ankles. The patient is placed in the anatomic position. Note that the patient is standing on a raised platform so that the ankles are shown.

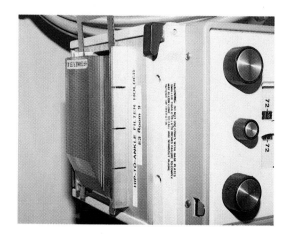

Fig. 6-199 Special filter for lower limb projections. The filter enables the hips, knees, and ankles to be demonstrated on one radiograph.

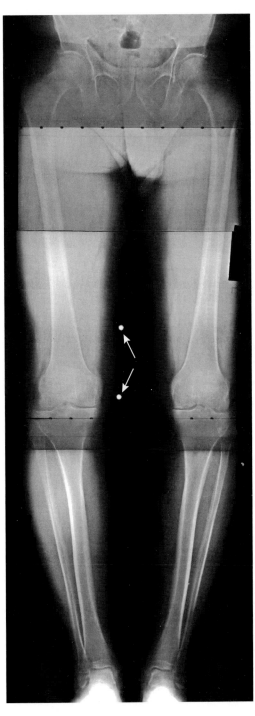

Fig. 6-200 Lower limbs: hips, knees, and ankles. *Arrows* point to magnification marker taped to knee

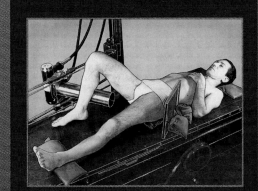

PELVIS AND UPPER FEMORA

7

RIGHT Axiolateral hip, 1949.

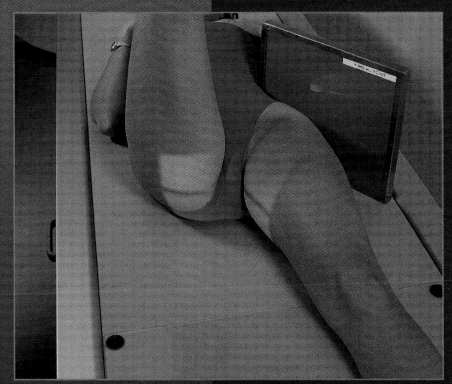

LEFT Axiolateral hip, 1999.

PROJECTIONS, POSITIONS & METHODS

Page	Essential	Anatomy	Projection	Position	Method
332	⚜	Pelvis and upper femora	AP		
334		Pelvis and upper femora	Lateral	R or L	
336		Pelvis and hip joints	Axial		CHASSARD-LAPINÉ
338	⚜	Femoral necks	AP oblique		MODIFIED CLEAVES
340		Femoral necks	Axiolateral		ORIGINAL CLEAVES
342	⚜	Hip	AP		
344	⚜	Hip	Lateral (mediolateral)		LAUENSTEIN; HICKEY
346	⚜	Hip	Axiolateral		DANELIUS-MILLER
348		Hip	Axiolateral		CLEMENTS-NAKAYAMA
350		Hip	Axiolateral		LEONARD-GEORGE
352		Hip	Axiolateral		FRIEDMAN
354		Hip	PA oblique	RAO or LAO	HSIEH
356		Hip	Mediolateral oblique	RAO or LAO	LILIENFELD
358		Acetabulum	PA axial oblique	RAO or LAO	TEUFEL
358		Acetabulum	AP oblique	RPO or LPO	JUDET
359		Acetabulum	Axiolateral		DUNLAP, SWANSON, and PENNER
360		Anterior pelvic bones	PA		
361		Anterior pelvic bones	AP axial		TAYLOR
362		Anterior pelvic bones	Superoinferior axial		LILIENFELD
363		Anterior pelvic bones	PA axial		STAUNIG
364		Ilium	AP and PA oblique	RPO and LPO, RAO and LAO	

Icons in the Essential column indicate projections frequently performed in the United States and Canada. Students should be competent in these projections.

The *pelvis* serves as a base for the trunk and a girdle for the attachment of the lower limbs. The pelvis consists of four bones: two *hip bones,* the *sacrum,* and the *coccyx.* The *pelvic girdle* is composed of only the two hip bones, however.

Hip Bone

The *hip bone* is often referred to as the *os coxae,* and some textbooks continue to refer to it as the *innominate bone.* The most widely used term is *hip bone.*

The hip bone consists of the *ilium, pubis,* and *ischium* (Figs. 7-1 and 7-2). These three bones join together to form the *acetabulum,* the cup-shaped socket that receives the head of the femur. The ilium, pubis, and ischium are separated by cartilage in youth but become fused into one bone in adulthood.

ILIUM

The *ilium* consists of a *body* and a broad, curved portion called the *ala.* The body of the ilium forms approximately two fifths of the acetabulum superiorly (Fig. 7-3). The ala projects superiorly from the body to form the prominence of the hip. The ala has three borders: anterior, posterior, and superior. The anterior and posterior borders present four prominent projections:

- Anterior superior iliac spine
- Anterior inferior iliac spine
- Posterior superior iliac spine
- Posterior inferior iliac spine

The *anterior superior iliac spine (ASIS)* is an important and frequently used radiographic positioning reference point. The superior margin extending from the ASIS to the posterior superior iliac spine is called the *iliac crest.* The medial surface of the wing contains the *iliac fossa* and is separated from the body of the bone by a smooth, arc-shaped ridge, the *arcuate line,* which forms a part of the circumference of the pelvic brim. The arcuate line passes obliquely, inferiorly, and medially to its junction with the pubis. The inferior and posterior portions of the wing present a large, rough surface, the *auricular surface,* for articulation with the sacrum. This articular surface and the articular surface of the adjacent sacrum have irregular elevations and depressions that cause a partial interlock of the two bones. Below this surface the ilium curves inward, forming the *greater sciatic notch.*

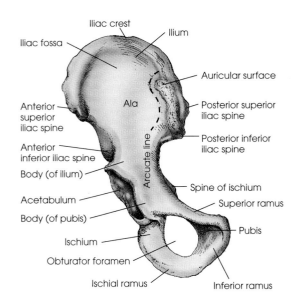

Fig. 7-1 Anterior aspect of right hip bone.

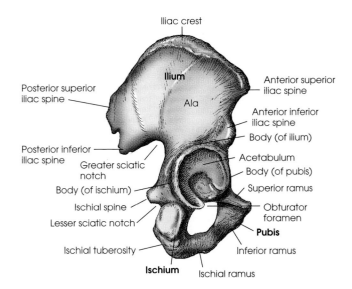

Fig. 7-2 Lateral aspect of right hip bone.

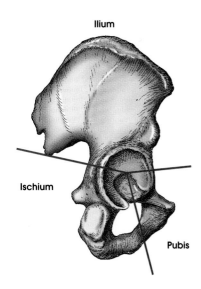

Fig. 7-3 Lateral aspect of right hip bone showing its three parts.

PUBIS

The *pubis* consists of a *body,* the *superior ramus,* and the *inferior ramus.* The body of the pubis forms approximately one fifth of the acetabulum anteriorly (see Fig. 7-3). The superior ramus projects inferiorly and medially from the acetabulum to the midline of the body. There the bone curves inferiorly and then posteriorly and laterally to join the ischium. The lower prong is termed the *inferior ramus.*

ISCHIUM

The *ischium* consists of a *body* and the *ischial ramus.* The body of the ischium forms approximately two fifths of the acetabulum posteriorly (see Fig. 7-3). It projects posteriorly and inferiorly from the acetabulum to form an expanded portion called the *ischial tuberosity.* When the body is in a seated-upright position, its weight rests on the two ischial tuberosities. The ischial ramus projects anteriorly and medially from the tuberosity to its junction with the inferior ramus of the pubis. By this posterior union the rami of the pubis and ischium enclose the *obturator foramen.* At the superoposterior border of the body is a prominent projection called the *ischial spine.* Just below the ischial spine is an indentation, the *lesser sciatic notch.*

Proximal Femur

The *femur* is the longest, strongest, and heaviest bone in the body. The proximal end of the femur consists of a *head,* a *neck,* and two large processes: the *greater* and *lesser trochanters* (Fig. 7-4). The smooth, rounded head is connected to the femoral body by a pyramid-shaped neck and is received into the acetabular cavity of the hip bone. A small depression at the center of the head, the *fovea capitis,* attaches to the ligamentum capitis femoris (Fig. 7-5). The neck is constricted near the head but expands to a broad base at the *body* of the bone. The neck projects medially, superiorly, and anteriorly from the body. The trochanters are situated at the junction of the body and the base of the neck. The greater trochanter is at the superolateral part of the femoral body, and the lesser trochanter is at the posteromedial part. The prominent ridge extending between the trochanters at the base of the neck on the posterior surface of the body is called the *intertrochanteric crest.* The less prominent ridge connecting the trochanters anteriorly is called the *intertrochanteric line.* The femoral neck and the intertrochanteric crest are two common sites of fractures in the elderly. The superior portion of the greater trochanter projects above the neck and curves slightly posteriorly and medially.

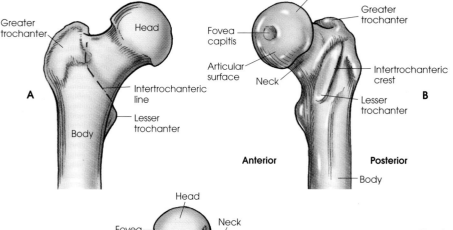

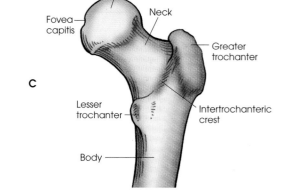

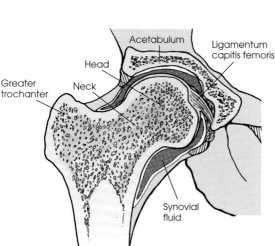

Fig. 7-4 Proximal right femur. **A,** Anterior aspect. **B,** Medial aspect. Note that the body is positioned 15 to 20 degrees posterior from the head. **C,** Posterior aspect.

Fig. 7-5 Hip joint. Coronal section of proximal femur in acetabulum.

The angulation of the neck of the femur varies considerably with age, sex, and stature. In the average adult the neck projects anteriorly from the body at an angle of approximately 15 to 20 degrees and superiorly at an angle of approximately 120 to 130 degrees to the long axis of the femoral body (Fig. 7-6). The longitudinal plane of the femur is angled about 10 degrees from vertical. In youth the latter angle is wider; that is, the neck is more vertical in position. In wide pelvises the angle is narrower, placing the neck in a more horizontal position.

Articulations of the Pelvis

A summary of the three joints of the pelvis and upper femora is contained in Table 7-1 and Fig. 7-7, and a description follows. The articulation between the acetabulum and the head of the femur (the hip joint) is a *synovial ball-and-socket* joint that permits free movement in all directions. The knee and ankle joints are hinge joints; thus the wide range of motion of the lower limb depends on the ball-and-socket joint of the hip. Because the knee and ankle joints are hinge joints, medial and lateral rotations of the foot cause rotation of the entire limb, which is centered at the hip joint.

TABLE 7-1
Joints of the pelvis and upper femora

| Joint | Structural classification | | Movement |
	Tissue	Type	
Hip joint	Synovial	Ball and socket	Freely movable
Pubic symphysis	Cartilaginous	Symphysis	Slightly movable
Sacroiliac	Synovial	Irregular gliding*	Slightly movable

*Some anatomists term this a *synovial fibrous joint.*

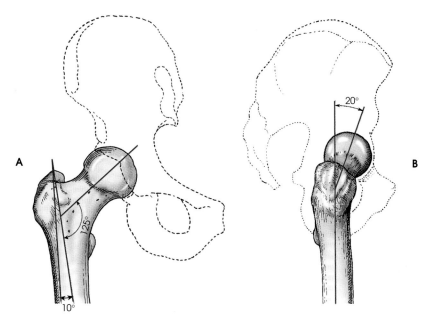

Fig. 7-6 A, Anterior aspect of right femur. **B**, Lateral aspect of right femur.

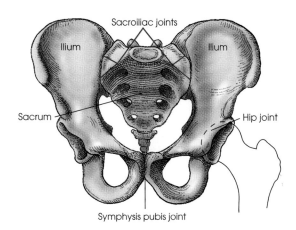

Fig. 7-7 Joints of the pelvis and upper femora.

TABLE 7-2

Female and male pelvis characteristics

Feature	Female	Male
Shape	Wide, shallow	Narrow, deep
Bony structure	Light	Heavy
Superior aperture (inlet)	Oval	Round
Inferior aperture (outlet)	Wide	Narrow

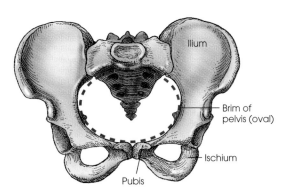

Fig. 7-8 Female pelvis.

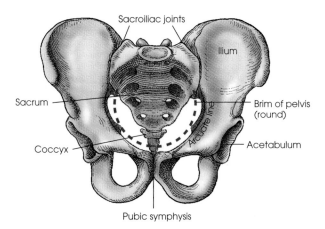

Fig. 7-9 Male pelvis.

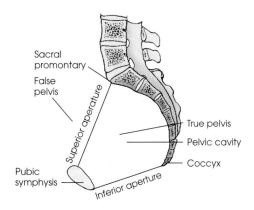

Fig. 7-10 Midsagittal section showing inlet and outlet of true pelvis.

The pubes of the hip bones articulate with each other at the anterior midline of the body, forming a joint called the *pubic symphysis.* The pubic symphysis is a *cartilaginous symphysis* joint.

The right and left ilia articulate with the sacrum posteriorly at the *sacroiliac* joints. The sacroiliac articulations are *synovial irregular gliding* joints. Because the bones of the sacroiliac joints interlock, movement is very limited or nonexistent.

Pelvis

The female pelvis (Fig. 7-8) is lighter in structure than the male pelvis (Fig. 7-9). It is wider and shallower, and the inlet is larger and more oval shaped. The sacrum is wider, it curves more sharply posteriorly, and the sacral promontory is flatter. The width and depth of the pelvis vary with stature and gender (Table 7-2). The female pelvis is shaped for childbearing and delivery.

The pelvis is divided into two portions by an oblique plane that extends from the upper anterior margin of the sacrum to the upper margin of the pubic symphysis. The boundary line of this plane is called the *brim of the pelvis* (see Figs. 7-8 and 7-9). The region above the brim is called the *false* or *greater pelvis,* and the region below the brim is called the *true* or *lesser pelvis.*

The brim forms the *superior aperture,* or *inlet,* of the true pelvis. The *inferior aperture,* or *outlet,* of the true pelvis is measured from the tip of the coccyx to the inferior margin of the pubic symphysis in the anteroposterior direction and between the ischial tuberosities in the horizontal direction. The region between the inlet and the outlet is called the *pelvic cavity* (Fig. 7-10).

When the body is in the upright or seated position, the brim of the pelvis forms an angle of approximately 60 degrees to the horizontal plane. This angle varies with other body positions; the degree and direction of the variation depend on the lumbar and sacral curves.

Localizing Anatomic Structures

The bony landmarks used in radiography of the pelvis and hips are as follows:
- Iliac crest
- ASIS
- Pubic symphysis
- Greater trochanter of the femur
- Ischial tuberosity
- Tip of the coccyx

Most of these points are easily palpable, even in hypersthenic patients (Fig. 7-11). However, because of the heavy muscles immediately above the iliac crest, care must be exercised in locating this structure to avoid *centering errors*. It is advisable to have the patient inhale deeply; while the muscles are relaxed during expiration, the radiographer should palpate for the highest point of the iliac crest.

The highest point of the greater trochanter, which can be palpated immediately below the depression in the soft tissues of the lateral surface of the hip, is in the same horizontal plane as the midpoint of the hip joint and the coccyx. The most prominent point of the greater trochanter is in the same horizontal plane as the pubic symphysis (see Fig. 7-11).

The greater trochanter is most prominent laterally and more easily palpated when the lower leg is medially rotated. When properly used, medial rotation facilitates localization of hip and pelvis centering points and avoids distortion of the proximal end of the femur during radiography. Improper rotation of the lower leg can rotate the pelvis. Consequently, the positioning of the lower leg is important in radiography of the hip and pelvis; the feet must be immobilized in the correct position to avoid distortion of the image. Traumatic injuries or pathologic conditions of the pelvis or lower limb may rule out the possibility of medial rotation.

The pubic symphysis can be palpated on the midsagittal plane and on the same horizontal plane as the greater trochanters. By placing the fingertips at this location and performing a brief downward palpation with the hand flat, palm down, and fingers together, the radiographer can locate the superior margin of the pubic symphysis. To avoid possible embarrassment or misunderstanding, the radiographer should advise the patient in advance that this and other palpations of pelvic landmarks are part of normal procedure and necessary for an accurate examination. When carried out in an efficient and professional manner with respect for the patient's condition, such palpations are generally well tolerated.

The hip joint can be located by palpating the ASIS and the superior margin of the pubic symphysis (Fig. 7-12). The midpoint of a line drawn between these two points is directly above the center of the dome of the acetabular cavity. A line drawn at right angles to the midpoint of the first line lies parallel to the long axis of the femoral neck of an average adult in the anatomic position. The femoral head lies 1½ inches (3.8 cm) distal and the femoral neck is 2½ inches (6.4 cm) distal to this point.

For accurate localization of the femoral neck in atypical patients or in those in whom the limb is not in the anatomic position, a line is drawn between the ASIS and the superior margin of the pubic symphysis, and a second line is drawn from a point 1 inch (2.5 cm) inferior to the greater trochanter to the midpoint of the previously marked line. The femoral head and neck lies along this line (see Fig. 7-12).

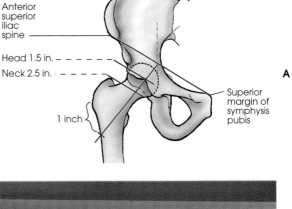

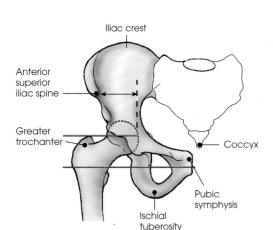

Fig. 7-11 Bony landmarks and localization planes of pelvis.

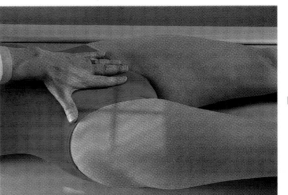

Fig. 7-12 **A,** Method of localizing the right hip joint and long axis of femoral neck. **B,** Suggested method of localizing the right hip. Left thumb is on ASIS, and second finger is on superior margin of pubic symphysis. Note central ray is positioned 1.5 inches distal to the center of a line drawn between the ASIS and the pubic symphysis.

SUMMARY OF ANATOMY*

Pelvis
hip bones (2)
sacrum
coccyx
pelvic girdle

Hip bone
ilium
pubis
ischium
acetabulum

Ilium
body
wing
superior spine
inferior spine
anterior superior iliac
  spine (ASIS)
anterior inferior iliac
  spine
posterior superior
  iliac spine
posterior inferior iliac
  spine

iliac crest
iliac fossa
arcuate line
auricular surface
greater sciatic notch

Pubis
body
superior ramus
inferior ramus

Ischium
body
ischial ramus
ischial tuberosity
obturator foramen
ischial spine
lesser sciatic notch

**Femur (proximal
  aspect)**
head
neck
body
fovea capitis

greater trochanter
lesser trochanter
intertrochanteric
  crest
intertrochanteric line

Articulations
hip
pubic symphysis
sacroiliac joints

Pelvis
brim of the pelvis
greater or false pelvis
lesser or true pelvis
superior aperture or
  inlet
inferior aperture or
  outlet
pelvic cavity

*See *Addendum* at the end of the volume for a summary of the changes in the anatomic terms used in this edition.

Radiation Protection

Protection of the patient from unnecessary radiation is a professional responsibility of the radiographer (see Chapter 1 for specific guidelines). In this chapter the *Shield gonads* statement at the end of the *Position of part* section indicates that the patient is to be protected from unnecessary radiation by restricting the radiation beam using proper collimation. In addition, placing lead shielding between the gonads and the radiation source is appropriate when the clinical objectives of the examination are not compromised (Figs. 7-13 and 7-14).

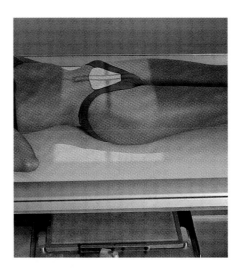

Fig. 7-13 Female AP pelvis with gonad shield.

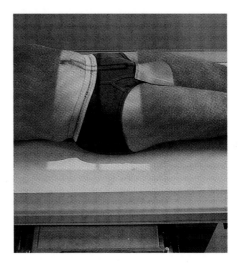

Fig. 7-14 Male AP pelvis with gonad shield.

▲ AP PROJECTION

Image receptor: 35 × 43 cm (14 × 17 inch) crosswise

Position of patient
- Place the patient on the table in the supine position.

Position of part
- Center the midsagittal plane of the body to the midline of the grid, and adjust it in a true supine position.
- Flex the elbows, and rest the hands on the upper chest.

- Unless contraindicated because of trauma or pathologic factors, medially rotate the feet and lower limbs about 15 to 20 degrees to place the femoral necks parallel with the plane of the cassette (Figs. 7-15 and 7-16). Medial rotation is easier for the patient to maintain if the knees are supported. The heels should be placed about 8 to 10 inches (20 to 24 cm) apart.
- Immobilize the legs with a sandbag across the ankles, if needed.
- Check the distance from the ASIS to the tabletop on each side to be sure that the pelvis is not rotated.

- If a soft tissue abnormality (swelling or atrophy) is causing rotation of the pelvis, elevate one side of the pelvis on a radiolucent pad to overcome the rotation.
- Center the cassette midway between the ASIS and the pubic symphysis. The cassette will be about 2 inches (5 cm) inferior to the ASIS and 2 inches (5 cm) superior to the pubic symphysis in average-sized patients (Fig. 7-17).
- If the pelvis is deep, palpate for the crest of the ilium and adjust the position of the cassette so that its upper border will project 1 to 1½ inches (2.5 to 3.8 cm) above the crest of the ilium.
- *Shield gonads.*
- *Respiration:* Suspend.

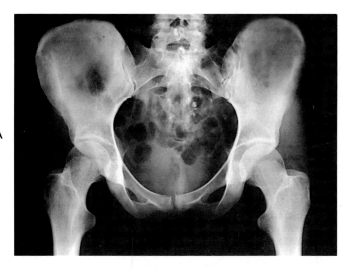
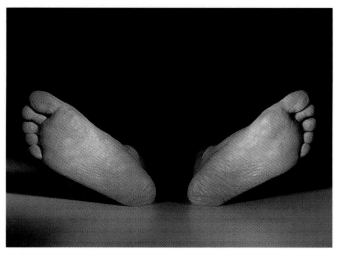

Fig. 7-15 A, AP pelvis with femoral necks and trochanters poorly positioned because of lateral rotation of the limbs. **B,** Feet and lower limbs in their natural laterally rotated tabletop position, causing poor profile of the proximal femora in **A.**

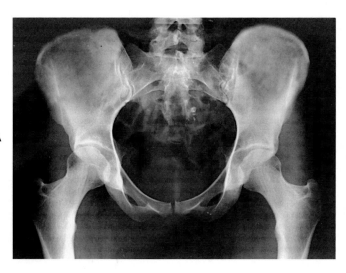
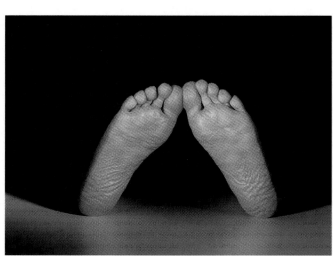

Fig. 7-16 A, AP pelvis with femoral necks and trochanters in correct position. **B,** Feet and lower limbs medially rotated 15 to 20 degrees, correctly placed with the upper femora in correct profile in **A.**

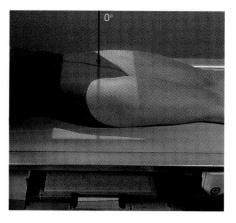

Fig. 7-17 AP pelvis.

Central ray
- Perpendicular to the midpoint of the cassette

Structures shown
The resulting image shows an AP projection of the pelvis and of the head, neck, trochanters, and proximal one third or one fourth of the shaft of the femora (Fig. 7-18).

EVALUATION CRITERIA
The following should be clearly demonstrated:
- Entire pelvis along with the proximal femora
- Lesser trochanters, if seen, demonstrated on the medial border of the femora

- Femoral necks in their full extent without superimposition
- Greater trochanters in profile
- Both ilia equidistant to the edge of the radiograph
- Both greater trochanters equidistant to the edge of the radiograph
- Lower vertebral column centered to the middle of the radiograph
- Symmetric obturator foramina
- Ischial spines equally demonstrated
- Symmetric iliac alae
- Sacrum and coccyx aligned with the pubic symphysis

Congenital dislocation of the hip
Martz and Taylor[1] recommended two AP projections of the pelvis for demonstration of the relationship of the femoral head to the acetabulum in patients with congenital dislocation of the hip. The first projection is obtained with the central ray directed perpendicular to the pubic symphysis to detect any lateral or superior displacement of the femoral head. The second projection is obtained with the central ray directed to the pubic symphysis at a cephalic angulation of 45 degrees (Fig. 7-19). This angulation casts the shadow of an anteriorly displaced femoral head above that of the acetabulum and the shadow of a posteriorly displaced head below that of the acetabulum.

---

[1]Martz CD, Taylor CC: The 45-degree angle roentgenographic study of the pelvis in congenital dislocation of the hip, *J Bone Joint Surg* 36A:528, 1954.

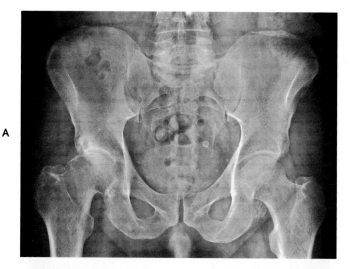

A

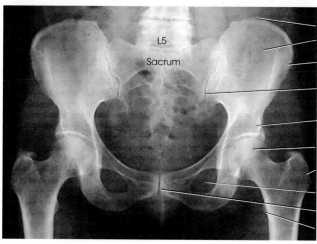

B

L5

Sacrum

Iliac crest
Ala

Anterior superior
iliac spine

Sacroiliac joint

Anterior inferior
iliac spine

Femoral head

Greater trochanter

Obturator foramen

Pubic symphysis

Lesser trochanter

Fig. 7-18 A, Male AP pelvis. **B,** Female AP pelvis.

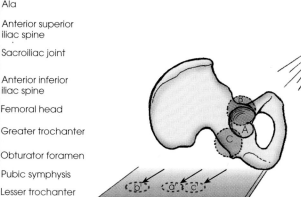

Fig. 7-19 Special projection taken for congenital dislocation of the hip.

LATERAL PROJECTION
Right or Left position

Image receptor: 35 × 43 cm (14 × 17 inch) lengthwise

Position of patient
- Place the patient in the lateral recumbent, dorsal decubitus, or upright position.

Position of part
Recumbent position
- When the patient can be placed in the lateral position, center the midcoronal plane of the body to the midline of the grid.
- Extend the thighs enough to prevent the femora from obscuring the pubic arch.
- Place a support under the lumbar spine, and adjust it to place the vertebral column parallel with the tabletop (Fig. 7-20). If the vertebral column is allowed to sag, it will tilt the pelvis in the longitudinal plane.

- Adjust the pelvis in a true lateral position, with the ASISs lying in the same vertical plane.
- Place one knee directly over the other knee. A pillow or other support between the knees promotes stabilization and patient comfort.
- Berkebile, Fischer, and Albrecht[1] recommended a dorsal decubitus lateral projection of the pelvis for demonstration of the "gull-wing sign" in cases of fracture dislocation of the acetabular rim and posterior dislocation of the femoral head.

[1] Berkebile RD, Fischer DL, Albrecht LF: The gull-wing sign: value of the lateral view of the pelvis in fracture dislocation of the acetabular rim and posterior dislocation of the femoral head, *Radiology* 84:937, 1965.

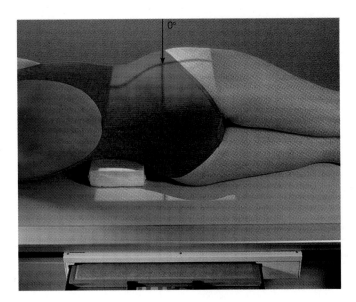

Fig. 7-20 Lateral pelvis.

Upright position

- Place the patient in the lateral position in front of a vertical grid device, and center the midcoronal plane of the body to the midline of the grid.
- Have the patient stand straight, with the weight of the body equally distributed on the feet so that the midsagittal plane is parallel with the plane of the cassette.
- If the limbs are of unequal length, place a support of suitable height under the foot of the short side.
- Have the patient grasp the side of the stand for support.
- *Shield gonads.*
- *Respiration:* Suspend.

Central ray

- Perpendicular to a point centered at the level of the soft tissue depression just above the greater trochanter (approximately 2 inches [5 cm]) and to the midpoint of the image receptor

COMPUTED RADIOGRAPHY

The higher kilovolt (peak) (kVp) used for this projection requires that the collimation be very close. Scattered and primary radiation reaching the cassette phosphor may cause computer artifacts.

Structures shown

The resulting image shows a lateral radiograph of the lumbosacral junction, sacrum, coccyx, and superimposed hip bones and upper femora (Fig. 7-21).

EVALUATION CRITERIA

The following should be clearly demonstrated:

- Entire pelvis and the proximal femora.
- Sacrum and coccyx.
- Superimposed posterior margins of the ischium and ilium.
- Superimposed femora.
- Superimposed acetabular shadows. The larger circle of the fossa (farther from the cassette) will be equidistant from the smaller circle of the fossa nearer the cassette throughout their circumference.
- Pubic arch unobscured by the femora.

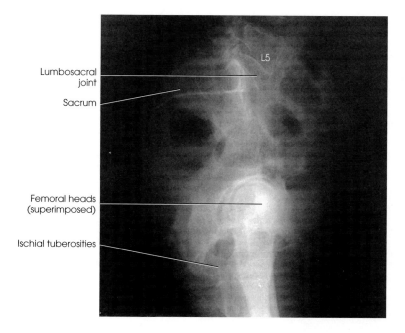
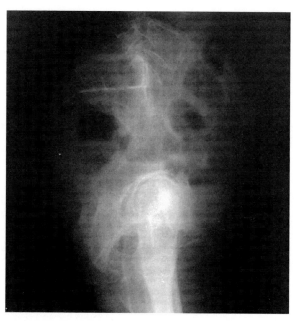

Fig. 7-21 Lateral pelvis.

AXIAL PROJECTION
CHASSARD-LAPINÉ METHOD[1]

Chassard and Lapiné[1] devised this method for the purpose of measuring the horizontal, or biischial, diameter in pelvimetry. Some radiographers use this method to determine the relationship of the femoral head to the acetabulum, and others employ it to demonstrate the opacified rectosigmoid portion of the colon.

---

[1]Chassard, Lapiné: Ètude radiographique de l'arcade pubienne chez la femme enceinte; une nouvelle méthode d'appréciation du diamètre bi-ischiatique, *J Radiol Electrol* 7:113, 1923.

NOTE: This examination is contraindicated for patients with a suspected fracture or pathologic condition.

Image receptor: 35 × 43 cm (14 × 17 inch) crosswise

Position of patient

Seat the patient well back on the end or side of the radiographic table so that the posterior surface of the knees is in contact with the edge of the table.

Position of part

- If the patient is seated at the side of the table, place the longitudinal axis of the cassette perpendicular to the midsagittal plane. If the patient is seated on the end of the table, center the midsagittal plane of the body to the midline of the grid. If needed, place a stool or other suitable support under the feet (Fig. 7-22).
- To prevent the thighs from limiting flexion of the body too greatly, have the patient abduct them as far as the end of the table permits.
- Instruct the patient to lean directly forward until the pubic symphysis is in close contact with the table; the vertical axis of the pelvis will be tilted forward approximately 45 degrees. The average patient can achieve this degree of flexion without strain.
- Have the patient grasp the ankles to aid in maintaining the position.
- *Shield gonads.*
- *Respiration:* Suspend.

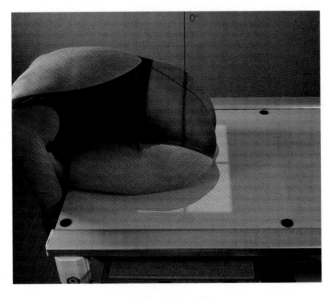

Fig. 7-22 Axial pelvis.

Central ray

- Perpendicular through the lumbosacral region at the level of the greater trochanters.
- When flexion of the body is restricted, direct the central ray anteriorly, perpendicular to the coronal plane of the pubic symphysis.

Structures shown

The resulting image shows an axial projection of the pelvis, demonstrating the relationship between the femoral heads and the acetabula, the pelvic bones, and any opacified structure within the pelvis (Fig. 7-23).

The following should be clearly demonstrated:

- Femoral heads and acetabula
- Entire pelvis along with the proximal femora
- Symmetric hip bones
- Greater trochanters equidistant to the sacrum

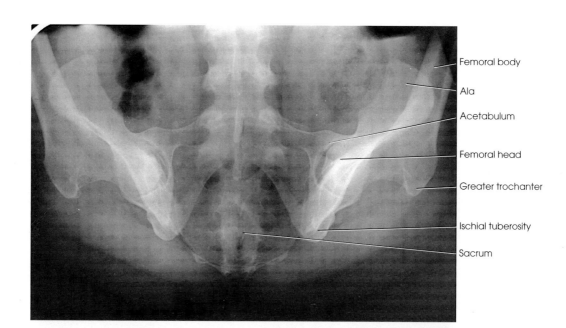

Femoral body

Ala

Acetabulum

Femoral head

Greater trochanter

Ischial tuberosity

Sacrum

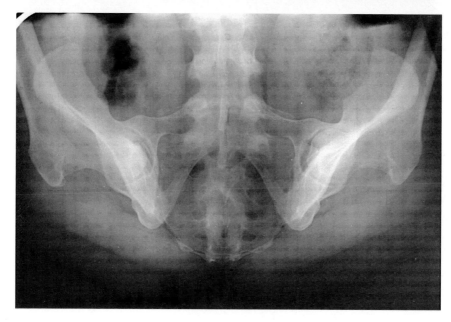

Fig. 7-23 Axial pelvis.

Pelvis and hip joints

337

AP OBLIQUE PROJECTION
MODIFIED CLEAVES METHOD

Image receptor: 35 × 43 cm (14 × 17 inch) crosswise

This projection is often called the bilateral "frog leg" position.

NOTE: This examination is contraindicated for the patient suspected of having a fracture or other pathologic disease.

Position of patient
- Place the patient in the supine position.

Position of part
- Center the midsagittal plane of the body to the midline of the grid.
- Flex the patient's elbows, and rest the hands on the upper chest.
- Adjust the patient so that the pelvis is not rotated. This can be achieved by placing the two ASISs equidistant from the radiographic table.
- Place a compression band across the patient well above the hip joints for stability, if needed.

Bilateral projection
Step 1
- Have the patient flex the hips and knees and draw the feet up as much as possible (i.e., enough to place the femora in a nearly vertical position if the affected side permits).
- Instruct the patient to hold this position, which is relatively comfortable, while the x-ray tube and cassette are adjusted.
Step 2
- Center the cassette 1 inch (2.5 cm) superior to the pubic symphysis.
Step 3
- Abduct the thighs as much as possible, and have the patient turn the feet inward to brace the soles against each other for support. According to Cleaves, the angle may vary between 25 and 45 degrees, depending on how vertical the femora can be placed.
- Center the feet to the midline of the grid (Fig. 7-24).
- If possible, abduct the thighs approximately 45 degrees from the vertical plane to place the long axes of the femoral necks parallel with the plane of the cassette.
- Check the position of the thighs, being careful to abduct them to the same degree.

Unilateral projection
- Adjust the body position to center the ASIS of the affected side to the midline of the grid.
- Have the patient flex the hip and knee of the affected side and draw the foot up to the opposite knee as much as possible.
- After adjusting the perpendicular central ray and positioning the cassette tray, have the patient brace the sole of the foot against the opposite knee and abduct the thigh laterally approximately 45 degrees (Fig. 7-25). The pelvis may rotate slightly.
- *Shield gonads.*
- *Respiration:* Suspend.

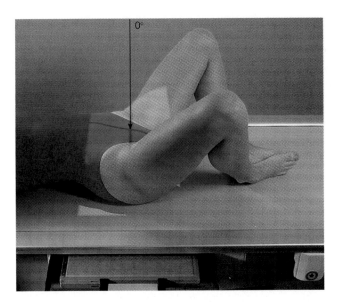

Fig. 7-24 AP oblique femoral necks with perpendicular central ray: modified Cleaves method.

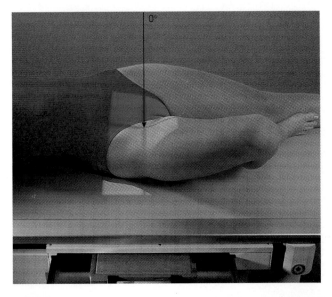

Fig. 7-25 Unilateral AP oblique femoral neck: modified Cleaves method.

Pelvis and upper femora

Central ray

- Perpendicular to enter the patient's midsagittal plane at the level 1½ inch (3.8 cm) superior to the pubic symphysis. For the unilateral position, direct the central ray to the femoral neck (see Fig. 7-12).

Structures shown

The bilateral resulting image shows an AP oblique projection of the femoral heads, necks, and trochanteric areas projected onto one radiograph for comparison (Figs. 7-26 to 7-28).

EVALUATION CRITERIA

The following should be clearly demonstrated:

- No rotation of the pelvis, as evidenced by a symmetric appearance.
- Acetabulum, femoral head, and femoral neck.
- Lesser trochanter on the medial side of the femur.
- Femoral neck without superimposition by the greater trochanter. Excess abduction causes the greater trochanter to obstruct the neck.
- Femoral axes extended from the hip bones at equal angles.

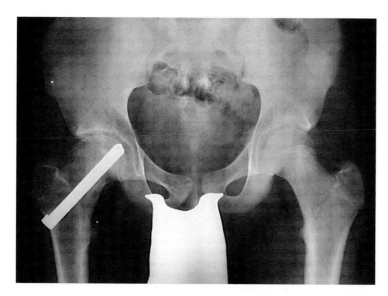

Fig. 7-26 AP femoral necks. Note the fixation device in the right hip as well as the male gonad shield.

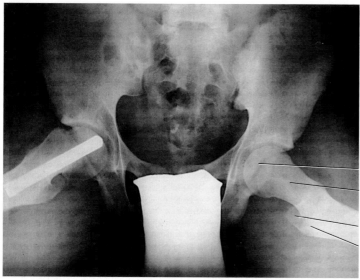

Femoral head

Femoral neck

Greater trochanter

Lesser trochanter

Fig. 7-27 AP oblique femoral necks: modified Cleaves method (same patient as in Fig. 7-26).

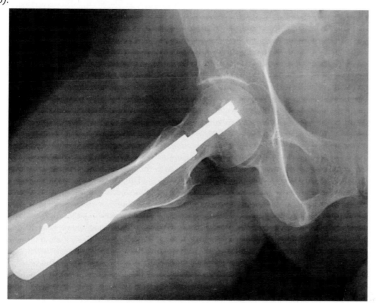

Fig. 7-28 AP oblique femoral neck: modified Cleaves method.

AXIOLATERAL PROJECTION
ORIGINAL CLEAVES METHOD[1]

NOTE: This examination is contraindicated for patients with suspected fracture or pathologic condition.

Image receptor: 35×43 cm (14×17 inch) crosswise

---

[1]Cleaves EN: Observations on lateral views of the hip, *Am J Roentgen* 34:964, 1938.

Position of patient
- Place the patient in the supine position.

Position of part

NOTE: This is the same part position as the modified Cleaves method previously described. The projection can be performed unilaterally or bilaterally.

- Before having the patient abduct the thighs (described in step 3 on p. 338), direct the x-ray tube parallel to the long axes of the femoral shafts (Fig. 7-29).
- Adjust the cassette so the midpoint coincides with the central ray.
- *Shield gonads.*
- *Respiration:* Suspend.

Central ray
Parallel with the femoral shafts. According to Cleaves,[1] the angle may vary between 25 and 45 degrees, depending on how vertical the femora can be placed.

---

[1]Cleaves EN: Observations on lateral views of the hip, *Am J Roentgen* 34:964, 1938.

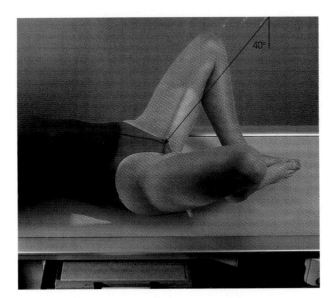

Fig. 7-29 Axiolateral femoral necks: Cleaves method.

Structures shown

The resulting image shows an axiolateral projection of the femoral heads, necks, and trochanteric areas (Fig. 7-30).

EVALUATION CRITERIA

The following should be clearly demonstrated:

- Axiolateral projections of the femoral necks
- Femoral necks without overlap from the greater trochanters

- Small parts of the lesser trochanters on the posterior surfaces of the femurs
- Small amount of the greater trochanters on both the posterior and anterior surfaces of the femurs
- Both sides equidistant from the edge of the radiograph
- Greater amount of the proximal femur on a unilateral examination
- Femoral neck angles approximately 15 to 20 degrees superior to the femoral bodies.

Congenital dislocation of the hip

The diagnosis of congenital dislocation of the hip in newborns has been discussed in numerous articles. Andren and von Rosén[1] described a method based on certain theoretic considerations. Their method requires accurate and judicious application of the positioning technique to make an accurate diagnosis. The Andren-von Rosén approach involves taking a bilateral hip projection with both legs forcibly abducted to at least 45 degrees with appreciable inward rotation of the femora. Knake and Kuhns[2] described the construction of a device that controlled the degree of abduction and rotation of both limbs. They reported that the device essentially eliminated and greatly simplified the positioning difficulties, thereby reducing the number of repeat examinations.

[1]Andren L, von Rosén S: The diagnosis of dislocation of the hip in newborns and the primary results of immediate treatment, *Acta Radiol* 49:89, 1958.
[2]Knake JE, Kuhns LR: A device to aid in positioning for the Andren-von Rosén hip view, *Radiology* 117:735, 1975.

A

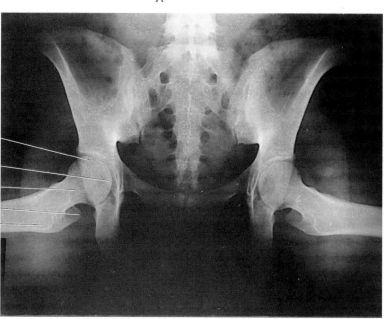

Femoral head
Femoral head within acetabulum
Femoral neck
Greater trochanter
Lesser trochanter

B

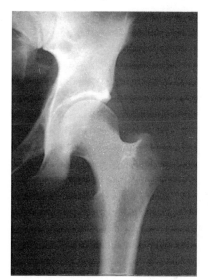

C

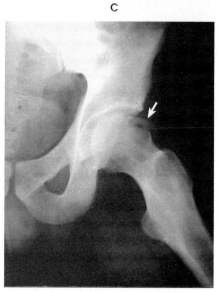

Fig. 7-30 Axiolateral femoral necks: Cleaves method. **A,** Bilateral examination. **B** and **C,** Unilateral hip examination of a patient who fell. No fractures were seen on the initial AP hip radiograph **(B)**, and a second projection using the Cleaves method was performed. A chip fracture of the femoral head (*arrow*) was seen **(C)**. At least two projections are required in trauma diagnoses.

☀ AP PROJECTION

Image receptor: 24 × 30 cm (10 × 12 inches) lengthwise

Position of patient
- Place the patient in the supine position.

Position of part
- Adjust the patient's pelvis so it is not rotated. This is accomplished by placing the ASISs equidistant from the table (Figs. 7-31 and 7-32).
- Place the patient's arms in a comfortable position.
- Medially rotate the lower limb and foot approximately 15 to 20 degrees to place the femoral neck parallel with the plane of the cassette, unless this maneuver is contraindicated or other instructions are given.
- Place a support under the knee and a sandbag across the ankle. This makes it easier for the patient to maintain this position.
- *Shield gonads.*
- *Respiration:* Suspend.

Central ray
- Perpendicular to the femoral neck. Using one half of the localizing technique previously described (see Fig. 7-12), place the central ray approximately 2½ inches (6.4 cm) distal on a line drawn perpendicular to the midpoint of a line between the ASIS and the pubic symphysis.
- Center the cassette to the central ray.
- Make any necessary adjustments in the cassette size and central ray point when an entire orthopedic device is to be shown on one image.

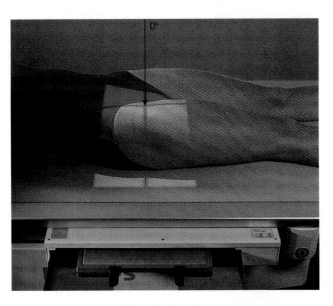

Fig. 7-31 AP hip.

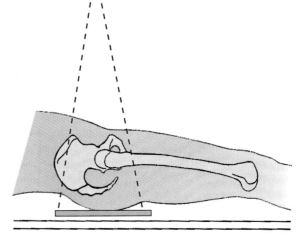

Fig. 7-32 AP hip.

Structures shown

The resulting image shows the head, neck, trochanters, and proximal one third of the body of the femur (Fig. 7-33).

In the initial examination of a hip lesion, whether traumatic or pathologic in origin, the AP projection is often obtained using an image receptor large enough to include the entire pelvic girdle and upper femora. Progress studies may be restricted to the affected side.

EVALUATION CRITERIA

The following should be clearly demonstrated:

■ Femoral head, penetrated and seen through the acetabulum.
■ Regions of the ilium and pubic bones adjoining the pubic symphysis.
■ Any orthopedic appliance in its entirety.
■ Hip joint.
■ Greater trochanter in profile.
■ Entire long axis of the femoral neck not foreshortened.
■ Proximal one third of the femur.

■ Lesser trochanter is usually not projected beyond the medial border of the femur, or only a very small amount of the trochanter is seen.

NOTE: Trauma patients who have sustained severe injury are not usually transferred to the radiographic table but are radiographed on the stretcher or bed. After the localization point has been established and marked, one assistant should be on each side of the stretcher to grasp the sheet and lift the pelvis just enough for placement of the cassette while a third person supports the injured limb. Any necessary manipulation of the limb must be made by a physician.

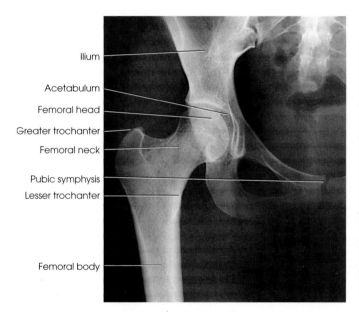
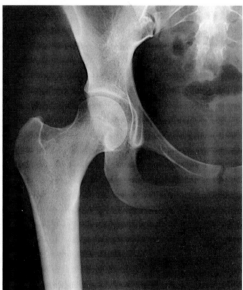

Ilium
Acetabulum
Femoral head
Greater trochanter
Femoral neck
Pubic symphysis
Lesser trochanter
Femoral body

Fig. 7-33 AP hip.

☀ LATERAL PROJECTION
Mediolateral
LAUENSTEIN AND HICKEY METHODS

NOTE: This examination is contraindicated for patients with a suspected fracture or pathologic condition.

The Lauenstein and Hickey methods are used to demonstrate the hip joint and the relationship of the femoral head to the acetabulum. This position is similar to the previously described modified Cleaves method.

Image receptor: 24 × 30 cm (10 × 12 inch) crosswise

Position of patient
• From the supine position, rotate the patient slightly toward the affected side to an oblique position. The degree of obliquity will depend on how much the patient can abduct the leg.

Position of part
• Adjust the patient's body, and center the affected hip to the midline of the grid.
• Ask the patient to flex the affected knee and draw the thigh up to a position at nearly a right angle to the hip bone.
• Keep the body of the affected femur parallel to the table.
• Extend the opposite limb and support it at hip level and under the knee.
• Rotate the pelvis no more than necessary to accommodate flexion of the thigh and to avoid superimposition of the affected side (Fig. 7-34).
• *Shield gonads.*
• *Respiration:* Suspend.

Central ray
• Perpendicular through the hip joint, which is located midway between the ASIS and the pubic symphysis for the Lauenstein method (Fig. 7-35) and at a cephalic angle of 20 to 25 degrees for the Hickey method (Fig. 7-36).
• Center the cassette to the central ray.

Structures shown
The resulting image shows a lateral projection of the hip, including the acetabulum, the proximal end of the femur, and the relationship of the femoral head to the acetabulum (see Figs. 7-35 and 7-36).

EVALUATION CRITERIA
The following should be clearly demonstrated:
- Hip joint centered to the radiograph
- Hip joint, acetabulum, and femoral head
- Femoral neck overlapped by the greater trochanter in the Lauenstein method
- With cephalic angulation in the Hickey method, the femoral neck free of superimposition

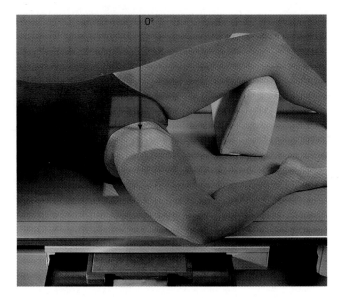

Fig. 7-34 Mediolateral hip: Lauenstein method.

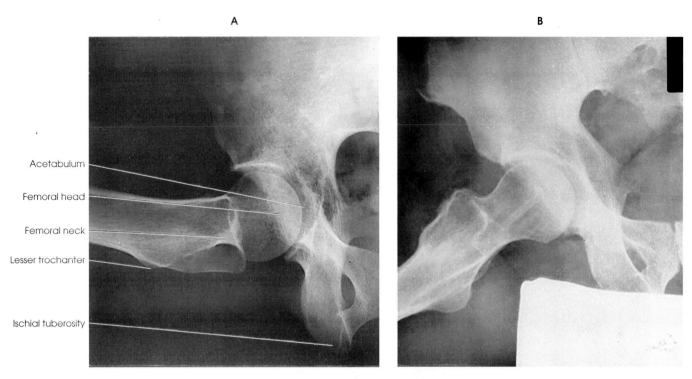

Acetabulum

Femoral head

Femoral neck

Lesser trochanter

Ischial tuberosity

Fig. 7-35 A, Mediolateral hip with perpendicular central ray: Lauenstein method.
B, Mediolateral hip with perpendicular central ray using male gonad (contact) shield.

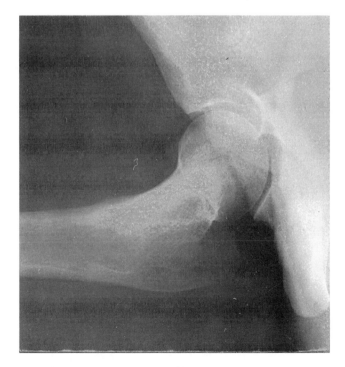

Fig. 7-36 Mediolateral hip with 20-degree cephalad angulation: Hickey method.

AXIOLATERAL PROJECTION
DANELIUS-MILLER METHOD

Image receptor: 24 × 30 cm (10 × 12 inch) lengthwise

Position of patient
- Place the patient in the supine position.

Position of part
- When examining a patient who is thin or who is lying on a soft bed, elevate the pelvis on a firm pillow or folded sheets sufficiently to center the most prominent point of the greater trochanter to the midline of the cassette. The support must not extend beyond the lateral surface of the body; otherwise it will interfere with the placement of the cassette.
- When the pelvis is elevated, support the affected limb at hip level on sandbags or firm pillows.

- Flex the knee and hip of the unaffected side to elevate the thigh in a vertical position.
- Rest the unaffected leg on a suitable support that will not interfere with the central ray. Special support devices are available.
- Adjust the pelvis so that it is not rotated (Figs. 7-37 and 7-38).
- Unless contraindicated, grasp the heel and medially rotate the foot and lower limb of the affected side about 15 or 20 degrees. A sandbag may be used to hold the leg and foot in this position, and a small support can be placed under the knee. The manipulation of patients with unhealed fractures should be performed by a physician.

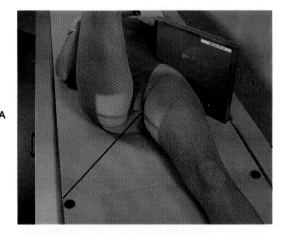
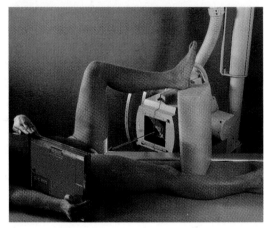

Fig. 7-37 A, Axiolateral hip: Danelius-Miller method, cassette supported with sandbags. **B,** Same projection, patient holding cassette. Note that the foot is on a footrest.

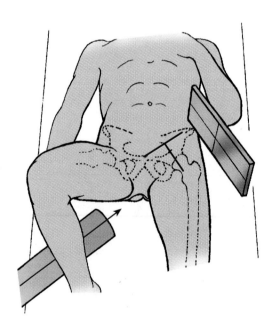

Fig. 7-38 Axiolateral hip: Danelius-Miller method.

Position of cassette

- Place the cassette in the vertical position with its upper border in the crease above the iliac crest.
- Angle the lower border away from the body until the cassette is exactly parallel with the long axis of the femoral neck.
- Support the cassette in this position with sandbags or a vertical cassette holder. These are the preferred methods. Alternatively, the patient may support the cassette with the hand.
- Be careful to position the grid so that the lead strips are in the horizontal position.
- *Shield gonads.*
- *Respiration:* Suspend.

Central ray

- Perpendicular to the long axis of the femoral neck. The central ray enters midthigh and passes through the femoral neck about 2½ inches (6.4 cm) below the point of intersection of the localization lines described previously (see Fig. 7-12).

COMPUTED RADIOGRAPHY

Both dense and nondense body areas will be exposed. The kVp must be sufficient to penetrate the dense area. Collimation must be very close to keep unnecessary radiation from reaching the cassette phosphor.

Structures shown

The resulting image shows the acetabulum, head, neck, and trochanters of the femur (Fig. 7-39).

EVALUATION CRITERIA

The following should be clearly demonstrated:

- Femoral neck without overlap from the greater trochanter
- Small amount of the lesser trochanter on the posterior surface of the femur
- Small amount of the greater trochanter on the anterior and posterior surfaces of the proximal femur when the femur is properly inverted
- Soft tissue shadow of the unaffected thigh not overlapping the hip joint or proximal femur
- Hip joint with the acetabulum
- Any orthopedic appliance in its entirety
- Ischial tuberosity below the femoral head

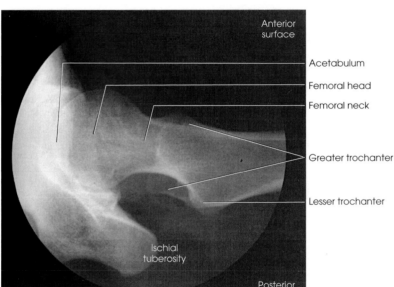
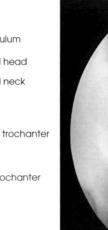
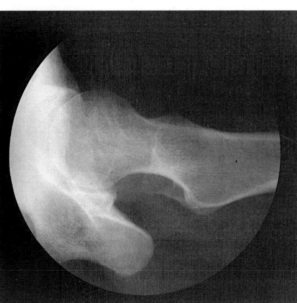

Fig. 7-39 Axiolateral hip: Danelius-Miller method.

Pelvis and upper femora

AXIOLATERAL PROJECTION
CLEMENTS-NAKAYAMA MODIFICATION[1]

When the patient has bilateral hip fractures, bilateral hip arthroplasty (plastic surgery of the hip joints), or limitation of movement of the unaffected leg, the Danelius-Miller method cannot be used. Clements and Nakayama[1] described a modification using a 15-degree posterior angulation of the central ray (Fig. 7-40).

[1]Clements RS, Nakayama HK: Radiographic methods in total hip arthroplasty, *Radiol Technol* 51:589, 1980.

Image receptor: 24 × 30 cm (10 × 12 inch)

Position of patient
- Position the patient supine on the radiographic table with the affected side near the edge of the table.

Position of part
- For this position, do not rotate the lower limb internally. Instead, the limb remains in a neutral or slightly externally rotated position.
- Support a grid cassette on the Bucky tray so that its lower margin is below the patient. Position the grid so the lines run parallel with the floor.
- Adjust the grid parallel to the axis of the femoral neck and tilt its top back 15 degrees.
- *Shield gonads.*
- *Respiration:* Suspend.

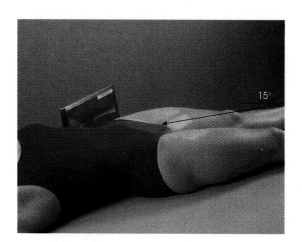

Fig. 7-40 Axiolateral hip: Clements-Nakayama method.

Central ray

- Directed 15 degrees posteriorly and aligned perpendicular to the femoral neck and grid cassette

Structures shown

This leg position demonstrates a lateral hip image because the central ray is angled 15 degrees posterior instead of the toes being medially rotated. The resulting image shows the acetabulum and the proximal femur, including the head, neck, and trochanters in lateral profile. The Clements-Nakayama modification (Fig. 7-41) can be compared to the Danelius-Miller approach described previously (Fig. 7-42).

EVALUATION CRITERIA

The following should be clearly demonstrated:

- Hip joint with the acetabulum
- Femoral head, neck, and trochanters
- Any orthopedic appliance in its entirety

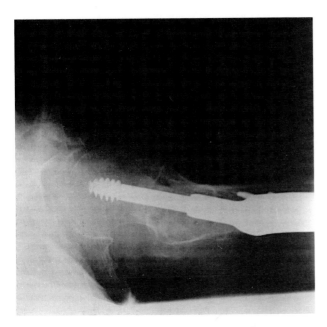

Fig. 7-41 Clements-Nakayama method with 15-degree central ray angulation in the same patient as in Fig. 7-42.

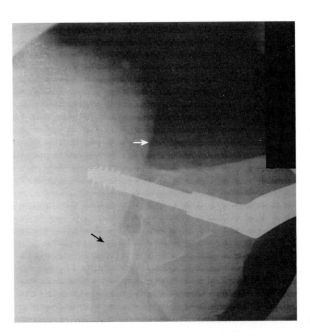

Fig. 7-42 Postoperative Danelius-Miller method used for a patient who was unable to flex the unaffected hip. The contralateral thigh (*arrows*) is obscuring the femoral head and acetabular area.

AXIOLATERAL PROJECTION
LEONARD-GEORGE METHOD

Image receptor: 8 × 10 inch (18 × 24 cm) curved cassette preferred for reduced part-film distance

Position of patient
• Place the patient in the supine position.

Position of part
• If necessary, elevate the patient's pelvis on a small, firm pillow or folded sheets to center the hip to the vertically placed curved cassette.
• Support the affected limb at hip level on pillows or sandbags when the pelvis is elevated.
• Flex the hip and knee of the unaffected side (if they are not immobilized), and abduct the thigh to accommodate the position of the curved cassette.
• The affected limb is usually in abduction in a cast or a splint. If not and if possible, abduct the leg enough to accurately place the curved cassette.
• Place the cassette in the vertical position well up between the thighs and center it to the femoral neck of the affected side (Figs. 7-43 and 7-44).
• If the limb can be safely moved, grasp the heel and internally rotate the foot and lower limb about 15 or 20 degrees to overcome the anteversion of the femoral neck.
• *Shield gonads.*
• *Respiration:* Suspend.

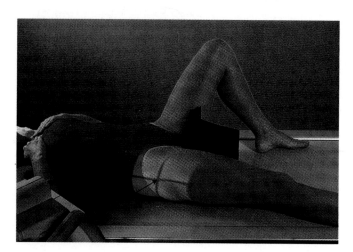

Fig. 7-43 Axiolateral hip with curved cassette: Leonard-George method.

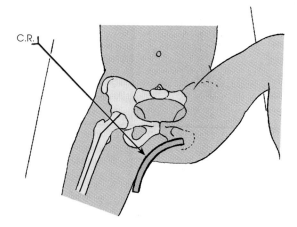

Fig. 7-44 Axiolateral hip with curved cassette: Leonard-George method.

Central ray

• Lateromedially and perpendicular to the long axis of the femoral neck. The central ray enters the lateral surface of the hip above the soft tissue depression just above the greater trochanter.

Structures shown

The resulting image shows the acetabulum, head, neck, and trochanteric area of the femur (Fig. 7-45). Because of the convexity of the cassette, the femoral head and trochanteric areas are somewhat elongated.

EVALUATION CRITERIA

The following should be clearly demonstrated:

■ Femoral neck without overlapping from the trochanters
■ Small amount of the lesser trochanter on the posterior surface of the femur
■ Small amount of the greater trochanter on the anterior and posterior surfaces of the proximal femur when the femur is properly placed
■ Hip joint with the acetabulum

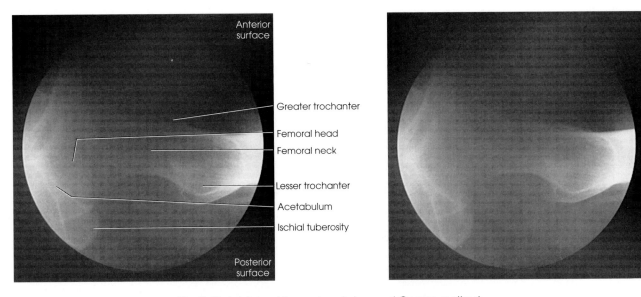

Fig. 7-45 Axiolateral femoral neck: Leonard-George method.

Pelvis and upper femora

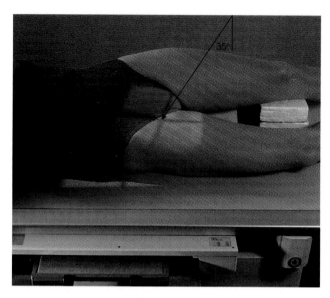

Fig. 7-46 Axiolateral hip with central ray angulation of 35 degrees: Friedman method.

AXIOLATERAL PROJECTION
FRIEDMAN METHOD

NOTE: This examination is contraindicated for patients with a suspected fracture or pathologic condition.

Image receptor: 24 × 30 cm (10 × 12 inch) lengthwise

Position of patient

* Have the patient lie in the lateral recumbent position on the affected side.
* Center the midcoronal plane of the body to the midline of the radiographic table.

Position of part

* Extend the affected limb and adjust it in a lateral position.
* Roll the upper side of the patient's limb gently posteriorly, approximately 10 degrees, and place a support under the knee to support it at hip level. The affected femur does not change position if it is properly immobilized; the pelvis rotates from the femoral head (Fig. 7-46).

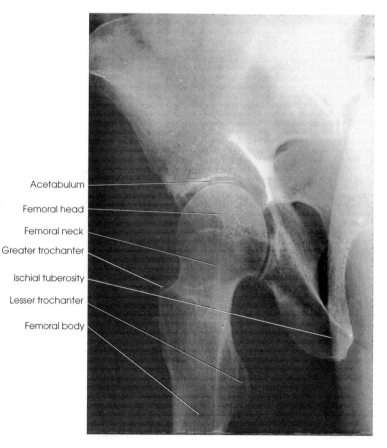
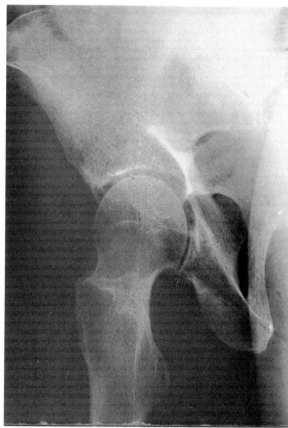

Acetabulum
Femoral head
Femoral neck
Greater trochanter
Ischial tuberosity
Lesser trochanter
Femoral body

Fig. 7-47 Axiolateral hip with central ray angulation of 35 degrees: Friedman method.

- With the cassette in the Bucky tray, adjust its position so that the midpoint of the cassette coincides with the central ray.
- *Shield gonads.*
- *Respiration:* Suspend.

Central ray

- Directed to the femoral neck at an angle of 35 degrees cephalad (Fig. 7-47).
- Kisch[1] recommended that the central ray be angled 15 or 20 degrees cephalad for this position (Fig. 7-48).

Structures shown

The resulting image shows an axiolateral projection of the head, neck, trochanters, and proximal body (shaft) of the femur.

---

[1]Kisch E: Eine neue Methode für röntgenolische Darstellung des Hüftgelenks in frontaler Ebene, *Fortschr Roentgenstr* 27:309, 1920.

The following should be clearly demonstrated:

- Moderately distorted femoral head, neck, and trochanters because of the angulation of the x-ray beam
- Hip joint

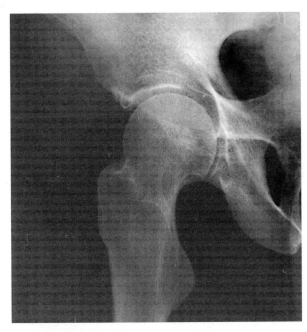

Fig. 7-48 Axiolateral hip with central ray angulation of 20 degrees: Friedman method.

PA OBLIQUE PROJECTION

HSIEH METHOD[1]

RAO or LAO position

Hsieh[1] recommended this projection for demonstrating posterior dislocations of the femoral head in cases other than acute fracture dislocations.

Image receptor: 24 × 30 cm (10 × 12 inch) lengthwise

Position of patient

• Place the patient with a suspected posterior hip dislocation in the semiprone position, and center the affected hip to the midline of the radiographic table.

[1]Hsieh CK: Posterior dislocation of the hip, *Radiology* 27:450, 1936.

Position of part

• Elevate the unaffected side approximately 40 to 45 degrees and have the patient support the body on the flexed knee and forearm of the elevated side.
• Adjust the position of the body to place the posterior surface of the affected iliac bone over the midline of the grid (Fig. 7-49).
• With the cassette in the Bucky tray, adjust its position so that the center of the cassette will lie at the level of the superior border of the greater trochanter.
• *Shield gonads.*
• *Respiration:* Suspend.

Central ray

• Perpendicular to the midpoint of the cassette passing between the posterior surface of the iliac blade and the dislocated femoral head

Structures shown

The resulting image shows a PA oblique projection of the ilium, hip joint, and proximal femur (Fig. 7-50).

The following should be clearly demonstrated:

■ Hip joint near the center of the radiograph
■ Acetabulum and femoral head
■ Superimposed soft tissue of buttock over the area of the femoral neck
■ Urist[1] recommended a right or left posterior oblique position (AP projection) for demonstration of the posterior rim of the acetabulum in acute fracture-dislocation injuries of the hip. For this projection, the patient is adjusted from the supine position. The injured hip is elevated 60 degrees to place the posterior rim of the acetabulum in profile, and the body is adjusted to center the sagittal plane passing through the ASIS to the midline of the table. The cassette is centered at the level of the upper border of the greater trochanter. The central ray is directed perpendicular to the midpoint of the cassette (Fig. 7-51).

[1]Urist MR: Fracture-dislocation of the hip joint, *J Bone Joint Surg* 30A:699, 1948.

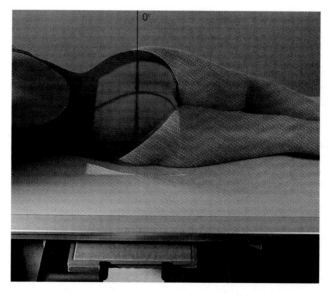

Fig. 7-49 PA oblique hip, LAO position: Hsieh method.

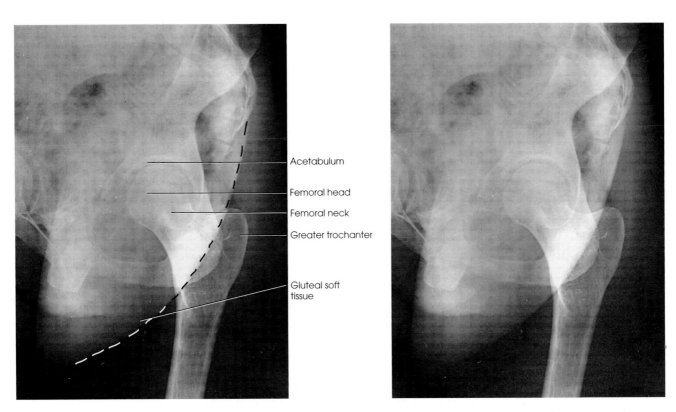

Acetabulum

Femoral head

Femoral neck

Greater trochanter

Gluteal soft tissue

Fig. 7-50 PA oblique hip: Hsieh method. No dislocation is seen.

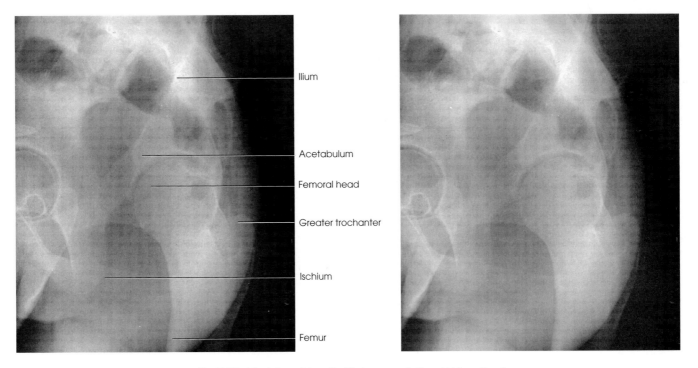

Ilium

Acetabulum

Femoral head

Greater trochanter

Ischium

Femur

Fig. 7-51 AP oblique hip with 60-degree rotation: Urist method.

MEDIOLATERAL OBLIQUE PROJECTION
LILIENFELD METHOD
RAO or LAO position

NOTE: This examination is contraindicated for patients with a suspected fracture or pathologic condition.

Image receptor: 24 × 30 cm (10 × 12 inch) lengthwise

Position of patient

- Have the patient lie in the lateral recumbent position on the affected side.

Position of part

- Center the midcoronal plane of the body to the midline of the grid.
- Fully extend the affected thigh, adjust it in a true lateral position, and immobilize it with sandbags.
- Roll the upper side gently forward approximately 15 degrees or just enough to separate the two sides of the pelvis.
- Support the limb at hip level on sandbags.
- If the affected side is well immobilized and the upper side is gently rolled forward, the affected hip will not change position; the pelvis will rotate from the femoral head (Fig. 7-52).
- With the cassette in the Bucky tray, adjust its position so that the center point of the cassette lies at the level of the greater trochanter.
- *Shield gonads.*
- *Respiration:* Suspend.

Central ray

- Perpendicular to the midpoint of the cassette, traversing the affected hip joint

Structures shown

The resulting image shows a mediolateral oblique projection of the ilium, acetabulum, and proximal femur (Fig. 7-53).

EVALUATION CRITERIA

The following should be clearly demonstrated:

- Hip joint near the center of the radiograph
- Femoral head and acetabulum
- Unaffected hip and acetabulum not overlapping the same structures of the side of interest

NOTE: Because the Lilienfeld projection is not used with patients who have an acute hip injury, these patients can be comfortably, safely, and satisfactorily examined in the position described by Colonna.[1] Positioning is approximately the same as for the Lilienfeld method except that the patient is placed *on the unaffected side* and adjusted to center the uppermost hip to the midline of the radiographic table. Colonna recommended that the uppermost side—the affected side—be rotated about 17 degrees anteriorly from the true lateral position. He stated that this degree of rotation separates the shadows of the hip joints and gives the optimum projection of the slope of the acetabular roof and the depth of the socket (Fig. 7-54).

[1]Colonna PC: A diagnostic roentgen view of the acetabulum, *Surg Clin North Am* 33:1565, 1953.

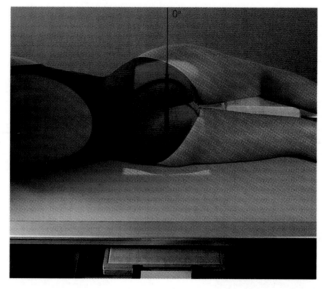

Fig. 7-52 Mediolateral oblique hip, LAO position: Lilienfeld method.

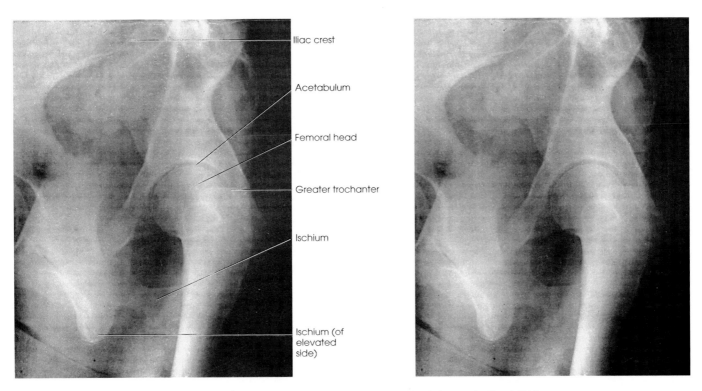

Fig. 7-53 Mediolateral oblique hip: Lilienfeld method demonstrating left hip.

Iliac crest

Acetabulum

Femoral head

Greater trochanter

Ischium

Ischium (of elevated side)

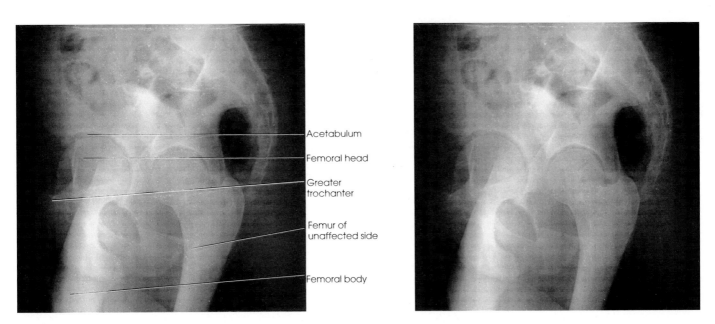

Fig. 7-54 Colonna method of patient positioning, demonstrating elevated right hip.

Acetabulum

Femoral head

Greater trochanter

Femur of unaffected side

Femoral body

PA AXIAL OBLIQUE PROJECTION
TEUFEL METHOD
RAO or LAO position

Image receptor: 18 × 24 cm (8 × 10 inch) lengthwise

Position of patient
• Have the patient lie in a semiprone position on the affected side.

Position of part
• Align the body, and center the hip being examined to the midline of the grid.
• Elevate the unaffected side so that the anterior surface of the body forms a 38-degree angle from the table (Fig. 7-55).

• Have the patient support the body on the forearm and flexed knee of the elevated side.
• With the cassette in the Bucky tray, adjust the position of the cassette so that its midpoint coincides with the central ray.
• *Shield gonads.*
• *Respiration:* Suspend.

Central ray
• Directed through the acetabulum at an angle of 12 degrees cephalad. The central ray enters the body at the inferior level of the coccyx and approximately 2 inches (5 cm) lateral to the midsagittal plane toward the side being examined.

Structures shown
The resulting image shows the fovea capitis and particularly the superoposterior wall of the acetabulum (Fig. 7-56).

EVALUATION CRITERIA
The following should be clearly demonstrated:
■ Hip joint and acetabulum near the center of the radiograph
■ Femoral head in profile to show the concave area of the fovea capitis
■ Superoposterior wall of the acetabulum

AP OBLIQUE PROJECTION
JUDET METHOD[1]
RPO or LPO position

Judet, Judet, and Letournel[1] described two 45-degree posterior oblique positions that are useful in diagnosing fractures of the acetabulum: the internal oblique (affected side up) position and the external oblique (affected side down) position. In both positions a perpendicular central ray is directed through the acetabulum.

---

[1]Judet R, Judet J, Letournel E: Fractures of the acetabulum: classification and surgical approaches for open reduction, *J Bone Joint Surg* 46A:1615, 1964.

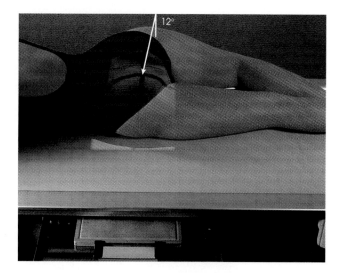

Fig. 7-55 PA axial oblique acetabulum: Teufel method.

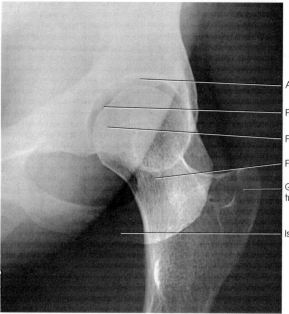
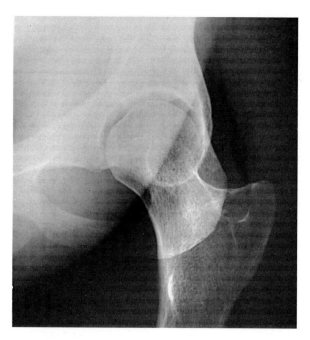

Acetabulum

Fovea capitis

Femoral head

Femoral neck

Greater trochanter

Ischium

Fig. 7-56 PA axial oblique acetabulum: Teufel method.

AXIOLATERAL PROJECTION

DUNLAP, SWANSON, AND PENNER METHOD[1]

NOTE: This method uses two exposures that are made on the same image receptor while the patient remains in position. *The patient should not move between the first and second exposures* while the central ray and image receptor are recentered.

---

[1]Dunlap K, Swanson AB, Penner RS: Studies of the hip joint by means of lateral acetabular roentgenograms, *J Bone Joint Surg* 38A:1218, 1956.

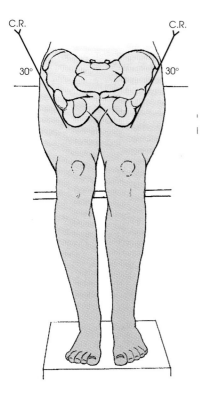

Fig. 7-57 Axiolateral acetabulum.

Image receptor: 18 × 43 cm (7 × 17 inch) or 35 × 43 cm (14 × 17 inch) crosswise for bilateral examination of adults. Close collimation is used to restrict the radiation to the adjacent half of the cassette, or lead may be taped to the cassette.

Position of patient

- Place the patient in the seated-upright position on the side of the radiographic table.

Position of part

- Ask the patient to move back far enough to place the posterior surface of the knees in contact with the edge of the radiographic table (Fig. 7-57).
- Prepare the image receptor for recentering by aligning the midpoint of one half of the image receptor to the midsagittal plane.
- Mark the position of the grid so that it can be moved back to this position for the second exposure without disturbing the patient's position; then center the opposite half of the cassette to the midsagittal plane of the body for the first exposure.
- Ask the patient to sit upright with thighs together.
- Have the patient cross the arms over the chest so that they are away from the crests of the ilia.
- *Shield gonads.*
- *Respiration:* Suspend.

Central ray

- Directed to the crest of the ilium at a medial angle of 30 degrees, first from one side and then from the other
- Dunlap, Swanson, and Penner[1] stated that although the plane of the acetabulum forms an angle of 35 degrees with the sagittal plane in the average adult and an angle of 32 degrees in most children, a central ray angulation of 30 degrees results in the least superimposition of parts.

Structures shown

The resulting image shows the acetabula in profile, projected from a plane at right angles to the frontal projection, as well as the relationship of the femoral heads to the acetabula. The femoral heads, necks, and trochanters are seen from a nearly frontal plane because the position of the femora changes little between the supine and the seated-upright positions (Fig. 7-58).

EVALUATION CRITERIA

The following should be clearly demonstrated:

- Acetabula in profile
- Ilium, ischium, and pubic bones not overlapping the acetabular region
- Acetabula and hip joints near the center of the image

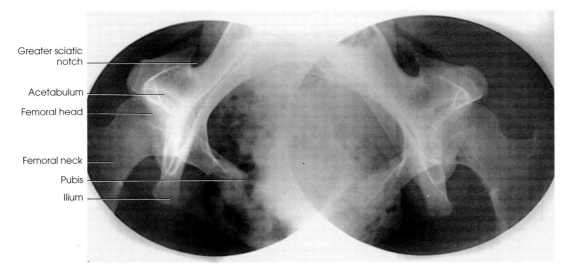

Greater sciatic notch

Acetabulum
Femoral head

Femoral neck
Pubis
Ilium

Fig. 7-58 Axiolateral acetabulum.

Pelvis and upper femora

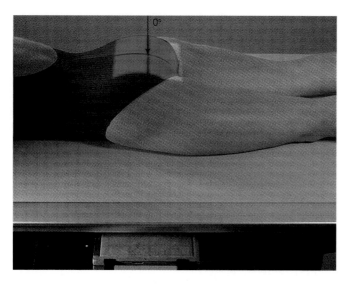

Fig. 7-59 PA pelvic bones.

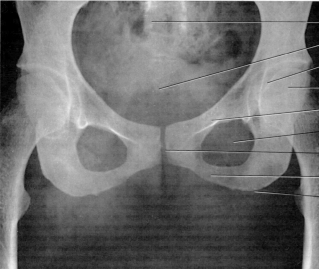

- Sacrum
- Coccyx
- Acetabulum
- Femoral head
- Superior pubic ramus
- Obturator foramen
- Pubic symphysis
- Inferior pubic ramus
- Ischial tuberosity

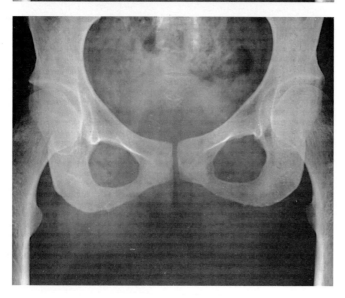

Fig. 7-60 PA pelvic bones.

PA PROJECTION

Image receptor: 18 × 24 cm (8 × 10 inch) crosswise

Position of patient
- Place the patient in the prone position, and center the midsagittal plane of the body to the midline of the grid.

Position of part
- With the cassette in the Bucky tray, center the cassette at the level of the greater trochanters. This positioning also centers the cassette to the pubic symphysis (Fig. 7-59).
- *Shield gonads.*
- *Respiration:* Suspend.

Central ray
- Perpendicular to the midpoint of the cassette. The central ray enters the distal coccyx and exits the pubic symphysis.

Structures shown
The resulting image shows a PA projection of the pubic symphysis and ischia, including the obturator foramina (Fig. 7-60).

EVALUATION CRITERIA
The following should be clearly demonstrated:
- Pubic and ischial bones not magnified or superimposing the sacrum or coccyx
- Pubic and ischial bones near the center of the radiograph
- Hip joints
- Symmetric obturator foramina

AP AXIAL PROJECTION
TAYLOR METHOD

Image receptor: 24×30 cm (10×12 inch) crosswise

Position of patient
• Place the patient in the supine position.

Position of part
• Center the midsagittal plane of the patient's body to the midline of the grid, and adjust the pelvis so that it is not rotated. The ASISs should be equidistant from the table (Fig. 7-61).
• With the cassette in the Bucky tray, adjust the tray's position so the midpoint of the cassette will coincide with the central ray.
• *Shield gonads.*
• *Respiration:* Suspend.

Central ray
Males
• Directed 20 to 35 degrees cephalad and centered to a point 2 inches (5 cm) distal to the superior border of the pubic symphysis.
Females
• Directed 30 to 45 degrees cephalad and centered to a point 2 inches (5 cm) distal to the upper border of the pubic symphysis.

Structures shown
The resulting image shows an elongated projection of the pubic and ischial rami (Figs. 7-62 and 7-63).

EVALUATION CRITERIA
The following should be clearly demonstrated:
■ Pubic and ischial bones magnified with pubic bones superimposed over the sacrum and coccyx
■ Symmetric obturator foramina
■ Pubic and ischial rami near the center of the radiograph
■ Hip joints

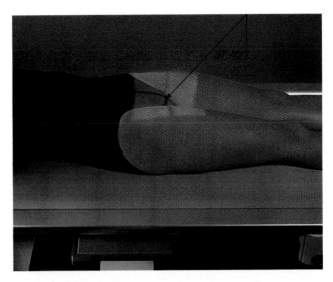

Fig. 7-61 AP axial pelvic bones: Taylor method.

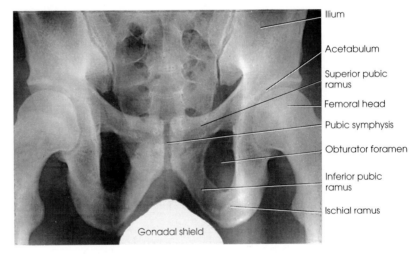

Fig. 7-62 Male AP axial pelvic bones: Taylor method.

Ilium

Acetabulum

Superior pubic ramus

Femoral head

Pubic symphysis

Obturator foramen

Inferior pubic ramus

Ischial ramus

Gonadal shield

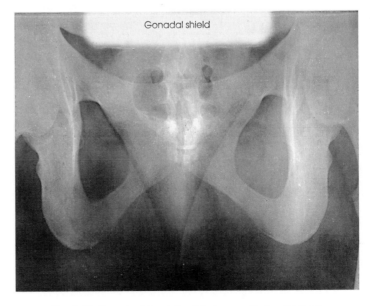

Gonadal shield

Fig. 7-63 Female AP axial pelvic bones: Taylor method.

SUPEROINFERIOR AXIAL PROJECTION
LILIENFELD METHOD

Image receptor: 8 × 10 inch (18 × 24 cm) crosswise

Position of patient
- Place the patient on the radiographic table in a seated-upright position.

Position of part
- Center the midsagittal plane of the patient's body to the midline of the grid.
- Flex the knees slightly and support them to relieve strain. If the travel of the cassette tray is great enough to permit centering near the end of the table, have the patient sit so that the legs can hang over and the feet can rest on a suitable support.
- Adjust the pelvis so that the ASISs are equidistant from the table.
- Have the patient extend the arms for support, lean backward 45 or 50 degrees, and then arch the back, if possible, to place the pubic arch in a vertical position (Fig. 7-64).
- With the cassette in the Bucky tray, center it at the level of the greater trochanters.
- *Shield gonads.*
- *Respiration:* Suspend.

Central ray
- Perpendicular to the midpoint of the image receptor and entering 1½ inches (3.8 cm) superior to the pubic symphysis

Structures shown
The resulting image shows a superoinferior axial projection of the anterior pubic and ischial bones and the pubic symphysis. (Fig. 7-65).

EVALUATION CRITERIA
The following should be clearly demonstrated:
- Medially superimposed superior and inferior rami of the pubic bones
- Nearly superimposed lateral two thirds of the pubic and ischial bones
- Symmetric pubes and ischia
- Pubic and ischial bones centered to the radiograph
- Hip joints
- Anterior pelvic bones

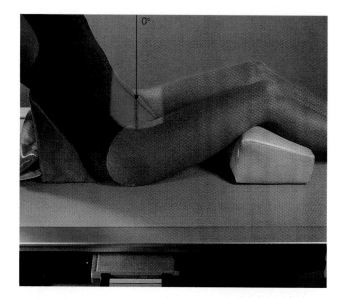

Fig. 7-64 Superoinferior axial pelvic bones: Lilienfeld method.

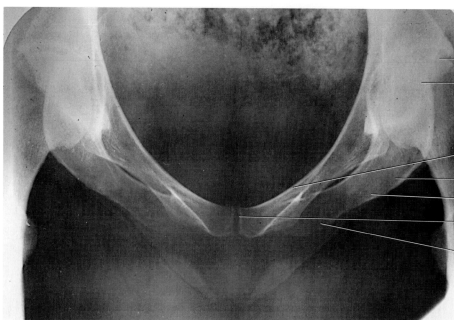

Acetabulum

Femoral head

Superior pubic ramus

Ischial tuberosity

Ischial ramus

Pubic symphysis

Inferior pubic ramus

Fig. 7-65 Superoinferior axial pelvic bones: Lilienfeld method.

PA AXIAL PROJECTION
STAUNIG METHOD

Image receptor: 8 × 10 inch (18 × 24 cm) crosswise

Position of patient
- Place the patient in the prone position.

Position of part
- Center the midsagittal plane of the body to the midline of the radiographic table.
- Adjust the body so that the pelvis is not rotated.
- With the cassette in the Bucky tray, adjust its position so that the midpoint of the cassette will coincide with the central ray (Fig. 7-66).
- *Shield gonads.*
- *Respiration:* Suspend.

Central ray
- Directed 35 degrees cephalad exiting the pubic symphysis on the midsagittal plane anteriorly at the level of the greater trochanters

Structures shown
The resulting image shows a PA axial projection of the pubic and ischial bones and the pubic symphysis. The appearance of this radiograph will be nearly identical to the superoinferior axial projection discussed previously.

EVALUATION CRITERIA
The following should be clearly demonstrated:
- Medially superimposed superior and inferior rami of the pubic bones
- Nearly superimposed lateral two thirds of the pubic and ischial bones
- Symmetric pubes and ischia
- Pubic and ischial bones centered to the radiograph
- Hip joints

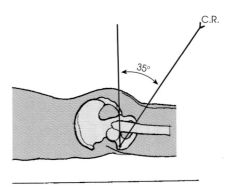

Fig. 7-66 PA axial anterior pelvic bones: Staunig method.

AP AND PA OBLIQUE PROJECTIONS

Image receptor: 24 × 30 cm (10 × 12 inch) lengthwise

RPO and LPO positions
Position of patient
- Place the patient in the supine position.

Position of part
- Center the sagittal plane passing through the hip joint of the affected side to the midline of the grid.

- Elevate the *unaffected* side approximately 40 degrees to place the broad surface of the wing of the affected ilium parallel with the plane of the cassette.
- Support the elevated shoulder, hip, and knee on sandbags.
- Adjust the position of the uppermost limb to place the ASISs in the same transverse plane (Fig. 7-67).
- Center the cassette at the level of the ASIS.
- *Shield gonads.*
- *Respiration:* Suspend.

RAO and LAO positions
Position of patient
- Place the patient in the prone position.

Position of part
- Center the sagittal plane passing through the hip joint of the affected side to the midline of the grid.
- Elevate the *unaffected* side about 40 degrees to place the affected ilium perpendicular to the plane of the cassette.
- Have the patient rest on the forearm and flexed knee of the elevated side.
- Adjust the position of the uppermost thigh to place the iliac crests in the same horizontal plane.
- Center the cassette at the level of the ASIS (Fig. 7-68).
- *Shield gonads.*
- *Respiration:* Suspend.

Central ray
- Perpendicular to the midpoint of the cassette

Structures shown
The AP oblique image shows an unobstructed projection of the ala and sciatic notches and a profile image of the acetabulum (Fig. 7-69).

The PA oblique image shows the ilium in profile and the femoral head within the acetabulum (Fig. 7-70).

EVALUATION CRITERIA
The following should be clearly demonstrated:
- Entire ilium
- Hip joint, proximal femur, and sacroiliac joint
  AP oblique projection
- Broad surface of the iliac wing without rotation
  PA oblique projection
- Ilium in profile

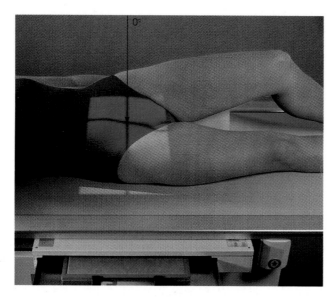

Fig. 7-67 AP oblique ilium, RPO.

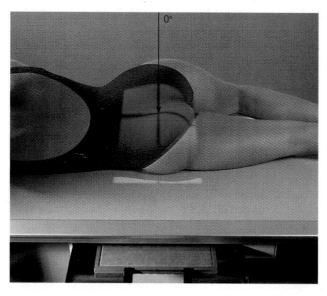

Fig. 7-68 PA oblique ilium, LAO.

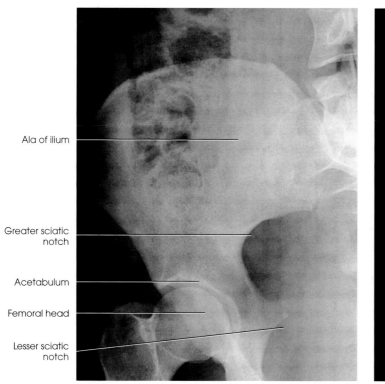
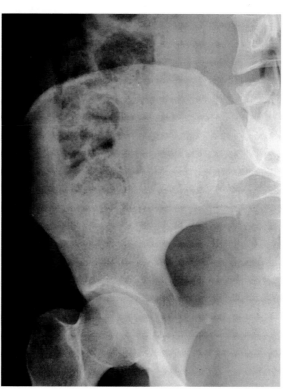

Ala of ilium

Greater sciatic notch

Acetabulum

Femoral head

Lesser sciatic notch

Fig. 7-69 AP oblique ilium, RPO.

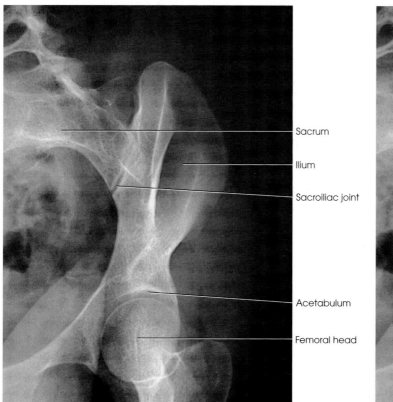
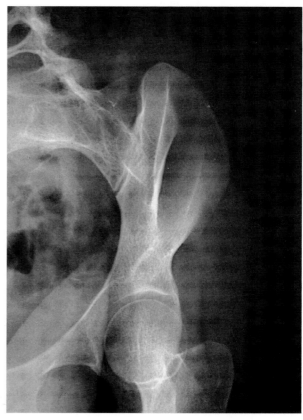

Sacrum

Ilium

Sacroiliac joint

Acetabulum

Femoral head

Fig. 7-70 PA oblique ilium, LAO.

VERTEBRAL COLUMN

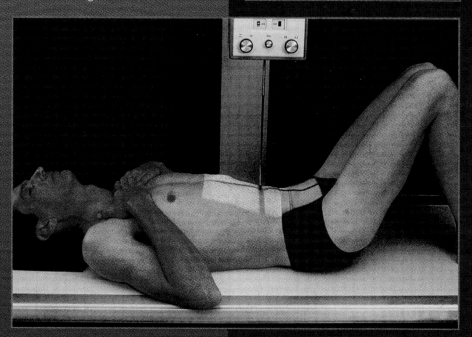

RIGHT Performance of lumbosacral junction, 1949.

BELOW Lumbosacral junction performed with close collimation and lead shielding, 1999.

PROJECTIONS, POSITIONS & METHODS

Page	Essential	Anatomy	Projection	Position	Method
384		Atlanto-occipital articulation	AP oblique	R and L head rotations	
386		Atlanto-occipital articulation	PA		
388	✵	Atlas and axis	AP	Open mouth	
387	✵	Dens	AP		FUCHS
390		Atlas and dens	PA		JUDD
391		Dens	AP axial oblique rotations	R or L head rotations	KASABACH
392		Atlas and axis	Lateral	R or L	
394	✵	Cervical vertebrae	AP axial		
396	✵	Cervical vertebrae	Lateral	R or L	GRANDY
398	✵	Cervical vertebrae	Lateral	R or L, hyperflexion or hyperextension	
400	✵	Cervical intervertebral foramina	AP axial oblique	RPO and LPO	
402		Cervical intervertebral foramina	AP oblique	Hyperflexion and hyperextension	
402	✵	Cervical intervertebral foramina	PA axial oblique	RAO and LAO	
404		Cervical vertebrae	AP		OTTONELLO
406		Cervical and upper thoracic vertebrae: *vertebral arch* (*pillars*)	AP axial		
408		Cervical and upper thoracic vertebrae: *vertebral arch* (*pillars*)	AP axial oblique	R and L head rotations	
409		Cervical and upper thoracic vertebrae: *vertebral arch* (*pillars*)	PA axial oblique	R and L head rotations	
411	✵	Cervical vertebrae: *trauma*	Lateral	R or L, dorsal decubitus	
412	✵	Cervical vertebrae: *trauma*	AP axial		
413	✵	Cervical vertebrae: *trauma*	AP axial oblique	RPO and LPO	

AP, anteroposterior; *PA,* posteroanterior; *R,* right; *L,* left; *RPO,* right posterior oblique; *LPO,* left posterior oblique.
Icons in the Essential column indicate projections that are frequently performed in the United States and Canada. Students should be competent in these projections.

PROJECTIONS, POSITIONS & METHODS

Page	Essential	Anatomy	Projection	Position	Method
414	♠	Cervicothoracic region	Lateral	R or L upright	TWINING
416	♠	Cervicothoracic region	Lateral	R or L recumbent	PAWLOW, MODIFIED PAWLOW
418	♠	Thoracic vertebrae	AP		
420	♠	Thoracic vertebrae	Lateral	R or L	
423		Zygapophyseal joints	AP oblique	LAO and LPO	
423		Zygapophyseal joints	PA oblique	RAO and RPO	
426	♠	Lumbar-lumbosacral vertebrae	AP		
428		Lumbar-lumbosacral vertebrae	PA		
430	♠	Lumbar-lumbosacral vertebrae	Lateral	R or L, recumbent or upright	
432	♠	L5-S1 lumbosacral junction	Lateral	R or L	
434	♠	Zygapophyseal joints	AP oblique	RPO and LPO	
436		Zygapophyseal joints	PA oblique	RAO and LAO	
438		Intervertebral foramen: fifth-lumbar	PA axial oblique	RAO and LAO	KOVACS
440	♠	Lumbosacral junction and sacroiliac joints	AP axial		
440		Lumbosacral junction and sacroiliac joints	PA axial		
442	♠	Sacroiliac joints	AP oblique	RPO and LPO	
444		Sacroiliac joints	PA oblique	RAO and LAO	
446		Pubic symphisis	PA		CHAMBERLAIN
448	♠	Sacrum and coccyx	AP axial (sacrum)		
449	♠	Sacrum and coccyx	AP axial (coccyx)		
451	♠	Sacrum and coccyx	Lateral (sacrum)	R or L	
451	♠	Sacrum and coccyx	Lateral (coccyx)	R or L	
452		Sacral vertebral canal and sacroiliac joints	Axial		NÖLKE
454		Lumbar intervertebral disks	PA	R and L bending	WEIGHT- BEARING
458	♠	Thoracolumbar spine: scoliosis	PA, lateral		FERGUSON
460		Lumbar spine: spinal fusion	AP	R and L bending	
462		Lumbar spine: spinal fusion	Lateral	R or L, hyperflexion and hyperextension	

Vertebral Column

The *vertebral column,* or *spine,* forms the central axis of the skeleton and is centered in the midsagittal plane of the posterior part of the trunk. The vertebral column has many functions: it encloses and protects the spinal cord; it acts as a support for the trunk; it supports the skull superiorly; and it provides for attachment for the deep muscles of the back and the ribs laterally. The upper limbs are supported indirectly via the ribs, which articulate with the sternum. The sternum in turn articulates with the shoulder girdle. The vertebral column articulates with each hipbone at the sacroiliac joints. This articulation supports the vertebral column and transmits the weight of the trunk through the hip joints and to the lower limbs.

The vertebral column is composed of small segments of bone called *vertebrae.* Disks of fibrocartilage are interposed between the vertebrae and act as cushions. The vertebral column is held together by ligaments, and it is jointed and curved so that it has considerable flexibility and resilience.

In early life the vertebral column usually consists of 33 small, irregularly shaped bones. These bones are divided into five groups and named according to the region they occupy (Fig. 8-1). The most superior seven vertebrae occupy the region of the neck and are termed *cervical vertebrae.* The succeeding 12 bones lie in the dorsal, or posterior, portion of the thorax and are called the *thoracic vertebrae.* The five vertebrae occupying the region of the loin are termed *lumbar vertebrae.* The next five vertebrae, located in the pelvic region, are termed *sacral vertebrae.* The terminal vertebrae, also in the pelvic region, vary from three to five in number in the adult and are called the *coccygeal vertebrae.*

The 24 vertebral segments in the upper three regions remain distinct throughout life and are termed the *true* or movable vertebrae. The pelvic segments in the two lower regions are called *false* or fixed vertebrae because of the change they undergo in adults. The sacral segments usually fuse into one bone called the *sacrum,* and the coccygeal segments, referred to as the *coccyx,* also fuse into one bone.

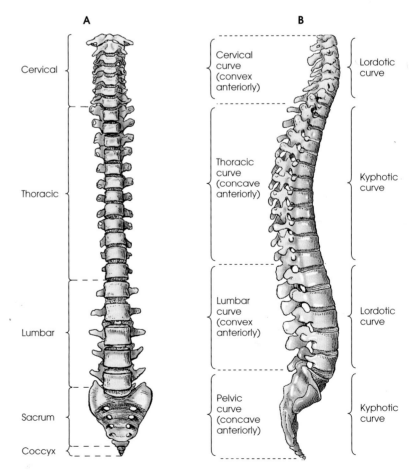

Fig. 8-1 A, Anterior aspect of vertebral column. **B,** Lateral aspect of vertebral column, showing regions and curvatures.

Vertebral Curvature

Viewed from the side, the vertebral column has four curves that arch anteriorly and posteriorly from the midcoronal plane of the body. The *cervical, thoracic, lumbar,* and *pelvic curves* are named for the regions they occupy.

In this text the vertebral curves are discussed in reference to the *anatomic position* and are referred to as "convex anteriorly" or "concave anteriorly." Because physicians and surgeons evaluate the spine from the posterior aspect of the body, convex and concave terminology can be the exact opposites. For example, when viewed posteriorly, the normal lumbar curve can correctly be referred to as "concave posteriorly." Whether the curve is described as "convex anteriorly" or "concave posteriorly," the curvature of the patient's spine is the same. The cervical and lumbar curves, which are convex anteriorly, are called *lordotic* curves. The thoracic and pelvic curves are concave anteriorly and are called *kyphotic* curves (see Fig. 8-1, *B*). The cervical and thoracic curves merge smoothly.

The lumbar and pelvic curves join at an obtuse angle termed the *lumbosacral angle.* The acuity of the angle in the junction of these curves varies in different patients. The thoracic and pelvic curves are called *primary curves* because they are present at birth. The cervical and lumbar curves are called *secondary* or *compensatory curves* because they develop after birth. The cervical curve, which is the least pronounced of the curves, develops when the child begins to hold the head up at about 3 or 4 months of age and begins to sit alone at about 8 or 9 months of age. The lumbar curve develops when the child begins to walk at about 1 to 1½ years of age. The lumbar and pelvic curves are more pronounced in females, who therefore have a more acute angle at the lumbosacral junction.

Any abnormal increase in the anterior concavity (or posterior convexity) of the thoracic curve is termed *kyphosis* (Fig. 8-2, *B*). Any abnormal increase in the anterior convexity (or posterior concavity) of the lumbar or cervical curve is termed *lordosis.*

In frontal view the vertebral column varies in width in several regions (see Fig. 8-1). Generally the width of the spine gradually increases from the second cervical vertebra to the superior part of the sacrum and then decreases sharply. A *slight* lateral curvature is sometimes present in the upper thoracic region. The curve is to the right in right-handed persons and to the left in left-handed persons. For this reason, lateral curvature of the vertebral column is believed to be the result of muscle action and to be influenced by occupation. An abnormal lateral curvature of the spine is called *scoliosis.* This condition also causes the vertebrae to rotate toward the concavity. The vertebral column then develops a second or compensatory curve in the opposite direction to keep the head centered over the feet (Fig. 8-2, *A*).

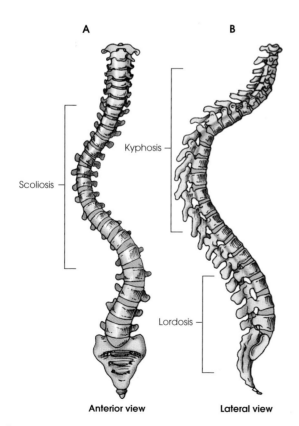

Anterior view   Lateral view

Fig. 8-2 A, Scoliosis, lateral curvature of the spine. **B,** Kyphosis, increased convexity of the thoracic spine. Lordosis, increased concavity of the lumbar spine.

Typical Vertebra

A typical vertebra is composed of two main parts—an anterior mass of bone called the *body* and a posterior ringlike portion called the *vertebral arch* (Figs. 8-3 and 8-4). The vertebral body and arch enclose a space called the *vertebral foramen*. In the articulated column the vertebral foramina form the *vertebral canal.*

The body of the vertebra is approximately cylindric in shape and is composed largely of cancellous bony tissue covered by a layer of compact tissue. From the superior aspect the posterior surface is flattened, and from the lateral aspect the anterior and lateral surfaces are concave. The superior and inferior surfaces of the bodies are flattened and covered by a thin plate of *articular cartilage.*

In the articulated spine the vertebral bodies are separated by *intervertebral disks.* These disks account for approximately one fourth of the length of the vertebral column. Each disk has a central mass of soft, pulpy, semigelatinous material called the *nucleus pulposus,* which is surrounded by an outer fibrocartilaginous disk called the *annulus fibrosus.* It is fairly common for the pulpy nucleus to rupture or protrude into the vertebral canal, thereby impinging on a spinal nerve. This condition is called *herniated nucleus pulposus (HNP),* or more commonly *slipped disk.* HNP most often occurs in the lumbar region as a result of improper body mechanics, and it can cause considerable discomfort and pain.

The vertebral arch (see Figs. 8-3 and 8-4) is formed by two *pedicles* and two *laminae* that support four articular processes, two transverse processes, and one spinous process. The pedicles are short, thick processes that project posteriorly, one from each side, from the superior and lateral parts of the posterior surface of the vertebral body. The superior and inferior surfaces of the pedicles, or roots, are concave. These concavities are called *vertebral notches.* By articulation with the vertebrae above and below, the notches form *intervertebral foramina* for the transmission of spinal nerves and blood vessels. The broad, flat *laminae* are directed posteriorly and medially from the pedicles.

The *transverse processes* project laterally and slightly posteriorly from the junction of the pedicles and laminae. The *spinous process* projects posteriorly and inferiorly from the junction of the laminae in the posterior midline. A congenital defect of the vertebral column in which the laminae fail to unite posteriorly at the midline is called *spina bifida.* In serious cases of spina bifida the spinal cord may protrude from the affected individual's body.

Four articular processes, two superior and two inferior, arise from the junction of the pedicles and laminae to articulate with the vertebrae above and below (see Fig. 8-4). The articulating surfaces of the four articular processes are covered with fibrocartilage and are called *facets.* In a typical vertebra, each *superior articular process* has an articular facet on its posterior surface, and each *inferior articular process* has an articular facet on the anterior surface. The planes of the facets vary in direction in the different regions of the vertebral column and often vary within the same vertebra. The articulations between the articular processes of the vertebral arches are referred to as *zygapophyseal joints.* Some texts refer to these joints as *interarticular facet joints.*

The movable vertebrae, with the exception of the first and second cervical vertebrae, are similar in general structure. However, each group has certain distinguishing characteristics that must be considered in radiography of the vertebral column.

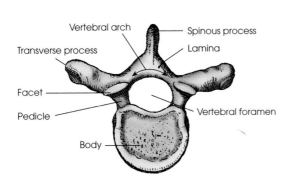

Fig. 8-3 Superior aspect of a thoracic vertebra, showing structures common to all vertebral regions.

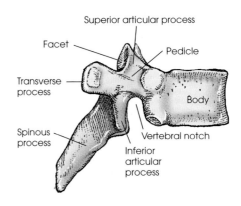

Fig. 8-4 Lateral aspect of a thoracic vertebra, showing structures common to all vertebral regions.

Cervical Vertebrae

The first two cervical vertebrae are atypical in that they are structurally modified to join the skull. The seventh vertebra is slightly modified to join the thoracic spine. Atypical and typical vertebrae are described in the following sections.

ATLAS

The *atlas,* the first cervical vertebra, is a ringlike structure with no body and a very short spinous process (Fig. 8-5). The atlas consists of an *anterior arch,* a *posterior arch,* two *lateral masses,* and two transverse processes. The anterior and posterior arches extend between the lateral masses. The ring formed by the arches is divided into anterior and posterior portions by a ligament called the *transverse atlantal ligament.* The anterior portion of the ring receives the dens (odontoid process) of the axis, and the posterior portion transmits the proximal spinal cord.

The transverse processes of the atlas are longer than those of the other cervical vertebrae, and they project laterally and slightly inferiorly from the lateral masses. Each lateral mass bears a superior and an inferior articular process. The superior processes lie in a horizontal plane, are large and deeply concave, and are shaped to receive the condyles of the occipital bone of the cranium.

AXIS

The *axis,* the second cervical vertebra (Figs. 8-6 and 8-7), has a strong conical process arising from the upper surface of its body. This process, called the *dens* or *odontoid process,* is received into the anterior portion of the atlantal ring to act as the pivot or body for the atlas. At each side of the dens on the superior surface of the vertebral body are the superior articular processes, which are adapted to join with the inferior articular processes of the atlas. These joints, which differ in position and direction from the other cervical zygapophyseal joints, are clearly visualized in an anteroposterior (AP) projection if the patient is properly positioned. The inferior articular processes of the axis have the same direction as those of the succeeding cervical vertebrae. The laminae of the axis are broad and thick. The spinous process is horizontal in position.

SEVENTH VERTEBRA

The seventh cervical vertebra, termed the *vertebra prominens,* has a long, prominent spinous process that projects almost horizontally to the posterior. The spinous process of this vertebra is easily palpable at the posterior base of the neck. It is convenient to use this process as a guide in localizing other vertebrae.

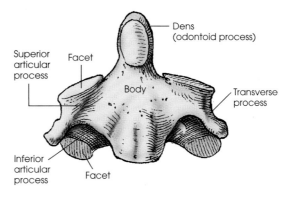

Fig. 8-6 Anterior aspect of axis (C2).

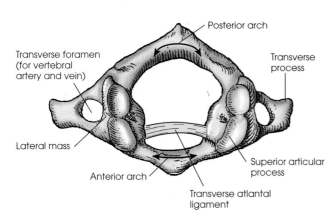

Fig. 8-5 Superior aspect of atlas (C1).

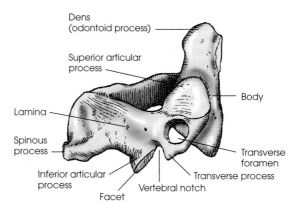

Fig. 8-7 Lateral aspect of axis (C2).

TYPICAL CERVICAL VERTEBRA

The *typical cervical vertebra* has a small, transversely located, oblong body with slightly elongated anteroinferior borders (Figs. 8-8 and 8-9). The result is anteroposterior overlapping of the bodies in the articulated column. The transverse processes of the typical cervical vertebra arise partly from the sides of the body and partly from the vertebral arch. These processes are short and wide, are perforated by the *transverse foramina* for the transmission of the vertebral artery and vein, and present a deep concavity on their upper surfaces for the passage of the spinal nerves. All cervical vertebrae contain three foramina: the right and left transverse foramina and the vertebral foramen.

The pedicles of the typical cervical vertebra project laterally and posteriorly from the body, and their superior and inferior vertebral notches are nearly equal in depth. The laminae are narrow and thin. The spinous processes are short, have bifid tips, and are directed posteriorly and slightly inferiorly. Their palpable tips lie at the level of the interspace below the body of the vertebra from which they arise.

The superior and inferior articular processes are located posterior to the transverse processes at the point where the pedicles and laminae unite. Together the processes form short, thick columns of bone called *articular pillars.* The fibrocartilaginous articulating surfaces of the articular pillars contain facets. The zygapophyseal facet joints of the second through seventh cervical vertebrae lie at right angles to the midsagittal plane and are clearly demonstrated in a lateral projection (Fig. 8-10).

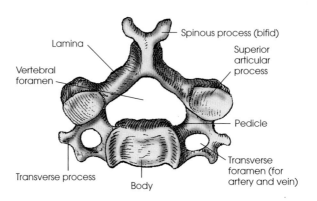

Fig. 8-8 Superior aspect of typical cervical vertebra.

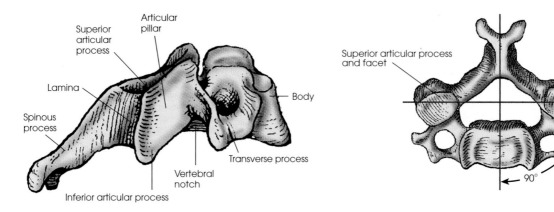

Fig. 8-9 Lateral aspect of typical cervical vertebra.

Fig. 8-10 Direction of cervical zygapophyseal joints.

The intervertebral foramina of the cervical region are directed anteriorly at a 45-degree angle from the midsagittal plane of the body (Figs. 8-11 and 8-12). The foramina are also directed at a 15-degree inferior angle to the horizontal plane of the body. Accurate radiographic demonstration of these foramina requires a 15-degree longitudinal angulation of the central ray and a 45-degree medial rotation of the patient (or a 45-degree medial angulation of the central ray). A lateral projection is necessary to demonstrate the cervical zygapophyseal joints. The positioning rotations required for demonstrating the intervertebral foramina and zygapophyseal joints of the cervical spine are summarized in Table 8-1.

TABLE 8-1

Positioning rotations needed for demonstration of intervertebral foramina and zygapophyseal joints

Area of spine	Intervertebral foramina	Zygapophyseal joint
Cervical spine	45 degrees oblique AP—side up PA—side down	Lateral
Thoracic spine	Lateral	70 degrees* AP—side up PA—side down
Lumbar spine	Lateral	30 to 50 degrees* AP—side down PA—side up

*From the anatomic position.

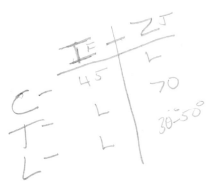

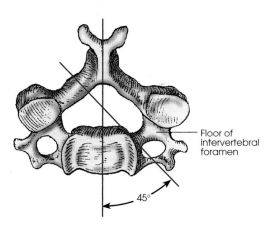

Fig. 8-11 Direction of cervical intervertebral foramina.

Floor of intervertebral foramen

45°

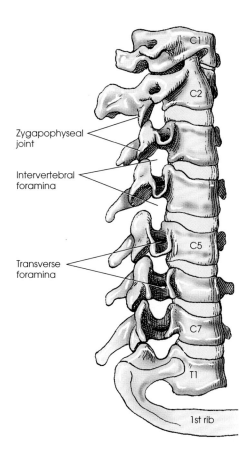

C1
C2
Zygapophyseal joint
Intervertebral foramina
C5
Transverse foramina
C7
T1
1st rib

Fig. 8-12 Anterior oblique of cervical vertebrae, showing intervertebral transverse foramina and zygapophyseal joints.

Thoracic Vertebrae

The bodies of the thoracic vertebrae increase in size from the first to the twelfth vertebrae. They also vary in form, with the superior thoracic bodies resembling cervical bodies and the inferior thoracic bodies resembling lumbar bodies. The bodies of the typical (third through ninth) thoracic vertebrae are approximately triangular in form (Figs. 8-13 and 8-14). These vertebral bodies are deeper posteriorly than anteriorly, and their posterior surface is concave from side to side.

The posterolateral margins of each thoracic body have *costal facets* for articulation with the heads of the ribs (Fig. 8-15). The body of the first thoracic vertebra presents a whole costal facet near its superior border for articulation with the head of the first rib and presents a *demifacet* (half facet) on its inferior border for articulation with the head of the second rib. The

bodies of the second through eighth thoracic vertebrae contain demifacets both superiorly and inferiorly. The ninth thoracic vertebrae has only a superior demifacet. Finally, the tenth, eleventh, and twelfth thoracic vertebral bodies have a single whole facet at the superior margin for articulation with the eleventh and twelfth ribs (Table 8-2).

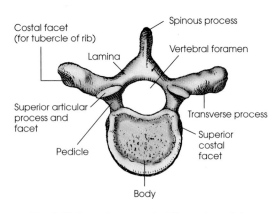

Fig. 8-13 Superior aspect of thoracic vertebra.

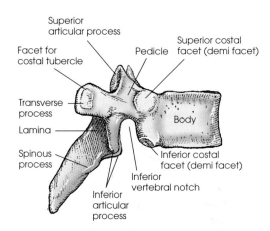

Fig. 8-14 Lateral aspect of thoracic vertebra.

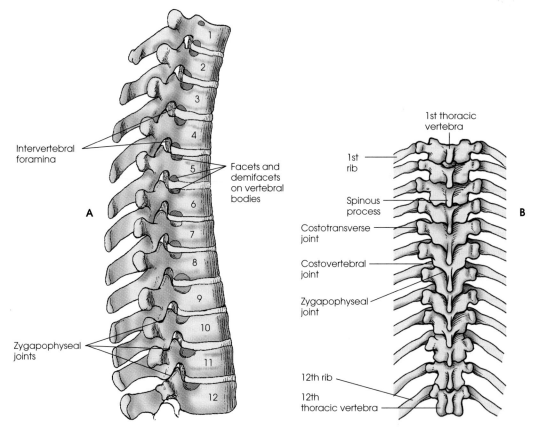

Fig. 8-15 Thoracic spine. **A,** Posterior oblique aspect showing zygapophyseal joints, intervertebral foramina, and facets and demifacets (see Table 18-2). **B,** Posterior aspect showing attachment of ribs and joints.

TABLE 8-2

Costal facets and demifacets

Vertebrae	Vertebral Border	Facet/Demifacet*
T1	Superior	Whole facet
	Inferior	Demifacet
T2-T8	Superior	Demifacet
	Inferior	Demifacet
T9	Superior	Demifacet
	Inferior	None
T10-T12	Superior	Whole facet
	Inferior	None

*On *each side* of a vertebral body.

The transverse processes of the thoracic vertebrae project obliquely, laterally, and posteriorly. With the exception of the eleventh and twelfth pairs, each process has on the anterior surface of its extremity a small concave facet for articulation with the tubercle of a rib. The laminae are broad and thick, and they overlap the subjacent lamina. The spinous processes are long. From the fifth to the ninth vertebrae the spinous process project sharply inferiorly and overlap each other, but they are less vertical above and below this region. The palpable tip of each spinous process of the fifth to ninth thoracic vertebrae corresponds in position to the interspace *below* the vertebra from which it projects.

The zygapophyseal joints of the thoracic region angle (except the inferior articular processes of the twelfth vertebra) anteriorly approximately 15 to 20 degrees to form an angle of 70 to 75 degrees (open anteriorly) to the midsagittal plane of the body (see Figs. 8-15 and 8-16). For radiographic demonstration of the zygapophyseal joints of the thoracic region, the patient's body must be rotated 70 to 75 degrees from the anatomic position or 15 to 20 degrees from the lateral position.

The intervertebral foramina of the thoracic region are perpendicular to the midsagittal plane of the body (see Figs. 8-15 and 8-17). These foramina are clearly demonstrated radiographically with the patient in a true lateral position (see Table 8-1). During inspiration the ribs are elevated. The arms must also be raised enough to elevate the ribs, which otherwise cross the intervertebral foramina.

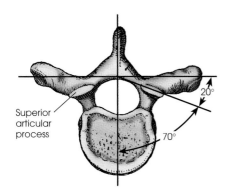

Fig. 8-16 Direction of thoracic zygapophyseal joints.

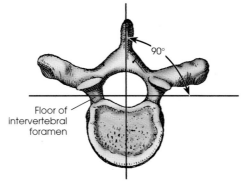

Fig. 8-17 Direction of thoracic intervertebral foramina.

Lumbar Vertebrae

The lumbar vertebrae have large, bean-shaped bodies that increase in size from the first to the fifth vertebra in this region. The lumbar bodies are deeper anteriorly than posteriorly, and their superior and inferior surfaces are flattened or slightly concave (Fig. 8-18). At their posterior surface these vertebrae are flattened anteriorly to posteriorly, and they are transversely concave. The anterior and lateral surfaces are concave from the top to the bottom (Fig. 8-19).

The transverse processes of lumbar vertebrae are smaller than those of the thoracic vertebrae. The superior three pairs are directed almost exactly laterally, whereas the inferior two pairs are inclined slightly superiorly. The lumbar pedicles are strong and are directed posteriorly; the laminae are thick. The spinous processes are large, thick, and blunt, and they have an almost horizontal projection posteriorly. The palpable tip of each spinous process corresponds in position with the interspace below the vertebra from which it projects. The *mamillary process* is a smoothly rounded projection on the back of each superior articular process. The *accessory process* is at the back of the root of the transverse process.

The laminae lie posterior to the pedicles and transverse processes. The part of the lamina between the superior and inferior articular processes is called the *pars interarticularis.*

The body of the fifth lumbar segment is considerably deeper in front than behind, which gives it a wedge shape that adapts it for articulation with the sacrum. The intervertebral disk of this joint is also more wedge shaped than the disks in the interspaces above the lumbar region. The spinous process of the fifth lumbar vertebra is smaller and shorter, and the transverse processes are much thicker than those of the upper lumbar vertebrae.

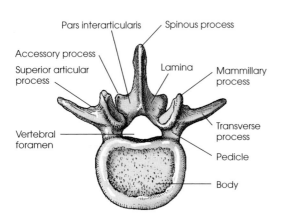

Fig. 8-18 Superior aspect of lumbar vertebra.

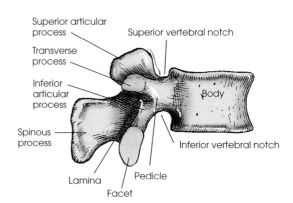

Fig. 8-19 Lateral aspect of lumbar vertebra.

The zygapophyseal joints of the lumbar region (Figs. 8-20 and 8-21) are inclined posteriorly from the coronal plane, forming an angle (open posteriorly) of 30 to 50 degrees to the midsagittal plane of the body. These joints can be demonstrated radiographically by rotating the body from the anatomic position.

The intervertebral foramina of the lumbar region are situated at right angles to the midsagittal plane of the body, except the fifth, which turns slightly anteriorly (Fig. 8-22). The superior four pairs of foramina are demonstrated radiographically with the patient in a true lateral position; the last pair requires slight obliquity of the body (see Table 8-1).

Spondylolysis is an acquired bony defect occurring in the pars interarticularis, the area of the lamina between the two articular processes. The defect may occur on one or both sides of the vertebra, resulting in a condition termed *spondylolisthesis*. This condition is characterized by the anterior displacement of one vertebra over another, generally the fifth lumbar over the sacrum. Spondylolisthesis almost exclusively involves the lumbar spine.

Spondylolisthesis is of radiologic importance because oblique-position radiographs demonstrate the "neck" area of the "Scottie dog" (i.e., the pars interarticularis). (Oblique positions involving the lumbar spine, including the "Scottie dog," are presented later in this chapter, starting with Fig. 8-104.)

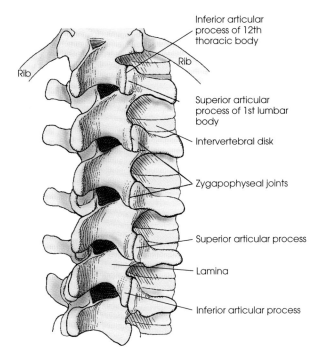

Fig. 8-20 Right posterior oblique view of lumbar vertebrae, showing zygapophyseal joints.

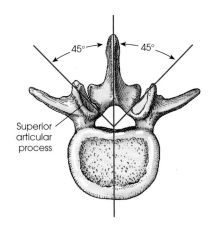

Fig. 8-21 Direction of lumbar zygapophyseal joints.

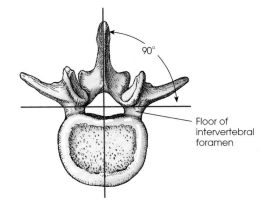

Fig. 8-22 Superior aspect showing direction of lumbar intervertebral foramina.

Sacrum

The *sacrum* is formed by fusion of the five sacral vertebral segments into a curved, triangular bone (Figs. 8-23, 8-24, and 8-25). The sacrum is wedged between the iliac bones of the pelvis, with its broad base directed obliquely, superiorly, and anteriorly and its apex directed posteriorly and inferiorly. Although the size and degree of curvature of the sacrum vary considerably in different patients, the bone is normally longer, narrower, more evenly curved, and more vertical in position in males than in females. The female sacrum is more acutely curved, with its greatest curvature in the lower half of the bone; it also lies in a more oblique plane, which results in a sharper angle at the junction of the lumbar and pelvic curves.

The superior portion of the first sacral segment remains distinct and resembles the vertebrae of the lumbar region (see Fig. 8-25). The superior surface of the *base* of the sacrum corresponds in size and shape to the inferior surface of the last lumbar segment, with which it articulates to form the lumbosacral junction. The concavities on the upper surface of the pedicles of the first sacral segment and the corresponding concavities on the lower surface of the pedicles of the last lumbar segment form the last pair of intervertebral foramina. The *superior articular processes* of the first sacral segment articulate with the inferior articular processes of the last lumbar vertebra to form the last pair of zygapophyseal joints.

At its superior anterior margin the base of the sacrum has a prominent ridge termed the *sacral promontory.* Directly behind the bodies of the sacral segments is the *sacral canal,* which is the continuation of the vertebral canal. The sacral canal is contained within the bone and transmits the sacral nerves. The anterior and posterior walls of the sacral canal are each perforated by four pairs of *pelvic sacral foramina* for the passage of the sacral nerves and blood vessels.

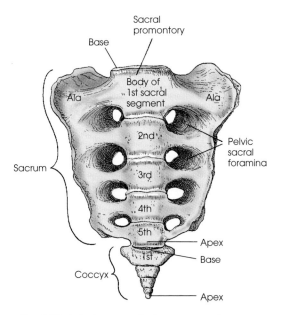

Fig. 8-23 Anterior aspect of sacrum and coccyx.

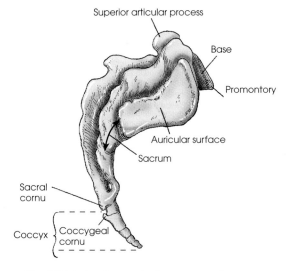

Fig. 8-24 Lateral aspect of sacrum and coccyx.

On each side of the sacral base is a large, winglike lateral mass called the *ala* (Fig. 8-26). At the superoanterior part of the lateral surface of each ala is the *auricular surface,* a large articular process for articulation with similarly shaped processes on the iliac bones of the pelvis.

The inferior surface of the *apex* of the sacrum (Fig. 8-27) has an oval facet for articulation with the coccyx and the *sacral cornua,* two processes that project inferiorly from the posterolateral aspect of the last sacral segment to join the *coccygeal cornua.*

Coccyx

The *coccyx* is composed of three to five (usually four) rudimentary *vertebrae* that have a tendency to fuse into one bone in the adult (see Figs. 8-23 and 8-24). The coccyx diminishes in size from its *base* inferiorly to its *apex.* From its articulation with the sacrum it curves inferiorly and anteriorly, often deviating from the midline of the body. The *coccygeal cornua* project superiorly from the posterolateral aspect of the first coccygeal segment to join the sacral cornua.

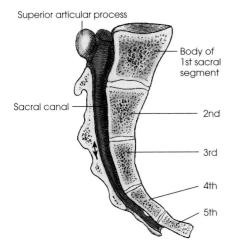

Fig. 8-25 Sagittal section of sacrum.

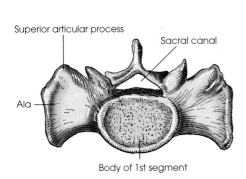

Fig. 8-26 Base of sacrum.

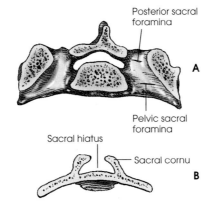

Fig. 8-27 Transverse sections of sacrum.
A, Section through superior sacral portion.
B, Section through inferior sacral portion.

Vertebral Articulations

The joints of the vertebral column are summarized in Table 8-3. A detailed description follows.

The vertebral articulations consist of two types of joints: (1) *intervertebral* joints, which are between the two vertebral bodies and are *cartilaginous-symphysis* joints that permit only slight movement of individual vertebrae but considerable motility for the column as a whole, and (2) *zygapophyseal* joints, which are between the articulation processes of the vertebral arches and are *synovial gliding* joints that permit free movements. The movements permitted in the vertebral column by the combined action of the joints are flexion, extension, lateral flexion, and rotation.

The articulations between the atlas and the occipital bone are *synovial ellipsoidal* joints and are called the *atlanto-occipital* articulations. The anterior arch of the atlas rotates about the dens of the axis to form the *atlantoaxial* joint, which is both a synovial gliding articulation and a *synovial pivot* articulation (see Table 8-3).

In the thoracic region, the heads of the ribs articulate with the bodies of the vertebrae to form the *costovertebral* joints, which are synovial gliding articulations. The tubercles of the ribs and the transverse processes of the thoracic vertebrae articulate to form *costotransverse* joints, which are also synovial gliding articulations.

The articulations between the sacrum and the two ilia—the *sacroiliac* joints—were discussed in Chapter 7.

TABLE 8-3

Joints of the vertebral column

| Joint | Structural classification | | Movement |
	Tissue	Type	
Atlanto-occipital	Synovial	Ellipsoidal	Freely movable
Atlantoaxial			
Lateral (2)	Synovial	Gliding	Freely movable
Medial (1-dens)	Synovial	Pivot	Freely movable
Intervertebral	Cartilaginous	Symphysis	Slightly movable
Zygapophyseal	Synovial	Gliding	Freely movable
Costovertebral	Synovial	Gliding	Freely movable
Costotransverse	Synovial	Gliding	Freely movable

Vertebral column (spine)
vertebrae (24)
  cervical (7)
  thoracic (12)
  lumbar (5)
  sacral
  coccygeal
true vertebrae
false vertebrae
sacrum
coccyx

Vertebral curvature
curves
  cervical
  thoracic
  lumbar
  pelvic
lordotic curve
kyphotic curve
lumbosacral angle
primary curves
secondary or
  compensatory curves

Typical vertebra
body
vertebral arch
vertebral foramen
vertebral canal
articular cartilage plate
intervertebral disks
nucleus pulposus
annulus fibrosus
pedicles
vertebral notches
intervertebral foramina
laminae
transverse processes
spinous process
facets
superior articular
  processes
inferior articular
  processes
zygapophyseal joints
  (interarticular facet
  joints)

Cervical vertebrae
atlas (first)
  anterior arch
  posterior arch
  lateral masses
  transverse atlantal
    ligament
axis (second)
  dens (odontoid
    process)
cervical (seventh)
  vertebra prominens
typical cervical vertebra
  transverse foramina
  articular pillars

Thoracic vertebrae
costal facets
demifacets

Lumbar vertebrae
mammillary process
accessory process
pars interarticularis

Sacrum
base
superior articular
  processes
sacral promontory
sacral canal
pelvic sacral foramina
ala
auricular surface
apex
sacral cornua

Coccyx
base
apex
coccygeal cornua

Vertebral articulations
atlanto-occipital
atlantoaxial
  lateral (2)
  medial (1-dens)
costovertebral
costotransverse
intervertebral
zygapophyseal

*See *Addendum* at the end of the volume for a summary of the changes in the anatomic terms used in this edition.

Vertebral articulations

Radiation Protection

The radiographer has a professional responsibility to protect patients from unnecessary radiation (see Chapter 1 for specific guidelines). In this chapter the *Shield gonads* statement at the end of the *Position of part* sections indicates that the patient is to be protected from unnecessary radiation by restricting the radiation beam through proper collimation. The placement of lead shielding between the gonads and the radiation source is also appropriate when the clinical objectives of the examination are not compromised.

For any procedure discussed in this chapter, contact gonad shields can be used to protect male patients. Female gonad shields can only be used when the ovaries do not lie within the area of interest.

AP OBLIQUE PROJECTION
R and L head rotations

Image receptor: 8 × 10 inch (18 × 24 cm)

Position of patient
- Place the patient in the supine position.
- Center the midsagittal plane of the body to the midline of the grid, and adjust the shoulders to lie in the same horizontal plane.
- Place a support under the patient's knees for comfort.

Position of part
- Place the cassette in the Bucky tray, and adjust the patient's head so that the midpoint of the cassette is 1 inch (2.5 cm) lateral to the midsagittal plane of the head at the level of the external acoustic meatus (EAM).
- Rotate the head 45 to 60 degrees *away* from the side being examined (Fig. 8-28).
- Adjust the flexion of the neck to place the infraorbitomeatal line (IOML) perpendicular to the cassette.
- *Shield gonads.*
- *Respiration:* Suspend.

Central ray
- Perpendicular to the midpoint of the cassette. It enters 1 inch (2.5 cm) anterior to the EAM and emerges at the atlanto-occipital articulation.

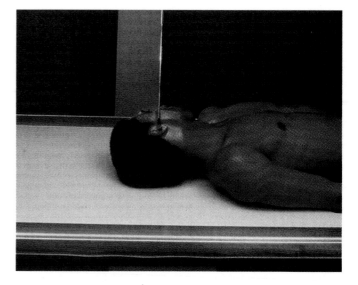

Fig. 8-28 AP oblique atlanto-occipital joint.

Structures shown

The resulting image shows an AP oblique projection of the atlanto-occipital articulation, with the joint being shown between the orbit and the ramus of the mandible. Both sides should be examined for comparison (Fig. 8-29).

The dens of the axis is also well demonstrated in this position. Therefore it can be used for this purpose when a patient cannot be adjusted in the open-mouth position.

The following should be clearly demonstrated:

■ Open atlanto-occipital articulation
■ Dens

NOTE: Buetti[1] recommended a position for the atlanto-occipital articulations wherein the head is turned 45 to 50 degrees to one side and, with the mouth wide open, the chin is drawn down as much as the open mouth allows. The central ray is then directed vertically through the open mouth to the dependent mastoid tip.

---

[1]Buetti C: Zur Darstellung der Atlanto-Epistropheal-Gelenke bzw. der Procc. ransversi atlantis und epistrophei, *Radiol Clin North Am* 20:168, 1951.

Mastoid air cells   External acoustic meatus   Atlanto-occipital articulation   Dens

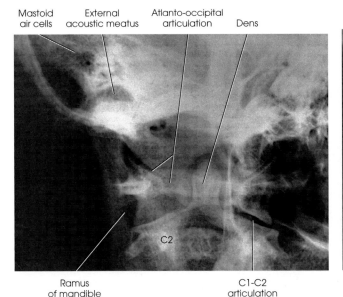
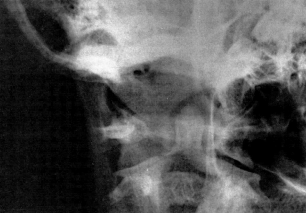

C2

Ramus of mandible

C1-C2 articulation

Fig. 8-29 AP oblique atlanto-occipital joint.

Atlanto-Occipital Articulations

PA PROJECTION

Image receptor: 8 × 10 inch (18 × 24 cm) crosswise

Position of patient

- Place the patient in the prone position.
- Center the midsagittal plane of the body to the midline of the grid.
- If the patient is thin, place a small, firm pillow under the chest to relieve strain in holding the position.
- Flex the patient's elbows, place the arms in a comfortable position, and adjust the shoulders to lie in the same horizontal plane.

Position of part

- Rest the patient's forehead and nose on the table, and adjust the head so that the midsagittal plane is perpendicular to the midline of the grid (Fig. 8-30).
- Adjust the flexion of the neck to place the orbitomeatal line (OML) perpendicular to the plane of the cassette; center the cassette at or slightly below the level of the infraorbital margins.
- *Shield gonads.*
- *Respiration:* Suspend.

Central ray

- Perpendicular to the midpoint of the cassette. It enters the back of the neck on the midsagittal plane and exits at the level of the infraorbital margins.

Structures shown

The resulting image shows a PA projection of the atlanto-occipital joints projected through the maxillary sinuses (Fig. 8-31).

EVALUATION CRITERIA

The following should be clearly demonstrated:

- Open bilateral atlanto-occipital articulations
- Mandibular condyles equidistant from the midline

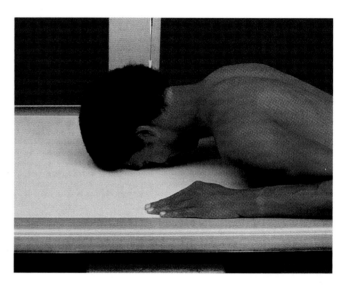

Fig. 8-30 PA atlanto-occipital articulations.

Mastoid air cells   Air-filled maxillary sinus   Roof of orbit   Atlanto-occipital joints

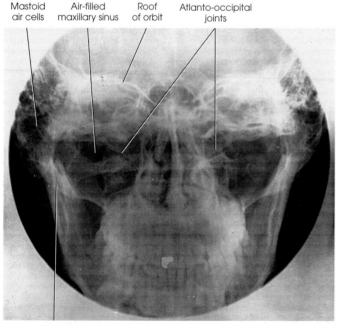
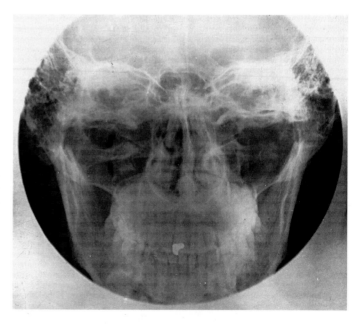

Mandibular ramus

Fig. 8-31 PA atlanto-occipital articulations.

♠ AP PROJECTION
FUCHS METHOD

Fuchs[1] has recommended the AP projection for demonstration of the dens when its upper half is not clearly shown in the open-mouth position. This patient position must not be attempted if fracture or degenerative disease of the upper cervical region is suspected.

Image receptor: 8 × 10 inch (18 × 24 cm) crosswise

Position of patient

• Place the patient in the supine position.
• Center the midsagittal plane of the body to the midline of the grid.
• Place the arms along the sides of the body, and adjust the shoulders to lie in the same horizontal plane.
• Place a support under the patient's knees for comfort.

Position of part

• Place the cassette in the Bucky tray, and center the cassette to the level of the tips of the mastoid processes.
• Extend the chin until the tip of the chin and the tip of the mastoid process are vertical (Fig. 8-32).
• Adjust the head so that the midsagittal plane is perpendicular to the plane of the grid.
• *Shield gonads.*
• *Respiration:* Suspend.

---

[1]Fuch AW: Cervical vertebrae (part 1), *Radiogr Clin Photogr* 16:2, 1940.

Central ray

• Perpendicular to the midpoint of the cassette; it enters the neck on the midsagittal plane just distal to the tip of the chin.

Structures shown

The resulting image shows an AP projection of the dens lying within the circular foramen magnum (Fig. 8-33).

EVALUATION CRITERIA

The following should be clearly demonstrated:

■ Entire dens within the foramen magnum
■ Symmetry of the mandible, cranium, and vertebrae, indicating no rotation of the head or neck

Smith and Abel[1] described a method for demonstrating the laminae and articular facets of the upper cervical vertebrae. They slightly extend the patient's neck, and the mouth is opened wide. The central ray is directed 35 degrees caudad and centered to C3. The exposure is made with the head passively rotated 10 degrees to the side, thereby removing the mandible from the overlying areas of interest.

---

[1]Smith G, Abel M: Visualization of the posterolateral elements of the upper cervical vertebrae in the anteroposterior projection, *Radiology* 115:219, 1975.

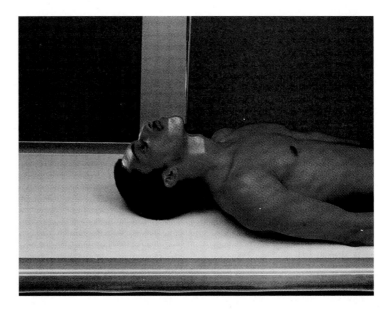

Fig. 8-32 AP dens: Fuchs method.

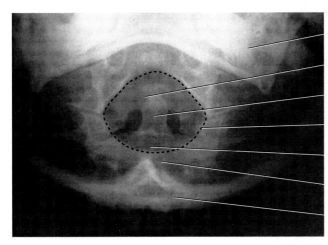

Mandible

Anterior arch of atlas

Dens

Foramen magnum

Body of axis

Posterior arch of atlas

Occipital bone

Fig. 8-33 AP dens: Fuchs method.

▲ AP PROJECTION
Open mouth

The open-mouth technique was described by Albers-Schönberg[1] in 1910 and by George[2] in 1919.

Image receptor: 8 × 10 inch (18 × 24 cm)

Position of patient

- Place the patient in the supine position.
- Center the midsagittal plane of the body to the midline of the grid.
- Place the patient's arms along the sides of the body, and adjust the shoulders to lie in the same horizontal plane.
- Place a support under the patient's knees for comfort.

---

[1]Albers-Schönberg HE: *Die Röntgentechnik,* ed 3, Hamburg, 1910, Gräfe & Sillem.
[2]George AW: Method for more accurate study of injuries to the atlas and axis, *Boston Med Surg J* 181:395, 1919.

Position of part

- Place the cassette in the Bucky tray, and center the cassette at the level of the axis.
- Adjust the patient's head so that the midsagittal plane is perpendicular to the plane of the table (Figs. 8-34 and 8-35).
- Select the exposure factors, and move the x-ray tube into position so that any minor change can be made quickly after the final adjustment of the patient's head. Although this position is not easy to hold, the patient is usually able to co-operate fully unless he or she is kept in the final, strained position too long.
- Have the patient open the mouth as wide as possible, and then adjust the head so that a line from the lower edge of the upper incisors to the tip of the mastoid process is perpendicular to the cassette. A small support under the back of the head may be needed to facilitate opening of the mouth while proper alignment of the upper incisors and mastoid tips is maintained.
- *Shield gonads.*
- *Respiration:* Instruct the patient to keep the mouth wide open and to softly phonate "ah" during the exposure. This will place the tongue in the floor of the mouth so that it is not projected on the atlas and axis and will prevent movement of the mandible.

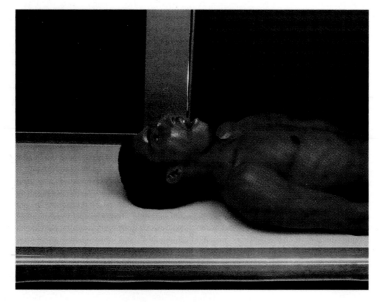

Fig. 8-34 AP atlas and axis.

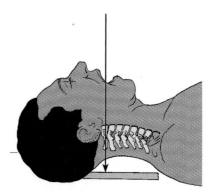

Fig. 8-35 Open-mouth spine alignment.

Atlas and Axis

Central ray
- Perpendicular to the center of the cassette and entering the midpoint of the open mouth

Structures shown

The resulting image demonstrates an AP projection of the atlas and axis through the open mouth (Fig. 8-36).

If the patient has a deep head or a long mandible, the entire atlas is not demonstrated. When the exactly superimposed shadows of the occlusal surface of the upper central incisors and the base of the skull are in line with those of the tips of the mastoid processes, the position cannot be improved.

If the patient cannot open the mouth, tomography may be required (Fig. 8-37).

The following should be clearly demonstrated:
- Dens, atlas, axis, and articulations between the first and second cervical vertebrae
- Entire articular surfaces of the atlas and axis (to check for lateral displacement)
- Superimposed occlusal surface of the upper central incisors and the base of the skull
- Wide-open mouth
- Shadow of the tongue not projected over the atlas and axis
- Mandibular rami equidistant from dens

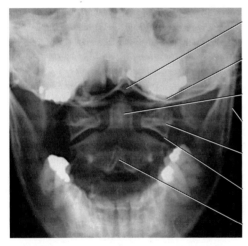

Occipital base

Occlusal surface of teeth

Dens (odontoid process)

Mandibular ramus

Lateral mass of atlas

Inferior articular process of atlas

Spinous process of axis

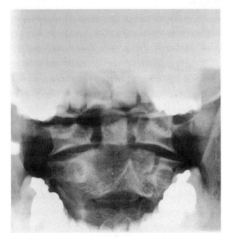

Fig. 8-36 A, Open-mouth atlas and axis.
B, Same projection, showing fracture of the left lateral mass of axis (*arrow*).

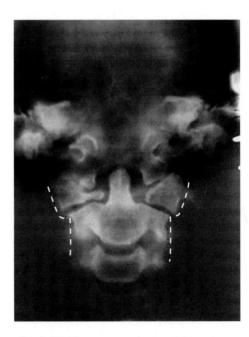

Fig. 8-37 AP upper cervical vertebrae tomogram of a patient who fell and landed on his head. A bursting-type Jefferson fracture caused outward displacement of both lateral masses of the atlas. A tomogram is often necessary to demonstrate the upper cervical area in trauma patients who cannot move their heads or open their mouths.

PA PROJECTION
JUDD METHOD

NOTE: The radiographer must not attempt this position with a patient who has an unhealed fracture or who has a degenerative disease or suspected fracture of the upper cervical region.

Image receptor: 8 × 10 inch (18 × 24 cm) crosswise

Position of patient
- Place the patient in the prone position.
- Center the midsagittal plane of the body to the midline of the grid.
- Flex the patient's elbows, place the arms in a comfortable position, and adjust the shoulders to lie in the same horizontal plane.

Position of part
- Have the patient extend the neck and rest the chin on the table.
- Place the cassette in the Bucky tray, and adjust the cassette so that the midpoint is centered to the throat at the level of the upper margin of the thyroid cartilage (Fig. 8-38).
- Adjust the head so that the chin and mastoid tips are vertical or the OML is approximately 37 degrees to the plane of the cassette (Fig. 8-39).
- Adjust the midsagittal plane to be perpendicular to the table.
- *Shield gonads.*
- *Respiration:* Suspend.

Central ray
- Perpendicular to the midpoint of the cassette. It enters on the midsagittal plane just distal to the level of the mastoid tips.

Structures shown
The resulting image demonstrates a PA projection of the dens and atlas as seen through the foramen magnum (Fig. 8-40).

EVALUATION CRITERIA
The following should be clearly demonstrated:
- Entire dens within foramen magnum
- Anterior and posterior arches of atlas
- No rotation of head or neck

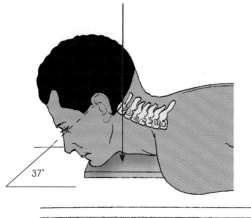

Fig. 8-38 PA atlas and dens: Judd method.

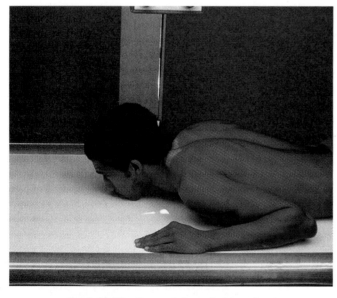

Fig. 8-39 PA dens.

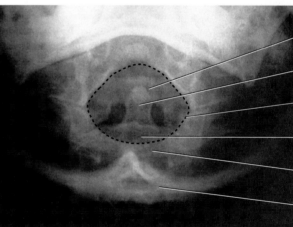

Anterior arch of atlas

Dens (odontoid process)

Foramen magnum

Body of axis

Posterior arch of atlas

Occipital bone

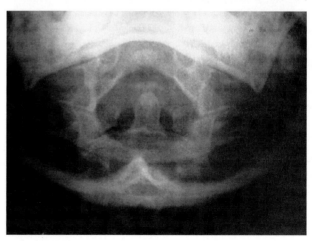

Fig. 8-40 PA atlas and dens: Judd method.

Dens

AP AXIAL OBLIQUE PROJECTION
KASABACH METHOD
R or L head rotations

NOTE: The head of a patient who has a possible fracture or degenerative disease must *not* be rotated. Kasabach[1] recommended that the entire body, rather than only the head, be rotated.

Image receptor: 8 × 10 inch (18 × 24 cm)

Position of patient
- Place the patient in the supine position.
- Center the midsagittal plane of the body to the midline of the grid.
- Place the arms along the sides of the body, and adjust the shoulders to lie in the same horizontal plane.
- Place a support under the patient's knees for comfort.

Position of part
- Place the cassette in the Bucky tray, and center the cassette to the midsagittal plane at the level of the mastoid tip.
- Rotate the head either right or left approximately 40 to 45 degrees. Adjust the head so that the IOML is perpendicular to the plane of the table (Fig. 8-41).
- For right-angle images of the dens, make one exposure with the head turned to the right and one exposure with the head turned to the left.
- *Shield gonads.*
- *Respiration:* Suspend.

Central ray
- Angled 10 to 15 degrees caudad. Center to a point midway between the outer canthus and the EAM.

Structures shown
The resulting image shows an AP axial oblique projection of the dens and was recommended by Kasabach[1] for use in conjunction with the AP and lateral projections (Fig. 8-42).

[1]Kasabach HH: A roentgenographic method for the study of the second cervical vertebra, *AJR* 42:782, 1939.

NOTE: Herrmann and Stender[1] described a position for demonstrating the atlanto-occipital–dens relationship: the head is adjusted as for the Kasabach method, and the central ray is then directed vertically midway between the mastoid processes at the level of the atlanto-occipital joints.

[1]Herrmann E, Stender H: Ein einfache Aufnahmetechnik zur Darstellung der Dens Axis, *Fortschr Roentgenstr* 96:115, 1962.

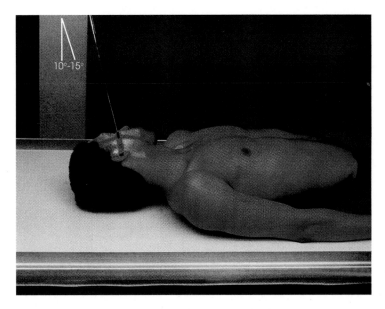

Fig. 8-41 AP axial oblique dens: Kasabach method.

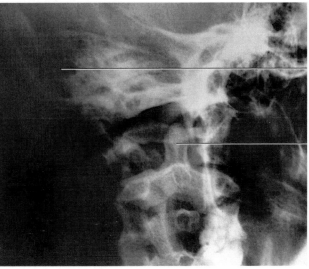

Mastoid air cells (side up)

Dens

Fig. 8-42 AP axial oblique dens: Kasabach method.

LATERAL PROJECTION
R or L position

Image receptor: 8 × 10 inch (18 × 24 cm)

Position of patient
- Place the patient in the supine position.
- Place the arms along the sides of the body, and adjust the shoulders to lie in the same horizontal plane.
- Place a sponge or pad under the patient's head unless traumatic injury has been sustained, in which case the neck should not be moved.

Position of part
- With the cassette in the vertical position and in contact with the upper neck, center it at the level of the atlantoaxial articulation (1 inch [2.5 cm] distal to the tip of the mastoid process).
- Adjust the cassette so that it is parallel with the midsagittal plane of the neck, and then support the cassette in position (Fig. 8-43).
- Extend the neck slightly so that the shadow of the mandibular rami does not overlap that of the spine.
- Adjust the head so that the midsagittal plane is perpendicular to the table.
- *Shield gonads.*
- *Respiration:* Suspend.

Central ray
- Perpendicular to a point 1 inch (2.5 cm) distal to the adjacent mastoid tip. A grid and close collimation should be used to minimize secondary radiation.

Structures shown
The resulting image demonstrates a lateral projection of the atlas and axis. The atlanto-occipital articulations are also demonstrated (Fig. 8-44). Because of the short *object-to-image receptor distance (OID)*, better definition is obtained with this technique than with the customary method of performing the lateral examination of the cervical vertebrae using a 72-inch (183-cm) *source-to-image receptor distance (SID).*

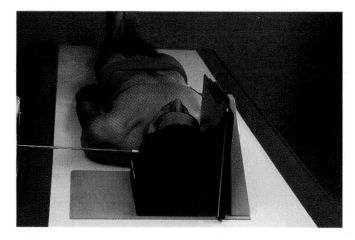

Fig. 8-43 Lateral atlas and axis.

EVALUATION CRITERIA

The following should be clearly demonstrated:

- Upper cervical vertebrae
- Superimposed laminae of the axis and superimposed posterior arches of the atlas
- Neck extended so the mandibular rami does not overlap the axis or atlas
- Nearly superimposed rami of the mandible

NOTE: Pancoast, Pendergrass, and Schaeffer[1] recommended that the head be rotated slightly to prevent superimposition of the laminae of the atlas. They further recommended a slight horizontal tilt of the head for demonstration of the arches of the atlas.

[1]Pancoast HK, Pendergrass EP, Schaeffer JP: *The head and neck in roentgen diagnosis,* Springfield, Ill, 1940, Charles C Thomas.

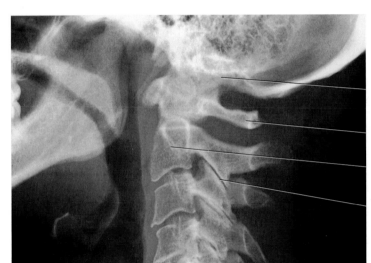

Atlantooccipital articulation

Posterior arch atlas

Body of axis

Zygapophyseal joint

A

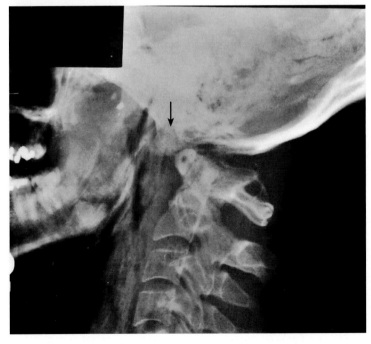

B

Fig. 8-44 A, Lateral atlas and axis. **B,** Lateral atlas and axis on a patient involved in a snowmobile accident. Complete anterior dislocation of the cranium on the atlas narrowed the foramen magnum, causing sudden death. *Arrow* points to the occipital condyle.

AP AXIAL PROJECTION

Image receptor: 8 × 10 inch (18 × 24 cm) lengthwise

Position of patient
- Place the patient in the supine or upright position with the back against the cassette holder.
- Adjust the patient's shoulders to lie in the same horizontal plane to prevent rotation.

Position of part
- Center the midsagittal plane of the patient's body to the midline of the table or vertical grid device.
- Extend the chin enough so that a line from the upper occlusal plane to the mastoid tips is perpendicular to the tabletop. This prevents superimposition of the mandible and midcervical vertebrae (Figs. 8-45 and 8-46).
- Center the cassette at the level of C4.
- Adjust the head so that the midsagittal plane is in straight alignment and perpendicular to the cassette.
- Provide support for the head of any patient who has a pronounced lordotic curvature. This support helps compensate for the curvature and reduce image distortion.
- *Shield gonads.*
- *Respiration:* Suspend.

Central ray
- Directed through C4 at an angle of 15 to 20 degrees cephalad. The central ray enters at or slightly inferior to the most prominent point of the thyroid cartilage.

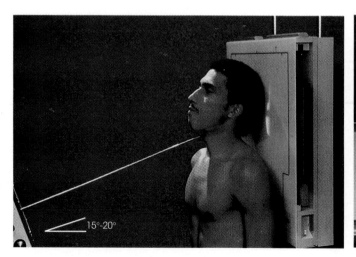

Fig. 8-45 AP axial cervical vertebrae: upright.

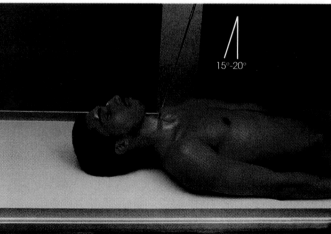

Fig. 8-46 AP axial cervical vertebrae: recumbent.

Cervical Vertebrae

Structures shown

The resulting image shows the lower five cervical bodies and the upper two or three thoracic bodies, the interpediculate spaces, the superimposed transverse and articular processes, and the intervertebral disk spaces (Fig. 8-47).

This projection is also used to demonstrate the presence or absence of cervical ribs.

EVALUATION CRITERIA

The following should be clearly demonstrated:

- Area from C3 to the axis and surrounding soft tissue
- Shadows of the mandible and occiput superimposed over the atlas and most of the axis
- Open intervertebral disk spaces
- Spinous processes equidistant to the pedicles
- Mandibular angles equidistant to the vertebrae

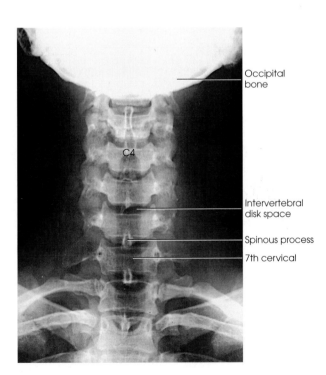
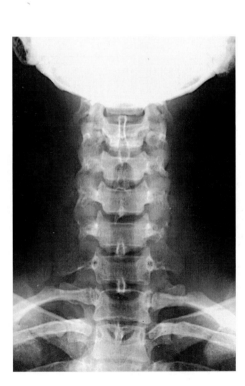

Occipital bone

C4

Intervertebral disk space

Spinous process

7th cervical

Fig. 8-47 AP axial cervical vertebrae.

♠ LATERAL PROJECTION
GRANDY METHOD[1]
R or L position

Image receptor: 8 × 10 inch (18 × 24 cm) lengthwise

SID: A 60- to 72-inch (152- to 183-cm) SID is recommended because of the increased OID. A longer distance helps demonstrate C7.

Position of patient
- Place the patient in a lateral position, either seated or standing, before a vertical grid device.
- Have the patient sit or stand straight, and adjust the height of the cassette so that it is centered at the level of C4.

[1]Grandy CC: A new method for making radiographs of the cervical vertebrae in the lateral position, *Radiology* 4:128, 1925.

Position of part
- Center the coronal plane that passes through the mastoid tips to the midline of the cassette.
- Move the patient close enough to the vertical grid device to permit the adjacent shoulder to rest against the device for support (Fig. 8-48). This projection may be performed without the use of a grid.
- Rotate the shoulders anteriorly or posteriorly according to the natural kyphosis of the back: if the patient is round shouldered, rotate the shoulder anteriorly; otherwise, rotate them posteriorly.
- Adjust the shoulders to lie in the same horizontal plane, depress them as much as possible, and immobilize them by attaching one small sandbag to each *wrist*. The sandbags should be of equal weight.
- Alternatively, place a long strip of gauze bandage under the patient's feet or, if the patient is seated, under the rungs of the stool. Have the patient grasp one end of the gauze in each hand and pull. This allows depression of the shoulders, according to the needs of the radiographer.

- Be careful to ensure that the patient does not elevate the shoulder.
- Adjust the patient's body in a true lateral position with the long axis of the cervical vertebrae parallel to the plane of the cassette.
- Elevate the chin slightly, or have the patient protrude the mandible to prevent superimposition of the mandibular rami and the spine. At the same time and with the midsagittal plane of the head vertical, ask the patient to look steadily at one spot on the wall. This helps maintain the position of the head.
- *Shield gonads.*
- *Respiration:* Suspend respiration at the end of full expiration to obtain maximum depression of the shoulders.

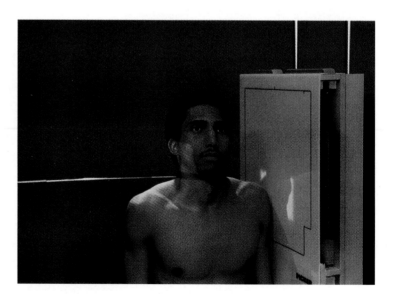

Fig. 8-48 Lateral cervical vertebrae: Grandy method.

Central ray

- Horizontal and perpendicular to C4. With such centering, the magnified outline of the shoulder *farthest* from the cassette is be projected below the lower cervical vertebrae.

Structures shown

The resulting image demonstrates a lateral projection of the cervical bodies and their interspaces, the articular pillars, the lower five zygapophyseal joints, and the spinous processes (Fig. 8-49). Depending on how well the shoulders can be depressed, a good lateral projection must include C7; sometimes T1 and T2 can also be seen.

EVALUATION CRITERIA

The following should be clearly demonstrated:

- All seven cervical vertebrae and at least one third of the T1. (Otherwise a separate radiograph of the cervicothoracic region is recommended.)
- Neck extended so that mandibular rami are not overlapping the atlas or axis.
- Superimposed or nearly superimposed rami of the mandible.
- No rotation or tilt of the cervical spine indicated by superimposed open zygapophyseal joints. The foramina should appear uniform in size and contour.
- C4 in the center of the radiograph.
- Bone and soft tissue detail.

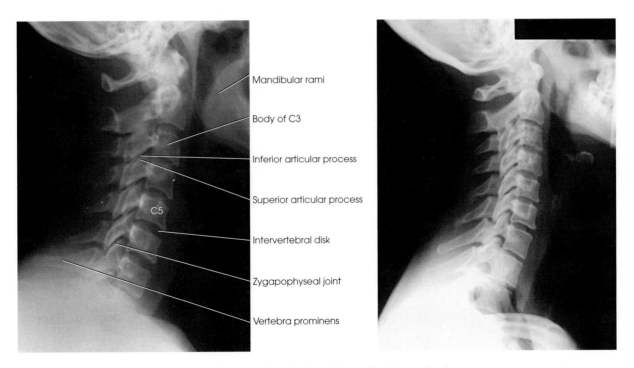

Mandibular rami

Body of C3

Inferior articular process

Superior articular process

C5

Intervertebral disk

Zygapophyseal joint

Vertebra prominens

Fig. 8-49 Lateral cervical vertebrae: Grandy method.

▲ LATERAL PROJECTION
R or L position
Hyperflexion and hyperextension

NOTE: This procedure must not be attempted until cervical spine pathology or fracture has been ruled out.

Functional studies of the cervical vertebrae in the lateral position are performed to demonstrate normal anteroposterior movement or an absence of movement resulting from trauma or disease. The spinous processes are elevated and widely separated in the hyperflexion position and are depressed in close approximation in the hyperextension position.

Image receptor: 24 × 30 cm (10 × 12 inch) lengthwise

SID: A 60- to 72-inch (152- to 183-cm) SID is recommended because of the increased OID. A longer distance helps demonstrate C7.

Position of patient
- Place the patient in a lateral position, either seated or standing, before a vertical grid device.
- Have the patient sit or stand straight, and adjust the height of the cassette so that it is centered at the level of C4.

Position of part
- Move the patient close enough to the vertical grid device to permit the adjacent shoulder to rest against the grid for support.
- Keep the midsagittal plane of the patient's head and neck parallel with the plane of the cassette.
- Alternatively, perform the projection without using a grid.

Hyperflexion
- Ask the patient to drop the head forward and then draw the chin as close as possible to the chest so that the cervical vertebrae are placed in a position of *hyperflexion* (forced flexion) for the first exposure (Fig. 8-50).

Hyperextension
- Ask the patient to elevate the chin as much as possible so that the cervical vertebrae are placed in a position of *hyperextension* (forced extension) for the second exposure (Fig. 8-51).
- *Shield gonads.*
- *Respiration:* Suspend.

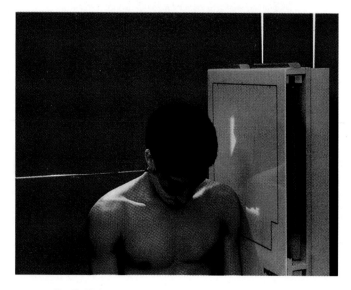

Fig. 8-50 Lateral cervical vertebrae: hyperflexion.

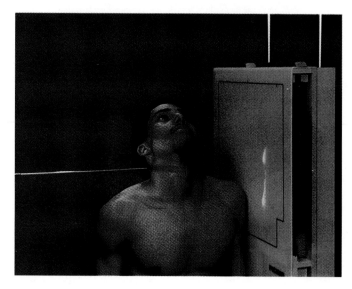

Fig. 8-51 Lateral cervical vertebrae: hyperextension.

Central ray

• Horizontal and perpendicular to C4

Structures shown

The resulting images show the motility of the cervical spine when hyperflexed (Fig. 8-52) and hyperextended (Fig. 8-53). The intervertebral disks and the zygapophyseal joints are also shown.

The following should be clearly demonstrated:

Hyperflexion
■ Body of the mandible almost vertical for hyperflexion in the normal patient
■ All seven spinous processes

Hyperextension
■ Body of the mandible almost horizontal in the normal patient
■ All seven cervical vertebrae in true lateral position

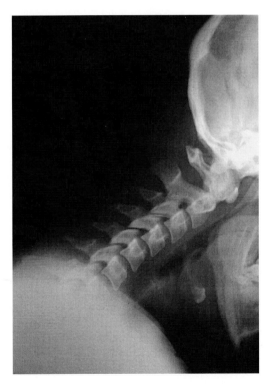

Fig. 8-52 Hyperflexion lateral cervical spine.

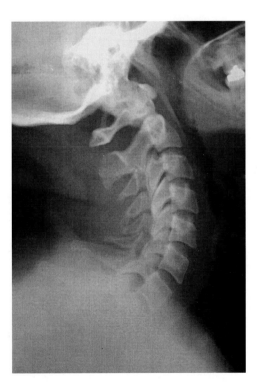

Fig. 8-53 Hyperextension lateral cervical spine.

⚜ AP AXIAL OBLIQUE PROJECTION
RPO and LPO positions

Oblique projections for demonstrating the cervical intervertebral foramina were first described by Barsóny and Koppenstein.[1,2] Both sides are examined for comparison.

[1]Barsóny T, Koppenstein E: Eine neue Method zur Röntgenuntersuchung der Halswirbelsäule, *Fortschr Roentgenstr* 35:593, 1926.
[2]Barsóny T, Koppenstein E: Beitrag zur Aufnahmetechnik der Halswirbelsäule; Darstellung der Foramina intervertebralia, *Röntgenpraxis* 1:245, 1929.

Image receptor: 8 × 10 inch (18 × 24 cm) lengthwise

SID: A 60- to 72-inch (152 to 183-cm) SID is recommended because of the increased OID.

Position of patient
- Place the patient in a supine or upright position facing the x-ray tube. The upright position (standing or seated) is preferable for the patient's comfort and makes it easier to position the patient.

Position of part
- Adjust the body (including the head) at a 45-degree angle, and center the cervical spine to the midline of the cassette.
- Center the cassette to the third cervical body (1 inch [2.5 cm] superior to the most prominent point of the thyroid cartilage) to compensate for the cephalic angulation of the central ray.

Upright position
- Ask the patient to sit or stand straight without strain and to rest the adjacent shoulder firmly against the vertical grid device for support.
- Ensure that the degree of body rotation is 45 degrees.
- While the patient looks straight ahead, elevate and, if needed, protrude the chin so that the mandible does not overlap the spine (Fig. 8-54). Turning the chin to the side causes slight rotation of the superior vertebrae and should be avoided.

Semisupine position
- Rotate the patient's head and body approximately 45 degrees.
- Center the cervical spine to the midline of the grid.
- Place suitable supports under the lower thorax and the elevated hip.
- Place a support under the patient's head, and adjust it so that the cervical column is horizontal.
- Check and adjust the 45-degree body rotation.
- Elevate the patient's chin and protrude the jaw as for the upright study (Fig. 8-55). Turning the chin to the side causes slight rotation of the superior vertebrae and should be avoided.
- *Shield gonads.*
- *Respiration:* Suspend.

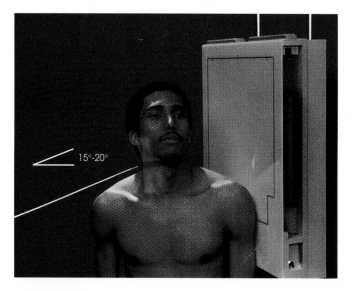

Fig. 8-54 Upright AP axial oblique right intervertebral foramina: LPO position.

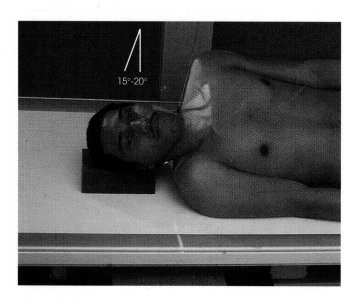

Fig. 8-55 Recumbent AP axial oblique left intervertebral foramina: RPO position.

Central ray

- Directed to C4 at a cephalad angle of 15 to 20 degrees so that the central ray coincides with the angle of the foramina

Structures shown

The resulting image shows the intervertebral foramina and pedicles *farthest* from the cassette and an oblique projection of the bodies and other parts of the cervical vertebrae (Fig. 8-56).

EVALUATION CRITERIA

The following should be clearly demonstrated:

- Open intervertebral foramina *farthest* from the cassette, from C2-C3 to C7-T1
- Open intervertebral disk spaces
- Uniform size and contour of the foramina
- Elevated chin that does not overlap the atlas and axis
- Occipital bone not overlapping the axis
- C1-C7 and T1

AP OBLIQUE PROJECTION
Hyperflexion and hyperextension

Boylston[1] suggested using functional studies of the cervical vertebrae in the oblique to demonstrate fractures of the articular processes as well as obscure dislocations and subluxations. When acute injury has been sustained, manipulation of the patient's head must be performed by a physician.

The patient is placed in a direct frontal body position facing the x-ray tube, with the shoulders held firmly against the grid device. The head is carefully rotated maximally to one side and kept in that position while the neck is flexed for the first exposure and extended for the second exposure. Both sides are examined for comparison.

---

[1]Boylston BF: Oblique roentgenographic views of the cervical spine in flexion and extension: an aid in the diagnosis of cervical subluxations and obscure dislocations, *J Bone Joint Surg* 39A:1302, 1957.

A

B

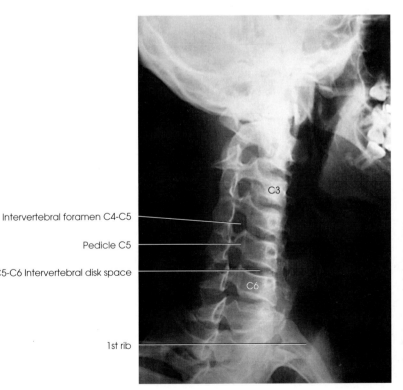 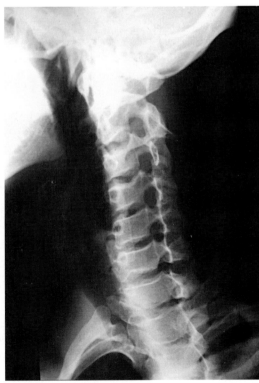

Intervertebral foramen C4-C5

Pedicle C5

C5-C6 Intervertebral disk space

1st rib

C3

C6

Fig. 8-56 AP axial oblique intervertebral foramina. **A,** LPO position demonstrating right side. **B,** RPO position demonstrating left side.

☀ PA AXIAL OBLIQUE PROJECTION
RAO and LAO positions

Image receptor: 8 × 10 inch (18 × 24 cm) lengthwise

SID: A 60- to 72-inch (152- to 183-cm) SID is recommended because of the increased OID.

Position of patient

• Place the patient prone or upright with the back toward the x-ray tube. For the patient's comfort and accurate adjustment of the part, the standing or seated-upright position is preferred.

Position of part

• Keeping one of the shoulder adjacent to the cassette, rotate the patient's entire body to a 45-degree angle to place the foramina parallel with the cassette. Center the cervical spine to the midline of the grid device.

• To allow for the caudal angulation of the central ray, center the cassette at the level of C5 (1 inch [2.5 cm] caudal to the most prominent point of the thyroid cartilage).

Upright position

• Ask the patient to sit or stand straight without strain; with the patient's arm hanging free, rest the adjacent shoulder against the grid device (Fig. 8-57).

• Ensure that the degree of body rotation is 45 degrees.

• With the midsagittal plane of the patient's head aligned with that of the spine, elevate and protrude the patient's chin slightly to prevent superimposition of the mandibular rami and the foramina. Turning the chin to the side causes slight rotation of the superior vertebrae and should be avoided.

Semiprone position

• With the patient's body at an angle of 45 degrees and the cervical spine centered to the midline of the grid, have the patient use the forearm and flexed knee of the elevated side to support the body and maintain the position.

• Adjust a suitable support under the patient's head to place the long axis of the cervical column parallel with the cassette.

• Check and adjust the degree of body rotation (Figs. 8-58 and 8-59).

• Adjust the position of the patient's head so that the midsagittal plane is aligned with the plane of the spine.

• Elevate and protrude the patient's chin just enough to prevent superimposition of the mandibular rami and the intervertebral foramina. Turning the chin to the side causes rotation of the superior vertebrae and should be avoided.

• *Shield gonads.*

• *Respiration:* Suspend.

Central ray

• Directed to C4 at an angle of 15 to 20 degrees caudad so that it coincides with the angle of the foramina

Structures shown

The resulting image shows the intervertebral foramina and pedicles *closest* to the cassette and an oblique projection of the bodies and other parts of the cervical column (Fig. 8-60).

EVALUATION CRITERIA

The following should be clearly demonstrated:

■ Open intervertebral foramina *closest* to the cassette, from the first and second cervical vertebrae to the seventh cervical and first thoracic vertebrae

■ Open intervertebral disk spaces

■ Elevated chin and protruded jaw so the angle of the mandible does not overlap the first and second cervical vertebrae

■ Occipital bone not overlapping the axis

■ All seven cervical and the first thoracic vertebrae

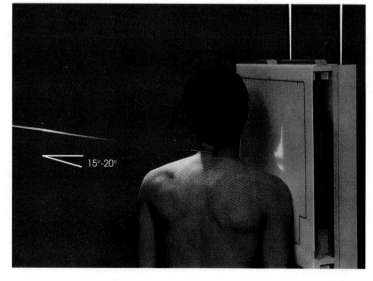

15°-20°

Fig. 8-57 PA axial oblique right intervertebral foramina: RAO position.

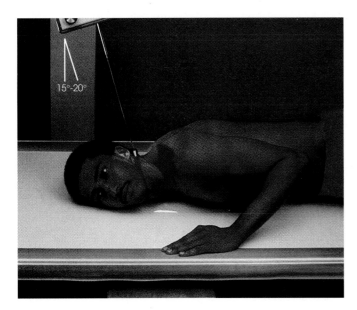

Fig. 8-58 PA axial oblique right intervertebral foramina: RAO position.

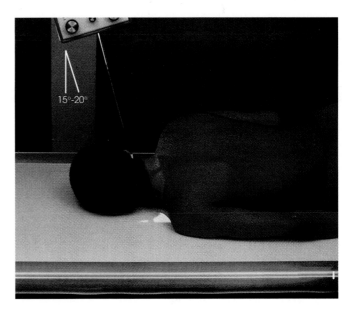

Fig. 8-59 PA axial oblique left intervertebral foramina: LAO position.

A

B

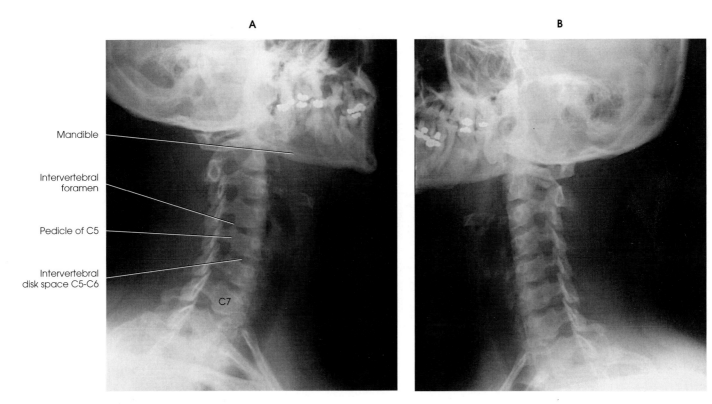

Mandible

Intervertebral foramen

Pedicle of C5

Intervertebral disk space C5-C6

C7

Fig. 8-60 PA axial oblique intervertebral foramina. **A,** RAO position demonstrating right side. **B,** LAO position demonstrating left side.

AP PROJECTION
OTTONELLO METHOD

With the Ottonello method the mandibular shadow is blurred or even obliterated by having the patient perform an even chewing motion of the mandible during the exposure. The patient's head must be rigidly immobilized to prevent movement of the vertebrae. The exposure time must be long enough to cover several complete excursions of the mandible.

Image receptor: 8 × 10 in (18 × 24 cm) lengthwise

Position of patient
- Place the patient in the supine position.
- Center the midsagittal plane of the body to the midline of the grid.
- Place the patient's arms along the sides of the body, and adjust the shoulders to lie in the same horizontal plane.
- Place a support under the knees for the patient's comfort.

Position of part
- Adjust the patient's head so that the midsagittal plane is aligned with the lower body and is perpendicular to the table.
- Elevate the patient's chin enough to place the occlusal surface of the upper incisors and the mastoid tips in the same vertical plane.
- Immobilize the head, and have the patient practice opening and closing the mouth until the mandible can be moved smoothly without striking the teeth together (Fig. 8-61).
- Place the cassette in a Bucky tray, and center the cassette at the level of C4.
- To blur the mandible, use an exposure technique with a low milliamperage (mA) and long exposure time (minimum of 1 second).
- *Shield gonads.*
- *Respiration:* Suspend.

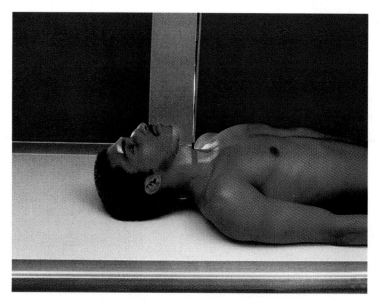

Fig. 8-61 AP cervical vertebrae: Ottonello method.

Cervical Vertebrae

Central ray

- Perpendicular to C4. The central ray enters at the most prominent point of the thyroid cartilage.

Structures shown

The resulting image shows an AP projection of the entire cervical column, with the mandible blurred if not obliterated (Figs. 8-62 and 8-63).

The following should be clearly demonstrated:

- All seven cervical vertebrae
- Blurred mandible with resultant visualization of the underlying atlas and axis

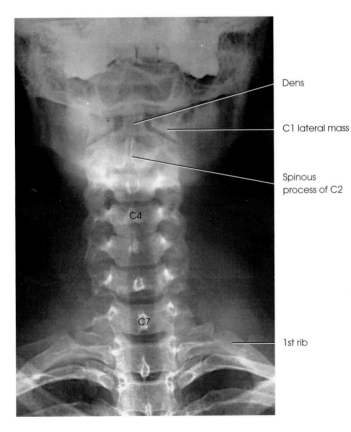

Dens

C1 lateral mass

Spinous process of C2

C4

C7

1st rib

Fig. 8-62 AP cervical spine: Ottonello method with chewing motion of the mandible and the use of a perpendicular central ray.

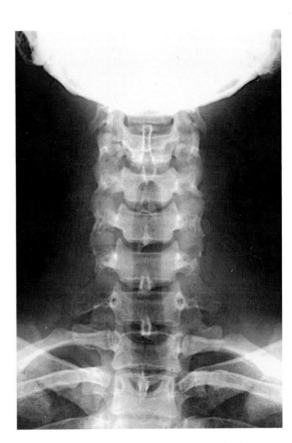

Fig. 8-63 Conventional AP axial cervical spine with stationary mandible and 15- to 20-degree cephalad angulation of the central ray.

Vertebral Arch (Pillars)
AP AXIAL PROJECTION[1]

NOTE: The procedure must not be attempted until cervical spine pathology or fracture has been ruled out.

The vertebral arch projections, sometimes referred to as *pillar* or *lateral mass* projections, are used to demonstrate the posterior elements of the cervical vertebrae, the upper three or four thoracic vertebrae, the articular processes and their facets, the laminae, and the spinous processes. The central ray angulations that are employed project the vertebral arch elements free of the anteriorly situated vertebral bodies and transverse processes. When the central ray angulation is correct, the resultant image resembles a hemisection of the vertebrae. In addition to frontal plane delineation of the articular pillars and facets, vertebral arch projections are especially useful for demonstrating the cervicothoracic spinous processes in patients with whiplash injury.[2]

Image receptor: 8 × 10 inch (18 × 24 cm) or 24 × 30 cm (10 × 12 inch)

[1]Dorland P, Frémont J: Aspect radiologique normal du rachis postérieur cervicodorsal (vue postérieure ascendante), *Semaine Hop* 1457, 1957.
[2]Abel MS: Moderately severe whiplash injuries of the cervical spine and their roentgenologic diagnosis, *Clin Orthop* 12:189, 1958.

Position of patient
- Adjust the patient in the supine position with the midsagittal plane of the body centered to the midline of the grid.
- Depress the patient's shoulders, and adjust them to lie in the same horizontal plane.

Position of part
- With the midsagittal plane of the head perpendicular to the table, *hyperextend* the patient's neck. The success of this projection depends on this hyperextension (Figs. 8-64 and 8-65).
- If the patient cannot tolerate hyperextension without undue discomfort, the oblique projection described in the next section is recommended.
- *Shield gonads.*
- *Respiration:* Suspend.

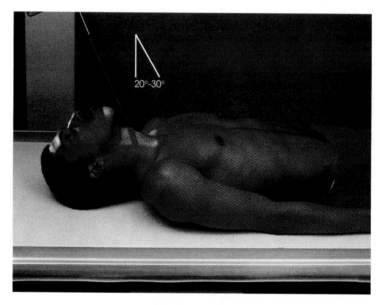

Fig. 8-64 AP axial vertebral arch.

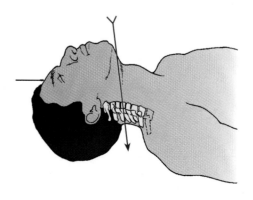

Fig. 8-65 AP axial vertebral arch.

Central ray

- Directed to C7 at an average angle of 25 degrees caudad (range: 20 to 30 degrees). The central ray enters the neck in the region of the thyroid cartilage.
- The degree of the central ray angulation is determined by the cervical lordosis. The goal is to have the central ray coincide with the plane of the articular facets so that a greater angle is required when the cervical curve is accentuated and a lesser angle is required when the curve is diminished
- To reduce an accentuated cervical curve and thus place C3-C7 in the same plane as the T1-T4, the originators[1] of this technique have suggested that a radiolucent wedge be placed under the patient's neck and shoulders, with the head extended somewhat over the edge of the wedge.

[1]Dorland P et al: Techniques d'examen radiologique de l'arc postérieur des vertebres cervicodorsales, *J Radiol* 39:509, 1958.

Structures shown

The resulting image demonstrates the posterior portion of the cervical and upper thoracic vertebrae, including the articular and spinous processes (Fig. 8-66).

EVALUATION CRITERIA

The following should be clearly demonstrated:

- Vertebral arch structures, especially the superior and inferior articulating processes (pillars), without overlapping of the vertebral bodies and transverse processes
- Articular processes
- Open zygapophyseal joints between the articular processes

NOTE: For a PA axial projection showing both sides on one cassette, rest the patient's head on the table with the neck fully extended and the midsagittal plane of the head perpendicular to the table. Direct the central ray at an average angle of 40 degrees cephalad (range: 35 to 45 degrees).

A

B

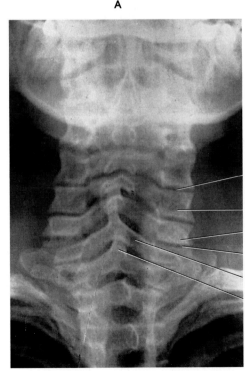
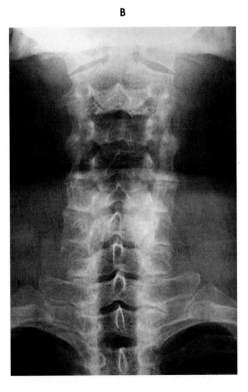

Zygapophyseal joint

Pillar or lateral mass

Inferior articular process

Superior articular process

Lamina

Spinous process

Fig. 8-66 AP axial. **A,** Central ray parallel with plateau of articular processes. **B,** Head fully extended but inadequate central ray angulation; central ray not parallel with zygapophyseal joints.

Vertebral Arch (Pillars)
AP AXIAL OBLIQUE PROJECTION
R and L head rotations[1]

These radiographic projections are used to demonstrate the vertebral arches or pillars when the patient cannot hyperextend the head for the AP or PA axial projection. Both sides are examined for comparison.

Image receptor: 8 × 10 inch (18 × 24 cm)

Position of patient
• Place the patient in the supine position.

[1]Dorland P et al: Techniques d'examen radiologique de l'arc postérieur des vertebres cervicodorsales, *J Radiol* 39:509, 1958.

Position of part
• Rotate the patient's head 45 to 50 degrees, turning the jaw away from the side of interest. A 45- to 50-degree rotation of the head usually demonstrates the articular processes of C2-C7 and T1. A rotation of as much as 60 to 70 degrees is sometimes required to demonstrate the processes of C6 and T1-T4 (Figs. 8-67 and 8-68).
• Position the cassette so that the top edge is at the level of the mastoid tip.
• *Shield gonads.*
• *Respiration:* Suspend.

Central ray
• Directed to exit the spinous process of C7 at an average angle of 35 degrees caudad (range: 30 to 40 degrees)

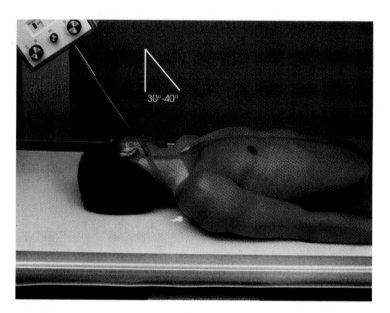

Fig. 8-67 AP axial oblique demonstrating right vertebral arches.

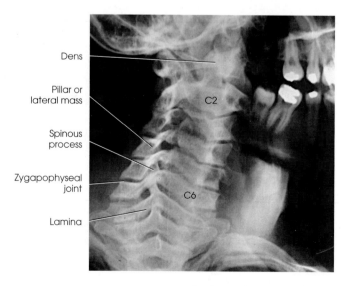
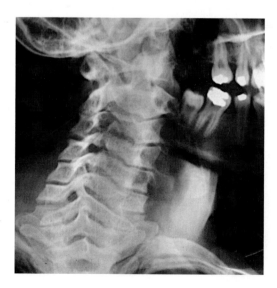

Dens

Pillar or lateral mass

Spinous process

Zygapophyseal joint

Lamina

C2

C6

Fig. 8-68 AP axial oblique demonstrating right vertebral arches.

Vertebral Arch (Pillars)
PA AXIAL OBLIQUE PROJECTIONS
R and L head rotations

Image receptor: 8 × 10 inch (18 × 24 cm)

Position of patient
- Unless contraindicated, place the patient in the prone position. For injured patients, the prone position seems to be more comfortable than the supine position.
- Center the midsagittal plane of the patient's body to the midline of the grid.
- When the patient is thin, place a pillow under the chest to obviate accentuation of the cervical curve.
- Depress the patient's shoulders and adjust them to lie in the same horizontal plane.

Position of part
- Rest the patient's head on one cheek, turning the jaw away from the side of interest. Adjust the head so that the midsagittal plane is at an angle of 45 degrees.
- To demonstrate the C2-C5, flex the patient's neck somewhat to reduce the cervical curve.
- To demonstrate C5-C7 and T1-T4, adjust the patient's head in moderate extension.
- Position the cassette so that its bottom edge is at the level of the tip of the C7 spinous process (Fig. 8-69).
- *Shield gonads.*
- *Respiration:* Suspend.

Central ray
- Directed to C7 at an average angle of 35 degrees cephalad (range: 30 to 40 degrees) and exiting at the level of the mandibular symphysis

Structures shown
The resulting AP and PA projections show the posterior arch and pillars of the cervical and upper thoracic vertebrae with open zygapophyseal articulations (see Figs. 8-68 and 8-70).

EVALUATION CRITERIA

The following should be clearly demonstrated:
- Vertebral arch structures, especially the superior and inferior articular processes, free of overlap of the vertebral bodies and transverse processes
- Articular processes and facets on the side of interest
- Open joints between the articular facets on the side of interest

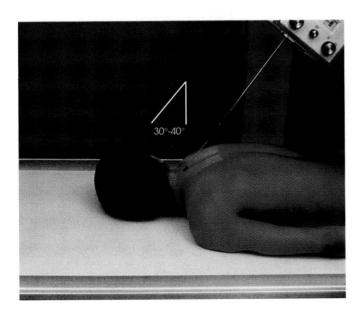

Fig. 8-69 PA axial oblique demonstrating left vertebral arches.

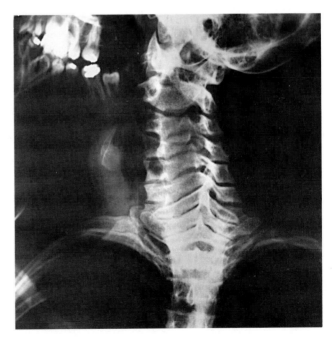

Fig. 8-70 PA axial oblique demonstrating left vertebral arches.

Adaptation of positions for trauma

The patient who has sustained a severe injury of the cervical spine and arrives by stretcher or bed should not be transferred to the radiographic table and must not be rotated. Unless a cervical collar is removed by a physician, it should always be left in place for the initial radiographs. To preclude the possibility of movement resulting in damage to the spinal cord by the sharp edge of a bone fragment or by a subluxated vertebra, a physician must perform any necessary manipulation of the patient's head.

If no specially equipped emergency room is available, the initial radiographic examination is performed with a mobile unit or in an examining room that is large enough to accommodate a stretcher or bed and the positioning of an x-ray tube for the required images.

Grid-front cassettes or a stationary grid is recommended for the AP and AP axial projections.

Shield gonads by placing a lead shield over the patient's pelvis. *Suspend respiration.*

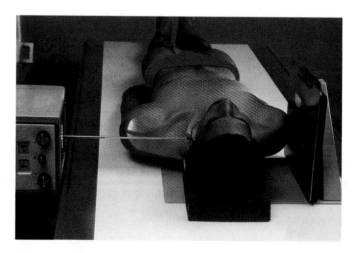

Fig. 8-71 Lateral cervical vertebrae: dorsal decubitus position.

Cervical Vertebrae: Trauma

☀ LATERAL PROJECTION
Dorsal decubitus position

The lateral projection, using a *horizontal* central ray, presents no problem because it requires little or no adjustment of the patient's head and neck.

The cassette is placed in the vertical position, with its lower portion in contact with the lateral aspect of the patient's shoulder, and centered to C4, and then immobilized. The central ray is directed horizontally to C4 (Figs. 8-71 and 8-72). Because of the increased OID, a 60- to 72-inch (152- to 183-cm) SID is recommended.

This radiograph must be reviewed by a physician before any further positioning is attempted.

For demonstration of the inferior cervical vertebra, the patient's shoulders must be fully depressed. Depending on the patient's condition, this can be done by looping a long strip of bandage around the patient's feet and flexing the knees slightly; then the other end of the bandage is attached to each of the patient's wrists, and the knees are extended to pull the shoulders down. If the patient's condition does not permit this maneuver, an assistant can depress the shoulders by applying symmetric traction on the arms, or a dorsal decubitus lateral projection (twining method) may be taken. To prevent additional injury to the patient, only qualified personnel should make any body adjustments. (A description of this projection using a mobile x-ray machine is presented in Chapter 30.)

NOTE: Although a grid is used in the lateral position photographs, it need not be used because of the increased OID. This increase in the OID creates an air gap that reduces the amount of scatter radiation reaching the cassette.

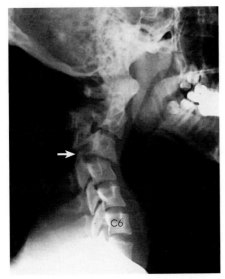

Fig. 8-72 Dorsal decubitus cervical spine performed on a trauma patient. Dislocation of the C3 and C4 articular processes (*arrow*). Note that C7 is not demonstrated well in most trauma patients.

✴ AP AXIAL PROJECTION

For an AP axial projection, the patient's head must be held (to prevent it from turning) and lifted enough for the cassette to be slipped into position without appreciable movement of the head and neck. If the patient is brought into the radiographic room on a backboard, the cassette may be placed under the board for the initial radiograph so that the patient's head is not moved.

AP axial projections with a 15- to 20-degree cephalad angulation of the central ray are obtained for demonstration of the vertebral bodies and their interspaces (Fig. 8-73).

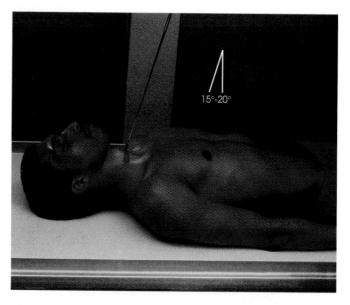

Fig. 8-73 AP axial cervical vertebrae: 15-degree grid technique.

⚕ AP AXIAL OBLIQUE PROJECTION
RPO and LPO positions

For demonstration of the pedicles and intervertebral foramina, the cassette must be positioned near the side *opposite* the one being examined so that its midpoint coincides with the 45-degree lateromedial angulation of the central ray.

The cassette may be placed directly under the patient or backboard. The backboard or the patient's head must be lifted slightly. The cassette is held so that its midpoint is at the level of C4, and it is then gently slid under the patient's head just far enough that it is centered under the adjacent mastoid process. This centering places the midline of the cassette approximately 3 inches (7.6 cm) lateral to the median sagittal plane of the neck.

The central ray is directed from the opposite side to C4 at a compound angle of 45 degrees medial and 15 to 20 degrees cephalad (Figs. 8-74 to 8-76). The compound angle used for this projection requires a nongrid technique to prevent grid cutoff from affecting the image.

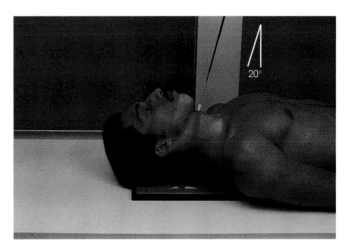

Fig. 8-75 AP axial oblique cervical vertebrae showing 20-degree cephalad central ray angulation and 45-degree medial central ray angulation: nongrid technique.

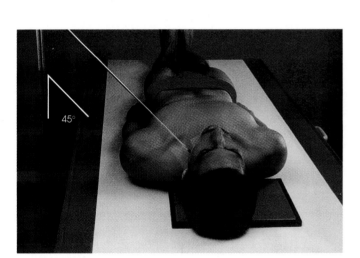

Fig. 8-74 AP axial oblique cervical vertebrae showing 45-degree medial central ray angulation and 20-degree cephalad angulation: nongrid technique.

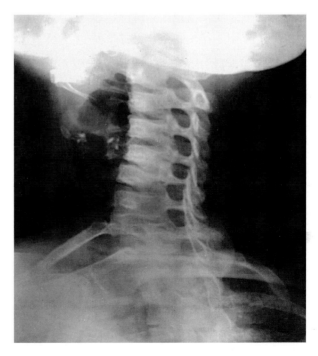

Fig. 8-76 Resultant nongrid AP axial oblique cervical vertebrae demonstrating left structures.

▲ LATERAL PROJECTION

TWINING METHOD
R or L position
Upright

This projection is often called the "swimmer's lateral" projection.

Image receptor: 24 × 30 cm (10 × 12 inch) lengthwise

Position of patient

• Place the patient in a lateral position, either seated or standing, against a vertical grid device.

Position of part

• Center the midcoronal plane of the body to the midline of the grid.
• Move the patient close enough to the grid device so that the shoulder can rest firmly against the grid for support.
• Elevate the arm that is adjacent to the vertical grid device to a vertical position, flex the elbow, and rest the forearm on the patient's head.
• Adjust the height of the cassette so that it is centered at the level of C7-T1, which will be at the level of the vertebral prominence posteriorly.
• Adjust the patient's head and body into a true lateral position, with the midsagittal plane parallel to the plane of the cassette (Fig. 8-77).

• Depress the patient's shoulder that is farthest from the cassette as much as possible, and move this shoulder anteriorly. Then move the shoulder closest to the cassette posteriorly.
• The goal is to have one shoulder placed slightly anterior and the other slightly posterior, with simultaneous elevation of one shoulder and depression of the opposite one. This shoulder placement is sufficient to prevent the humeral heads from being superimposed over the vertebrae.
• *Shield gonads.*
• *Respiration:* Suspend.
• If the patient can cooperate and can be immobilized, a long exposure time (low mA) should be used while the patient takes shallow breaths. Shallow breathing blurs the lung anatomy.

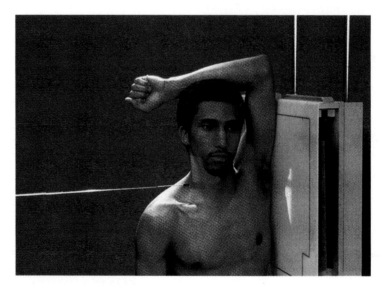

Fig. 8-77 Upright lateral cervicothoracic region: Twining method.

Central ray
- Directed to the interspace of C7 and T1: (1) perpendicular if the shoulder is well depressed or (2) at a caudal angle of 5 degrees if the shoulder cannot be well depressed.

COMPUTED RADIOGRAPHY

Both dense and nondense body areas will be exposed. The kilovolts (peak) (kVp) must be sufficient to penetrate the dense area. Collimation must be very close to keep unnecessary radiation from reaching the cassette phosphor.

Structures shown
The resulting image demonstrates a lateral projection of the lower cervical and upper thoracic vertebrae between the two shoulders (Fig. 8-78).

EVALUATION CRITERIA
The following should be clearly demonstrated:
- Lateral vertebrae, not appreciably rotated
- Shoulders separated from each other
- Area from approximately C5 to T4
- X-ray penetration of the shoulder region

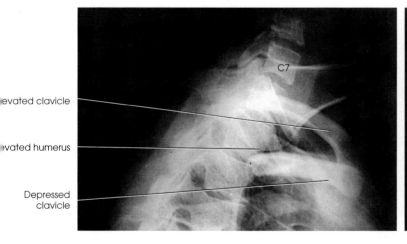
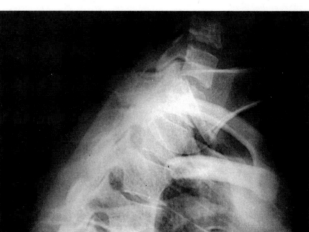

Fig. 8-78 Lateral cervicothoracic region: Twining method.

LATERAL PROJECTION
PAWLOW METHOD AND
MODIFIED PAWLOW METHOD[1]
R or L position
Recumbent

This projection is also called the "swimmer's lateral" projection It is most often performed with either a lateral cervical or lateral thoracic projection when the shoulders superimpose the vertebrae in the area of interest.

Image receptor: 24 × 30 cm (10 × 12 inch)

Position of patient
- Place the patient in a lateral recumbent position, with the head elevated on the patient's arm, sandbags, or a small, firm pillow.

---

[1]Monda, LA: Modified Pawlow projection for the upper thoracic spine, *Radiol Technol* 68:117, 1996.

Position of part
- Center the midcoronal plane of the patient's body to the midline of the grid.
- Adjust the support under the patient's head, and place another support under the lower thorax so that the long axis of the cervicothoracic vertebrae is horizontal.
- Grasp the arm on which the patient is lying, and extend it above the head. Move the humeral head posteriorly.
- Place the top arm at the patient's side, and immobilize it by having the patient grab the posterior thigh. Move the humeral head anteriorly.
- Adjust the body into a true lateral position (Fig. 8-79).
- Center the cassette at the level of the interspace of C7-T1 which is located 2 inches (5 cm) above the jugular notch.
- *Shield gonads.*
- *Respiration:* Suspend.

Central ray
- Directed to the interspace of C7 and T1 at an angle of 3 to 5 degrees caudad.
- Monda[1] modified the central ray by angling it 5 to 15 degrees *cephalad*.

COMPUTED RADIOGRAPHY
Both dense and nondense body areas will be exposed. The kVp must be sufficient to penetrate the dense area. Collimation must be very close to keep unnecessary radiation from reaching the cassette phosphor.

Structures shown
The resulting image shows a lateral projection of the cervicothoracic vertebrae between the shoulders (Fig. 8-80).

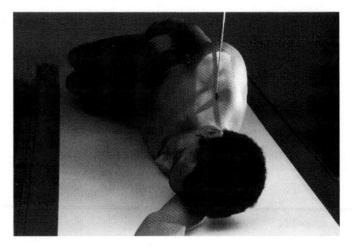

Fig. 8-79 Recumbent lateral cervicothoracic region: Pawlow method.

Cervicothoracic Region

EVALUATION CRITERIA

The following should be clearly demonstrated:

■ Lateral vertebrae not appreciably rotated
■ Shoulders separated from each other
■ Area from approximately C5 to T5
■ X-ray penetration of the shoulder region

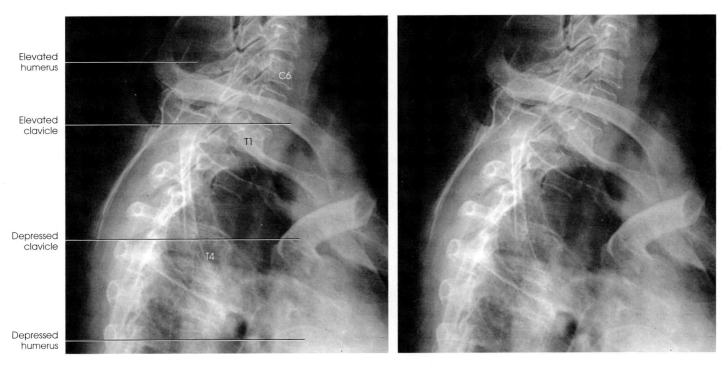

Elevated humerus

Elevated clavicle

Depressed clavicle

Depressed humerus

Fig. 8-80 Lateral cervicothoracic region: Pawlow method.

AP PROJECTION

Image receptor: 35 × 43 cm (14 × 17 inch) or 18 × 43 cm (7 × 17 inch) lengthwise

Position of patient
- Place the patient in the supine or upright position.
- Place the patient's arms along the sides of the body, and adjust the shoulders to lie in the same horizontal plane.
- If the patient is supine, let the head rest directly on the table or on a thin pillow to avoid accentuating the thoracic kyphosis.
- If the upright position is used, ask the patient to sit or stand up as straight as possible.

Position of part
- Center the midsagittal plane of the body to the midline grid.
- If the supine position is used, further reduce the thoracic kyphosis by flexing the patient's hips and knees enough to place the back in contact with the table. Adjust the thighs in a vertical position, and immobilize the feet with sandbags (Fig. 8-81).
- If the patient's limbs cannot be flexed, support the knees to relieve strain and invert the feet slightly.
- When the upright position is used, have the patient stand so that weight is equally distributed on the feet to prevent rotation of the vertebral column.
- If the patient's lower limbs are of unequal length, place a support of correct height under the foot of the shorter side.
- Center the cassette at the level of the seventh thoracic vertebra. Depending on the stature of the patient, the anterior localization point lies halfway between the jugular notch and the xyphoid process. The superior edge of the cassette should lie 1½ to 2 inches (3.8 to 5 cm) above the shoulders.
- *Shield gonads.*
- *Respiration:* The patient may be allowed to take shallow breaths during the exposure unless breathing is labored; in this case, respiration is suspended at the end of full expiration to obtain a more uniform density.

Central ray
- Perpendicular to T7 approximately halfway between the jugular notch and the xyphoid process (see Fig. 8-81).
- Collimate closely to the spine.
- As suggested by Fuchs,[1] a more uniform density of the thoracic vertebrae can be obtained if the "heel effect" of the tube is used (Fig. 8-82). With the tube positioned so that the cathode end is toward the feet, the greatest percentage of radiation goes through the thickest part of the thorax. A variety of wedge filters are available to assist in providing an even density of the entire thoracic spine.

Structures shown
The resulting image shows an AP projection of the thoracic bodies, intervertebral disk spaces, transverse processes, costovertebral articulations, and surrounding structures (see Fig. 8-82).

In many radiology departments a full 35 × 43 cm (14 × 17 inch) projection of the thoracic spine and chest is routinely performed, in particular for trauma patients. These larger-field projections are typically done using a thoracic filter. The larger field gives the radiologist a better look at the ribs, shoulder, diaphragm, and lungs (see Fig. 8-82, *C*).

EVALUATION CRITERIA
The following should be clearly demonstrated:
- All 12 vertebrae
- Wide latitude of exposure (or two radiographs can be taken for the upper and lower vertebrae).
- X-ray beam collimated to the thoracic spine as shown in Fig. 8-82
- Spinous processes at the midline of the patient
- Vertebral column aligned to the middle of the radiograph
- Ribs, shoulders, lungs, and diaphragm if a 35 × 43 cm (14 × 17 inch) image receptor is used

[1]Fuchs AW: Thoracic vertebrae, *Radiogr Clin Photogr* 17:2, 1941.

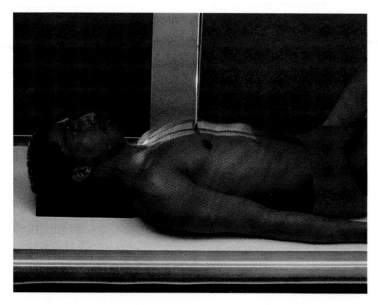

Fig. 8-81 AP thoracic vertebrae.

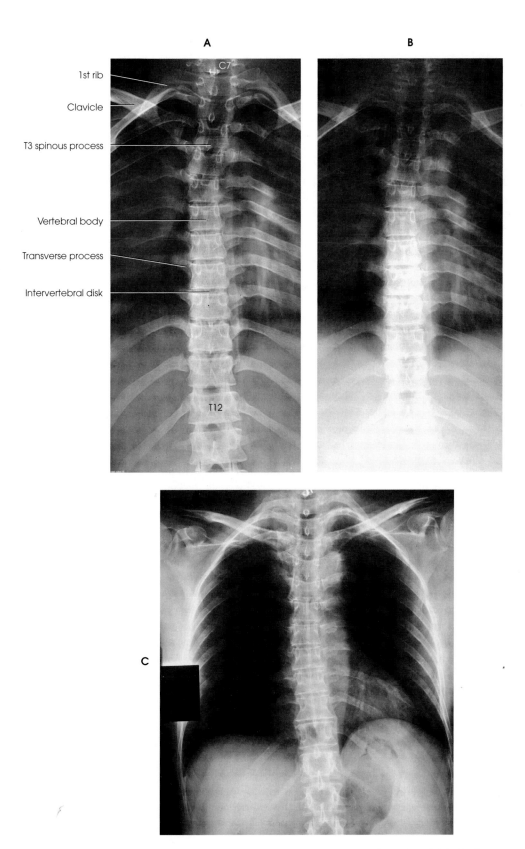

1st rib

Clavicle

T3 spinous process

Vertebral body

Transverse process

Intervertebral disk

C7

T12

A

B

C

Fig. 8-82 A, Cathode end of x-ray tube over lower thorax (more uniform density). **B,** Cathode end of x-ray tube over upper thorax (nonuniform density). **C,** Entire thorax projection.

🔺 LATERAL PROJECTION
R or L position

Image receptor: 35 × 43 cm (14 × 17 inch) or 18 × 43 cm (7 × 17 inch) lengthwise

Position of patient
- Place the patient in a lateral position, either recumbent or upright.
- If possible, use the left lateral position to place the heart closer to the cassette. This minimizes overlapping of the vertebrae by the heart.
- Oppenheimer[1] recommended the use of an upright position to reproduce the physiologic conditions and reported that the patient should be allowed to stand in a normal position. No attempt should be made to force the patient into an unwanted position, especially one involving straightening of the vertebral column.
- Have the patient dressed in an open-backed gown so that the vertebral column can be exposed for adjustment of the position.

Recumbent position
- Place a firm pillow under the patient's head to keep the long axis of the vertebral column horizontal.
- Flex the patient's hips and knees to a comfortable position.
- Center the *posterior half* of the thorax to the midline of the grid at the level of T7 (Fig. 8-83). The superior edge of the image receptor should lie 1½ to 2 inches (3.8 to 5 cm) above the relaxed shoulders.
- With the patient's knees exactly superimposed to prevent rotation of the pelvis, place a small sandbag between the knees.

[1]Oppenheimer A: The apophyseal intervertebral articulations roentgenologically considered, *Radiology* 30:724, 1938.

- Adjust the patient's arms at right angles to the long axis of the body to elevate the ribs enough to clear the intervertebral foramina. This placement of the arms gives a clear projection of the vertebrae distal to the level of the scapulohumeral joints. Drawing the arms forward or extending them to more than a right-angle position carries the scapulae forward, where they will superimpose over the upper thoracic vertebrae.
- If the long axis of the vertebral column is not horizontal, elevate the lower or upper thoracic region with a radiolucent support (Fig. 8-84, *A*). This is the *preferred method.*
- Adjust the body in a true lateral position.
- When necessary to support the patient, apply a compression band across the trochanteric area of the pelvis.

Upright position
- Have the patient stand or sit straight without strain, and adjust the height of the vertical grid device so that the midpoint of the cassette is at the level of T7.
- Center the *posterior half* of thorax to the midline of the grid. Move the patient close enough to the grid so that the adjacent shoulder can be firmly rested against the grid front for support.
- Ensure that the patient's body weight is equally distributed on the feet. If the limbs are of unequal length, place a support of correct height under the foot of the shorter side.
- Adjust the patient's body so that the long axis of the vertebral column is parallel with the plane of the cassette.

- Elevate the patient's ribs by raising the arms to a position at right angles to the long axis of the body, and support the arms in this position. An IV stand is very useful for this purpose. Place the stand in front of the patient, and immobilize it with sandbags. Then, placing one of the patient's hands on the other (for correct alignment of the arms), have the patient grasp the IV stand at the correct height (Fig. 8-85). This support of the upper limbs usually furnishes sufficient immobilization.
- *Shield gonads.*
- *Respiration:* Make the exposure with the patient breathing normally. This obliterates or at least diffuses the vascular markings and ribs. If the patient's breathing is labored, make the exposure at the end of expiration.

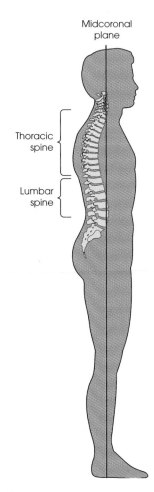

Fig. 8-83 Lateral view of the body, demonstrating the midcoronal plane. Note that the plane divides the thorax in half and thoracic vertebrae lie in the posterior half. Centering for lateral thoracic vertebrae is on the posterior half of the thorax.

Central ray

- Perpendicular to the center of the cassette at the level of T7 (lower margin of the scapula). The central ray enters the *posterior half* of the thorax.
- If the vertebral column is not elevated to a horizontal plane when the patient is in a recumbent position, angle the tube to direct the central ray perpendicular to the long axis of the thoracic column and then center it at the level of T7. An average angle of 10 degrees cephalad is sufficient in most female patients; an average angle of 15 degrees is satisfactory in most male patients because of their greater shoulder width (Fig. 8-84, *B*).

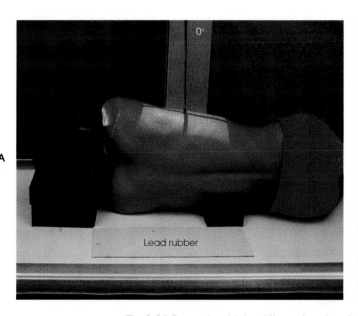

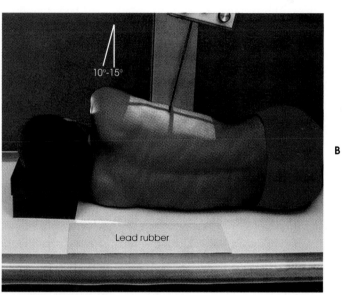

Fig. 8-84 Recumbent lateral thoracic spine. **A,** Support placed under lower thoracic region; perpendicular central ray. **B,** No support under lower thoracic spine; central ray angled 10 to 15 degrees cephalad.

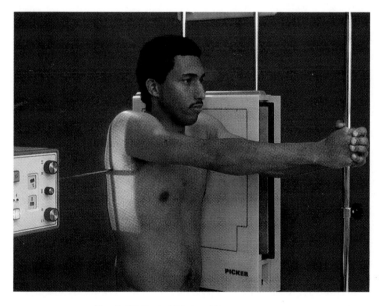

Fig. 8-85 Upright lateral thoracic spine.

Thoracic vertebrae

Thoracic Vertebrae

Improving radiographic quality

The quality of the radiographic image can be improved if a sheet of leaded rubber is placed on the table behind the patient (see Fig. 8-84). The lead absorbs the scatter radiation coming from the patient and prevents table scatter from affecting the image. Scatter radiation serves only to decrease the quality of the radiograph and blacken the spinous processes. More important with automatic exposure control (AEC), the scatter radiation coming from the patient is often sufficient to terminate the exposure prematurely. The resulting image may be underexposed because of the effect of the scatter radiation on the AEC device. For the same reason, close collimation is necessary for lateral spine radiographs. This is critically important when using computed radiography.

Structures shown

The resulting image is a lateral projection of the thoracic bodies that demonstrates their interspaces, the intervertebral foramina, and the lower spinous processes. Because of the overlapping shoulders the upper vertebrae may not be demonstrated in this position (Fig. 8-86). If the upper thoracic area is the area of interest, a "swimmer's lateral" may be included with the examination. The younger the patient, the easier it is to show the upper thoracic bodies.

EVALUATION CRITERIA

The following should be clearly demonstrated:

- Vertebrae clearly seen through rib and lung shadows.
- Twelve thoracic vertebrae centered on the image receptor. Superimposition of the shoulders on the upper vertebrae may cause underexposure in this area. The number of vertebrae visualized depends on the size and shape of the patient.
- Ribs superimposed posteriorly to indicate that the patient was not rotated.
- Open intervertebral disk spaces.
- Wide latitude of exposure.
- X-ray beam tightly collimated to reduce scatter radiation.

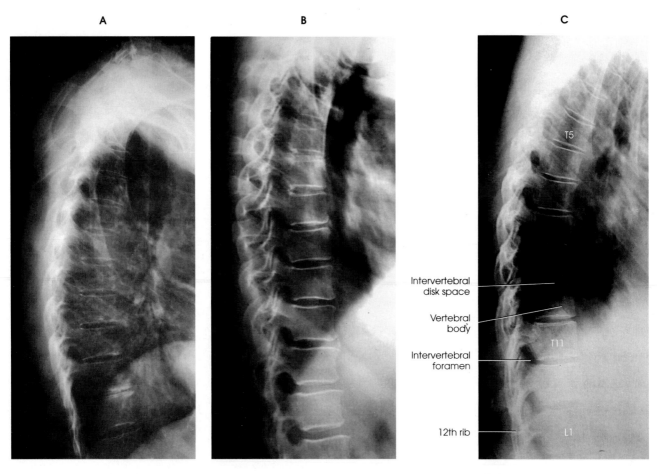

Fig. 8-86 Lateral thoracic spine. **A,** Suspended respiration for an exposure of 0.75 second. **B,** Normal breathing for an exposure of 7.5 seconds. **C,** Lateral thoracic spine with breathing technique.

AP OR PA OBLIQUE PROJECTION
RAO and LAO or RPO and LPO
Upright and recumbent positions

The thoracic zygapophyseal joints are examined using PA oblique projections as recommended by Oppenheimer[1] or using AP oblique projections as recommended by Fuchs.[2] The joints are well demonstrated with either projection. The AP obliques demonstrate the joints *farthest* from the cassette, and the PA obliques demonstrate the joints *closest* to the cassette. Although the difference in OID between the two projections is not great, the same rotation technique is used bilaterally.

Image receptor: 35 × 43 cm (14 × 17 inch)

[1]Oppenheimer A: The apophyseal intervertebral articulations roentgenologically considered, *Radiology* 30:724, 1938.
[2]Fuchs AW: Thoracic vertebrae (part 2), *Radiogr Clin Photogr* 17:42, 1941.

Upright position
Position of patient

- Place the patient, standing or sitting upright, in a lateral position before a vertical grid.

Position of part

- Rotate the body slightly anterior (PA oblique) or posterior (AP oblique) so that the coronal plane forms an angle of 70 degrees from the plane of the cassette (the midsagittal plane forms an angle of 20 degrees with the cassette).
- Center the patient's vertebral column to the midline of the grid, and have the patient rest the adjacent shoulder firmly against it for support.
- Adjust the height of the grid to center the cassette to T7.
- For the PA oblique, flex the elbow of the arm adjacent to the grid and rest the hand on the hip. For the AP oblique, the arm adjacent to the grid is brought forward to avoid superimposing the humerus on the upper thoracic vertebrae.

- For the AP oblique, have the patient grasp the side of the grid device with the outer hand (Fig. 8-87). For the AP oblique, have the patient place the outer hand on the hip.
- Adjust the patient's shoulders to lie in the same horizontal plane.
- Have the patient stand straight to place the long axis of the vertebral column parallel with the cassette.
- The weight of the patient's body must be equally distributed on the feet, and the head must not be turned laterally.
- *Shield gonads.*
- *Respiration:* Suspend the end of expiration.

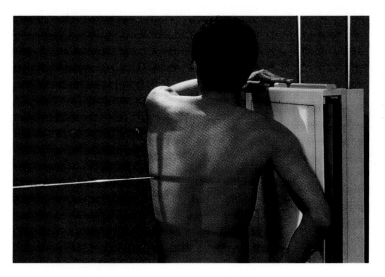
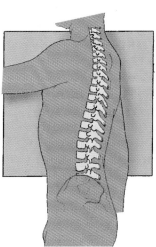

Fig. 8-87 PA oblique zygapophyseal joints: RAO for joints closest to film.

Image receptor: 35 × 43 cm (14 × 17 in) or 18 × 43 cm (7 × 17 in)

Recumbent position
Position of patient
- Place the patient in a lateral recumbent position.
- Elevate the head on a firm pillow so that its midsagittal plane is continuous with that of the vertebral column.
- Flex the patient's hips and knees to a comfortable position.

Position of part
- For anterior (PA oblique) rotation, place the lower arm behind the back and the upper arm forward with the hand on the table for support (Fig. 8-88).
- For posterior (AP oblique) rotation, adjust the lower arm at right angles to the long axis of the body, flex the elbow, and place the hand under or beside the head. Place the upper arm posteriorly and support it (Fig. 8-89).
- Rotate the body slightly, either anteriorly or posteriorly as preferred, so that the coronal plane forms an angle of 70 degrees with the horizontal (20 degrees with the vertical).
- Center the vertebral column to the midline of the grid.
- Center the cassette at the level of T7.

- If needed, apply a compression band across the hips, but be careful not to change the position.
- *Shield gonads.*
- *Respiration:* Suspend at the end of expiration.

Central ray
- Perpendicular to the cassette exiting or entering T7

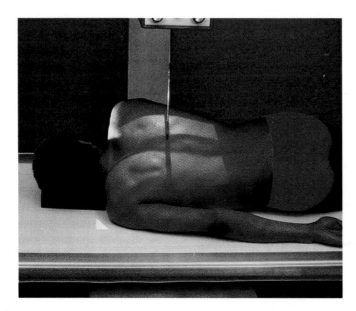

Fig. 8-88 PA oblique zygapophyseal joints: LAO for joints closest to film.

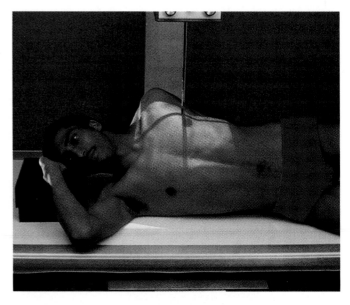

Fig. 8-89 AP oblique zygapophyseal joints: RPO for joints farthest from film.

Zygapophyseal Joints

Structures shown

The resulting images show oblique projections of the zygapophyseal joints (arrows on Figs. 8-90 and 8-91). The number of joints shown depends on the thoracic curve. A greater degree of rotation from the lateral position is required to show the joints at the proximal and distal ends of the region in patients with an accentuated dorsal kyphosis. The inferior articular processes of T12, having an inclination of about 45 degrees, are not shown in this projection.

EVALUATION CRITERIA

The following should be clearly demonstrated:

■ All twelve thoracic vertebrae
■ Zygapophyseal joints closest to the cassette on PA obliques and the joints farthest from the film on AP obliques
■ Wide exposure latitude

NOTE: The AP oblique projection gives an excellent demonstration of the cervicothoracic spinous processes and is used for this purpose when the patient cannot be satisfactorily positioned for a direct lateral projection.

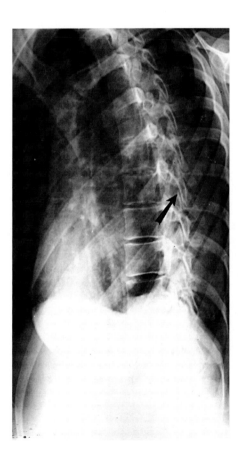

Fig. 8-90 Upright PA oblique zygapophyseal joints: LAO position. The arrow indicates the articulation that is closest to the cassette.

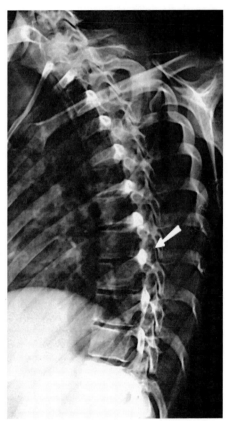

Fig. 8-91 Recumbent AP oblique zygapophyseal joints: RPO position. The arrow indicates the articulation that is farthest from the cassette.

♠ AP PROJECTION
PA PROJECTION (OPTIONAL)

If possible, gas and fecal material should be cleared from the intestinal tract for the examination of bones lying within the abdominal and pelvic regions. The urinary bladder should be emptied just before the examination to eliminate superimposition caused by secondary radiation generated within the filled bladder.

An AP or PA projection may be used, but the AP projection is more commonly employed.

Special positioning

- If a patient is having *severe* back pain, place a footboard on the radiographic table and stand the table upright before beginning the examination.
- Have the patient stand on the footboard, and position the part for the projection.
- Turn the table to the horizontal position for the exposure and return it to the upright position for the next projection.
- Although this procedure takes a few minutes, the patient will appreciate its ability to minimize pain.

AP Projection

The AP projection is generally used for recumbent examinations. The extended limb position accentuates the lordotic curve. This in turn increases the angle between the vertebral bodies and the divergent rays, with resultant distortion of the bodies and poor delineation of the intervertebral disk spaces (Figs. 8-92 and 8-93). In the AP projection the lordotic curve can be reduced and the intervertebral disk spaces clearly delineated by flexing the patient's hips and knees enough to place the back in firm contact with the radiographic table (Figs. 8-94 and 8-95).

Image receptor: 35 × 43 cm (14 × 17 inch) or 30 × 35 cm (11 × 14 in) for general survey examinations

SID: 48 inches (122 cm) is recommended to reduce distortion, more completely open the intervertebral joint spaces, and improve the overall quality of the examination.

Position of patient

- Examine the lumbar or lumbosacral spine with the patient recumbent or upright.
- Because acute back disorders are excruciatingly painful, examine ambulatory patients in the upright position whenever possible to reduce the physical discomfort associated with the examination.

Position of part

- For AP projections in the supine position, center the midsagittal plane of the patient's body to the midline of the grid.
- Adjust the patient's shoulders and hips to lie in the same horizontal plane.
- Flex the patient's elbows, and place the hands on the upper chest so that the forearms do not lie within the exposure field.
- When a soft tissue abnormality (atrophy or swelling) causes rotation of the pelvis, adjust a radiolucent support under the lower pelvic side.
- Reduce lumbar lordosis by flexing the patient's hips and knees enough to place the back in firm contact with the table (see Fig. 8-95).

Cassette centering

- For demonstration of the lumbar spine and sacrum, center the 35 × 43 cm (14 × 17 inch) cassette at the level of the iliac crests (L4).
- Carefully palpate the crest of the ilium. It is possible to be misled by the contour of the heavy muscles and fatty tissue lying above the bone.
- For demonstration of only the lumbar spine, center the 30 × 35 cm (11 × 14 inch) cassette 1½ inches (3.8 cm) above the iliac crest (L3).
- *Shield gonads.*
- *Respiration:* Suspend at the end of expiration.

Central ray

- Perpendicular to the midsagittal plane at the level of the iliac crests (L4) for a *lumbosacral* examination or 1½ inches (3.8 cm) above the iliac crests (L3) for a *lumbar* examination.

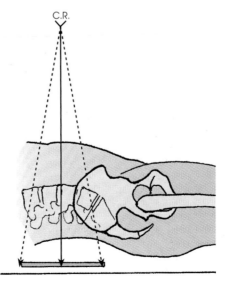

C.R.

Fig. 8-92 Lumbar spine demonstrating intervertebral disk spaces are not parallel; diverging central ray.

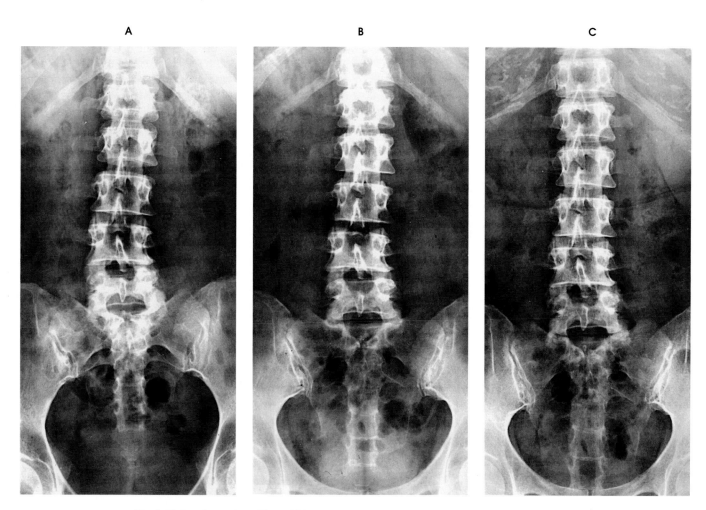

Fig. 8-93 Lumbar spine: AP and PA comparison on same patient. **A,** AP with limbs extended. **B,** AP with limbs flexed. **C,** PA.

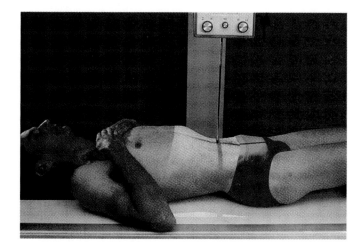

Fig. 8-94 AP lumbar spine with limbs extended, creating increased lordotic curve.

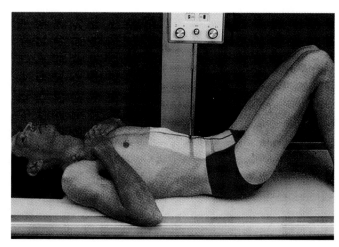

Fig. 8-95 AP lumbar spine with limbs flexed, decreasing lordotic curve.

PA projection (optional)

Because the PA projection presents the concave side of the lordotic curve toward the x-ray tube, it places the intervertebral disk spaces at an angle closely paralleling the divergence of the beam of radiation (see Figs. 8-96 and 8-93, *C*). For this reason the PA projection is sometimes used for upright studies of the lumbar and lumbosacral spine. The position does not increase the OID, except in the patient with a large abdomen. When used in the recumbent position, the PA projection has the advantage of being more comfortable for the patient with a painful back, especially an emaciated patient. An additional advantage of the PA projection is that the gonad dose can be significantly less than with the AP projection.[1]

Position of part

- Center the midsagittal plane of the body to the midline of the grid.
- Flex the patient's elbows, and then adjust the arms and forearms in a comfortable, bilaterally symmetric position.
- Adjust the patient's shoulders and hips to lie in the same horizontal plane, and have the patient rest the head *on the chin* to prevent rotation of the spine.

[1]Heriard JB, Terry JA, Arnold AL: Achieving dose reduction in lumbar spine radiography. *Radiol Technol* 65:97, 1993.

Structures shown, AP and PA

The resulting image shows the lumbar bodies, intervertebral disk spaces, interpediculate spaces, laminae, and spinous and transverse processes (Figs. 8-97 and 8-98). When the larger cassette is used, the images include one or two of the lower thoracic vertebrae, the sacrum coccyx, and the pelvic bones. Because of the angle at which the last lumbar segment joins the sacrum, this lumbosacral disk space is not shown well in the AP projection. The positions used for this purpose are described in the next several sections.

Many radiologists request or prefer that the AP projection be performed with the collimator open to the cassette size. This provides additional information about the abdomen, in particular when the projection is done for trauma purposes. The larger field enables visualization of the liver, kidney, spleen, and psoas muscle margins along with air or gas patterns (Fig. 8-97, *B*).

The following should be clearly demonstrated:

- Area from the lower thoracic vertebrae to the sacrum
- X-ray beam collimated to the lateral margin of the psoas muscles
- No artifact across the midabdomen from any elastic in the patient's underclothing
- X-ray penetration of all vertebral structures
- Open intervertebral joints
- Sacroiliac joints equidistant from the vertebral column
- Symmetric vertebrae, with spinous processes centered to the bodies

C.R.

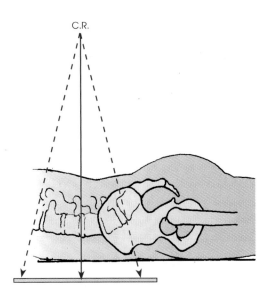

Fig. 8-96 Lumbar spine showing intervertebral disk spaces nearly parallel with divergent PA x-ray beam.

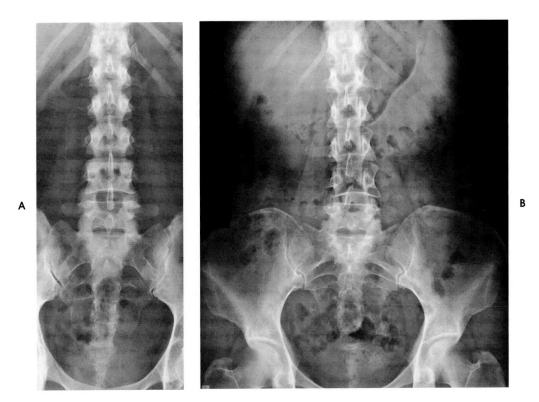

Fig. 8-97 AP lumbosacral spine. **A,** Close collimation technique. **B,** Collimation opened to cassette size 35 × 43 cm (14 × 17 inch) to show the abdomen along with the lumbar spine.

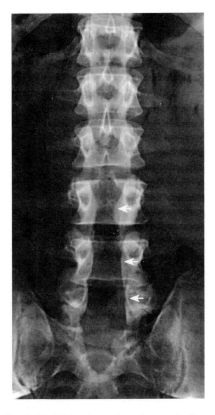

Fig. 8-98 AP lumbar spine demonstrating spina bifida (*arrows*).

LATERAL PROJECTION
R or L position

Image receptor: 35 × 43 cm (14 × 17 inch) or 30 × 35 cm (11 × 14 inch) for general survey examinations

Position of patient

- For the lateral position, use the same body position (recumbent or upright) as for the AP or PA projection.
- Have the patient dressed in an open-backed gown so that the spine can be exposed for final adjustment of the position.

Position of part
Recumbent position

- Ask the patient to turn onto the affected side and flex hips and knees to a comfortable position.
- When examining a thin patient, adjust a suitable pad under the dependent hip to relieve pressure.
- Align the midcoronal plane of the body to the midline of the grid. Remember that no matter how large the patient, the long axis of the body of the lumbar spine is situated in the midcoronal plane (Fig. 8-99).
- Adjust the pillow under the head to place the midsagittal plane of the patient's head in alignment with that of the spine.
- With the patient's elbow flexed, adjust the dependent arm at right angles to the body.
- To prevent rotation, exactly superimpose the knees and place a small sandbag between them.
- Place a suitable radiolucent support under the lower thorax, and adjust it so that the long axis of the spine is *horizontal* (Fig. 8-100, *A*). This is the *preferred method* of positioning the spine.
- Be certain that the midcoronal plane passing through the hips and shoulders is vertical.
- When using a 35 × 43 cm (14 × 17 inch) cassette, center it at the level of the crest of the ilium (L4). With a 30 × 35 cm (11 × 14 inch) cassette, center it 1½ inches (3.8 cm) above the crest.
- *Shield gonads.*
- *Respiration:* Suspend at the end of expiration.

Upright position

- Ask the patient to turn to the affected side and center the midcoronal plane of the body to the midline of the grid.
- Achieve immobilization by having the patient grasp an IV stand with both hands at shoulder height.
- Ensure that the patient stands straight. Patients with severe low back pain tend to relieve their discomfort by tilting the pelvis anteriorly and superiorly.
- Be certain that the patient's weight is equally distributed on the feet.

Central ray
Recumbent position

- Perpendicular to the level of the crest of the ilium (L4) when using a 35 × 43 cm (14 × 17 in) cassette for the lumbosacral spine, or 1½ inches (3.8 cm) above the crest (L3) if a 30 × 35 cm (11 × 14 in) cassette is used for the lumbar spine only. The central ray enters the midcoronal plane (Fig. 8-100, *A*).
- When the spine cannot be adjusted so that it is horizontal, angle the central ray caudad so that it is perpendicular to the long axis (Fig. 8-100, *B*). The degree of central ray angulation depends on the angulation of the lumbar column and the breadth of the pelvis. In most instances an average caudal angle of 5 degrees for men and 8 degrees for women with a wide pelvis is used.

Upright position

- Perpendicular to the cassette using the same centering points described for the recumbent position.

Because of the higher kVp used for this projection, the collimation must be very close. Scattered and primary radiation reaching the cassette phosphor may cause computer artifacts. The tabletop should be covered with a lead sheet.

Structures shown

The resulting image shows the lumbar bodies and their interspaces, the spinous processes, and the lumbosacral junction (Fig. 8-101). This projection gives a profile image of the intervertebral foramina of L1-4. The L5 intervertebral foramina (right and left) are not usually well visualized in this projection because of their oblique direction. Consequently, oblique projections are used for these foramina.

EVALUATION CRITERIA

The following should be clearly demonstrated:

- Area from the lower thoracic vertebrae to the coccyx using a 35 × 43 cm (14 × 17 in) image receptor
- Area from the lower thoracic vertebrae to the sacrum using a 30 × 35 cm (11 × 14 in) image receptor
- Open intervertebral disk spaces
- Superimposed posterior margins of each vertebral body
- Vertebrae aligned down the middle of the radiograph
- Nearly superimposed crests of the ilia when the x-ray beam is not angled
- Spinous processes

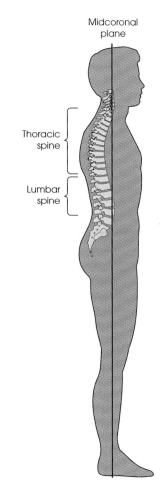

Fig. 8-99 Lateral view of the body demonstrating the midcoronal plane. Note that the plane goes through the lumbar bodies.

Improving radiographic quality

The quality of the radiographic image can be improved if a sheet of leaded rubber is placed on the table behind the patient (see Fig. 8-100). The lead absorbs scatter radiation coming from the patient and also prevents table scatter. Scatter radiation serves only to decrease the quality of the radiograph and to blacken the spinous processes. More important is that with AEC, scatter radiation coming from the patient is often sufficient to prematurely terminate the exposure. As a result, the image may be underexposed. For the same reason, close collimation is necessary for lateral spine radiographs. Scattered radiation control is critically important when using computed radiography.

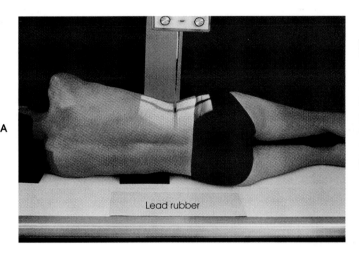

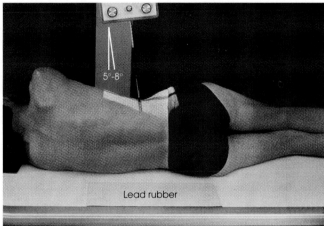

Fig. 8-100 Lateral lumbar spine. **A,** Horizontal spine and perpendicular central ray. **B,** Spine is angled and central ray directed caudad to be perpendicular to the long axis of the spine.

A

B

T12

Body L2

Intervertebral disk space

Intervertebral foramen

L4

Crest of ilium

Lumbosacral interspace

Sacrum

Fig. 8-101 A, Lateral lumbar spine, 30 × 35 cm (11 × 14 inch) cassette. **B,** Lateral lumbosacral spine, 35 × 43 cm (14 × 17 inch) cassette.

Lumbar-lumbosacral vertebrae

431

▲ LATERAL PROJECTION
R or L position

Image receptor: 8 × 10 inch (18 × 24 cm)

Position of patient
- Examine the L5-S1 lumbosacral region with the patient in the lateral recumbent position

Position of part
- With the patient in the recumbent position, adjust the pillow to place the midsagittal plane of the head in the same plane with the spine.

- Adjust the midcoronal plane of the body (passing through the hips and shoulders) to a vertical position.
- Flex the patient's elbow, and adjust the dependent arm in a position at right angles to the body (Fig. 8-102, *A*).
- If possible, fully extend the patient's hips for this study.
- As described for the lateral projection, place a radiolucent support under the lower thorax and adjust it so that the long axis of the spine is *horizontal* (see Fig. 8-102, *A*). This is the *preferred method.*
- Superimpose the knees exactly, and place a support between them.
- *Shield gonads.*
- *Respiration:* Suspend.

COMPUTED RADIOGRAPHY

The higher kVp used for this projection requires the use of very close collimation. Computer artifacts may be caused by scattered and primary radiation that could reach the cassette phosphor. Therefore the top of the radiography table should be covered by a lead sheet. If collimation is done correctly, no primary radiation should reach the cassette.

Central ray
- The elevated anterior superior iliac spine (ASIS) is easily palpated and found in all patients when lying on their side. The ASIS provides a standardized and accurate reference point from which to center the L5-S1 junction.
- Center on a coronal plane 2 inches (5 cm) posterior to the ASIS and 1½ inches (3.8 cm) inferior to the iliac crest.

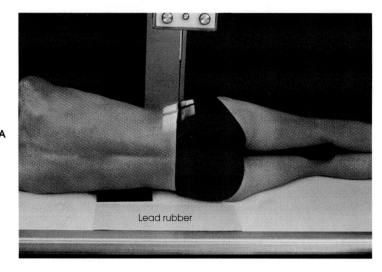

A

Lead rubber

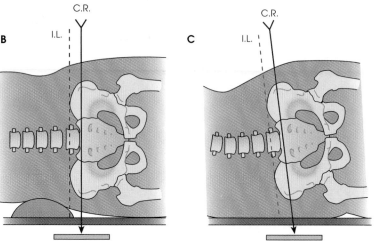

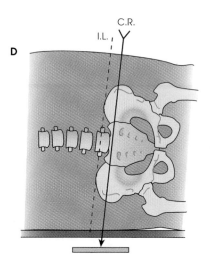

B   C.R.   I.L.

C   C.R.   I.L.

D   C.R.   I.L.

Fig. 8-102 A, Lateral L5-S1. **B,** Optimal L5-S1 joint position. The lower abdomen is blocked to place the spine parallel with the cassette. The interiliac *(IL)* line is perpendicular, and the central ray *(CR)* is perpendicular. **C,** Typical lumbar spine curvature. If blocking cannot be used, angle the CR caudad and parallel to the IL. **D,** Typical lumbar spine position in a patient with a large waist. The IL demonstrates that the CR must be angled cephalad to open the joint space.

(Modified from Francis C: Method improves consistency in L5-S1 joint space films, *Radiol Technol* 63:302, 1992.)

- Center the cassette to the central ray.
- Use close collimation.
- When the spine is not in the true horizontal position, the central ray is angled 5 degrees caudally for male patients and 8 degrees caudally for female patients.
- Francis[1] identified an alternate technique to demonstrate the open L5-S1 interspace when the spine is not horizontal:
  1. With the patient in the lateral position, locate both iliac crests.
  2. Draw an imaginary line between the two points (the interiliac line).
  3. Adjust central ray angulation to be parallel with the interiliac line (Fig. 8-102, *B*, *C*, and *D*).

Structures shown

The resulting image shows a lateral projection of the lumbosacral junction, the lower one or two lumbar vertebrae, and the upper sacrum (Fig. 8-103).

---

[1]Francis C: Method improves consistency in L5-S1 joint space films. *Radiol Technol* 63:302, 1992.

EVALUATION CRITERIA

The following should be clearly demonstrated:

- Open lumbosacral joint
- Collimated x-ray beam that includes all of L5 and the upper sacrum
- Lumbosacral joint in the center of the exposure area
- Crests of the ilia closely superimposing each other when the x-ray beam is not angled

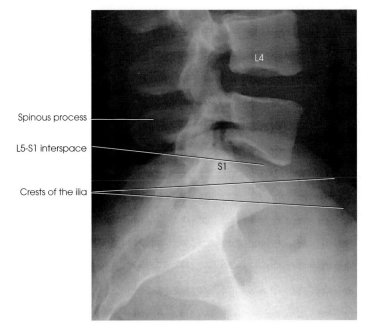
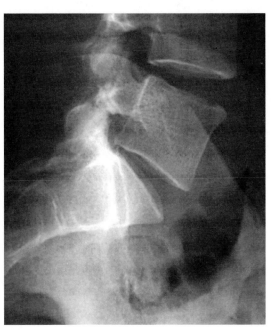

Fig. 8-103 Lateral L5-S1.

Spinous process

L5-S1 interspace

Crests of the ilia

L4

S1

Zygapophyseal Joints

AP OBLIQUE PROJECTION
RPO and LPO positions

The articular processes of the lumbar vertebrae form an angle of 30 to 50 degrees, and those between the last lumbar vertebra and the sacrum form an angle of 30 degrees to the midsagittal plane in the majority of patients. However, the angulation varies from patient to patient and from side to side in the same patient. For comparison, radiographs are generally obtained from both sides.

Image receptor: 35 × 43 cm (14 × 17 inch) or 30 × 35 cm (11 × 14 inch) lengthwise; 8 × 10 inch (18 × 24 cm) for the last zygapophyseal joint

Position of patient

• When oblique projections are indicated, they are generally performed immediately after the AP projection and in the same body position (recumbent or upright).

Position of part

• Have the patient turn from the supine position toward the affected side approximately 45 degrees to demonstrate the joints *closest* to the cassette (opposite the thoracic zygapophyseal joints).
• Adjust the patient's body so that the long axis of the patient is parallel with the long axis of the radiographic table.
• Center the patient's spine to the midline of the grid. In the oblique position the lumbar spine lies in the longitudinal plane that passes 2 inches (5 cm) medial to the elevated ASIS.

• Ask the patient to place the arms in a comfortable position. A support may be placed under the elevated shoulder, hip, and knee (Figs. 8-104 and 8-105).
• Check the degree of body rotation, and make any necessary adjustments. Adjust at an angle of 45 degrees for demonstration of the articular processes in the lumbar region and at an angle of 30 degrees for demonstration of the lumbosacral processes.
• *Shield gonads.*
• *Respiration:* Suspend at the end of expiration.

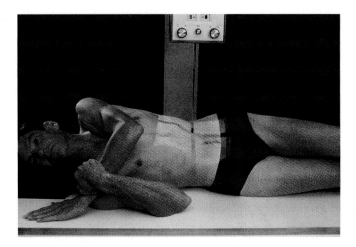

Fig. 8-104 AP oblique lumbar spine: RPO for right zygapophyseal joints.

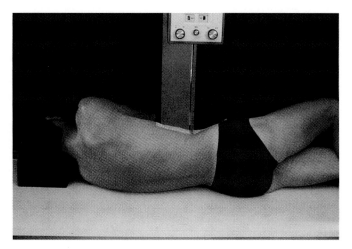

Fig. 8-105 AP oblique lumbar spine: LPO for left zygapophyseal joints.

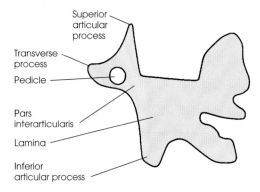

Fig. 8-106 Parts of "Scottie dog."

Zygapophyseal Joints

Central ray
- Perpendicular to the midpoint of the cassette as follows:

Lumbar region
- Enter 2 inches (5 cm) medial to the elevated ASIS and 1½ inches (3.8 cm) above the iliac crest (L3).

Fifth zygapophyseal joint
- Enter 2 inches (5 cm) medial to the elevated ASIS and then up to a point midway between the iliac crest and the ASIS.
- Center the cassette to the central ray.

Structures shown
The resulting image shows an oblique projection of the lumbar and/or lumbosacral spine, demonstrating the articular processes of the side *closest* to the cassette. Both sides are examined for comparison (Figs. 8-106 to 8-108).

When the body is placed in a 30- to 45-degree oblique position and the lumbar spine is radiographed, the articular processes and the zygapophyseal joints are demonstrated. When the patient has been properly positioned, images of the lumbar vertebrae have the appearance of "Scottie dogs." Fig. 8-106 identifies the different structures that comprise the "Scottie dog."

EVALUATION CRITERIA
The following should be clearly demonstrated:
- Area from the lower thoracic vertebrae to the sacrum.
- Zygapophyseal joints closest to the cassette—open and uniformly visible through the vertebral bodies.
  - When the joint is not well demonstrated and the pedicle is *anterior* on the vertebral body, the patient is not rotated enough.
  - When the joint is not well demonstrated and the pedicle is *posterior* on the vertebral body, the patient is rotated too much.
- Vertebral column parallel with the tabletop so that the T12-L1 and L1-L2 joint spaces remain open.

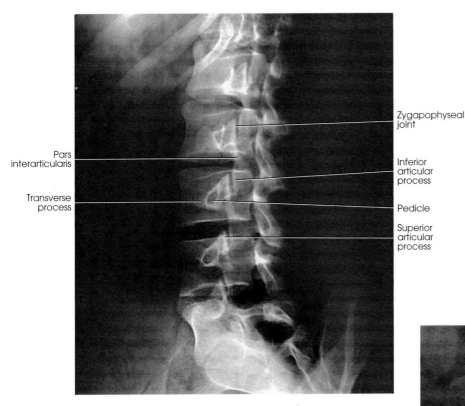

Pars interarticularis

Transverse process

Zygapophyseal joint

Inferior articular process

Pedicle

Superior articular process

Fig. 8-107 AP oblique lumbar spine: RPO for right zygapophyseal joints. (Note "Scottie dogs.")

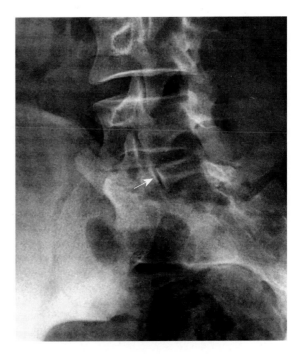

Fig. 8-108 AP oblique lumbar spine: RPO demonstrating L5 zygapophyseal joint (*arrows*) using a 30-degree position.

PA OBLIQUE PROJECTION
RAO and LAO positions

Image receptor: 35 × 43 cm (14 × 17 inch) or 30 × 35 cm (11 × 14 inch) lengthwise; 8 × 10 inch (18 × 24 cm) for the last zygapophyseal joint

Position of patient

- Examine the patient in the upright or recumbent prone position. The recumbent position is generally used because it facilitates immobilization.
- Greater ease in positioning the patient and a resultant higher percentage of success in duplicating results make the semiprone position preferable to the semisupine position. However, the OID is increased, which can affect resolution.

Position of part

- The joints *farthest* from the cassette are demonstrated with the PA oblique projection (opposite the thoracic zygapophyseal joints).
- From the prone position, have the patient turn to a semiprone position and support the body on the forearm and flexed knee.
- Align the body to center L3 to the midline of the grid (Fig. 8-109).
- Adjust the degree of body rotation to an angle of 45 degrees for the lumbar region and 30 degrees from the horizontal for the lumbosacral zygapophyseal joint.
- Center the cassette at the level of L3.
- To demonstrate the lumbosacral joint, position the patient as described above but center L5.
- *Shield gonads.*
- *Respiration:* Suspend at the end of expiration.

Central ray

- Perpendicular to enter the L3 (1 to 1½ inches [2.5 to 3.8 cm] above the crest of the ilium). The central ray enters the elevated side approximately 2 inches (5 cm) lateral to the palpable spinous process.

Structures shown

The resulting image shows an oblique projection of the lumbar or lumbosacral vertebrae, demonstrating the articular processes of the side *farther* from the cassette (Figs. 8-110, 8-111, and 8-112). The T12-L1 articulation between the twelfth thoracic and first lumbar vertebrae, having the same direction as those in the lumbar region, is shown on the larger cassette.

The fifth lumbosacral joint is usually well demonstrated in oblique positions (see Fig. 8-112).

When the body is placed in a 30- to 45-degree oblique position and the lumbar spine is radiographed, the articular processes and zygapophyseal joints are demonstrated. When the patient has been properly positioned, images of the lumbar vertebrae have the appearance of "Scottie dogs." Fig. 8-110 identifies the different structures that comprise the "Scottie dog."

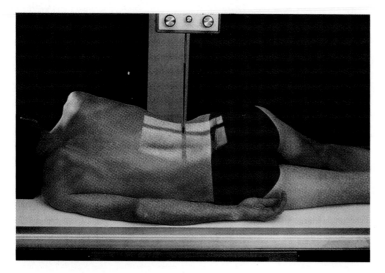

Fig. 8-109 PA oblique lumbar spine: LAO for right zygapophyseal joint.

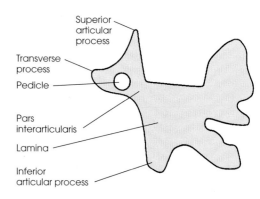

Superior articular process
Transverse process
Pedicle
Pars interarticularis
Lamina
Inferior articular process

Fig. 8-110 Parts of "Scottie dog."

Zygapophyseal Joints

EVALUATION CRITERIA

The following should be clearly demonstrated:

- Area from the lower thoracic vertebrae to the sacrum.
- Zygapophyseal joints *farthest* from the cassette:
  - □ When the joint is not well demonstrated and the pedicle is quite anterior on the vertebral body, the patient is not rotated enough.
  - □ When the joint is not well demonstrated and the pedicle is quite posterior on the vertebral body, the patient is rotated too much.
  - □ Vertebral column parallel with the tabletop so that the T12-L1 and L1-L2 joint spaces remain open.

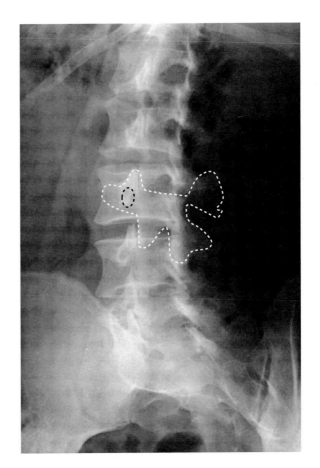

Fig. 8-111 PA oblique lumbar spine: LAO for right zygapophyseal joints. (Note "Scottie dogs.")

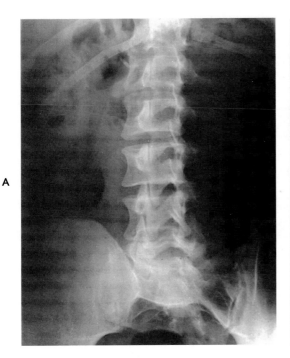

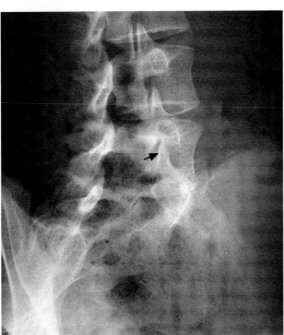

Fig. 8-112 PA oblique lumbar spine. **A,** LAO for right zygapophyseal joints. **B,** RAO for left L5 zygapophyseal joint *(arrow).*

Fifth Lumbar
PA AXIAL OBLIQUE PROJECTION
KOVÁCS METHOD[1]
RAO and LAO positions

Image receptor: 8 × 10 inch (18 × 24 cm) lengthwise.

Position of patient
- Place the patient in the lateral recumbent position lying on the side being examined.

---

[1]Kovács A: X-ray examination of the exit of the lowermost lumbar root, *Radiol Clin North Am* 19:6, 1950.

Position of part
- With the patient in the lateral position, align the body so that a plane passing 1½ inches (3.8 cm) posterior to the midcoronal plane is centered to the midline.
- Have the patient extend the upper arm and grasp the end of the radiographic table to maintain the thorax in the lateral position when the pelvis is rotated.
- Keeping the patient's thorax exactly lateral, rotate the pelvis 30 degrees anteriorly from the lateral position.
- Place a sandbag support under the flexed uppermost knee to prevent too much rotation of the hips (Fig. 8-113).
- Adjust the position of the cassette so that its midpoint coincides with the central ray.
- *Shield gonads.*
- *Respiration:* Suspend.

Central ray
- Directed along a straight line extending from the superior edge of the crest of the uppermost ilium through L5 to the inguinal region of the dependent side. Depending on the alignment of the spine, the central ray angulation may vary from 15 to 30 degrees caudad.

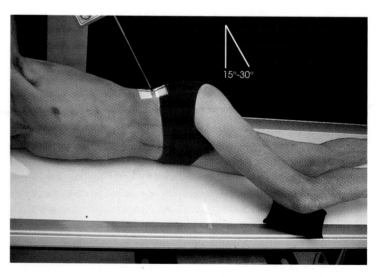

Fig. 8-113 PA axial oblique intervertebral foramen, L5, RAO: Kovacs method.

Vertebral column

Intervertebral Foramen

Structures shown

The resulting image shows the L5 intervertebral foramen. Both sides are examined for comparison.

The Kovács method (Figs. 8-114 and 8-115, *A*) is shown beside the lateral L5-S1 (Fig. 8-115, *B*) for comparison purposes.

EVALUATION CRITERIA

The following should be clearly demonstrated:

- Open L5 intervertebral foramen on the side closer to the cassette
- L5 intervertebral foramen in the center of the radiograph

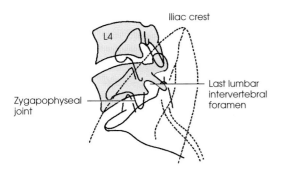

Fig. 8-114 PA axial oblique, intervertebral foramen, L5.

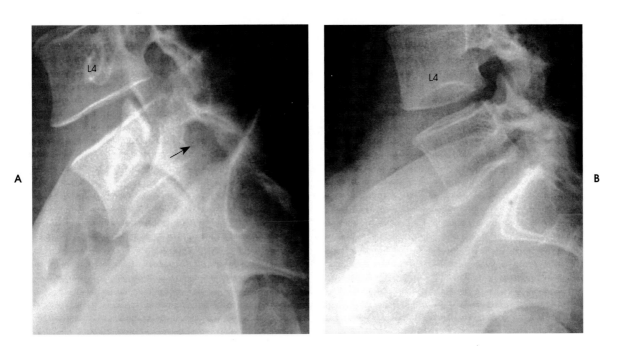

Fig. 8-115 **A,** PA axial oblique intervertebral foramen, L5, RAO: Kovacs method. Intervertebral foramen *(arrow).* **B,** Lateral L5-S1 in the same patient.

⚕ AP OR PA AXIAL PROJECTION

Image receptor: 8 × 10 inch (18 × 24 cm) or 24 × 30 cm (10 × 12 inch) lengthwise

Position of patient

- For the AP axial projection of the lumbosacral and sacroiliac joints, position the patient in the supine position.

Position of part

- With the patient supine and the midsagittal plane centered to the grid, extend patient's lower limbs or abduct the thighs and adjust in the vertical position (Fig. 8-116).
- Ensure that the pelvis is not rotated.
- *Shield gonads.*
- *Respiration:* Suspend.

Central ray

- Directed through the lumbosacral joint at an average angle of 30 to 35 degrees cephalad. The central ray enters about 1½ inches (3.8 cm) superior to the pubic symphysis on the midsagittal plane (Fig. 8-117).
- An angulation of 30 degrees in male patients and 35 degrees in female patients is usually satisfactory. By noting the contour of the lower back, unusual accentuation or diminution of the lumbosacral angle can be estimated and the central ray angulation can be varied accordingly.

Structures shown

The resulting image shows the lumbosacral joint and a symmetric image of both sacroiliac joints free of superimposition (Fig. 8-118).

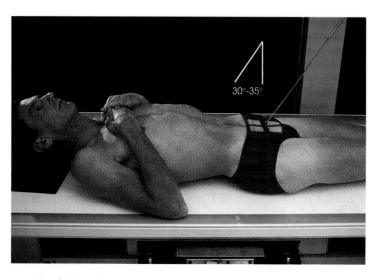

Fig. 8-116 AP axial lumbosacral junction and sacroiliac joints.

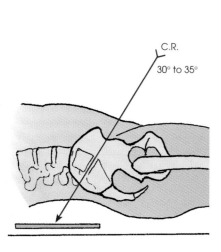

Fig. 8-117 AP axial sacroiliac joints.

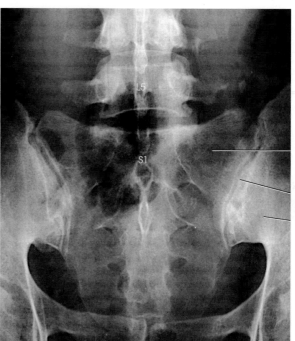

Fig. 8-118 AP axial lumbosacral junction and sacroiliac joints.

Vertebral column

EVALUATION CRITERIA

The following should be clearly demonstrated:

- Lumbosacral junction and sacrum
- Open intervertebral space between L5 and S1
- Both sacroiliac joints adequately penetrated

NOTE: The PA axial projection for the lumbosacral junction can be modified in accordance with the AP axial projection just described. With the patient in the prone position, the central ray is directed through the lumbosacral joint to the midpoint of the cassette at an average angle of 35 degrees caudad. The central ray enters the spinous process of L4 (Figs. 8-119 and 8-120).

Meese[1] recommended the prone position for examinations of the sacroiliac joints because their obliquity places them in a position more nearly parallel with the divergence of the beam of radiation. The central ray is directed perpendicularly and is centered at the level of the ASISs. It enters the midline of the patient about 2 inches (5 cm) distal to the spinous process of L5 (Fig. 8-121).

[1]Meese T: Die dorso-ventrale Aufnahme der Sacroiliacalgelenke, *Fortschr Roentgenstr* 85:601, 1956.

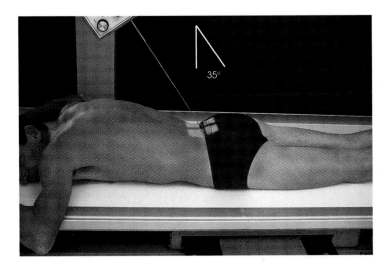

Fig. 8-119 PA axial lumbosacral junction and sacroiliac joints.

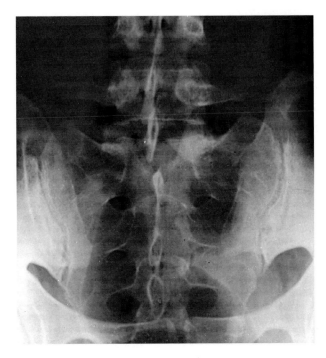

Fig. 8-120 PA axial lumbosacral junction and sacroiliac joints.

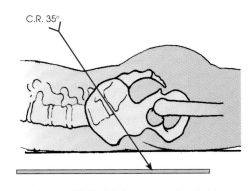

Fig. 8-121 PA bilateral sacroiliac joints.

AP OBLIQUE PROJECTION
RPO and LPO positions

Image receptor: 8 × 10 inch (18 × 24 cm) or 24 × 30 cm (10 × 12 inch) lengthwise. Both obliques are usually obtained for comparison.

Position of patient

- Place the patient in the supine position, and elevate the head on a firm pillow.

Position of part

- Use the LPO position to demonstrate the right joint and the RPO position to show the left joint. The side being examined is *farther* from the cassette.
- Elevate the side under examination approximately 25 to 30 degrees, and support the shoulder, lower thorax, and upper thigh (Figs. 8-122 and 8-123).
- Adjust the patient's body so that its long axis is parallel with the long axis of the radiographic table.
- Align the body so that a sagittal plane passing 1 inch (2.5 cm) medial to the ASIS of the elevated side is centered to the midline of the grid.
- Check the rotation at several points along the back.
- Center the cassette at the level of the ASIS.
- *Shield gonads.* Collimating close to the joint may shield the gonads in male patients. It may be difficult to use contact shielding in female patients.
- *Respiration:* Suspend.

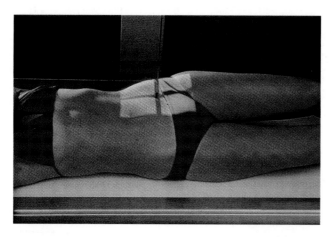

Fig. 8-122 AP oblique sacroiliac joint. RPO demonstrates left joint.

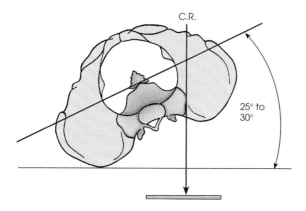

Fig. 8-123 Degree of obliquity required to demonstrate sacroiliac joint for an AP projection.

Central ray

• Perpendicular to the center of the cassette, entering 1 inch (2.5 cm) medial to the elevated ASIS

Structures shown

The resulting image shows the sacroiliac joint *farthest* from the cassette and an oblique projection of the adjacent structures. Both sides are examined for comparison (Fig. 8-124).

The following should be clearly demonstrated:

■ Open sacroiliac joint space with minimal overlapping of the ilium and sacrum

■ Joint centered on the radiograph

NOTE: An AP axial oblique can be obtained by positioning the patient as described above. For the AP axial oblique, the central ray is directed at an angle of 20 to 25 degrees cephalad, entering 1 inch (2.5 cm) medial and 1½ inches (3.8 cm) distal to the elevated ASIS (Fig. 8-125).

NOTE: Brower and Kransdorf[1] summarized difficulties in imaging the sacroiliac joints because of patient positioning and variability.

[1]Brower AC, Kransdorf MJ: Evaluation of disorders of the sacroiliac joint, *Appl Radiol* 21:31, 1992.

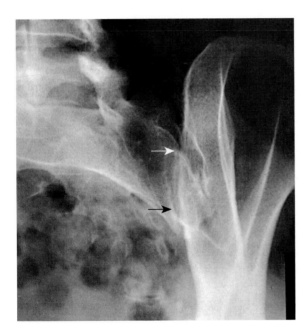

Fig. 8-124 AP oblique sacroiliac joint. RPO demonstrates left joint *(arrows)*.

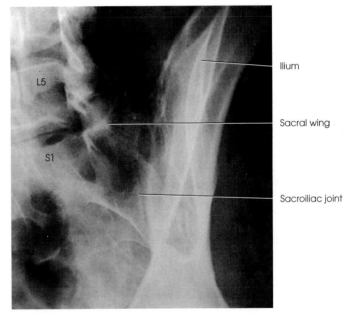

Fig. 8-125 AP axial oblique sacroiliac joint. RPO with 20-degree cephalad angulation demonstrates left joint.

PA OBLIQUE PROJECTION
RAO and LAO positions

Image receptor: 8 × 10 inch (18 × 24 cm) or 24 × 30 cm (10 × 12 inch) lengthwise. Both obliques are usually obtained for comparison.

Position of patient
- Place the patient in a semiprone position.
- Use the RAO position to demonstrate the right joint and the LAO position to show the left joint. The side being examined is *closer* to the cassette.
- Have the patient rest on the forearm and flexed knee of the elevated side.
- Place a small, firm pillow under the head.

Position of part
- Adjust the patient by rotating the side of interest toward the radiographic table until a body rotation of 25 to 30 degrees is achieved. The forearm and flexed knee usually furnish sufficient support for this position.
- Check the degree of rotation at several points along the anterior surface of the patient's body.
- Adjust the patient's body so that its long axis is parallel with the long axis of the table.

- Center the body so that a point 1 inch (2.5 cm) medial to the ASIS closest to the cassette is centered to the grid (Figs. 8-126 and 8-127).
- Center the cassette at the level of the ASIS.
- *Shield gonads.* Collimating close to the joint may shield the gonads in male patients. It may be difficult to use contact shielding in female patients.
- *Respiration:* Suspend.

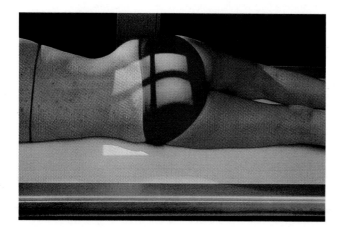

Fig. 8-126 PA oblique sacroiliac joint. LAO demonstrates left joint.

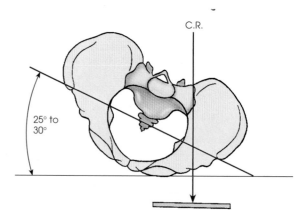

Fig. 8-127 Degree of obliquity required to demonstrate sacroiliac joint for a PA projection.

Central ray

- Perpendicular to the cassette and centered 1 inch (2.5 cm) medial to the ASIS closest to the cassette

Structures shown

The resulting image shows the sacroiliac joint *closest* to the cassette (Fig. 8-128).

EVALUATION CRITERIA

The following should be clearly demonstrated:

- Open sacroiliac joint space closest to the cassette or minimal overlapping of the ilium and sacrum
- Joint centered on the radiograph

NOTE: A PA axial oblique can be obtained by positioning the patient as described above. For the PA axial oblique, the central ray is directed 20 to 25 degrees caudad to enter the patient at the level of the transverse plane, pass $1^1/_2$ inches (3.8 cm) distal to the L5 spinous process, and exit at the level of the ASIS (Fig. 8-129).

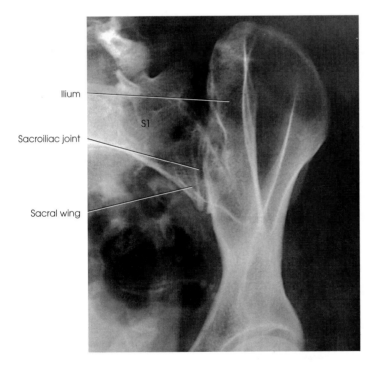

Ilium

S1

Sacroiliac joint

Sacral wing

Fig. 8-128 PA oblique sacroiliac joint. LAO demonstrates left joint.

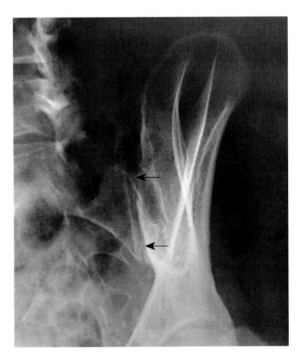

Fig. 8-129 PA axial oblique sacroiliac joint. LAO with 20-degree caudal central ray demonstrates left joint (*arrows*).

PA PROJECTION
CHAMBERLAIN METHOD FOR ABNORMAL SACROILIAC MOTION

Chamberlain[1] recommended the following projections in cases of sacroiliac slippage or relaxation:

1. A conventional lateral projection centered to the lumbosacral junction. Chamberlain suggested having this image made with the patient upright.
2. Two PA projections of the pubic bones, with the patient in the upright position and with weight-bearing on the alternate limbs to demonstrate pubic symphysis reaction by a change in the normal relation of the pubic bones in cases of sacroiliac slippage or relaxation.

This examination requires two blocks or supports approximately 6 inches (15 cm) high. The blocks are alternately removed to allow one leg to hang free.

Image receptor: 8 × 10 in (18 × 24 cm) lengthwise for each exposure

---

[1]Chamberlain WE: The symphysis pubis in the roentgen examination of the sacroiliac joint, *AJR* 24:621, 1930.

Position of patient

• Place the patient upright, facing the vertical grid device and standing on the two blocks.

Position of part

• Center the midsagittal plane of the body to the midline of the grid, and adjust the ASISs equidistant from the cassette.
• Have the patient grasp the sides of the device for steadiness. However, the device must not be used to support the patient's weight.
• If necessary, place a compression band across the pelvis to immobilize the patient but not to aid in supporting the weight of the body.
• Adjust the height of the grid, and center the cassette to the pubic symphysis.
• For the first exposure, remove one of the blocks so that one leg hangs free. The patient should be given good instructions about letting the leg hang with no muscular resistance.
• For the second exposure, replace the support under the foot that was hanging, and remove the opposite one, permitting the second leg to hang free. Chamberlain suggested that the identification marker be placed on the weight-bearing side (Fig. 8-130).
• *Shield gonads.*
• *Respiration:* Suspend.

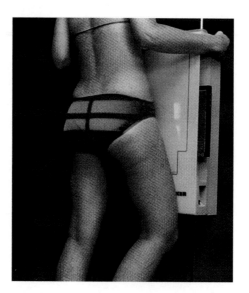

Fig. 8-130 PA symphysis pubis for demonstration of sacroiliac slippage.

Central ray
- Perpendicular and centered to the pubic symphysis.
- Use close collimation.

Structures shown
The two images show PA projections of the pubic symphysis. Abnormal motion of the sacroiliac joints is demonstrated by a change in the normal relation of the pubic bones to each other when the body weight is borne on one leg (Figs. 8-131 and 8-132).

EVALUATION CRITERIA
The following should be clearly demonstrated:
- Pubic symphysis in the center of the radiograph
- No rotation of the patient, indicated by symmetry of the pubic bones and obturator foramina
- Identification marker placed on the weight-bearing side

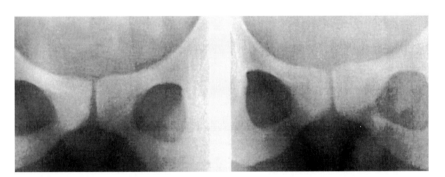

Fig. 8-131 PA pubic symphysis in a normal female patient.

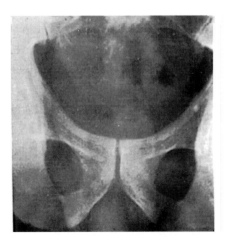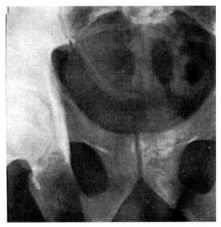

Fig. 8-132 PA pubic symphysis in a normal male patient.

▲ AP AND PA AXIAL PROJECTIONS

Because bowel content may interfere with the image, the colon should be free of gas and fecal material for examinations of the sacrum and coccyx. A physician's order for a bowel preparation may be needed. The urinary bladder should be emptied before the examination.

Image receptor: 24 × 30 cm (10 × 12 inch) for sacrum; 8 × 10 in (18 × 24 cm) for coccyx

Position of patient

- Place the patient in the supine position for the AP axial projection of the sacrum and coccyx so that the bones are as close as possible to the cassette. The supine position is most often used. The prone position can be used without appreciable loss of detail and is particularly appropriate for patients with a painful injury or destructive disease.

Position of part

- With the patient either supine or prone, center the midsagittal plane of the body to the midline of the table grid.
- Adjust the patient so that both ASISs are equidistant from the grid.
- Have the patient flex the elbows and place the arms in a comfortable, bilaterally symmetric position.
- Adjust the patient's shoulders to lie in the same horizontal plane.
- When the supine position is used, place a support under the patient's knees.
- *Shield gonads* on men. Women cannot be shielded for this projection.
- *Respiration:* Suspend.

Central ray

Sacrum

- With the patient supine, direct the central ray 15 degrees cephalad and center it to a point 2 inches (5 cm) superior to the pubic symphysis (Figs. 8-133 and 8-134).
- With the patient prone, angle the central ray 15 degrees caudad and center it to the clearly visible sacral curve (Fig. 8-135).

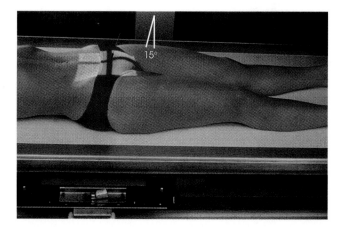

Fig. 8-133 AP axial sacrum.

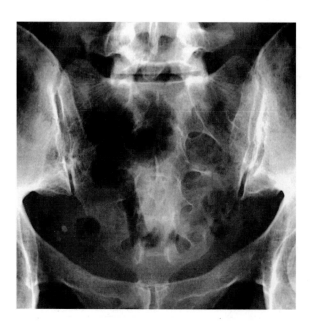

Fig. 8-134 AP axial sacrum.

Sacrum and Coccyx

Coccyx

- With the patient supine, direct the central ray 10 degrees caudad and center it to a point about 2 inches (5 cm) superior to the pubic symphysis (Figs. 8-136 and 8-137).
- With the patient prone, angle the central ray 10 degrees cephalad and center it to the easily palpable coccyx.
- Center the cassette to the central ray.

Structures shown

The resulting image demonstrates the sacrum or coccyx free of superimposition (see Figs. 8-134, 8-135, and 8-137).

EVALUATION CRITERIA

The following should be clearly demonstrated:

Sacrum
- Sacrum free of foreshortening, with the sacral curvature straightened
- Pubic bones not overlapping the sacrum
- Short-scale contrast
- No rotation of the sacrum, as indicated by symmetric alae
- Sacrum centered and seen in its entirety
- Tight collimation evident to improve the radiographic contrast
- Fecal material not overlapping the sacrum

Coccyx
- Coccygeal segments not superimposed
- Short-scale contrast on the radiograph
- No rotation
- Coccyx centered and seen in its entirety
- Tight collimation evident to improve the visibility

Radiation protection

- Because the ovaries lie within the exposure area, use close collimation for the female patient to limit the irradiated area and the amount of scatter radiation.
- For male patients, use gonad shielding in addition to close collimation.

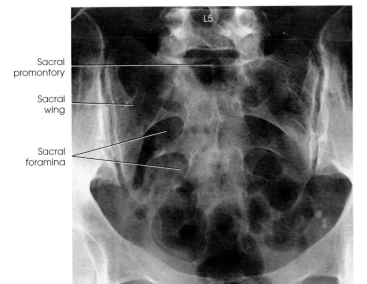

Sacral promontory

Sacral wing

Sacral foramina

L5

Fig. 8-135 PA axial sacrum.

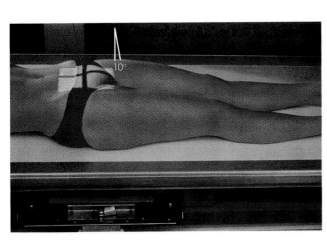

10°

Fig. 8-136 AP coccyx.

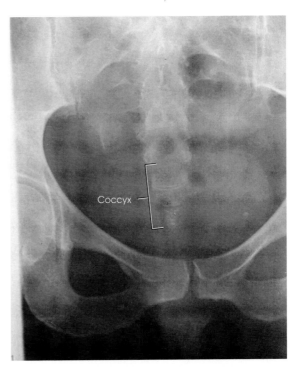

Coccyx

Fig. 8-137 AP coccyx.

⚜ LATERAL PROJECTIONS
R or L position

Image receptor: 24 × 30 cm (10 × 12 inch) for sacrum; 8 × 10 inch (18 × 24 cm) for coccyx, lengthwise

Position of patient
- Ask the patient to turn onto the indicated side and flex the hips and knees to a comfortable position.

Position of part
- Adjust the arms in a position at right angles to the body.
- Superimpose the knees, and if needed, place positioning sponges under and between the ankles and between the knees.
- Adjust a support under the body to place the long axis of the spine horizontal.
- Adjust the pelvis and shoulders so that the true lateral position is maintained (i.e., no rotation) (Figs. 8-138 and 8-139).
- To prepare for accurate positioning of the central ray, center the sacrum or coccyx to the midline of the grid.
- *Shield gonads.*
- *Respiration:* Suspend.

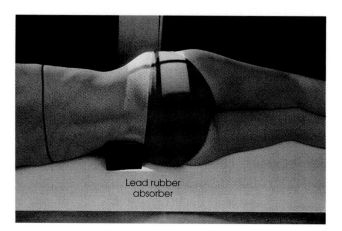

Fig. 8-138 Lateral sacrum.

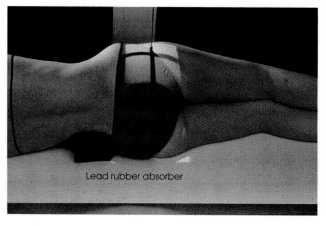

Fig. 8-139 Lateral coccyx.

Sacrum and Coccyx

Central ray
- The elevated ASIS is easily palpated and found on all patients when they are lying on their side. This provides a standardized reference point from which to center the sacrum and coccyx (Fig. 8-140).

Sacrum
- Perpendicular and directed to the level of the ASIS and to a point $3\frac{1}{2}$ inches (9 cm) posterior. This centering should work with most patients. The exact position of the sacrum depends on the pelvic curve.

Coccyx
- Perpendicular and directed toward a point $3\frac{1}{2}$ inches (9 cm) posterior to the ASIS and 2 inches (5 cm) inferior. This centering should work for most patients. The exact position of the coccyx depends on the pelvic curve.
- Center the cassette to the central ray.
- Use close collimation.

Structures shown
The resulting image shows a lateral projection of the sacrum or coccyx (Fig. 8-141).

EVALUATION CRITERIA
The following should be clearly demonstrated:
- Sacrum and coccyx seen clearly with short-scale contrast
- Use of tight collimation and a lead rubber absorber behind the sacrum
- Closely superimposed posterior margins of the ischia and ilia

Improving radiographic quality
The quality of the radiograph can be improved if a sheet of leaded rubber is placed on the table behind the patient (see Figs. 8-138 and 8-139). The lead absorbs the scatter radiation coming from the patient. Scatter radiation serves only to decrease the quality of the radiograph. More importantly, with AEC the scatter radiation coming from the patient is often sufficient to prematurely terminate the exposure, resulting in an underexposed radiograph. For the same reason, close collimation is necessary for lateral sacrum and coccyx images. This is critically important when using computed radiography.

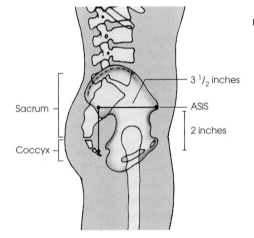

Fig. 8-140 Lateral sacrum, coccyx, and ilium (dashed outline) showing centering points. The ASIS provides a standardized reference point for central ray positioning

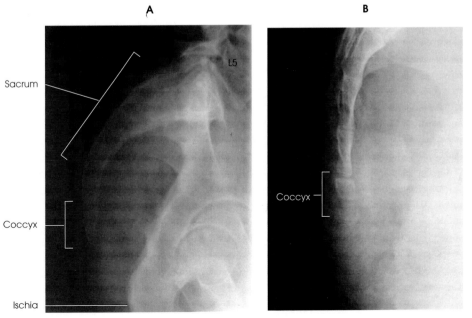

Fig. 8-141 A, Lateral sacrum. **B,** Lateral coccyx.

AXIAL PROJECTION
NÖLKE METHOD

Image receptor: 8 × 10 inch (18 × 24 cm) or 24 × 30 cm (10 × 12 inch) crosswise

Position of patient

- For examination of the sacral vertebral canal, seat the patient on the end of the radiographic table. The patient should sit far enough back to center the mid-coronal plane of the body to the horizontal axis of the Bucky tray.
- If the patient is too short to be comfortably seated far back on the end of the table, shift the cassette off center in the Bucky tray so that its midpoint coincides with the region of the canal to be examined (unless this is contraindicated by the use of AEC).
- Support the patient's feet on a chair or a stool.

Position of part

- Adjust the position of the patient's body so that the midsagittal plane is perpendicular to the midline of the grid.
- Have the patient lean forward enough that the upper, middle, or lower portion of the sacral vertebral canal is vertical.
- Be certain that the patient is not leaning laterally.
- Have the patient grasp the legs or ankles (depending on the degree of leaning) to maintain the position.
- Center the cassette to the vertically placed portion of the sacrum (Figs. 8-142 to 8-145).
- *Respiration:* Suspend.

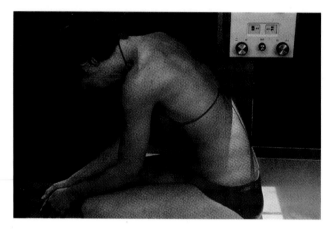

Fig. 8-142 Slight flexion.

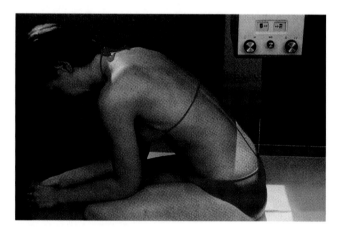

Fig. 8-144 Moderate flexion.

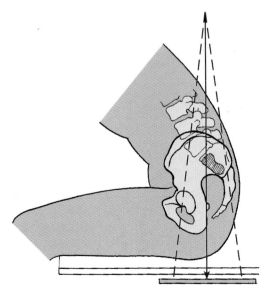

Fig. 8-143 Slight flexion alignment.

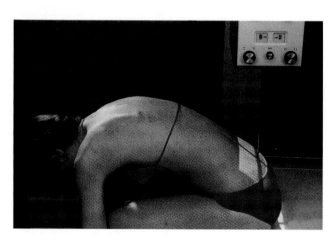

Fig. 8-145 Hyperflexion.

Central ray
- Perpendicular to the cassette and the long axis of the sacrum.
- Use close collimation.

Structures shown
The resulting image with the spine slightly flexed shows the lower sacral vertebral canal, the junction of the sacrum and coccyx, and the last lumbar vertebra (Fig. 8-146).

When the patient is leaning forward in a position of moderate flexion (see Fig. 8-144), the resultant image shows a cross section of the upper and lower sacral vertebral canal. The sacroiliac joints are also demonstrated (Fig. 8-147).

When the patient is leaning forward in a position of acute flexion (see Fig. 8-145), the resultant image shows the upper sacral vertebral canal projected into the angle formed by the ascending rami of the ischial bones just posterior to the pubic symphysis (Fig. 8-148). The spinous process of the last lumbar segment is projected across the shadow of the canal.

EVALUATION CRITERIA

The following should be clearly demonstrated:
- Sacral vertebral canal in the center of the exposure area
- No lateral rotation of the patient (sacral and pelvic structures are symmetric)

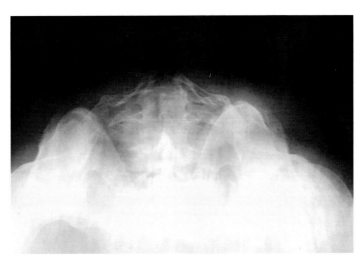

Fig. 8-146 Slight flexion.

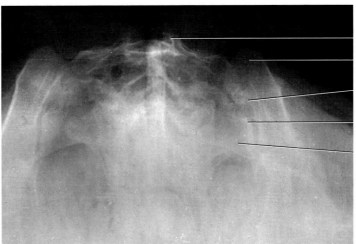

Sacral cornu

Ischial tuberosity

Obturator foramen

Sacroiliac joint

Inferior pubic ramus

Fig. 8-147 Moderate flexion.

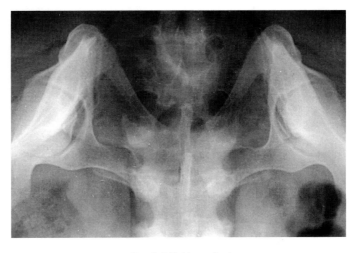

Fig. 8-148 Hyperflexion.

Sacral vertebral canal and sacroiliac joints

453

Lumbar Intervertebral Disks

PA PROJECTION
WEIGHT-BEARING METHOD
R and L bending

Image receptor: 35 × 43 cm (14 × 17 inch) lengthwise

Position of patient
- Perform this examination with the patient in the standing position. Duncan and Hoen[1] recommended that the PA projection be used because in this direction the divergent rays are more nearly parallel with the intervertebral disk spaces.

[1]Duncan W, Hoen T: A new approach to the diagnosis of herniation of the intervertebral disc, *Surg Gynecol Obstet* 75:257, 1942.

Position of part
- With the patient facing the vertical grid device, adjust the height of the grid to be at the level of L3.
- Adjust the patient's pelvis for rotation by ensuring that the ASISs are equidistant from the cassette.
- Center the midsagittal plane of the patient's body to the midline of the vertical grid device (Fig. 8-149).
- Let the patient's arms hang unsupported by the sides.
- Make one radiograph with the patient *bending* to the right and one with the patient *bending* to the left (see Fig. 8-149).
- Have the patient lean directly lateral as far as possible without rotation and without lifting the foot. The degree of bending must not be forced, and the patient must not be supported in position.
- Be certain that the midsagittal plane of the lower lumbar column and sacrum remains centered to the grid device as the upper portion moves laterally.
- *Shield gonads.*
- *Respiration:* Suspend.

Central ray
- Directed perpendicular to L3 at an angle of 15 to 20 degrees caudad or projected through the L4-L5 or L5-S1 interspaces, if these are the areas of interest.
- Use close collimation.

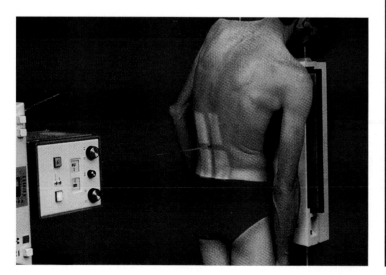 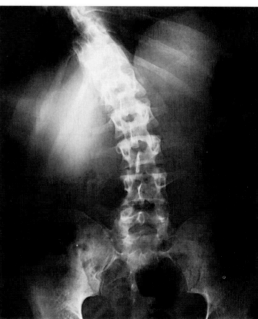

Fig. 8-149 PA lumbar intervertebral disks with right bending.

Lumbar Intervertebral Disks

Structures shown

The resulting images show bending PA projections of the lower thoracic region and the lumbar region for demonstration of the mobility of the intervertebral joints. In patients with disk protrusion, this type of examination is used to localize the involved joint as shown by limitation of motion at the site of the lesion (see Fig. 8-149).

EVALUATION CRITERIA

The following should be clearly demonstrated:

- Area from the lower thoracic interspaces to all of the sacrum
- No rotation of the patient in the bending position
- Bending direction correctly identified on the image with appropriate lead markers

Radiation protection

The PA projection is recommended over the AP projection whenever the clinical information provided by the examination is not compromised. With the PA projection the patient's gonad area and breast tissue receive significantly less radiation than when the AP projection is used. In addition, proper collimation reduces the radiation dose to the patient. Lead shielding material should be placed between the x-ray tube and the male patient's gonads to further protect this area from unnecessary radiation.

Scoliosis Radiography

Scoliosis is an abnormal lateral curvature of the vertebral column with some associated rotation of the vertebral bodies at the curve. This condition may be caused by disease, surgery, or trauma, but it is frequently idiopathic. Scoliosis is commonly detected in the adolescent years. If not detected and treated, it may progress to the point of debilitation.

Diagnosis and monitoring of scoliosis requires a series of radiographs that may include upright, supine, and bending studies. A typical scoliosis study might include the following projections:

- PA (or AP) upright
- PA (or AP) upright with lateral bending
- Lateral upright (with or without bending)
- PA (or AP) prone or supine

The PA (or AP) and lateral upright projections demonstrate the amount/degree of curvature that occurs with the force of gravity acting on the body (Fig. 8-150). Spinal fixation devices, such as Harrington rods, may also be evaluated. Bending studies are often used to differentiate primary from compensatory curves. Primary curves will not change when the patient bends; secondary curves will.

Because scoliosis is generally diagnosed and evaluated during the teenage years, proper radiographic techniques are important. Ideally, large film-screen systems and grids, such as 14 × 36 inches (35 × 90 cm), are used to demonstrate the entire spine with one exposure. The wide range of body-part thicknesses and specific gravities in the thoracic and abdominal areas necessitates the use of compensating filters.

A   B

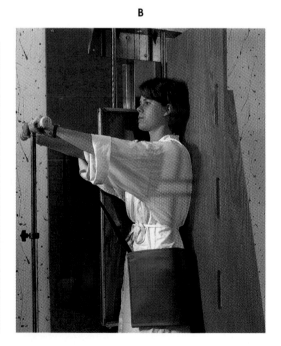

Fig. 8-150 Standing full spine radiography, using a 14 × 36 inch (35 × 90 cm) cassette. **A,** PA projection. **B,** Lateral projection.

RADIATION PROTECTION

In 1983 Frank et al[1] described the use of the PA projection for scoliosis radiography. Also in 1983, Frank and Kuntz[2] described a simple of method of protecting the breasts during scoliosis radiography. By 1986 the federal government had endorsed the use of these techniques in an article by Butler et al.[3]

Radiation protection is crucial. Collimation must be closely limited to irradiate only the thoracic and lumbar spine. The gonads should be shielded by placing a lead apron at the level of the ASISs between the patient and the x-ray tube. The breasts should be shielded with leaded rubber or leaded acrylic (Figs. 8-151 and 8-152), or the breast radiation exposure should be decreased by performing PA projections. Rare earth screens and high kVp techniques can also decrease the radiation dose.

---

[1]Frank ED et al: Use of the posteroanterior projection: a method of reducing x-ray exposure to specific radiosensitive organs, *Radiol Technol* 54:343, 1983.
[2]Frank ED, Kuntz JI: A simple method of protecting the breasts during upright lateral radiography for spine deformities, *Radiol Technol* 55:532, 1983.
[3]Butler PF et al: Simple methods to reduce patient exposure during scoliosis radiography, *Radiol Technol* 57:411, 1986.

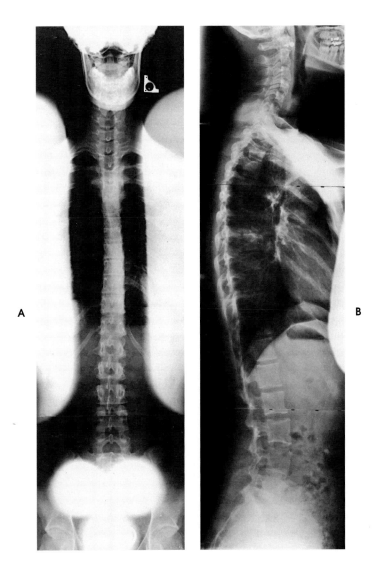

A B

Fig. 8-151 Standing full spine radiography. **A,** PA projection. Note the cloverleaf gonad shield and the bilateral breast shielding. **B,** Lateral projection. Note the breast shielding.

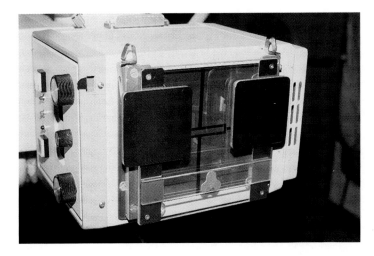

Fig. 8-152 Collimator face showing magnetically held breast shields and gonad shield.

(Courtesy Nuclear Associates, Carlyle, Pa.)

PA, OR LATERAL PROJECTIONS
FERGUSON METHOD[1]

The patient should be positioned to obtain a PA projection (in lieu of the AP projection) to reduce radiation exposure[2] to selected radiosensitive organs. The decision on whether to use a PA or AP projection is often determined by the physician or the institutional policy.

Image receptor: 14 × 36 inch (35 × 90 cm) or 35 × 43 cm (14 × 17 inch) lengthwise

Position of patient

- For a PA projection, place the patient in a seated or standing position in front of a vertical grid device.
- Have the patient sit or stand straight, and then adjust the height of the cassette to include about 1 inch (2.5 cm) of the iliac crests (Fig. 8-153).

[1]Ferguson AB: *Roentgen diagnosis of the extremities and spine,* New York, 1939, Harper & Row.
[2]Frank ED et al: Use of the posteroanterior projection: a method of reducing x-ray exposure to specific radiosensitive organs. *Radiol Technol* 54, 343, 1983.

Position of part

- For the first radiograph, adjust the patient in a normally seated or standing position to check the spinal curvature.
- Center the midsagittal plane of the patient's body to the midline of the grid.
- Allow the patient's arms to hang relaxed at the sides. If the patient is seated, flex the elbows and rest the hands on the lap (Fig. 8-154).
- Do not support the patient or use a compression band.
- *Shield gonads.*
- For the second radiograph, elevate the patient's hip or foot on the convex side of the primary curve approximately 3 or 4 inches (7.6 to 10.2 cm) by placing a block, a book, or sandbags under the buttock or foot (Fig. 8-155). Ferguson[1] specified that the elevation must be sufficient to make the patient expend some effort in maintaining the position.
- Do not support the patient in these positions.
- Do not employ a compression band.
- *Shield gonads.*
- *Respiration:* Suspend.

- Obtain additional radiographs (if needed) with elevation of the hip on the side *opposite* the major or primary curve (Fig. 8-156) or with the patient in a recumbent position (Fig. 8-157).

Central ray

- Perpendicular to the midpoint of the cassette

Structures shown

The resulting images show PA projections of the thoracic and lumbar vertebrae, which are used for comparison to distinguish the deforming or primary curve from the compensatory curve in patients with scoliosis (see Figs. 8-154 to 8-157).

EVALUATION CRITERIA

The following should be clearly demonstrated:

- Thoracic and lumbar vertebrae to include about 1 inch (2.5 cm) of the iliac crests
- Vertebral column aligned down the center of the radiograph
- Correct identification marker

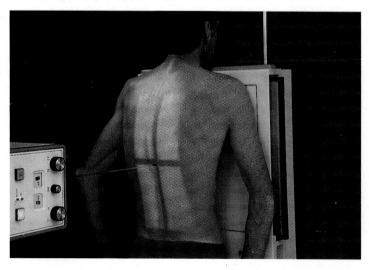

Fig. 8-153 PA thoracic and lumbar spine for scoliosis, upright.

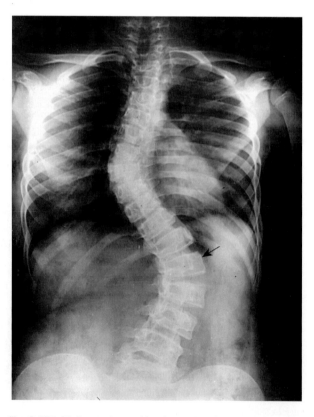

Fig. 8-154 PA thoracic and lumbar spine for scoliosis, upright, demonstrating structural (major or primary) curve *(arrow).*

Vertebral column

Thoracolumbar Spine: Scoliosis

NOTE: Another widely used scoliosis series consists of four images of the thoracic and lumbar spine: a direct PA projection with the patient standing, a direct PA projection with the patient prone, and PA projections with alternate right and left lateral flexion in the prone position. The right and left bending positions are described in the next section. For the scoliosis series, however, 35×43 cm (14×17 inch) cassettes are used and are placed to include about 1 inch (2.5 cm) of the crests of ilia.

NOTE: Young, Oestreich, and Goldstein[1] described their application of this scoliosis procedure in detail. They recommended the addition of a lateral position, made with the patient standing upright, to show spondylolisthesis or demonstrate exaggerated degrees of kyphosis or lordosis. Kittleson and Lim[2] described both the Ferguson and Cobb methods of measurement of scoliosis.

[1]Young LW, Oestreich AE, Goldstein LA: Roentgenology in scoliosis: contribution to evaluation and management, *Radiology* 97:778, 1970.
[2]Kittleson AC, Lim LW: Measurement of scoliosis, *AJR* 108:775, 1970.

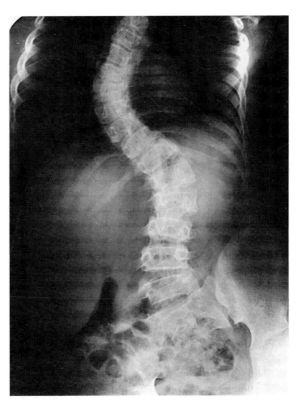

Fig. 8-155 PA thoracic and lumbar spine with left hip elevated.

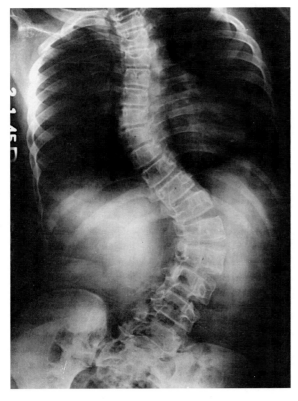

Fig. 8-156 PA thoracic and lumbar spine with right hip elevated.

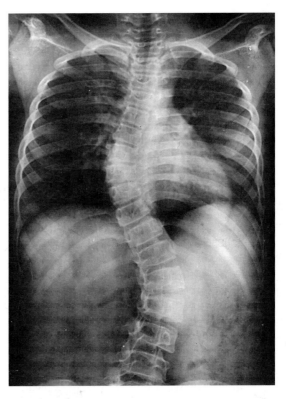

Fig. 8-157 PA thoracic and lumbar spine for scoliosis, prone.

AP PROJECTION
R and L bending

Image receptor: 24 × 30 cm (10 × 12 inch) or 35 × 43 cm (14 × 17 inch) lengthwise for each exposure

Position of patient
- Place the patient in the supine position, and center the midsagittal plane of the body to the midline of the grid.

Position of part
- Make the first radiograph with maximum right bending, and make the second radiograph with maximum left bending.
- To obtain equal bending force throughout the spine, cross the patient's leg on the opposite side to be flexed over the other leg. For example, a right bending requires the left leg to be crossed over the right.
- Move both of the patient's heels toward the side that is flexed. Immobilize the heels with sandbags.
- Move the shoulders directly lateral as far as possible without rotating the pelvis (Fig. 8-158).
- After the patient is in position, apply a compression band to prevent movement.
- *Shield gonads.*
- *Respiration:* Suspend.

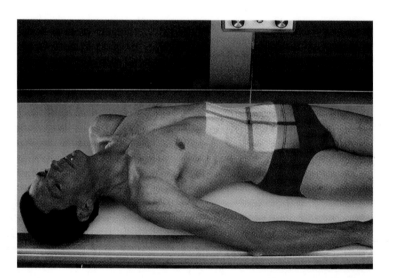

Fig. 8-158 AP lumbar spine, right bending.

Lumbar Spine: Spinal Fusion

Central ray

- Perpendicular to the level of the third lumbar vertebra, 1 to 1½ inches (2.5 to 3.8 cm) above the iliac crest on the midsagittal plane
- Center the cassette to the central ray

Structures shown

The resulting images show AP projections of the lumbar vertebrae, made in maximum right and left lateral flexion (Figs. 8-159 and 8-160). These studies are employed in patients with early scoliosis to determine the presence of structural change when bending to the right and left. The studies are also used to localize a herniated disk as shown by limitation of motion at the site of the lesion and to demonstrate whether there is motion in the area of a spinal fusion. The latter examination is usually performed 6 months after the fusion operation.

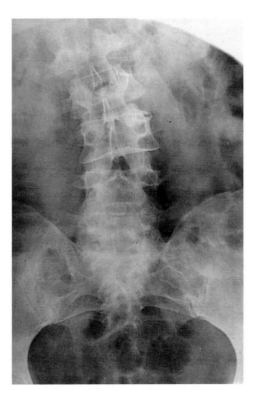

Fig. 8-159 AP lumbar spine, right bending spinal fusion series.

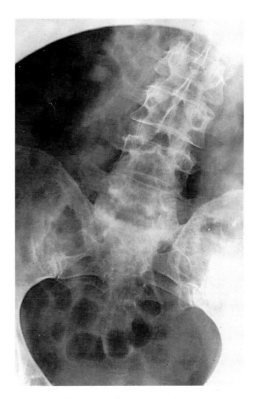

Fig. 8-160 AP lumbar spine, left bending spinal fusion series.

LATERAL PROJECTION
R or L position
Hyperflexion and hyperextension

Image receptor: 35 × 43 cm (14 × 17 inch) lengthwise for each exposure

Position of patient

- Adjust the patient in a lateral recumbent position.
- Center the midcoronal plane to the midline of the grid.

Position of part

- For the first radiograph, have the patient lean forward and draw the thighs up to forcibly flex the spine as much as possible (Fig. 8-161).
- For the second radiograph, have the patient lean the thorax backward and posteriorly extend the thighs and limbs as much as possible (Fig. 8-162).
- After the patient is in position, apply a compression band across the pelvis to prevent movement.
- Center the cassette at the level of the spinal fusion.
- *Shield gonads.*
- *Respiration:* Suspend.

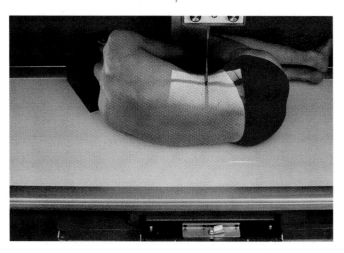

Fig. 8-161 Hyperflexion position.

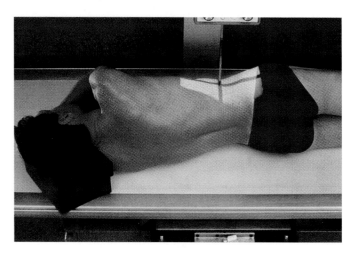

Fig. 8-162 Hyperextension position.

Vertebral column

Lumbar Spine: Spinal Fusion

Central ray
- Perpendicular to the spinal fusion area or L3

Structures shown
The resulting images show two lateral projections of the spine made in hyperflexion (Fig. 8-163) and hyperextension (Fig. 8-164) to determine whether motion is present in the area of a spinal fusion or to localize a herniated disk as shown by limitation of motion at the site of the lesion.

The following should be clearly demonstrated:
- Site of the spinal fusion in the center of the radiograph
- No rotation of the vertebral column (posterior margins of the vertebral bodies are superimposed)
- Hyperflexion and hyperextension identification markers correctly used for each respective projection

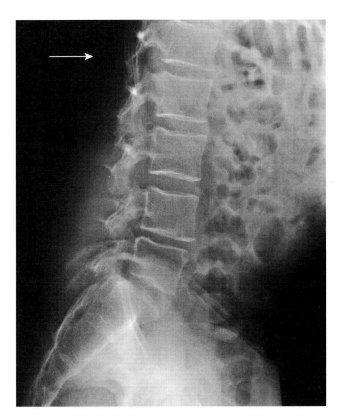

Fig. 8-163 Lateral with hyperflexion.

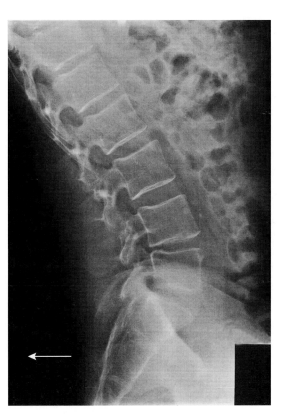

Fig. 8-164 Lateral with hyperextension.

9

BONY THORAX

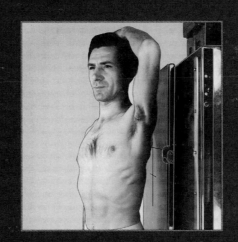

RIGHT: Axillary ribs, 1949.

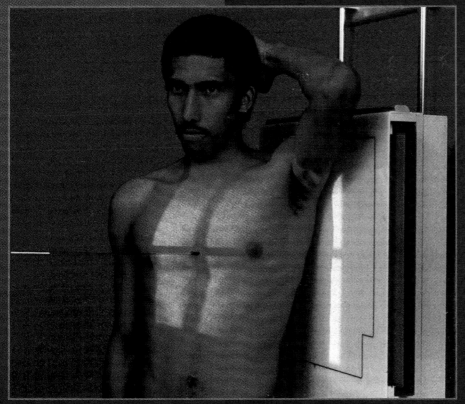

LEFT: AP oblique axillary ribs performed with close collimation, 1999.

PROJECTIONS, POSITIONS & METHODS

Page	Essential	Anatomy	Projection	Position	Method
476	✦	Sternum	PA oblique	RAO	
478		Sternum	PA oblique	Modified prone	MOORE
480	✦	Sternum	Lateral	R or L upright	
482	✦	Sternum	Lateral	R or L recumbent	
484	✦	Sternoclavicular articulations	PA		
485	✦	Sternoclavicular articulations	PA oblique	RAO or LAO	BODY ROTATION
486		Sternoclavicular articulations	PA oblique	RAO or LAO	CENTRAL RAY ANGULATION
488		Sternoclavicular articulations	Axiolateral		KURZBAUER
494	✦	Upper anterior ribs	PA		
496	✦	Posterior ribs	AP		
498	✦	Ribs: *axillary*	AP oblique	RPO or LPO	
500	✦	Ribs: *axillary*	PA oblique	RAO or LAO	
502		Costal joints	AP axial		

The icons in the Essential column indicate projections that are frequently performed in the United States and Canada. Students should be competent in these projections.

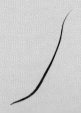

Bony Thorax

The *bony thorax* supports the walls of the pleural cavity and diaphragm used in respiration. The thorax is constructed so that the volume of the thoracic cavity can be varied during respiration. The thorax also serves to protect the heart and lungs.

The bony thorax is formed by the sternum, the 12 pairs of ribs, and the 12 thoracic vertebrae. The bony thorax protects the heart and lungs. Conical in shape, the bony thorax is narrower above than below, more wide than deep, and longer posteriorly than anteriorly.

Sternum

The *sternum,* or breastbone, is directed anteriorly and inferiorly and is centered over the midline of the anterior thorax (Figs. 9-1 to 9-3). A narrow, flat bone about 6 inches (15 cm) in length, the sternum consists of three parts: manubrium, body, and xiphoid process. The sternum supports the clavicles at the superior manubrial angles and provides attachment to the costal cartilages of the first seven pairs of ribs at the lateral borders.

The *manubrium,* the superior portion of the sternum, is quadrilateral in shape and is the widest portion of the sternum. At its center the superior border of the manubrium has an easily palpable concavity termed the *jugular notch.* In the upright position the jugular notch of the average person lies anterior to the interspace between the second and third thoracic vertebrae. The manubrium slants laterally and posteriorly on each side of the jugular notch, and an oval articular facet called

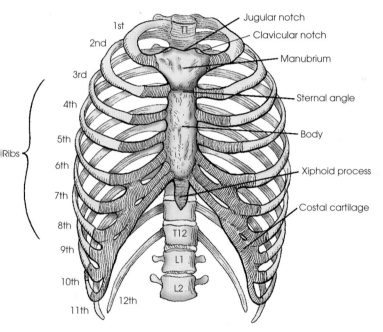

Fig. 9-1 Anterior aspect of bony thorax.

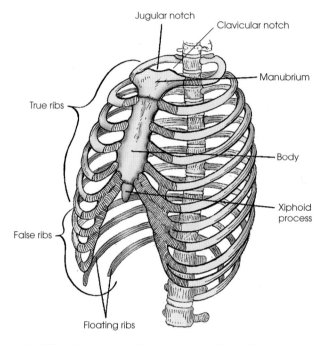

Fig. 9-2 Anterolateral oblique aspect of bony thorax.

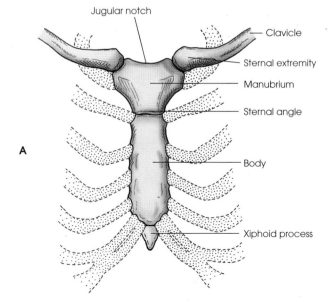

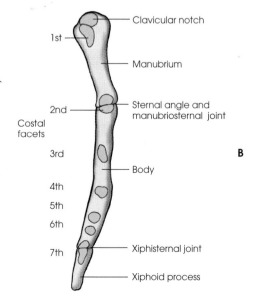

Fig. 9-3 A, Anterior aspect of sternum and sternoclavicular joints, B, Lateral sternum.

the *clavicular notch* articulates with the sternal extremity of the clavicle. On the lateral borders of the manubrium, immediately below the articular notches for the clavicles, are shallow depressions for the attachment of the cartilages of the first pair of ribs.

The *body* is the longest part of the sternum (4 inches [10.2 cm]) and is joined to the manubrium at the *sternal angle,* an obtuse angle that lies at the level of the junction of the second costal cartilage. Both the manubrium and the body contribute to the attachment of the second costal cartilage. The succeeding five pairs of costal cartilages are attached to the lateral borders of the body. The sternal angle is palpable; in the normally formed thorax, it lies anterior to the interspace between the fourth and fifth thoracic vertebrae when the body is upright.

The *xiphoid process,* the distal and smallest part of the sternum, is cartilaginous in early life and partially or completely ossifies, particularly the superior portion, in later life. The xiphoid process is variable in shape and often deviates from the midline of the body. In the normal thorax, the xiphoid process lies over the tenth thoracic vertebra and serves as a useful bony landmark for locating the superior portion of the liver and the inferior border of the heart.

Ribs

The 12 pairs of ribs are numbered consecutively superiorly to inferiorly (see Figs. 9-1, 9-2, and 9-4). The rib number corresponds to the thoracic vertebra to which it attaches. Each rib is a long, narrow, curved bone with an anteriorly attached piece of hyaline cartilage, the *costal cartilage.* The costal cartilages of the first through seventh ribs attach directly to the sternum. The costal cartilages of the eighth through tenth ribs attach to the costal cartilage of the seventh rib. The ribs are situated in an oblique plane slanting anteriorly and inferiorly so that their anterior ends lie 3 to 5 inches (7.6 to 12.5 cm) below the level of their vertebral ends. The degree of obliquity gradually increases from the first to the ninth rib and then decreases to the twelfth rib. The first seven ribs are called *true ribs* because they attach directly to the sternum. Ribs 8 to 12 are called *false ribs* because they do not attach directly to the sternum. The last two ribs (eleventh and twelfth ribs) are often called *floating ribs* because they are attached only to the vertebrae. The spaces between the ribs are referred to as the *intercostal spaces.*

The ribs vary in breadth and length. The first rib is the shortest and broadest; the breadth gradually decreases to the twelfth rib, the narrowest rib. The length increases from the first to the seventh rib and then gradually decreases to the twelfth rib.

A typical rib consists of a *head,* a flattened *neck,* a *tubercle,* and a *body* (Figs. 9-5 and 9-6). The ribs have *facets* on their heads for articulation with the vertebrae. On some ribs, the facet is divided into a superior and inferior portion for articulation with demifacets on the vertebral bodies. The tubercle also contains a facet for articulation with the transverse process of the vertebra. The eleventh and twelfth ribs do not have a neck or tubercular facets. The two ends of a rib are termed the *vertebral end* and the *sternal end.*

From the point of articulation with the vertebral body, the rib projects posteriorly at an oblique angle to the point of articulation with the transverse process. The rib turns laterally to the *angle* of the body, where the bone arches anteriorly, medially, and inferiorly in an oblique plane. Located along the inferior and internal border of each rib is the *costal groove,* which contains costal arteries, veins, and nerves. Trauma to the ribs can damage these neurovascular structures, causing pain and hemorrhage.

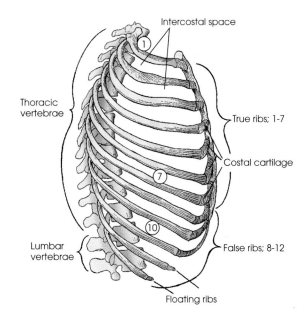

Fig. 9-4 Lateral aspect of bony thorax.

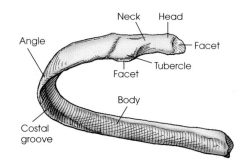

Fig. 9-5 Typical rib viewed from the posterior.

Bony Thorax Articulations

The eight joints of the bony thorax are summarized in Table 9-1. A detailed description follows.

The *sternoclavicular* joints are the only points of articulation between the upper limbs and the trunk (see Fig. 9-3). Formed by the articulation between the sternal extremity of the clavicles and the clavicular notches of the manubrium, these *synovial gliding* joints permit free movement (the gliding of one surface on the other). A circular disk of fibrocartilage is interposed between the articular ends of the bones in each joint, and the joints are enclosed in articular capsules.

TABLE 9-1
Joints of the bony thorax

| Joint | Structural classification | | Movement |
	Tissue	Type	
Sternoclavicular	Synovial	Gliding	Freely movable
Costovertebral:			
First through twelfth ribs	Synovial	Gliding	Freely movable
Costotransverse:			
First through tenth ribs	Synovial	Gliding	Freely movable
Costochondrial:			
First through tenth ribs	Cartilaginous	Synchondrosis	Immovable
Sternocostal:			
First rib	Cartilaginous	Synchondrosis	Immovable
Second through seventh ribs	Synovial	Gliding	Freely movable
Interchondral:			
Sixth through ninth ribs	Synovial	Gliding	Freely movable
Ninth through tenth ribs	Fibrous	Syndesmosis	Slightly movable
Manubriosternal	Cartilaginous	Symphysis	Slightly movable
Xiphisternal	Cartilaginous	Synchondrosis	Immovable

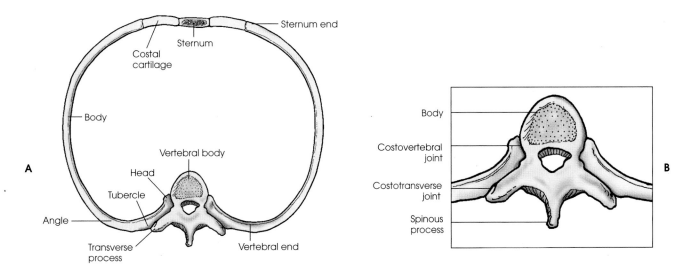

Fig. 9-6 A, Superior aspect of rib articulating with thoracic vertebra and sternum. **B,** Enlarged image of costovertebral articulations.

Posteriorly, the head of a rib is closely bound to the demifacets of two adjacent vertebral bodies to form a *synovial gliding* articulation called the *costovertebral* joint (see Figs. 9-6 and 9-7, *A*). The first, tenth, eleventh, and twelfth ribs each articulate with only one vertebral body.

The tubercle of a rib articulates with the anterior surface of the transverse process of the lower vertebra at the *costotransverse joint,* and the head of the rib articulates at the costovertebral joint. The head of the rib also articulates with the body of the same vertebra and articulates with the vertebra directly above. The costotransverse articulation is also a *synovial glid-*

ing articulation. The articulations between the tubercles of the ribs and the transverse processes of the vertebrae permit only superior and inferior movements of the first six pairs. Greater freedom of movement is permitted in the succeeding four pairs.

Costochondral articulations are found between the anterior extremities of the ribs and the costal cartilages (Fig. 9-7, *B*). These articulations are *cartilaginous synchondrosis* and allow no movement. The articulations between the costal cartilages of the true ribs and the sternum are called *sternocostal* joints. The first pair of ribs, rigidly attached to the sternum, form the first sternocostal joint. This is a *cartilaginous synchondrosis* type of joint, which allows no movement. The second through seventh sternocostal joints are considered *synovial gliding* joints and are freely movable. *Interchondral* joints are found between the costal cartilages of the sixth and seventh, seventh and eighth, and eighth and ninth ribs (Fig. 9-7, *C*). These interchondral joints are *synovial gliding* articulations. The interchondral articulation between the ninth and tenth ribs is *fibrous syndemosis* and only slightly movable.

The *manubriosternal* joint is *cartilaginous symphysis,* and the *xiphisternal* joints are *cartilaginous synchondrosis* joints that allow very little or no movement (Fig. 9-3, *B* and 9-7, *B* and *C*).

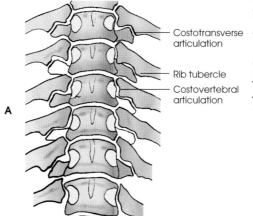

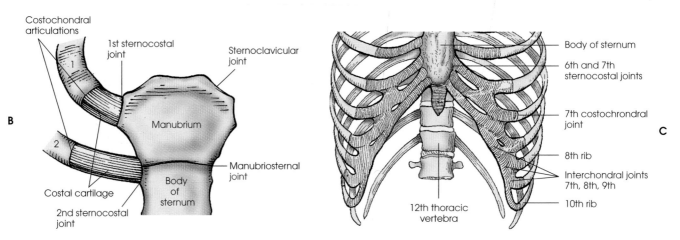

Fig. 9-7 Rib articulations. **A,** Anterior aspect of thoracic spine, showing costovertebral articulations. **B,** Anterior aspect of manubrium, sternum, and first two ribs, showing articulations. **C,** Lower sternum and ribs, showing intercostal, chondrocostal, and sternocostal joints.

RESPIRATORY MOVEMENT

The normal oblique orientation of the ribs changes very little during quiet respiratory movements; however, the degree of obliquity *decreases* with deep *inspiration* and *increases* with deep *expiration*. The first pair of ribs, which are rigidly attached to the manubrium, rotate at their vertebral ends and move with the sternum as one structure during respiratory movements.

On deep inspiration the anterior ends of the ribs are carried anteriorly, superiorly, and laterally, while their necks are rotated inferiorly (Fig. 9-8, *A*). On deep expiration the anterior ends are carried inferiorly, posteriorly, and medially, while the necks are rotated superiorly (Fig. 9-8, *B*). The last two pairs of ribs are depressed and held in position by the action of the diaphragm when the anterior ends of the upper ribs are elevated during respiration.

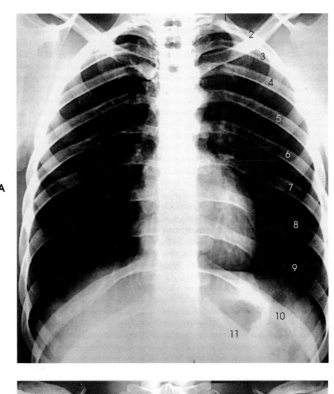

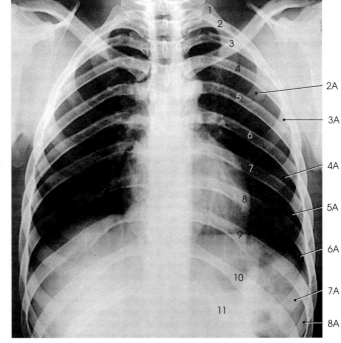

Fig. 9-8 Respiratory lung movement. **A,** Full inspiration with the posterior ribs numbered. **B,** Full expiration with the ribs numbered. The anterior ribs are labeled with a suffix.

DIAPHRAGM

The ribs located above the diaphragm are best examined radiographically through the air-filled lungs, whereas the ribs situated below the diaphragm must be examined through the upper abdomen. Because of the difference in penetration required for the two regions, the position and respiratory excursion of the diaphragm play a large role in radiography of the ribs.

The position of the diaphragm varies with body habitus: it is at a higher level in hypersthenic patients and at a lower level in hyposthenic patients (Fig. 9-9). In sthenic patients of average size and shape, the right side of the diaphragm arches posteriorly from the level of about the sixth or seventh costal cartilage to the level of the ninth or tenth thoracic vertebra when the body is in the upright position. The left side of the diaphragm lies at a slightly lower level. Because of the oblique location of both the ribs and the diaphragm, several pairs of ribs appear, on radiographs, to lie partly above and partly below the diaphragm.

The position of the diaphragm changes considerably with the body position, reaching its lowest level when the body is upright and its highest level when the body is supine. For this reason it is desirable to place the patient in the upright position for examination of the ribs above the diaphragm and in a recumbent position for examination of the ribs below the diaphragm.

The respiratory movement of the diaphragm averages about $1\frac{1}{2}$ inches (3.8 cm) between deep inspiration and deep expiration. The movement is less in hypersthenic patients and more in hyposthenic patients. Deeper inspiration or expiration, and therefore greater depression or elevation of the diaphragm, is achieved on the second respiratory movement than on the first. This greater movement should be taken into consideration when the ribs that lie at the diaphragmatic level are examined.

When the body is placed in the supine position, the anterior ends of the ribs are displaced superiorly, laterally, and posteriorly. For this reason the anterior ends of the ribs are less sharply visualized when the patient is radiographed in the supine position.

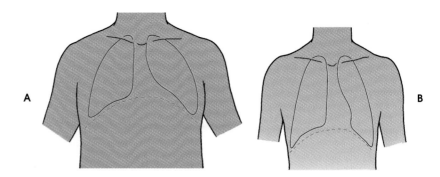

Fig. 9-9 Diaphragm position and body habitus. **A,** A hypersthenic patient has a higher positioned diaphragm. **B,** A hyposthenic patient has a lower positioned diaphragm.

BODY POSITION

Although in rib examinations it is desirable to take advantage of the effect that body position has on the position of the diaphragm, the effect is not of sufficient importance to justify subjecting a patient to a painful change from the upright position to the recumbent position or vice versa. Even minor rib injuries are painful, and slight movement frequently causes the patient considerable distress. Therefore, unless the change in position can be effected with a tilting radiographic table, patients with recent rib injury should be examined in the position in which they arrive in the radiology department. The ambulatory patient can be positioned for recumbent images with a minimum of discomfort by bringing the tilt table to the vertical position for each positioning change. The patient stands on the footboard, is comfortably adjusted, and is then lowered to the horizontal position.

TRAUMA PATIENTS

The first and usually the only requirement in the initial radiographic examination of a patient who has sustained severe trauma to the rib cage is to take AP and lateral projections of the chest. These projections are obtained not only to demonstrate the site and extent of rib injury but also to investigate the possibility of injury to the underlying structures by depressed rib fractures. Patients are examined in the position in which they arrive, usually recumbent on a stretcher. The recumbent position is necessary to demonstrate the presence of air or fluid levels using the decubitus technique.

SUMMARY OF ANATOMY*

Bony thorax	Ribs	Bony thorax articulations
sternum	costal cartilage	sternoclavicular
ribs (12)	true ribs	costovertebral
thoracic spine (12)	false ribs	costotransverse
	floating ribs	costochondral
Sternum	intercostal spaces	sternocostal
manubrium	head	interchondral
jugular notch	neck	manubriosternal
clavicular notch	tubercle	xiphisternal
body	body	
sternal angle	facets	
xiphoid process	vertebral end	
	sternal end	
	angle	
	costal groove	

*See *Addendum* at the end of the volume for a summary of the changes in the anatomic terms used in this edition.

Sternum

The position of the sternum with respect to the denser thoracic structures, both bony and soft, makes it one of the more difficult structures to radiograph satisfactorily. Few problems are involved in obtaining a lateral projection, but because of the location of the sternum directly anterior to the thoracic spine, an AP or PA projection provides little useful diagnostic information. To separate the vertebrae and sternum, it is necessary to rotate the body from the prone position or to angle the central ray medially. The exact degree of required angulation depends on the depth of the chest, with deep chests requiring less angulation than shallow chests (Fig. 9-10 and Table 9-2).

Angulation of the body or the central ray to project the sternum to the right of the thoracic vertebrae clears the sternum of the vertebrae but superimposes it over the posterior ribs and the lung markings (Fig. 9-11). If the sternum is projected to the left of the thoracic vertebrae, it is also projected over the heart and other mediastinal structures (Fig. 9-12). The superimposition of the homogeneous density of the heart can be used to advantage (compare Figs. 9-11 and 9-12).

The pulmonary structures, particularly in elderly persons and heavy smokers, can cast confusing markings over the sternum unless the motion of *shallow* breathing is used to eliminate them. If motion is desired, the exposure time should be long enough to cover several phases of shallow respiration (Figs. 9-13 and 9-14). The milliampere (mA) must be relatively low to achieve the desired milliampere-second (mAs).

If the female patient has large, pendulous breasts, they should be drawn to the sides and held in position with a wide bandage to prevent them from overlapping the sternum and to position the sternum closer to the cassette. This is particularly important in the lateral projection, in which the breast can obscure the inferior portion of the sternum.

Radiation Protection

Protection of the patient from unnecessary radiation is a professional responsibility of the radiographer (see Chapters 1 and 2 for specific guidelines). In this chapter the *Shield gonads* statement indicates that the patient is to be protected from unnecessary radiation by restricting the radiation beam using proper collimation. In addition, the placement of lead shielding between the gonads and the radiation source is appropriate when the clinical objectives of the examination are not compromised.

TABLE 9-2

Sternum: thickness and central ray angulation

Depth of thorax (cm)	Degree of tube angulation
15	22
16.5	21
18	20
19.5	19
21	18
22.5	17
24	16
25.5	15
27	14
28.5	13
30	12

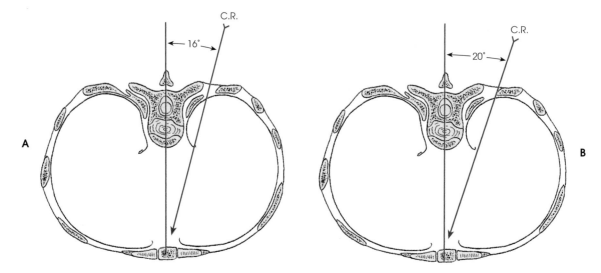

Fig. 9-10 A, Drawing of 24-cm chest. **B,** Drawing of 18-cm chest.

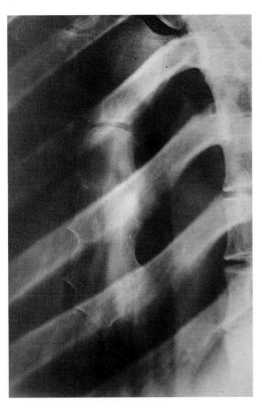

Fig. 9-11 PA oblique sternum, LAO position.

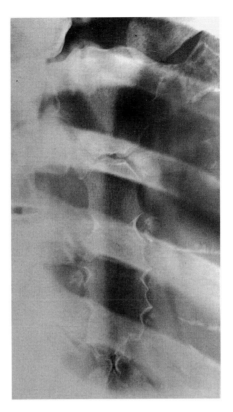

Fig. 9-12 PA oblique sternum, RAO position.

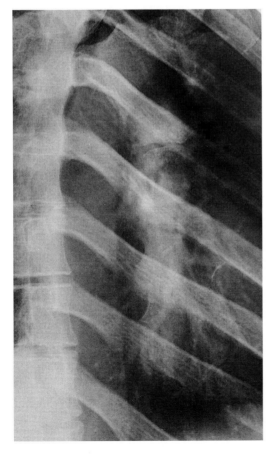

Fig. 9-13 Suspended respiration.

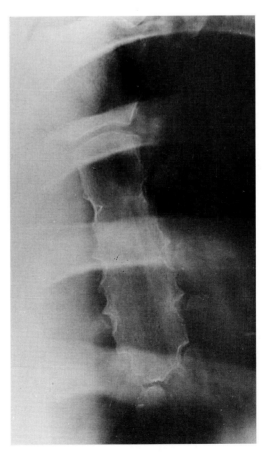

Fig. 9-14 Shallow breathing during exposure.

☀ PA OBLIQUE PROJECTION
RAO position

Image receptor: 24 × 30 cm (10 × 12 inch) lengthwise

SID: A 30-inch source-to-image receptor distance (SID) is recommended to blur the posterior ribs.

Position of patient
- With the patient prone, adjust the body into a right anterior oblique (RAO) position to use the heart for contrast as previously described.
- Have the patient support the body on the forearm and flexed knee.

Position of part
- Adjust the elevation of the left shoulder and hip so that the thorax is rotated just enough to prevent superimposition of the vertebrae and sternum.
- Estimate the amount of rotation with sufficient accuracy by placing one hand on the patient's sternum and the other hand on the thoracic vertebrae to act as guides while adjusting the degree of obliquity. The average rotation will be about 15 to 20 degrees (Fig. 9-15).
- Align the patient's body so that the long axis of the sternum is centered to the midline of the grid.
- Center the cassette midway between the jugular notch and the xiphoid process at the approximate level of the seventh thoracic vertebra.
- *Shield gonads.*
- *Respiration:* When breathing motion is to be used, instruct the patient to take slow, shallow breaths during the exposure. When a short exposure time is to be used, instruct the patient to suspend breathing at the end of expiration to obtain a more uniform density.

NOTE: On trauma patients, obtain this projection with the patient supine, and use the LPO position and an AP oblique projection.

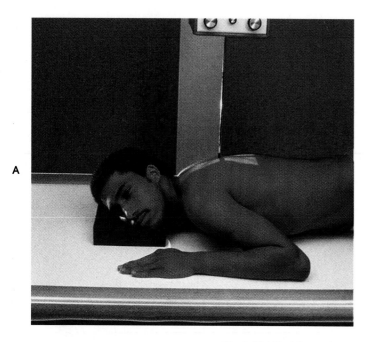

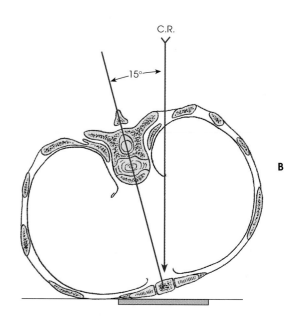

Fig. 9-15 PA oblique sternum, RAO position.

Central ray

- Perpendicular to the midsternum and entering the *elevated side* of the posterior thorax at the level of the seventh thoracic vertebra and approximately 1 inch (2.5 cm) lateral to the midsagittal plane

Structures shown

This image shows a slightly oblique projection of the sternum (Fig. 9-16). The detail demonstrated depends largely on the technical procedure employed. If breathing motion is used, the pulmonary markings will be obliterated.

EVALUATION CRITERIA

The following should be clearly demonstrated:

- Entire sternum from jugular notch to tip of the xiphoid process
- Reasonably good visibility of the sternum through the thorax, including blurred pulmonary markings if a breathing technique was used
- Minimally rotated sternum and thorax, as demonstrated by the following:
  □ Sternum projected just free of superimposition from vertebral column
  □ Minimally obliqued vertebrae to prevent excessive rotation of the sternum
  □ Lateral portion of the manubrium and sternoclavicular joint free of superimposition by the vertebrae
- Sternum projected over the heart

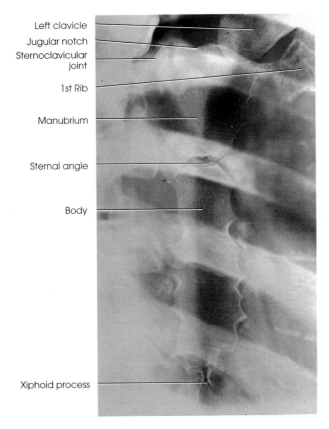

Left clavicle
Jugular notch
Sternoclavicular joint
1st Rib
Manubrium
Sternal angle
Body
Xiphoid process

Fig. 9-16 PA oblique sternum, RAO position.

PA OBLIQUE PROJECTION
MOORE METHOD[1]
Modified prone position

Image receptor: 24 × 30 cm (10 × 12 inch) lengthwise

SID: A 30-inch (76-cm) SID is recommended. This short distance assists in blurring the posterior ribs.

Radiography of the sternum can be difficult to perform on an ambulatory patient who is having acute pain. The alternative positioning method described by Moore[1] uses a modified prone position that makes it possible to produce a high-quality sternum image in a more comfortable manner for the patient.

[1]Moore TF: An alternative to the standard radiographic position for the sternum, *Radiol Technol* 60:133, 1988.

Position of patient
- Before positioning the patient, place the cassette *crosswise* in the Bucky tray. Place the x-ray tube at a 30-inch (76-cm) SID, angle it 25 degrees, and direct the central ray to the center of the cassette. The x-ray tube is positioned over the patient's right side.
- Place a marker on the tabletop near the patient's head to indicate the exact center of the cassette.
- Have the patient stand at the *side* of the radiographic table directly in *front* of the Bucky tray.
- Ask the patient to bend at the waist, and place the sternum in the center of the table directly over the prepositioned cassette.

Position of part
- Place the patient's arms above the shoulders and the palms down on the table. The arms then act as a support for the side of the head (Fig. 9-17, *left*).
- Ensure that the patient is in a true prone position and that the midsternal area is at the center of the radiographic table.
- *Shield gonads.*
- *Respiration:* A shallow breathing technique produces the best results. Instruct the patient to take slow, shallow breaths during the exposure. A low mA setting and an exposure time of 1 to 3 seconds is recommended. When a low mA setting and long exposure time technique cannot be used, instruct the patient to suspend respiration at the end of expiration to obtain a more uniform density.

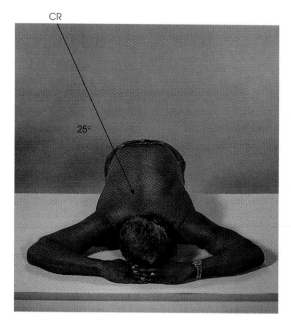
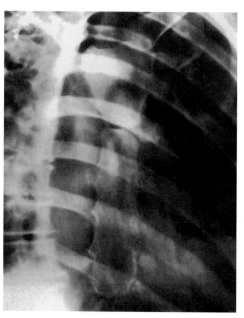

Fig. 9-17 PA oblique projection: Moore method.

Central ray

- The central ray will already have been angled 25 degrees and centered to the cassette. If patient positioning is accurate, the central ray enters at the level of T7 and approximately 2 inches (5 cm) to the right of the spine. This angulation places the sternum over the lung to maintain maximum contrast of the sternum.
- The x-ray tube angulation can be adjusted for extremely large or small patients. Large patients require *less* angulation, and thin patients require *more* than the standard 25-degree angle.

Structures shown

This image shows a slightly oblique projection of the sternum (Fig. 9-17, *right*). The degree of detail demonstrated depends largely on the technique used. If a breathing technique is used, the pulmonary markings will be obliterated.

The following should be clearly demonstrated:

- Entire sternum from the jugular notch to the tip of the xiphoid process
- Reasonably good visibility of the sternum through the thorax
- Blurred pulmonary markings if a breathing technique was used
- Blurred posterior ribs if a reduced SID was used
- Sternum projected free of superimposition from the vertebral column

☀ LATERAL PROJECTION
R or L position
Upright

Image receptor: 24 × 30 cm (10 × 12 inch) lengthwise

SID: Use a 72-inch (183-cm) SID to reduce magnification and distortion of the sternum.

Position of patient
- Place the patient in a lateral position, either seated or standing, before a vertical grid device.

Position of part
- Have the patient sit or stand straight.
- Rotate the shoulders posteriorly, and have the patient lock the hands behind the back.
- Center the sternum to the midline of the grid.
- Being careful to keep the midsagittal plane of the body vertical, place the patient close enough to the grid so that the shoulder can be rested firmly against it.
- Adjust the patient in a true lateral position so that the broad surface of the sternum is perpendicular to the plane of the cassette (Fig. 9-18).
- Large breasts on female patients should be drawn to the sides and held in position with a wide bandage so that their shadows do not obscure the lower portion of the sternum.
- Adjust the height of the cassette so that its upper border is $1\frac{1}{2}$ inches (3.8 cm) above the jugular notch.
- For a direct lateral projection of just the sternoclavicular region, center a vertically placed 8 × 10 inch (18 × 24 cm) cassette at the level of the jugular notch.
- *Shield gonads.*
- *Respiration:* Suspended deep inspiration. This provides sharper contrast between the posterior surface of the sternum and the adjacent structures.

Central ray
- Perpendicular to the center of the cassette and entering the lateral border of the midsternum

COMPUTED RADIOGRAPHY

Collimation must be very close to keep unnecessary radiation from reaching the cassette phosphor.

Structures shown
A lateral image of the entire length of the sternum shows the superimposed sternoclavicular joints and medial ends of the clavicles (Fig. 9-19, *A*). A lateral projection of only the sternoclavicular region is shown in Fig. 9-19, *B*.

EVALUATION CRITERIA
The following should be clearly demonstrated:
- Sternum in its entirety
- Manubrium free of superimposition by the soft tissue of the shoulders
- Sternum free of superimposition by the ribs
- Lower portion of the sternum unobscured by the breasts of a female patient (A second radiograph with increased penetration may be needed.)

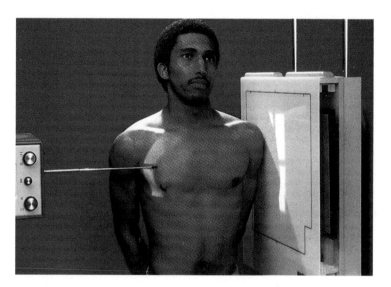

Fig. 9-18 Lateral sternum.

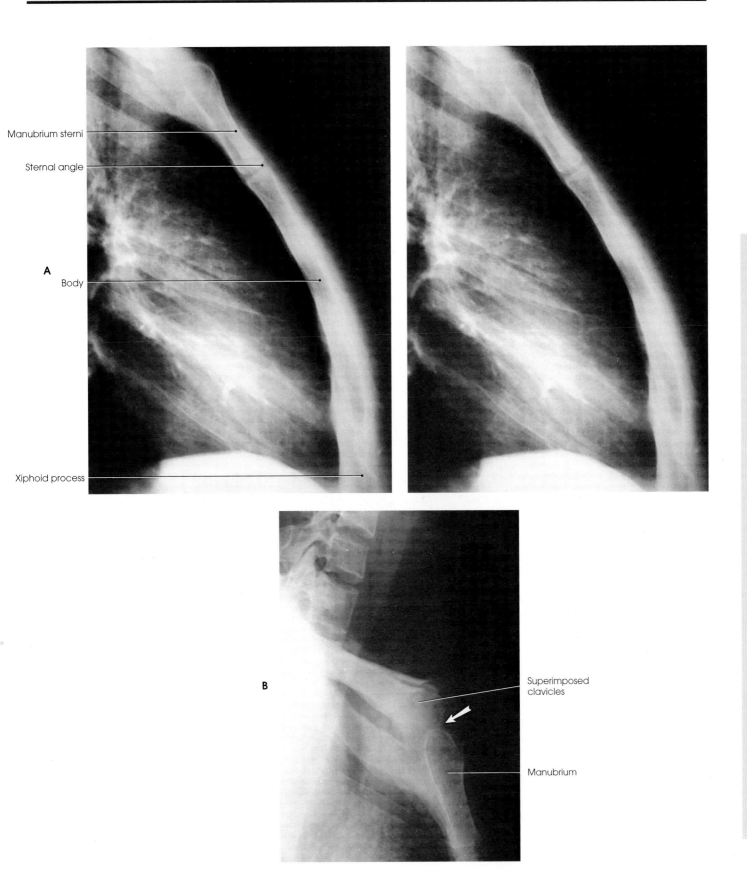

Manubrium sterni

Sternal angle

A

Body

Xiphoid process

B

Superimposed
clavicles

Manubrium

Fig. 9-19 A, Lateral sternum. **B,** Lateral sternoclavicular joint *(arrow).*

▲ LATERAL PROJECTION
R or L position
Recumbent

Image receptor: 24 × 30 cm (10 × 12 inch) lengthwise

SID: An SID of 72 inches (180 cm) is preferred. If this distance cannot be obtained with the overhead tube, the maximum allowed distance should be obtained.

Position of patient
- Place the patient in the lateral recumbent position.
- Flex the patient's hips and knees to a comfortable position.

Position of part
- Extend the patient's arms over the head to prevent them from overlapping the sternum.
- Rest the patient's head on the arms or on a pillow (Fig. 9-20).
- Place a support under the lower thoracic region to position the long axis of the sternum horizontally.
- Adjust the rotation of the patient's body so that the broad surface of the sternum is perpendicular to the plane of the cassette.
- Center the sternum to the midline of the grid.

- Apply a compression band across the hips for immobilization, if necessary.
- Adjust the height of the cassette so that its upper border is 1½ inches (3.8 cm) above the jugular notch.
- *Shield gonads.*
- *Respiration:* Suspend at the end of deep inspiration to obtain high contrast between the posterior surface of the sternum and the adjacent structures.

NOTE: Use the dorsal decubitus position for examination of a patient with severe injury. In this situation a grid-front cassette or a stationary grid should be used (Fig. 9-21). An SID of 72 inches (180 cm) can be used for this position.

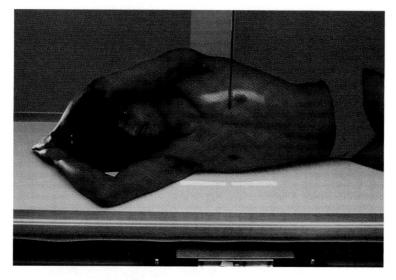

Fig. 9-20 Lateral sternum.

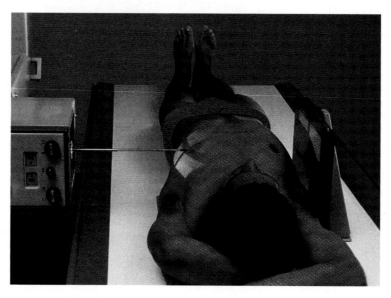

Fig. 9-21 Dorsal decubitus position for lateral sternum.

Central ray

- Perpendicular to the center of the cassette and entering the lateral border of the midsternum

COMPUTED RADIOGRAPHY

Collimation must be very close to keep unnecessary radiation from reaching the cassette phosphor.

Structures shown

The lateral aspect of the entire length of the sternum is shown (Fig. 9-22).

EVALUATION CRITERIA

The following should be clearly demonstrated:

- Lateral image of the sternum in its entirety
- Sternum free of superimposition by the soft tissues of the shoulders or arms
- Sternum free of superimposition by the ribs
- Inferior portion of the sternum unobscured by the breasts of a female patient (A second radiograph with increased penetration may be needed.)

Manubrium

Sternal angle

Body

Xiphoid process

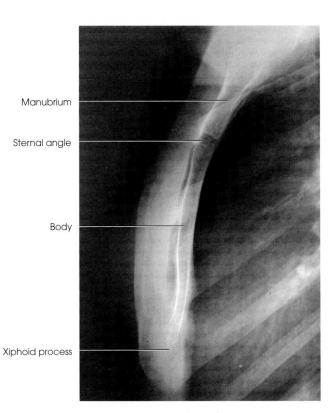
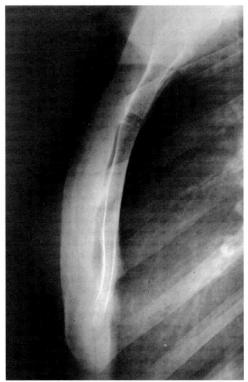

Fig. 9-22 Lateral sternum.

✹ PA PROJECTION

Image receptor: 8 × 10 inch (18 × 24 cm) crosswise

Position of patient
- Place the patient in the prone position.
- Center the midsagittal plane of the patient's body to the midline of the grid.
- Adapt the same procedure for use with the patient who is standing or seated upright.

Position of part
- Center the cassette at the level of the spinous process of the third thoracic vertebra, which lies posterior to the jugular notch.
- Place the patient's arms along the sides of the body with the palms facing upward.
- Adjust the shoulders to lie in the same transverse plane.
- For a bilateral examination, rest the patient's head on the chin and adjust it so that the midsagittal plane is vertical.

- For a unilateral projection, ask the patient to turn the head to face the affected side and rest the cheek on the table (Fig. 9-23). Turning the head rotates the spine slightly away from the side being examined and thus provides better visualization of the lateral portion of the manubrium.
- *Shield gonads.*
- *Respiration:* Suspend at the end of expiration to obtain a more uniform density.

Central ray
- Perpendicular to the center of the cassette and entering T3

Structures shown
A PA projection demonstrates the sternoclavicular joints and the medial portions of the clavicles (Figs. 9-24 and 9-25).

EVALUATION CRITERIA

The following should be clearly demonstrated:
- Both sternoclavicular joints and the medial ends of the clavicles
- Sternoclavicular joints through the superimposing vertebral and rib shadows
- No rotation present on a bilateral examination; slight rotation present on a unilateral examination

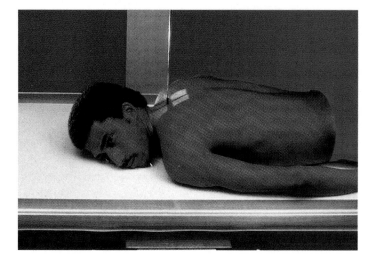

Fig. 9-23 Unilateral examination to demonstrate left sternoclavicular articulation.

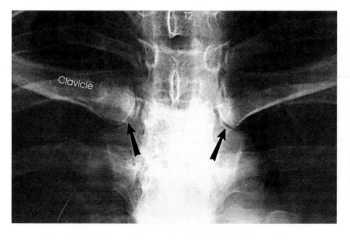

Fig. 9-24 Bilateral sternoclavicular joints *(arrows).*

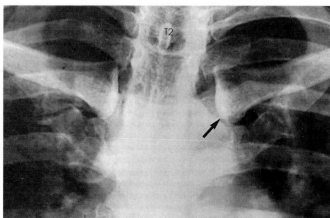

Fig. 9-25 Unilateral sternoclavicular joint *(arrow).*

Bony thorax

PA OBLIQUE PROJECTION
BODY ROTATION METHOD
RAO or LAO position

Image receptor: 8 × 10 inch (18 × 24 cm) crosswise

Position of patient
- Place the patient in a prone or seated-upright position.

Position of part
- Keeping the affected side adjacent to the cassette, position the patient at enough of an oblique angle to project the vertebrae well behind the sterno-clavicular joint closest to the cassette. The angle is usually about 10 to 15 degrees.
- Adjust the patient's position to center the joint to the midline of the grid.
- Adjust the shoulders to lie in the same transverse plane (Fig. 9-26).
- *Shield gonads.*
- *Respiration:* Suspend at the end of expiration to obtain a more uniform density.

Central ray
- Perpendicular to the sternoclavicular joint closest to the cassette. The central ray enters at the level of T2-T3 (about 3 inches [7.6 cm] distal to the vertebral prominens) and 1 to 2 inches (2.5 to 5 cm) lateral (toward the joint) from the midsagittal plane.
- Center the cassette to the central ray.

Structures shown
A slightly oblique image of the sterno-clavicular joint is demonstrated

EVALUATION CRITERIA
The following should be clearly demonstrated:
- Sternoclavicular joint of interest in the center of the radiograph, with the manubrium and the medial end of the clavicle included
- Open sternoclavicular joint space
- Sternoclavicular joint of interest directly in front of the vertebral column with minimal obliquity
- Reasonably good visibility of the sternoclavicular joint through the superimposing rib and lung fields

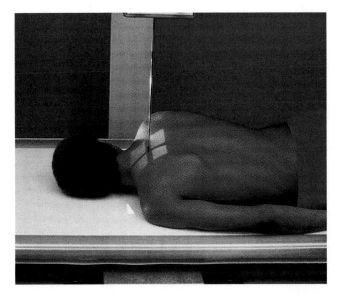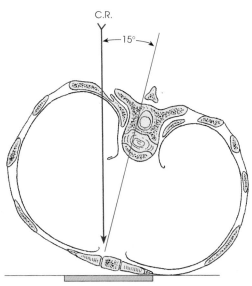

Fig. 9-26 PA oblique sternoclavicular joint, LAO position: body rotation method.

PA OBLIQUE PROJECTION
CENTRAL RAY ANGULATION
METHOD
Non-Bucky

Image Receptor: 8 × 10 inch (18 × 24 cm) lengthwise

NOTE: For this projection, the joint is closer to the cassette and less distortion is obtained than when the previously described body rotation method is used. A grid cassette placed on the tabletop also enables the joint to be projected with minimal distortion.

Position of patient
• Place the patient in the prone position on a grid cassette positioned directly under the upper chest.
• Center the grid to the level of the sternoclavicular joints.
• To avoid grid cutoff, place the grid on the radiographic table with its long axis running *perpendicular* to the long axis of the table.

Position of part
• Extend the patient's arms along the sides of the body with the palms of the hands facing upward.
• Adjust the shoulders to lie in the same transverse plane.
• Ask the patient to rest the head on the chin or to rotate the chin toward the side of the joint being radiographed (Fig. 9-27).

Central ray
• From the side opposite that being examined, direct to the midpoint of the cassette at an angle of 15 degrees toward the midsagittal plane. A small angle is satisfactory in examinations of sternoclavicular articulations because only a slight anteroposterior overlapping of the vertebrae and these joints occurs.
• The central ray should enter at the level of T2-T3 (about 3 inches [7.6 cm] distal to the vertebral prominens) and 1 to 2 inches (2.5 to 5 cm) lateral to the midsagittal plane.

Structures shown
A slightly oblique image of the sternoclavicular joint is demonstrated (Figs. 9-28 and 9-29).

EVALUATION CRITERIA
The following should be clearly demonstrated:
■ Sternoclavicular joint of interest in the center of the radiograph, with the manubrium and the medial end of the clavicle included
■ Open sternoclavicular joint space
■ Sternoclavicular joint of interest directly in front of the vertebral column with minimal obliquity
■ Reasonably good visibility of the sternoclavicular joint through the superimposing rib and lung fields

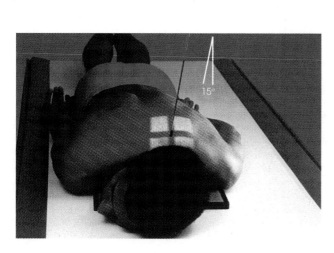
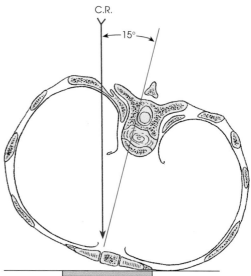

Fig. 9-27 PA oblique sternoclavicular joint: central ray angulation method.

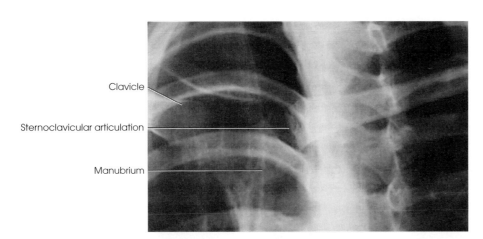

Clavicle

Sternoclavicular articulation

Manubrium

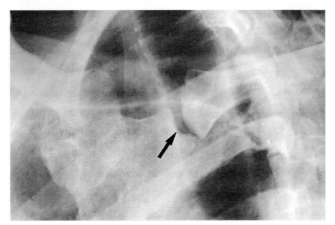

Fig. 9-28 PA oblique sternoclavicular joint, LAO position. The joint closest to cassette is shown *(arrow)*.

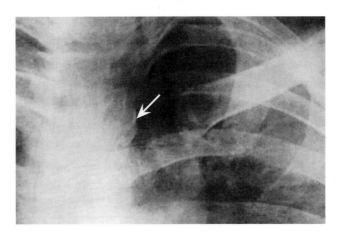

Fig. 9-29 Central ray angulation for sternoclavicular joint farthest from x-ray tube *(arrow)*.

AXIOLATERAL PROJECTION
KURZBAUER METHOD[1]

Image receptor: 8 × 10 inch (18 × 24 cm) lengthwise

Position of patient
- Have the patient lie in the lateral recumbent position on the affected side, with the sternoclavicular region centered to the midline of the grid.
- Flex the patient's hips and knees in a comfortable position.

---

[1]Kurzbauer R: The lateral projection in the roentgenography of the sternoclavicular articulation, *AJR* 56:104, 1946.

Position of part
- Have the patient fully extend the arm of the affected side and grasp the end of the radiographic table for support.
- Place the patient's other arm along the side of the body.
- Have the patient grasp the dorsal surface of the hip to hold the shoulder in a depressed position. The extension of the affected shoulder, along with the depression of the uppermost shoulder, prevents superimposition of the two articulations.
- Adjust the thorax to place the anterior surface of the manubrium perpendicular to the plane of the cassette (Figs. 9-30 and 9-31).
- Although the best result is obtained with the patient in the recumbent position, a comparable image can be made in the upright position if the patient cannot lie on the affected shoulder.
- *Shield gonads.*
- *Respiration:* Suspend at the end of full inspiration.

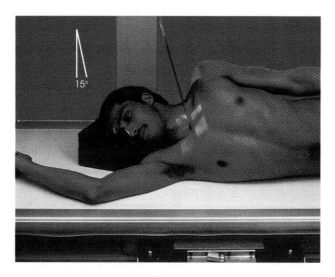

Fig. 9-30 Axiolateral sternoclavicular joint.

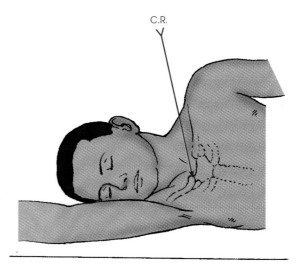

Fig. 9-31 Axiolateral sternoclavicular joint.

Sternoclavicular Articulations

Central ray

- Directed through the sternoclavicular articulation closest to the cassette at an angle of 15 degrees caudad.
- Center the cassette to the central ray.

Structures shown

This image shows an unobstructed axiolateral projection of the sternoclavicular articulation closest to the cassette (Fig. 9-32).

EVALUATION CRITERIA

The following should be clearly demonstrated:

- Sternoclavicular joint on affected side
- Sternoclavicular articulations, free of superimposition by the shoulders

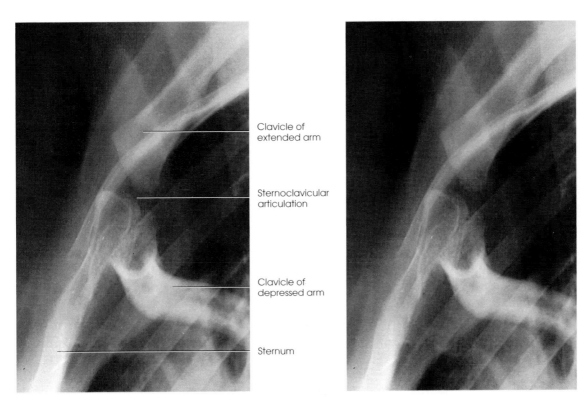

Clavicle of extended arm

Sternoclavicular articulation

Clavicle of depressed arm

Sternum

Fig. 9-32 Axiolateral sternoclavicular joint.

Ribs

In radiography of the ribs, a 35 × 43 cm (14 × 17 inch) cassette should be used to identify the ribs involved and to determine the extent of trauma or pathologic condition. A 28 × 36 cm (11 × 14 inch) cassette is often used with smaller patients. Projections can be made in recumbent and upright positions. If the area in question involves the first and last ribs, additional images may be required to better demonstrate the affected area (Fig. 9-33).

After the lesion is localized, the next step is to determine (1) the position required to place the affected rib region parallel with the plane of the cassette and (2) whether the radiograph should be made to include the ribs above or below the diaphragm.

The anterior portions of the ribs, usually referred to simply as the *anterior ribs*, are often examined with the patient facing the cassette for a PA projection (Fig. 9-34). The posterior portion of the ribs, or the *posterior ribs,* are more commonly radiographed with the patient facing the x-ray tube in the same manner as for an AP projection (Fig. 9-35).

The axillary portion of the ribs is best shown using an oblique projection. Because the lateral projection results in superimposition of the two sides, it is generally used only when fluid or air levels are evaluated after rib fractures.

When the ribs superimposed over the heart are involved, the body must be rotated to obtain a projection of the ribs free of the heart, or the radiographic exposure must be increased to compensate for the density of the heart. Although the anterior and posterior ends are superimposed, the left ribs are cleared of the heart when the LAO position (Fig. 9-36) or RPO position (Fig. 9-37) is used. These two body positions place the right-sided ribs parallel with the plane of the cassette and are reversed to obtain comparable projections of the left-sided ribs. Selection of technical factors that result in a short-scale radiograph are often used (about 70 kVp).

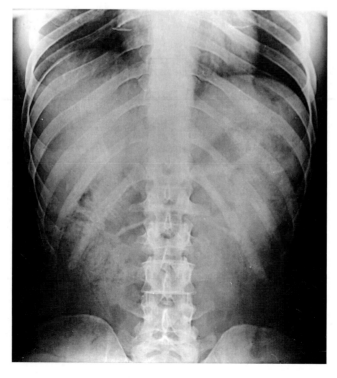

Fig. 9-33 AP lower ribs.

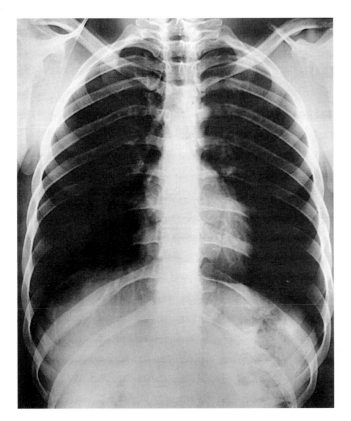

Fig. 9-34 PA ribs.

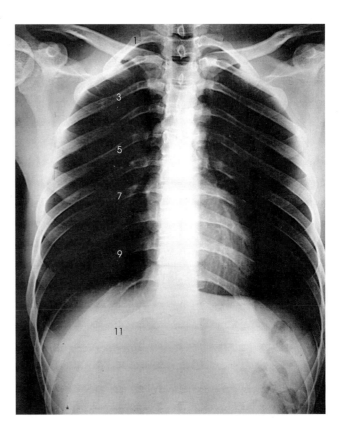

Fig. 9-35 AP upper ribs.

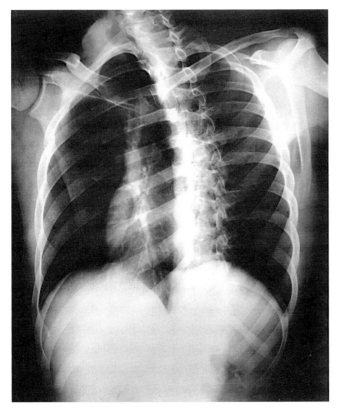

Fig. 9-36 PA oblique ribs, LAO position.

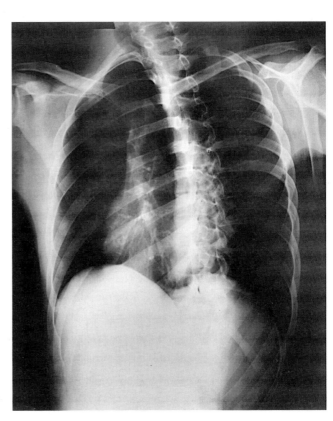

Fig. 9-37 AP oblique ribs, RPO position.

RESPIRATION

In radiography of the ribs the patient is usually examined with respiration suspended in either full inspiration or expiration. Occasionally, shallow breathing may be used to obliterate lung markings. If this technique is used, breathing must be shallow enough to ensure that the ribs are not elevated or depressed as described in the anatomy portion of this chapter. Examples of shallow breathing and suspended respiration are compared in Figs. 9-38 and 9-39.

Rib fractures can cause a great deal of pain and hemorrhage because of the closely related neurovascular structures. This situation commonly makes it difficult for the patient to breathe deeply for the required radiograph. Deeper inspiration will be attained if the patient fully understands the importance of expanding the lungs and if the exposure is made after the patient takes the second deep breath.

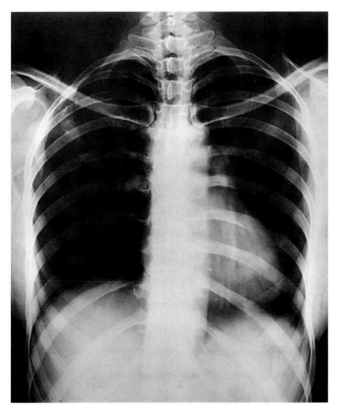

Fig. 9-38 Shallow breathing technique.

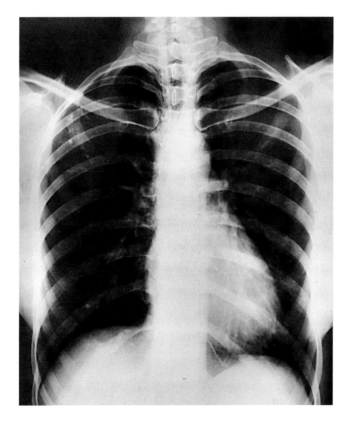

Fig. 9-39 Suspended respiration technique.

⚛ PA PROJECTION

Image receptor: 35 × 43 cm (14 × 17 inch) lengthwise

Position of patient
- Position the patient for a PA projection, either upright or recumbent.
- Because the diaphragm descends to its lowest level in the upright position, use the standing or seated-upright position for projections of the upper ribs when the patient's condition permits (Fig. 9-40). The upright position is also valuable for demonstrating fluid levels in the chest.

Position of part
- Center the midsagittal plane of the patient's body to the midline of the grid.
- To include the upper ribs, adjust the cassette position to project approximately 1½ inches (3.8 cm) above the upper border of the shoulders.
- Rest the patient's hands against the hips with the palms turned outward to rotate the scapulas away from the rib cage.
- Adjust the shoulders to lie in the same transverse plane.
- If the patient is prone, rest the head on the chin and adjust the midsagittal plane to be vertical (Fig. 9-41).
- To image affected ribs unilaterally, use a 30 × 35 cm (11 × 14 inch) cassette for contrast improvement.

- For hypersthenic patients with wide rib cages, include the entire lateral surface of the affected rib area on the radiograph. This may require moving the patient laterally to include all of the affected ribs.
- *Shield gonads.*
- *Respiration:* Suspend at *full inspiration* to depress the diaphragm as much as possible.

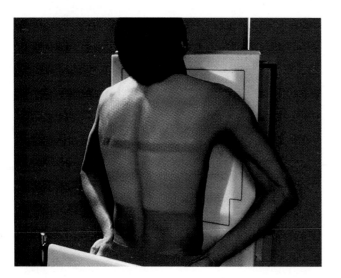

Fig. 9-40 PA ribs, upright position.

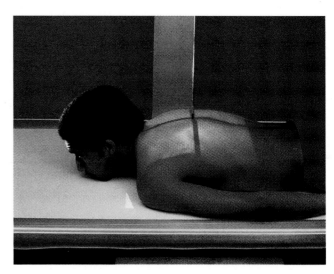

Fig. 9-41 PA ribs, recumbent position.

Upper Anterior Ribs

Central ray

- Perpendicular to the center of the cassette at the level of T7 for the upper ribs.
- A useful option for demonstrating the seventh, eighth, and ninth ribs is to angle the x-ray tube about 10 to 15 degrees caudad. This angulation aids in projecting the diaphragm below that of the affected ribs.

Structures shown

The PA projection best demonstrates the ribs above the diaphragm (Figs. 9-42 and 9-43).

EVALUATION CRITERIA

The following should be clearly demonstrated:

- First through ninth ribs in their entirety, with the posterior portions lying above the diaphragm
- First through seventh anterior ribs from both sides, in their entirety and above the diaphragm
- In a unilateral examination, ribs from the opposite side may not be entirely included
- Ribs visible through the lungs with sufficient contrast

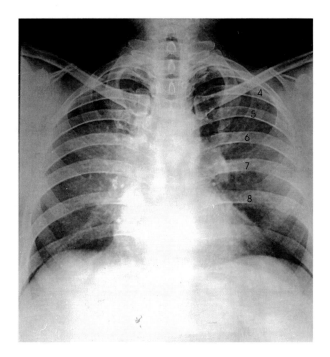

Fig. 9-42 PA ribs, normal centering.

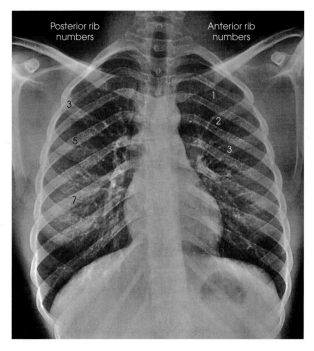

Fig. 9-43 PA ribs, with 10 to 15 degree caudal angulation.

☀ AP PROJECTION

Image receptor: 35 × 43 cm (14 × 17 inch) lengthwise

Position of patient
- Have the patient face the x-ray tube in either an upright or recumbent position.
- When the patient's condition permits, use the upright position to image ribs above the diaphragm and the supine position to image ribs below the diaphragm to permit gravity to assist in moving the patient's diaphragm.

Position of part
- Center the midsagittal plane of the patient's body to the midline of the grid.
Ribs above diaphragm
- Place the cassette lengthwise 1½ inches (3.8 cm) above the upper border of the *relaxed* shoulders.
- Rest the patient's hands, palms outward, against the hips. This position moves the scapula off the ribs. Alternatively, extend the arms to the vertical position with the hands under the head (Fig. 9-44).
- Adjust the patient's shoulders to lie in the same transverse plane, and rotate them forward to draw the scapulas away from the rib cage.
- *Shield gonads.*
- *Respiration:* Suspend at *full inspiration* to *depress* the diaphragm.

Ribs below diaphragm
- Place the cassette crosswise in the Bucky tray with the lower edge positioned at the level of the iliac crests. This positioning ensures inclusion of the lower ribs because of the divergent x-rays.
- Adjust the patient's shoulders to lie in the same transverse plane.
- Place the patient's arms in a comfortable position (Fig. 9-45).
- *Shield gonads.*
- *Respiration:* Suspend at *full expiration* to *elevate* the diaphragm.

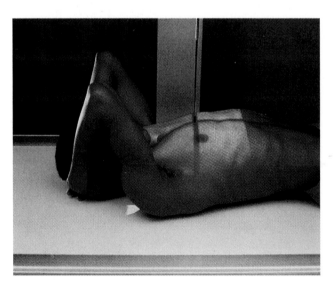

Fig. 9-44 AP ribs above diaphragm.

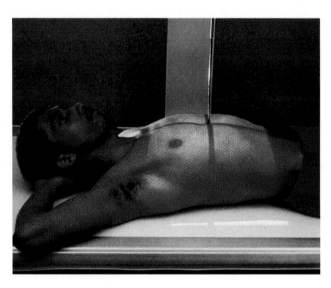

Fig. 9-45 AP ribs below diaphragm.

Posterior Ribs

Central ray

- Perpendicular to the cassette. If the cassette is positioned correctly, the central ray will be at the level of T7 for the upper projection. For the lower projection, the central ray will be at the level of T10 if the cassette is lengthwise and at T12 if the cassette is crosswise.

Structures shown

The AP projection shows the posterior ribs above or below the diaphragm, according to the region examined (Figs. 9-46 and 9-47).

EVALUATION CRITERIA

The following should be clearly demonstrated:

- For ribs above the diaphragm, first through tenth posterior ribs from both sides in their entirety
- For ribs below the diaphragm, eighth through twelfth posterior ribs on both sides in their entirety
- Ribs visible through the lungs or abdomen
- In a unilateral examination, ribs from the opposite side possibly not entirely included

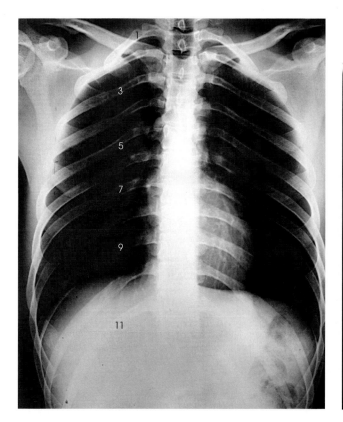

Fig. 9-46 AP ribs above diaphragm.

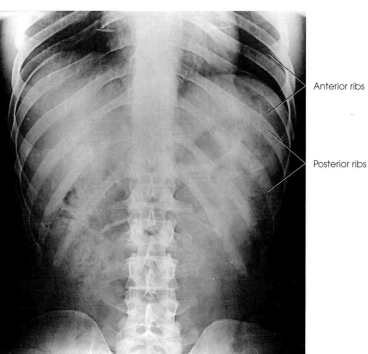

Anterior ribs

Posterior ribs

Fig. 9-47 AP lower ribs.

Axillary

✹ AP OBLIQUE PROJECTION
RPO or LPO position

Image receptor: 35 × 43 cm (14 × 17 inch) or 28 × 35 cm (11 × 14 inch) lengthwise

Position of patient
- Examine the patient in the upright or recumbent position.
- Unless contraindicated by the patient's condition, use the upright position to image ribs above the diaphragm and the recumbent position to image ribs below the diaphragm. Gravity assists by moving the diaphragm.

Position of part
- Position the patient's body for a 45-degree AP oblique projection using the RPO or LPO position. Place the *affected* side closest to the cassette.
- Center the affected side on a longitudinal plane drawn midway between the midsagittal plane and the lateral surface of the body.
- Position this plane to the midline of the grid.
- If the patient is in the recumbent position, support the elevated hip.
- Abduct the arm of the affected side, and elevate it to carry the scapula away from the rib cage.
- Rest the patient's hand on the head if the upright position is used (Fig. 9-48), or place the hand under or above the head if in the recumbent position is used (Fig. 9-49).

- Abduct the opposite limb with the hand on the hip.
- Center the cassette with the top 1½ inches (3.8 cm) above the upper border of the relaxed shoulder to image ribs above the diaphragm or with the lower edge of the cassette at the level of the iliac crest to image ribs below the diaphragm.
- *Shield gonads.*
- *Respiration:* Suspend at the end of *deep expiration* for ribs *below* the diaphragm and at the end of *full inspiration* for ribs *above* the diaphragm.

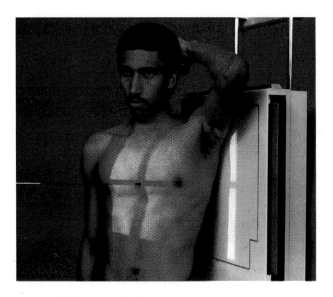

Fig. 9-48 Upright AP oblique ribs, LPO position.

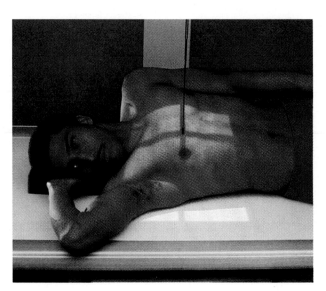

Fig. 9-49 Recumbent AP oblique ribs, RPO position.

Central ray

- Perpendicular to the center of the cassette. If the cassette is positioned correctly, the central ray will be at the level of T7 for the upper projection and at the level of T10 for the lower projection.

Structures shown

In these images the axillary portion of the ribs are projected free of superimposition (Fig. 9-50)

The following should be clearly demonstrated:

- Approximately twice as much distance between the vertebral column and the lateral border of the ribs on the affected side as is present on the unaffected side
- Axillary portion of the ribs free of superimposition
- First through tenth ribs visible above the diaphragm for upper ribs
- Eighth through twelfth ribs visible below the diaphragm for lower ribs
- Ribs visible through the lungs or abdomen according to the region examined

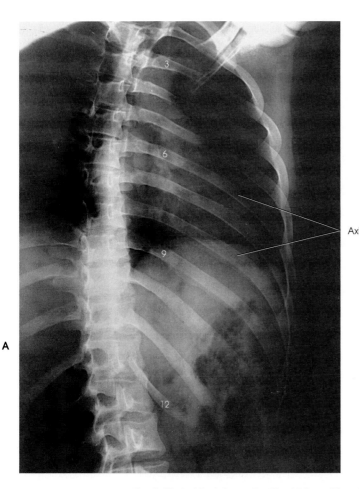

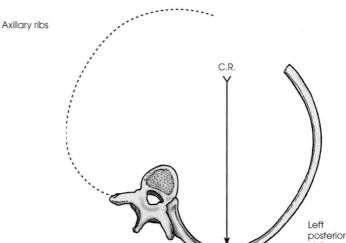

A

Axillary ribs

C.R.

Left posterior oblique

B

Fig. 9-50 A, AP oblique ribs. The LPO position demonstrates left-side ribs. **B,** Axial view (from feet upward) of the ribs and central ray, LPO position.

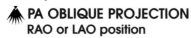

Axillary

⚛ PA OBLIQUE PROJECTION
RAO or LAO position

Image receptor: 35 × 43 cm (14 × 17 inch) or 28 × 35 cm (11 × 14 inch) lengthwise

Position of patient
- Examine the patient in the upright or recumbent position.
- Unless contraindicated by the patient's condition, use the upright position to image ribs above the diaphragm and the recumbent position to image ribs below the diaphragm. Gravity assists by moving the diaphragm.

Position of part
- Position the body for a 45-degree PA oblique projection using the RAO or LAO position. Place the affected side *away* from the cassette (Fig. 9-51).
- If the recumbent position is used, have the patient rest on the forearm and flexed knee of the elevated side (Fig. 9-52).
- Align the body so that a longitudinal plane drawn midway between the midline and the lateral surface of the body side up is centered to the midline of the grid.

- Center the cassette with the top 1½ inches (3.8 cm) above the upper border of the shoulder to image ribs above the diaphragm or with the lower edge of the cassette at the level of the iliac crest to image ribs below the diaphragm.
- *Shield gonads.*
- *Respiration:* Suspend at the end of *full expiration* for ribs *below* the diaphragm and at the end of *full inspiration* for ribs *above* the diaphragm.

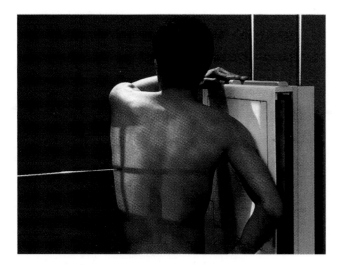

Fig. 9-51 Upright PA oblique ribs, RAO position.

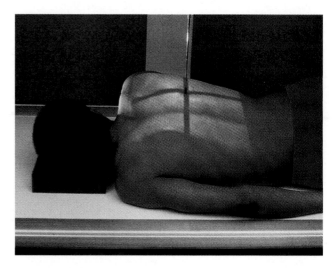

Fig. 9-52 Recumbent PA oblique ribs, LAO position.

Bony thorax

Central ray

- Perpendicular to the center of the cassette. If the cassette is positioned correctly, the central ray will be at the level of T7 for the upper projection and at the level of T10 for the lower projection.

Structures shown

- In these images the axillary portion of the ribs is projected free of bony superimposition (Fig. 9-53).

EVALUATION CRITERIA

The following should be clearly demonstrated:

- Approximately twice as much distance between the vertebral column and the lateral border of the ribs on the affected side as is present on the unaffected side
- Axillary portion of the ribs free of superimposition
- First through tenth ribs visible above the diaphragm for upper ribs
- Eighth through twelfth ribs visible below the diaphragm for lower ribs
- Ribs visible through the lungs or abdomen according to the region examined

A

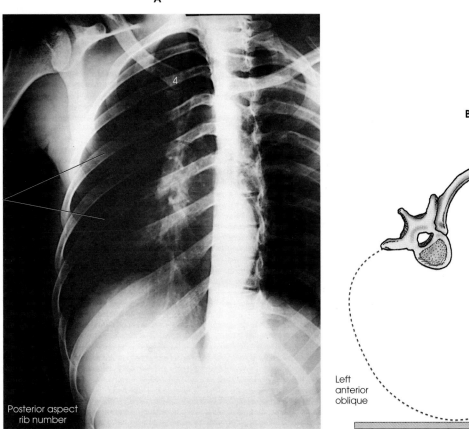

Axillary ribs

Posterior aspect
rib number

B

C.R.

Left
anterior
oblique

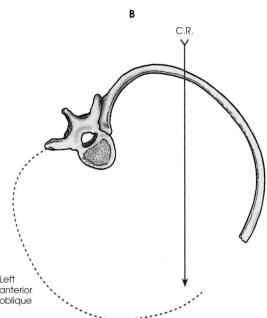

Fig. 9-53 A, PA oblique ribs. The LAO position demonstrates right side ribs. **B,** Axial view (from feet upward) of ribs and central ray with the patient in LAO position.

Costal Joints

AP AXIAL PROJECTION

This projection is recommended for demonstration of the costal joints in patients with rheumatoid spondylitis.

Image receptor: 30 × 35 cm (11 × 14 inch) lengthwise

Position of patient
- Place the patient in the supine position.
- Have the patient's head rest directly on the radiographic table to avoid accentuating the dorsal kyphosis.

Position of part
- Center the midsagittal plane to the midline of the grid.
- If the patient has pronounced dorsal kyphosis, extend the arms over the head; otherwise, place the arms along the sides of the body.
- Adjust the patient's shoulders to lie in the same transverse plane (Fig. 9-54).
- With the cassette in the Bucky tray, adjust its position so that the midpoint of the cassette coincides with the central ray.

- Apply compression across the thorax, if necessary.
- *Shield gonads.*
- *Respiration:* Suspend at the end of full inspiration because the lung markings are less prominent at this phase of breathing.

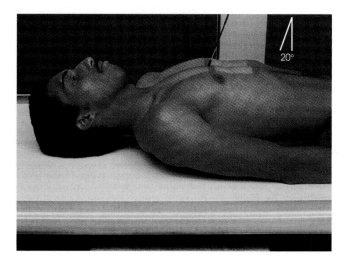

Fig. 9-54 AP axial costal joints.

Costal Joints

Central ray

- Directed 20 degrees cephalad and entering the midline about 2 inches (5 cm) above the xiphoid process.
- Increase the angulation of the central ray slightly (5 to 10 degrees) when examining patients who have pronounced dorsal kyphosis.

Structures shown

The costovertebral and costotransverse joints are demonstrated (Fig. 9-55).

EVALUATION CRITERIA

The following should be clearly demonstrated:

- Open costovertebral and costotransverse joints

NOTE: In large-boned patients the two sides may need to be examined separately to demonstrate the costovertebral joints. These projections are obtained by alternately rotating the body approximately 10 degrees medially; the elevated side is best demonstrated.

In their studies of the costal joints (costovertebral and costotransverse), Hohmann and Gasteiger[1] found that the central ray generally must be angled 30 degrees cephalad in the average patient. The central ray angulation is increased to 35 to 40 degrees when accentuated kyphosis is present. In patients with severe curvature of the spine, the pelvis is also elevated on a suitable support. For localized studies the central ray may be centered to T4 for the upper area and to T8 for the lower area.

---

[1]Hohmann D, Gasteiger W: Roentgen diagnosis of the costovertebral joints, *Fortschr Roentgenstr* 112:783,1970 (in German); Abstract, *Radiology* 98:481,1971.

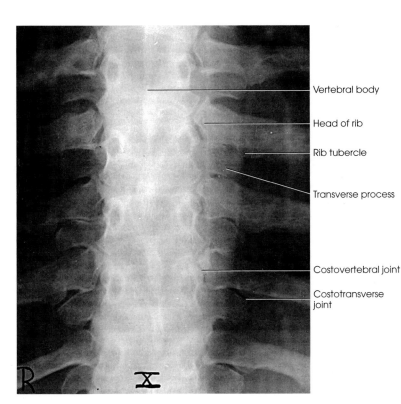
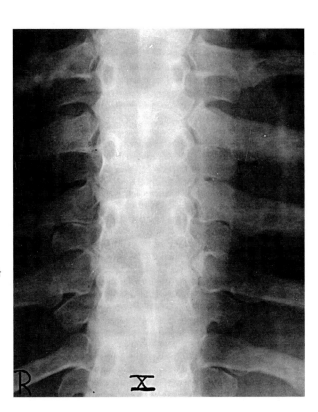

Vertebral body

Head of rib

Rib tubercle

Transverse process

Costovertebral joint

Costotransverse joint

Fig. 9-55 AP axial costal joints.

THORACIC VISCERA

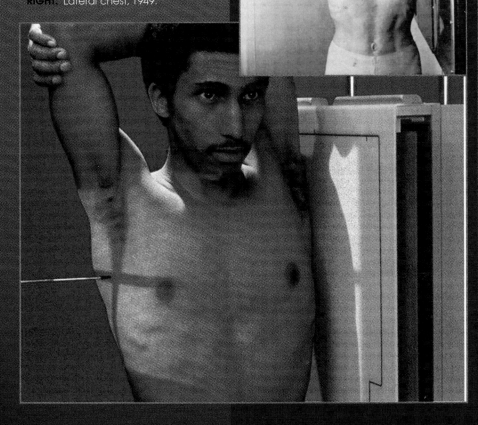

RIGHT: Lateral chest, 1949.

LEFT: Lateral chest performed with close collimation, 1999.

SUMMARY OF PROJECTIONS

PROJECTIONS, POSITIONS & METHODS

Page	Essential	Anatomy	Projection	Position	Method
518		Trachea	AP		
520		Trachea and superior mediastinum	Lateral	R or L	
522		Trachea and pulmonary apex	Axiolateral		TWINING
524	♠	Chest: *lungs and heart*	PA		
528	♠	Chest: *lungs and heart*	Lateral	R or L	
532	♠	Chest: *lungs and heart*	PA oblique	RAO and LAO	
536	♠	Chest: *lungs and heart*	AP oblique	RPO and LPO	
538	♠	Chest	AP		
540	♠	Pulmonary apices	AP axial	Lordotic	LINDBLOM
542		Pulmonary apices	PA axial		
544		Pulmonary apices	AP axial		
546		Pulmonary apices	PA axial	Lordotic	FLEISCHNER
548	♠	Lungs and pleurae	AP or PA	R or L lateral decubitus	
550	♠	Lungs and pleurae	Lateral	Ventral or dorsal decubitus	

Icons in the Essential column indicate projections frequently performed in the United States and Canada. Students should be competent in these projections.

Body Habitus

The general shape of the human body, or the *body habitus,* determines the size, shape, position, and movement of the internal organs. Fig. 10-1 outlines the general shape of the thorax in the four types of body habitus and how each appears on radiographs of the thoracic area.

Thoracic Cavity

The *thoracic cavity* is bounded by the walls of the thorax and extends from the *superior thoracic aperture,* where structures enter the thorax, to the *inferior thoracic aperture.* The *diaphragm* separates the thoracic cavity from the abdominal cavity. The anatomic structures that pass from the thorax to the abdomen go through openings in the diaphragm (Fig. 10-2).

The thoracic cavity contains the *lungs* and *heart,* organs of the *respiratory, cardiovascular,* and *lymphatic* systems, the *inferior portion of the esophagus,* and the *thymus gland.* Within the cavity are three separate chambers: a single *pericardial cavity* and the *right* and *left pleural cavities.* These cavities are lined by shiny, slippery, and delicate *serous membranes.* The space between the two pleural cavities is called the *mediastinum.* This area contains all the thoracic structures except the lungs and pleurae.

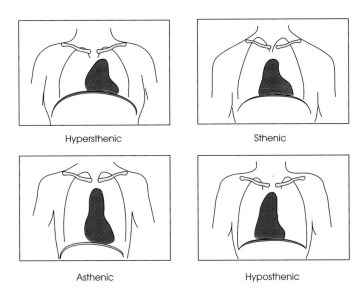

Hypersthenic

Sthenic

Asthenic

Hyposthenic

Fig. 10-1 Four types of body habitus. Note the general shape of the thorax, the size and shape of the lungs, and the position of the heart. A knowledge of this anatomy is helpful to accurately position for projections of the thorax.

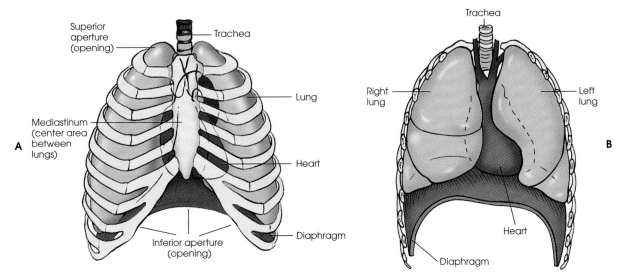

Fig. 10-2 A, Thoracic cavity. **B,** Thoracic cavity with anterior ribs removed.

Respiratory System

The *respiratory system* consists of the pharynx (described in Chapter 15), trachea, bronchi, and two lungs. The air passages of these organs communicate with the exterior through the pharynx, mouth, and nose, each of which, in addition to other described functions, is considered a part of the respiratory system.

TRACHEA

The *trachea* is a fibrous, muscular tube with 16 to 20 C-shaped cartilaginous rings embedded in its walls for greater rigidity (Fig. 10-3, *A*). It measures approximately $1/2$ inch (1.3 cm) in diameter and $4^1/_2$ inches (11 cm) in length, and its posterior aspect is flat. The cartilaginous rings are incomplete posteriorly and extend around the anterior two thirds of the tube. The trachea lies in the midline of the body, anterior to the esophagus in the neck. However, in the thorax the trachea is shifted slightly to the right of the midline as a result of the arching of the aorta. The trachea follows the curve of the vertebral column and extends from its junction with the larynx at the level of the sixth cervical vertebra inferiorly through the mediastinum to about the level of the space between the fourth and fifth thoracic vertebrae. The last tracheal cartilage is elongated and has a hooklike process, the *carina*, which extends posteriorly on its inferior surface. At the carina the trachea divides, or bifurcates, into two lesser tubes, the primary bronchi. One of these bronchi enters the right lung, and the other enters the left lung.

The *primary bronchi* slant obliquely inferiorly to their entrance into the lungs, where they branch out to form the right and left bronchial branches (Fig. 10-3, *B*). The *right primary bronchus* is shorter, wider, and more vertical than the *left primary bronchus*. Because of the more vertical position and greater diameter of the right main bronchus, foreign bodies entering the trachea are more likely to pass into the right bronchus than the left bronchus.

After entering the lung, each primary bronchus divides, sending branches to each lobe of the lung: three to the right lung and two to the left lung. These *secondary bronchi* further divide and decrease in caliber. The bronchi continue dividing into *tertiary bronchi*, then to smaller *bronchioles*, and end in minute tubes called the *terminal bronchioles* (see Fig. 10-3). The extensive branching of the trachea is commonly referred to as the *bronchial tree* because it resembles a tree trunk (see box).

SUBDIVISIONS OF THE BRONCHIAL TREE

Trachea
Primary bronchi
Secondary bronchi
Teritiary bronchi
Bronchioles
Terminal bronchioles

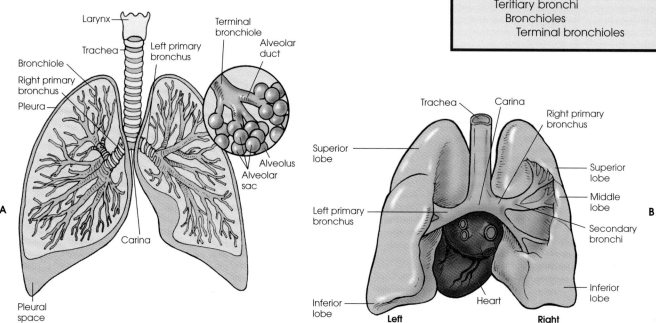

Fig. 10-3 A, Anterior aspect of respiratory system. **B,** Posterior aspect of heart, lungs, trachea, and bronchial trees.

ALVEOLI

The terminal bronchioles communicate with *alveolar ducts.* Each duct ends in several *alveolar sacs.* The walls of the alveolar sacs are lined with *alveoli* (see Fig. 10-3, *A*). Each lung contains millions of alveoli. Oxygen and carbon dioxide are exchanged by diffusion within the walls of the alveoli.

LUNGS

The *lungs* are the organs of respiration (Fig. 10-4). They make up the mechanism for introducing oxygen into the blood and removing carbon dioxide from the blood. The lungs are composed of a light, spongy, highly elastic substance, the *parenchyma,* and they are covered by a layer of serous membrane. Each lung presents a rounded *apex* that reaches above the level of the clavicles into the root of the neck and a broad *base* that, resting on the obliquely placed diaphragm, reaches lower in back and at the sides than in front. The right lung is about 1 inch (2.5 cm) shorter than the left lung because of the large space occupied by the liver, and it is broader than the left lung because of the position of the heart. The lateral surface of each lung conforms with the shape of the chest wall. The inferior surface of the lung is concave, fitting over the diaphragm, and the lateral margins are thin. During respiration the lungs move inferiorly for inspiration and superiorly for expiration (Fig. 10-5). During inspiration

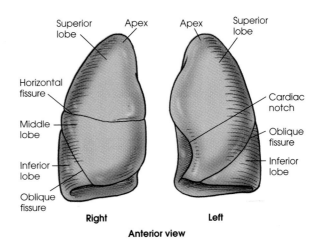

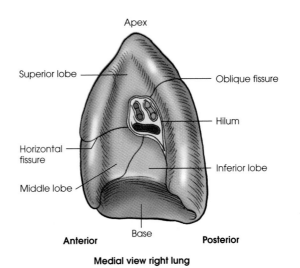

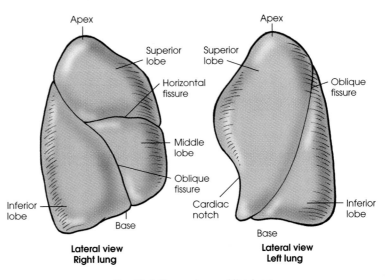

Fig. 10-4 Three views of the lung.

the lateral margins descend into the deep recesses of the parietal pleura. In radiology this recess is called the *costophrenic angle.* The mediastinal surface is concave with a depression, called the *hilum,* that accommodates the bronchi, pulmonary blood vessels, lymph vessels, and nerves. The inferior mediastinal surface of the left lung contains a concavity called the *cardiac notch.* This notch conforms to the shape of the heart.

Each lung is enclosed in a double-walled, serous membrane sac called the *pleura* (see Fig. 10-3, *A*). The inner layer of the pleural sac, called the *visceral pleura,* closely adheres to the surface of the lung, extends into the *interlobar fissures,* and is contiguous with the outer layer at the hilum. The outer layer, called the *parietal pleura,* lines the wall of the thoracic cavity occupied by the lung and closely adheres to the upper surface of the diaphragm. The two layers are moistened by *serous fluid* so that they move easily on each other. Thus the serous fluid prevents friction between the lungs and chest walls during respiration. The space between the two pleural walls is called the *pleural cavity.* Although the space is termed a *cavity,* the layers are actually in close contact.

Each lung is divided into *lobes* by deep fissures. The fissures lie in an oblique plane inferiorly and anteriorly from above, so that the lobes overlap each other in the AP direction. The *oblique fissures* divide the lungs into *superior* and *inferior lobes.* The superior lobes lie above and are anterior to the inferior lobes. The right superior lobe is further divided by a *horizontal fissure,* creating a *right middle lobe* (see Fig. 10-4). The left lung has no horizontal fissure and thus no middle lobe. The portion of the left lobe that corresponds in position to the right middle lobe is called the *lingula.* The lingula is a tongue-shaped process on the anteromedial border of the left lung. It fills the space between the chest wall and the heart.

Each of the five lobes divides into *bronchopulmonary segments* and subdivides into smaller units called *primary lobules.* The primary lobule is the anatomic unit of lung structure and consists of a terminal bronchiole with its expanded alveolar duct and alveolar sac.

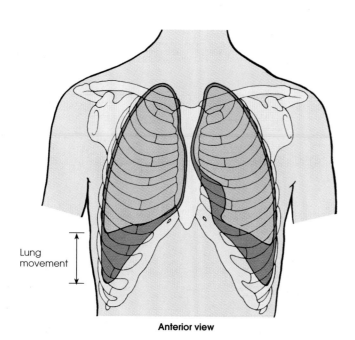

Lung movement

Anterior view

Fig. 10-5 Movement of the lungs during inspiration and expiration.

Mediastinum

The *mediastinum* is the area of the thorax bounded by the sternum anteriorly, the spine posteriorly, and the lungs laterally (Fig. 10-6). The structures associated with the mediastinum are as follows:

- Heart
- Great vessels
- Trachea
- Esophagus
- Thymus
- Lymphatics
- Nerves
- Fibrous tissue
- Fat

The *esophagus* is the part of the digestive canal that connects the pharynx with the stomach. It is a narrow, musculomembranous tube about 9 inches (23 cm) in length. Following the curves of the vertebral column, the esophagus descends through the posterior part of the mediastinum and then runs anteriorly to pass through the esophageal hiatus of the diaphragm.

The esophagus lies just in front of the vertebral column, with its anterior surface in close relation to the trachea, aortic arch, and heart. This makes the esophagus valuable in certain heart examinations. When the esophagus is filled with barium sulfate, the posterior border of the heart and aorta are outlined well in lateral and oblique projections (Fig. 10-7). Frontal, oblique, and lateral images are often used in examinations of the esophagus. Radiography of the esophagus is discussed later in this chapter.

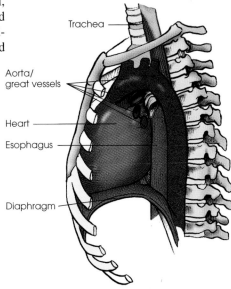

Fig. 10-6 Lateral view of the mediastinum, identifying the main structures.

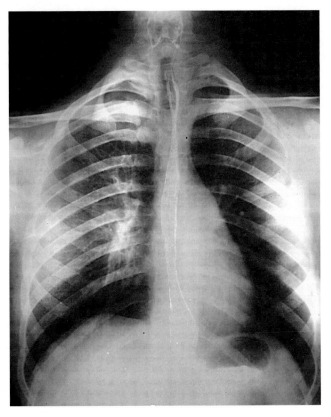

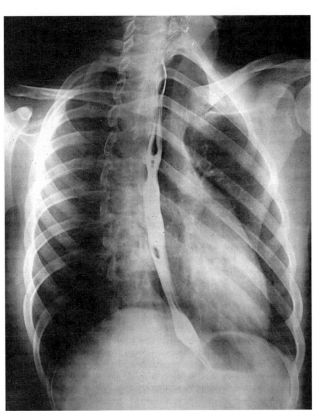

Fig. 10-7 A, PA projection of the esophagus with barium sulfate coating its walls. **B,** PA oblique projection with a barium-filled esophagus (RAO position).

The *thymus gland* is the primary control organ of the lymphatic system. It is responsible for producing the hormone *thymosin,* which plays a critical role in the development and maturation of the immune system. The thymus consists of two pyramid-shaped lobes that lie in the lower neck and superior mediastinum, anterior to the trachea and great vessels of the heart and posterior to the manubrium. The thymus reaches its maximum size at puberty and then gradually undergoes atrophy until it almost disappears (Figs. 10-8 and 10-9).

In older individuals, lymphatic tissue is replaced by fat. At its maximum development the thymus rests on the pericardium and reaches as high as the thyroid gland. When the thymus is enlarged in infants and young children, it can press on the retrothymic organs, displacing them posteriorly and causing respiratory disturbances. A radiographic examination may be made in both the AP and lateral projections. For optimal image contrast, exposures should be made at the end of full inspiration.

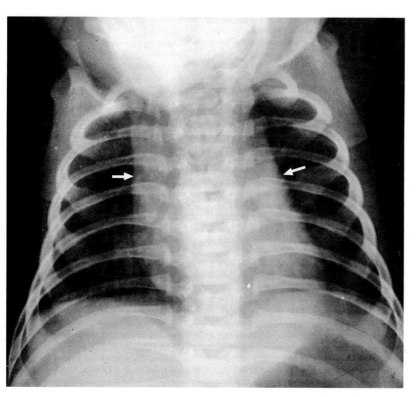

Fig. 10-8 PA chest radiograph showing mediastinal enlargement caused by hypertrophy of the thymus *(arrows).*

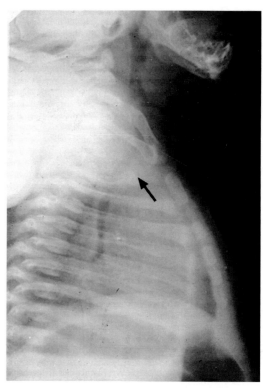

Fig. 10-9 Lateral chest radiograph demonstrating an enlarged thymus *(arrow).*

SUMMARY OF ANATOMY*

Body habitus
sthenic
asthenic
hyposthenic
hypersthenic

Thoracic cavity
superior thoracic
  aperature
inferior thoracic
  aperature
diaphragm
thoracic viscera
  lungs
  heart
  respiratory system
  cardiac system
  lymphatic system
  inferior esophagus
  thymus gland
  pericardial cavity
  pleural cavities
  serous membranes
  mediastinum

Respiratory system
pharynx
trachea
  carina
primary bronchi
  right primary
    bronchus
  left primary
    bronchus
    secondary
      bronchi
    tertiary bronchi
    bronchioles
    terminal
      bronchioles
bronchial tree

Alveoli
alveolar duct
alveolar sac
alveoli

Lungs
parenchyma
apex
base
costophrenic angles
hilum
cardiac notch

pleura
  visceral pleura
  parietal pleura
  serous fluid
  pleural cavity
lobes
  superior lobes
  inferior lobes
  right middle lobe
interlobar fissures
  oblique fissures (2)
  horizontal fissure
lingula
bronchopulmonary
  segments
primary lobules

Mediastinum
heart
great vessels
trachea
esophagus
thymus
lymphatics
nerves
fibrous tissue
fat

*See *Addendum* at the end of the volume for a summary of the changes in the anatomic terms used in this edition.

513

General Positioning Considerations

For radiography of the heart and lungs, the patient is placed in an *upright position* whenever possible to prevent engorgement of the pulmonary vessels and to allow gravity to depress the diaphragm. In the recumbent position, gravitational force causes the abdominal viscera and diaphragm to move superiorly; it compresses the thoracic viscera, which prevents full expansion of the lungs. Although the difference in diaphragm movement is not great in hyposthenic persons, it is marked in hypersthenic individuals. Figs. 10-10 and 10-11 illustrate the effect of body position in the same patient. The left lateral chest position (Fig. 10-12) is most commonly employed because it places the heart closer to the cassette, resulting in a less magnified heart image. Right and left lateral chest images are compared in Figs. 10-12 and 10-13.

A *slight amount of rotation* from the PA or lateral projections causes considerable distortion of the heart shadow. To prevent this distortion, the body must be carefully positioned and immobilized.

PA CRITERIA

For PA projections, procedures are as follows:
- Instruct the patient to sit or stand upright. If the standing position is used, the weight of the body must be equally distributed on the feet.
- Position the patient's head upright, facing directly forward.
- Have the patient depress the shoulders and hold them in contact with the grid device to carry the clavicles below the lung apices. Except in the presence of an upper thoracic scoliosis, a faulty body position can be detected by the asymmetric appearance of the sternoclavicular joints. Compare the clavicular margins in Figs. 10-14 and 10-15.

LATERAL CRITERIA

For lateral projections, procedures are as follows:
- Place the side of interest against the cassette holder.
- Have the patient stand so that the weight is equally distributed on the feet. The patient should not lean toward or away from the cassette holder.

- Raise the patient's arms to prevent the soft tissue of the arms from superimposing the lung fields
- Instruct the patient to face straight ahead and raise the chin.
- To determine rotation, examine the posterior aspects of the ribs. Radiographs without rotation show superimposed posterior ribs (see Figs. 10-12 and 10-13).

OBLIQUE CRITERIA

In oblique projections, the patient rotates the hips with the thorax and points the feet directly forward. The shoulders should lie in the same transverse plane on all radiographs.

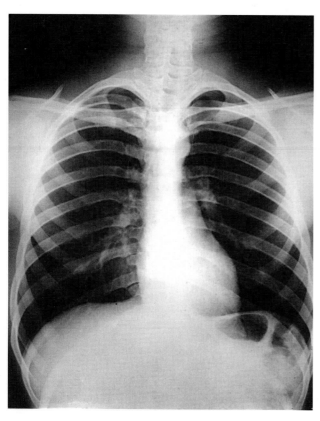

Fig. 10-10 Upright chest radiograph.

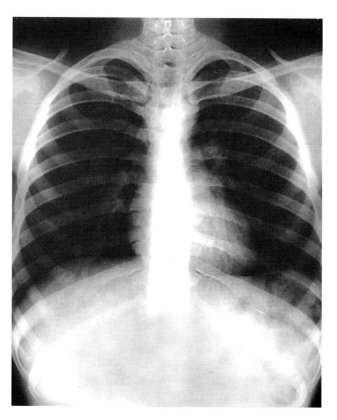

Fig. 10-11 Prone chest radiograph.

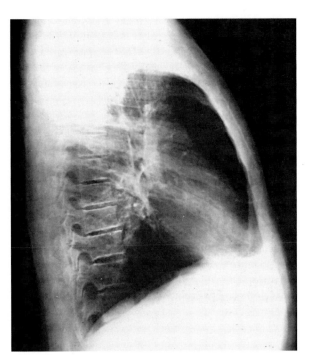

Fig. 10-12 Left lateral chest.

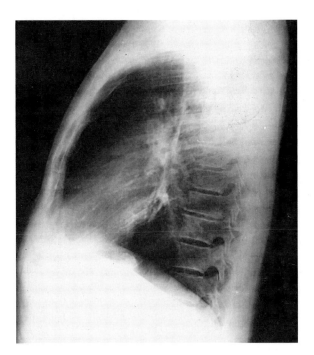

Fig. 10-13 Right lateral chest.

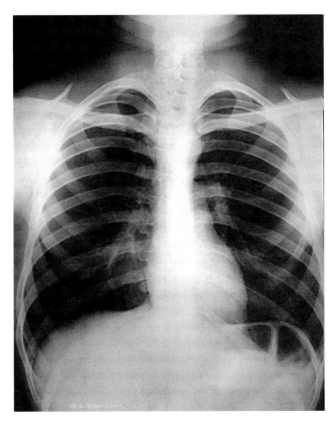

Fig. 10-14 PA chest without rotation.

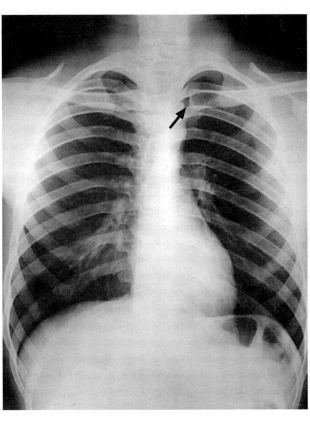

Fig. 10-15 PA chest with rotation *(arrow)*.

Breathing Instructions

During *normal inspiration,* the costal muscles pull the anterior ribs superiorly and laterally, the shoulders rise, and the thorax expands from front to back and from side to side. These changes in the height and AP dimension of the thorax must be considered when positioning the patient.

Deep inspiration causes the diaphragm to move inferiorly, resulting in elongation of the heart. Radiographs of the heart should therefore be obtained at the end of normal inspiration to prevent distortion. More air is inhaled during the second breath (and without strain) than during the first breath.

When a *pneumothorax* (gas or air in the pleural cavity) is suspected, one exposure is often made at the end of full inspiration and another at the end of full expiration to demonstrate small amounts of free air in the pleural cavity that might be obscured on the inspiration exposure (Figs. 10-16 and 10-17). Inspiration and expiration radiographs are also used to demonstrate the movement of the diaphragm, the occasional presence of a foreign body, and atelectasis (absence of air).

Technical Procedure

The projections required for an adequate demonstration of the thoracic viscera are usually requested by the attending physician and are determined by the clinical history of the patient. The PA projection of the chest is the most common projection and is used in all lung and heart examinations. Right and left oblique and lateral projections are also employed as required to supplement the PA projection. It is often necessary to improvise variations of the basic positions to project a localized area free of superimposed structures.

The exposure factors and accessories employed in examining the thoracic viscera depend on the radiographic characteristics of the individual patient's pathologic condition. Normally, chest radio- graphy uses a high kilovolt (peak) (kVp) to penetrate and demonstrate all thoracic anatomy on the radiograph. The kVp can be lowered if exposures are made without a grid.

However, if the selected kVp is too low, the radiographic contrast may be too high, resulting in few shades of gray. On such a radiograph the lung fields may appear properly penetrated, but the mediastinum appears underexposed. If the selected kVp is too high, the contrast may be too low, which does not allow for demonstration of the finer lung markings. Adequate kVp penetrates the mediastinum and demonstrates a faint shadow of the spine. Whenever possible, a minimum source-to-image receptor distance (SID) of 72 inches (183 cm) should be used to minimize magnification of the heart and to obtain greater recorded detail of the delicate lung structures (Fig. 10-18). A 120-inch (305-cm) SID is commonly used in radiography of the chest.

A grid technique is recommended for opaque areas within the lung fields and to demonstrate the lung structure through thickened pleural membranes (Figs. 10-19 and 10-20).

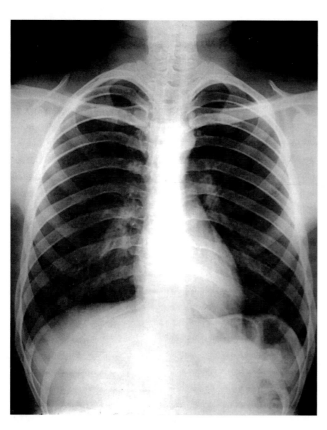

Fig. 10-16 PA chest during inspiration.

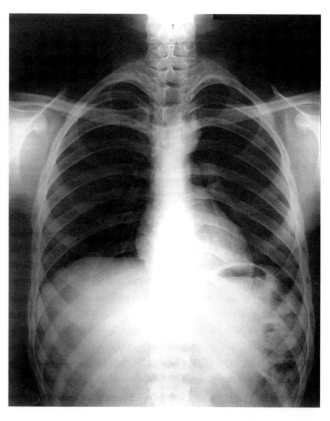

Fig. 10-17 PA chest during expiration.

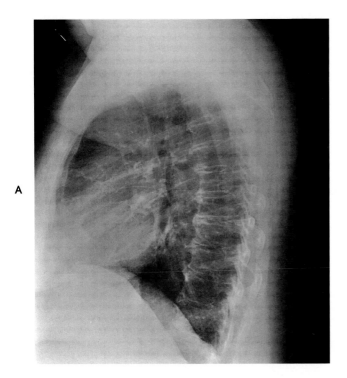

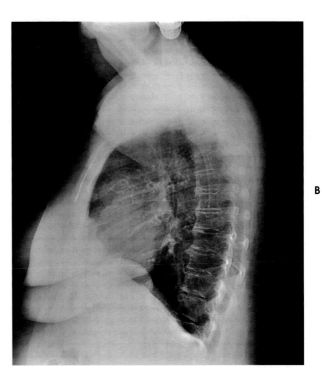

Fig. 10-18 A, Lateral chest radiograph performed at a 44-inch (112-cm) SID. **B,** Same patient's radiograph performed at a 72-inch (183-cm) SID. Note decreased magnification and greater recorded detail of lung structures.

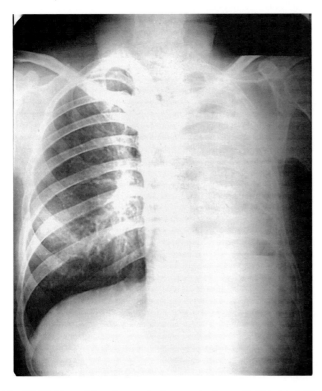

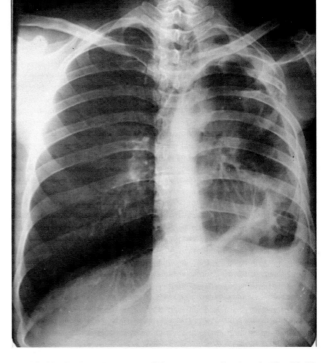

Fig. 10-19 Nongrid radiograph demonstrating a fluid-type pathologic condition in the same patient as in Fig. 10-20.

Fig. 10-20 Grid radiograph of the same patient as in Fig. 10-19.

Radiation Protection

Protection of the patient from unnecessary radiation is the professional responsibility of the radiographer (see Chapter 1 for specific guidelines). In this chapter the *Shield gonads* statement indicates that the patient is to be protected from unnecessary radiation by restricting the radiation beam using proper collimation. In addition, the placement of lead shielding between the gonads and the radiation source is appropriate when the clinical objectives of the examination are not compromised. An example of a properly placed lead shield is shown in Fig. 10-27.

AP PROJECTION

When preparing to radiograph the trachea for the AP projection, use a grid technique to minimize secondary radiation because the kVp must be high enough to penetrate both the sternum and the cervical vertebrae.

Image receptor: 24 × 30 cm (10 × 12 inch) lengthwise

Position of patient

- Examine the patient in either the supine or upright position.

Position of part

- Center the midsagittal plane of the body to the midline of the grid.
- Adjust the patient's shoulders to lie in the same transverse plane.
- Extend the patient's neck slightly, and adjust it so that the midsagittal plane is perpendicular to the plane of the cassette (Fig. 10-21).
- Center the cassette at the level of the manubrium.
- Collimate closely to the neck.
- *Shield gonads.*
- *Respiration:* Instruct the patient to inhale slowly *during* the exposure to ensure that the trachea is filled with air.

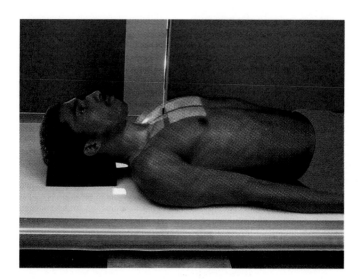

Fig. 10-21 AP trachea.

Central ray

- Perpendicular through the manubrium to the center of the cassette

Structures shown

An AP projection shows the outline of the air-filled trachea. Under normal conditions the trachea is superimposed on the shadow of the cervical vertebrae (Fig. 10-22).

The following should be clearly demonstrated:

- Area from the midcervical to the midthoracic region
- Air-filled trachea
- No rotation

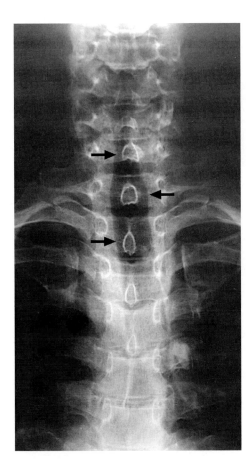

Fig. 10-22 AP trachea during inspiration demonstrating an air-filled trachea *(arrows)*.

LATERAL PROJECTION
R or L position

Image receptor: 24 × 30 cm (10 × 12 inch) or 30 × 35 cm (11 × 14 inch) lengthwise

Position of patient
- Place the patient in a lateral position, either seated or standing, before a vertical grid device. If the standing position is used, the weight of the patient's body must be equally distributed on the feet.

Position of part
- Instruct the patient to clasp the hands behind the body and then rotate the shoulders posteriorly as far as possible (Fig. 10-23). This will keep the superimposed shadows of the arms from obscuring the structures of the superior mediastinum. If necessary, immobilize the arms in this position with a wide bandage.
- Adjust the patient's position to center the trachea to the midline of the cassette. The trachea lies in the coronal plane that passes approximately midway between the jugular notch and the midcoronal plane.

- Adjust the height of the cassette so that the upper border is at or above the level of the laryngeal prominence.
- Readjust the position of the body, being careful to have the midsagittal plane vertical and parallel with the plane of the cassette.
- Extend the neck slightly.
- *Shield gonads.*
- *Respiration:* Make the exposure *during slow inspiration* to ensure that the trachea is filled with air.

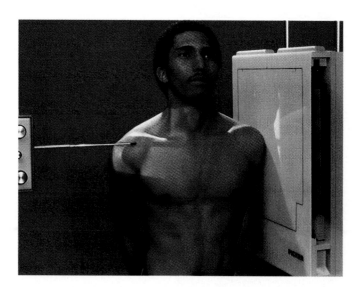

Fig. 10-23 Lateral trachea and superior mediastinum.

Central ray

- Horizontal through a point midway between the jugular notch and the midcoronal plane (Fig. 10-24, *A*) and through a point 4 to 5 inches (10.2 to 12.7 cm) lower for demonstration of the superior mediastinum (Fig. 10-24, *B*)

Structures shown

A lateral projection demonstrates the air-filled trachea and the regions of the thyroid and thymus glands. This projection, first described by Eiselberg and Sgalitzer,[1] is used extensively to demonstrate retrosternal extensions of the thyroid gland, thymic enlargement in infants (in the recumbent position), and the opacified pharynx and upper esophagus, as well as an outline of the trachea and bronchi. It is also used for foreign body localization.

[1]Eiselberg A, Sgalitzer DM: X-ray examination of the trachea and the bronchi, *Surg Gynecol Obstet* 47:53, 1928.

EVALUATION CRITERIA

The following should be clearly demonstrated:

- Area from the midcervical to the midthoracic region
- Trachea and superior mediastinum free of superimposition by the shoulders
- Air-filled trachea
- No rotation

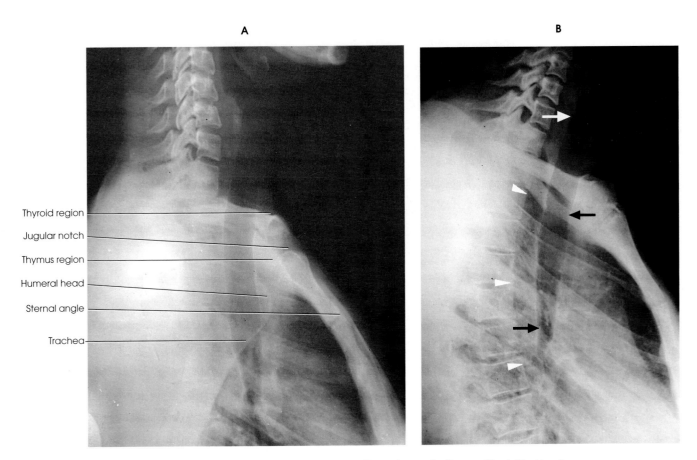

A

B

Thyroid region

Jugular notch

Thymus region

Humeral head

Sternal angle

Trachea

Fig. 10-24 A, Lateral superior mediastinum. **B,** Thoracic mediastinum with air-filled trachea *(arrows)* and esophagus *(arrowheads).*

AXIOLATERAL PROJECTION
TWINING METHOD
R or L position

This projection is used to obtain an axiolateral image of the apex of the lung nearest the cassette and the trachea and superior mediastinum in patients who cannot rotate their shoulders posteriorly enough for a true lateral projection.

Image receptor: 24 × 30 cm (10 × 12 inch) lengthwise

Position of patient

- Seat or stand the patient before a vertical grid device, with the affected side toward the cassette.

Position of part

- Elevate the arm adjacent to the cassette in extreme abduction, flex the elbow, and place the forearm across or behind the head.
- Center the cassette to the region of the trachea at the level of the axilla.
- Have the patient rest the shoulder firmly against the grid device for support.
- Depress the opposite shoulder as much as possible.
- Adjust the body in a true lateral position, with the midsagittal plane parallel with the plane of the cassette (Fig. 10-25).

- *Shield gonads.*
- *Respiration:* For the trachea, instruct the patient to inspire slowly *during* the exposure. For the lung apex, make the exposure at the end of *full inspiration.*

Central ray

- Directed to the center of the cassette through the adjacent supraclavicular impression at an angle of 15 degrees caudad

Structures shown

The axiolateral projection demonstrates the air-filled trachea and the apex of the lung closer to the cassette (Fig. 10-26).

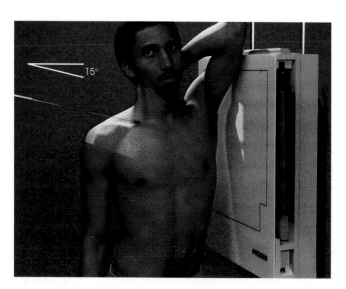

Fig. 10-25 Axiolateral trachea and pulmonary apex.

Trachea and Pulmonary Apex

EVALUATION CRITERIA

The following should be clearly demonstrated:

- Shoulders well separated from each other
- Area from the midcervical to the midthoracic region
- Air-filled trachea
- No rotation

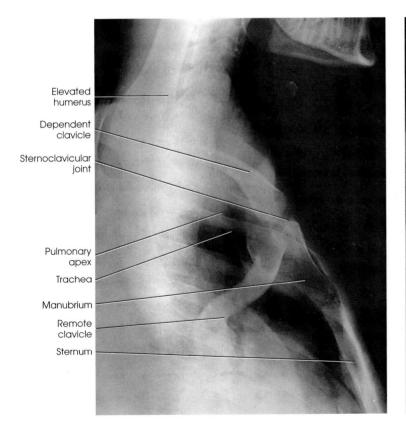
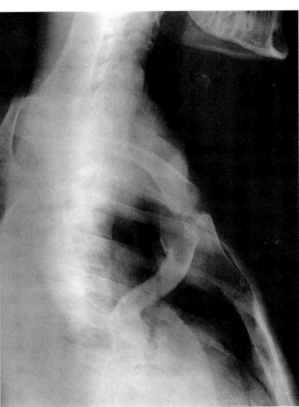

Elevated humerus

Dependent clavicle

Sternoclavicular joint

Pulmonary apex

Trachea

Manubrium

Remote clavicle

Sternum

Fig. 10-26 Axiolateral trachea and pulmonary apex.

Lungs and Heart
🦅 PA PROJECTION

Image receptor: 35 × 43 cm (14 × 17 inch) lengthwise, or crosswise for the hypersthenic patient

SID: A minimum SID of 72 inches (183 cm) is recommended to decrease magnification of the heart and increase recorded detail of the thoracic structures.

Position of patient

- If possible, always examine patients in the upright position, either standing or seated, so that the diaphragm is at its lowest position and engorgement of the pulmonary vessels is avoided.

Position of part

- Place the patient, with arms hanging at sides, before a vertical grid device.
- Adjust the height of the cassette so that its upper border is about $1\frac{1}{2}$ to 2 inches (3.8 to 5 cm) above the relaxed shoulders.
- Center the midsagittal plane of the patient's body to the midline of the cassette.
- Have the patient stand straight, with the weight of the body equally distributed on the feet.
- Extend the patient's chin upward or over the top of the grid device, and adjust the head so that the midsagittal plane is vertical.
- Ask the patient to flex the arms and to rest the *backs of the hands* low on the hips, below the level of the costophrenic angles. This maneuver rotates the scapulae laterally so that they are not superimposed over the lungs.
- Adjust the patient's shoulders to lie in the same transverse plane, and rotate them forward (Figs. 10-27 and 10-28).

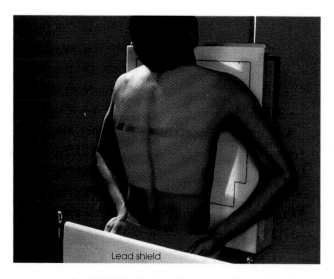

Fig. 10-27 Patient positioned for PA chest.

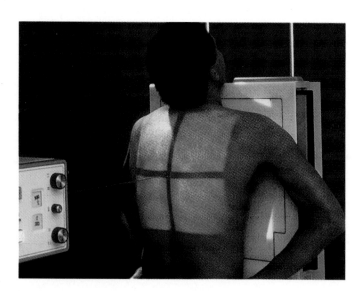

Fig. 10-28 PA chest.

- If an immobilization band is used, be careful not to rotate the body when applying the band. The least amount of rotation will result in considerable distortion of the heart shadow.
- If a female patient's breasts are large enough to be superimposed over the lower part of the lung fields, ask the patient to pull the breasts upward and laterally. Have the patient hold the breasts in place by leaning against the cassette holder (Figs. 10-29 and 10-30).
- *Shield gonads:* Place a lead shield between the x-ray tube and the patient's pelvis (see Fig. 10-27).

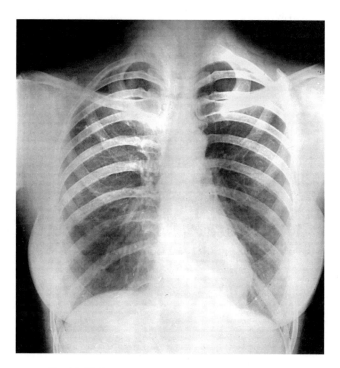

Fig. 10-29 Breasts superimposed over lower lungs.

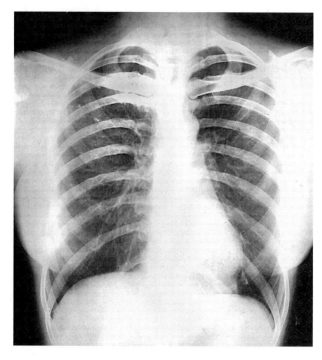

Fig. 10-30 Correct placement of breasts.

- *Respiration:* Full inspiration. The exposure is made after the *second* full inspiration to ensure maximum expansion of the lungs.
- For certain conditions, such as pneumothorax and the presence of a foreign body, radiographs are sometimes made at the end of full inspiration and expiration (Figs. 10-31 and 10-32).

Central ray

- Perpendicular to the midsagittal plane and the center of the cassette and entering at the level of T7.

A

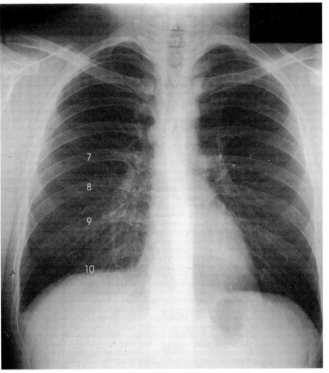

B

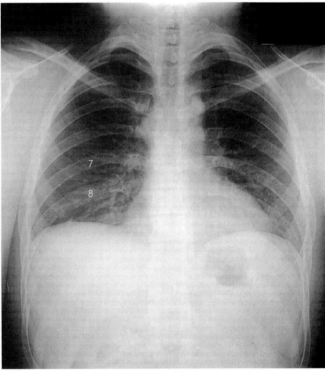

Fig. 10-31 A, Inspiration (posterior rib numbers). **B,** Expiration in the same patient (posterior rib numbers).

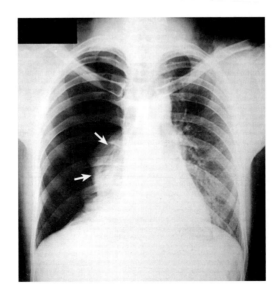

Fig. 10-32 PA chest during expiration. The patient had blunt trauma to the right chest. The left side is normal. Pneumothorax is seen on the entire right side, and a totally collapsed lung is seen near the hilum *(arrows).*

Structures shown

A PA projection of the thoracic viscera shows the air-filled trachea, the lungs, the diaphragmatic domes, the heart and aortic knob, and, if enlarged laterally, the thyroid or thymus gland (Figs. 10-33 and 10-34). The vascular markings are much more prominent on the projection made at the end of expiration. The bronchial tree is shown from an oblique angle. The esophagus is well demonstrated when it is filled with a barium sulfate suspension.

EVALUATION CRITERIA

The following should be clearly demonstrated:

- Entire lung fields from the apices to the costophrenic angles
- No rotation; sternal ends of the clavicles equidistant from the vertebral column
- Trachea visible in the midline
- Scapulae projected outside the lung fields
- Ten posterior ribs visible above the diaphragm
- Sharp outlines of heart and diaphragm
- Faint shadow of the ribs and superior thoracic vertebrae visible through the heart shadow
- Lung markings visible from the hilum to the periphery of the lung
- With inspiration and expiration chest images, diaphragm demonstrated on expiration at a higher level so that at least one fewer rib is seen within the lung field

NOTE: Inferior lobes of both lungs should be carefully checked for adequate penetration on women with large, pendulous breasts.

Cardiac studies with barium

PA chest radiographs are often obtained with the patient swallowing a bolus of barium sulfate to outline the posterior heart and aorta. The barium used in cardiac examinations should be thicker than that used for the stomach so that the contrast medium descends more slowly and adheres to the esophageal walls. The patient should hold the barium in the mouth until just before the exposure is made. Then the patient takes a deep breath and swallows the bolus of barium; at this time the exposure is made (see Fig. 10-6).

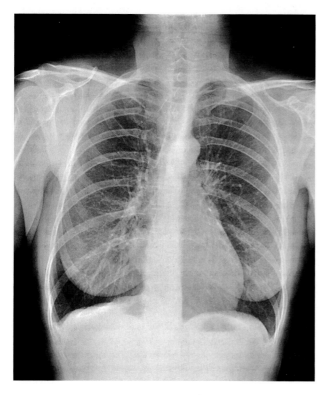

Fig. 10-33 PA chest in a female.

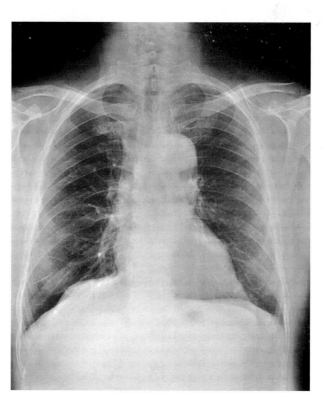

Fig. 10-34 PA chest in a male.

Lungs and Heart
🔺 LATERAL PROJECTION
R or L position

Image receptor: 35 × 43 cm (14 × 17 inch) lengthwise

SID: A minimum SID of 72 inches (183 cm) is recommended to decrease magnification of the heart and increase recorded detail of the thoracic structures.

Position of patient

- If possible, always examine the patient in the upright position, either standing or seated, so that the diaphragm is at its lowest position and engorgement of the pulmonary vessels is avoided.
- Turn the patient to a true lateral position, arms by the sides.
- To show the heart and left lung, use the left lateral position with the patient's left side against the cassette.
- Use the right lateral position to best demonstrate the right lung.

Position of part

- Adjust the position of the patient so that the midsagittal plane of the body is parallel with the cassette and the adjacent shoulder is touching the grid device.
- Center the thorax to the grid; the mid-coronal plane should be perpendicular and centered to the midline of the grid.
- Have the patient extend the arms directly upward, flex the elbows, and with the forearms resting on the elbows, hold the arms in position (Figs. 10-35 and 10-36).

- Place an IV stand in front of an unsteady patient. Have the patient extend the arms and grasp the stand as high as possible for support.
- Adjust the height of the cassette so that the upper border is about $1\frac{1}{2}$ to 2 inches (3.8 to 5 cm) above the shoulders.

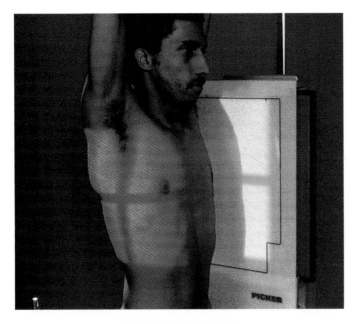

Fig. 10-35 Lateral chest.

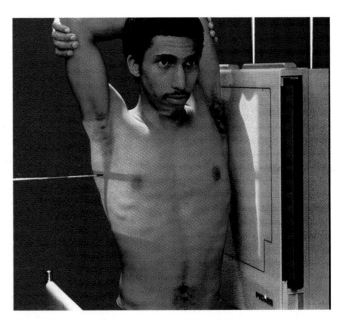

Fig. 10-36 Lateral chest.

- Recheck the position of the body; the midsagittal plane must be vertical. Depending on the width of the shoulders, the lower part of the thorax and hips may be a greater distance from the cassette, but this body position is necessary for a true lateral projection. Having the patient *lean* against the grid device (foreshortening) results in distortion of all thoracic structures (Fig. 10-37). *Forward bending* also results in distorted structural outlines (Fig. 10-38).
- *Shield gonads.*

- *Respiration:* Full inspiration. The exposure is made after the *second* full inspiration to ensure maximum expansion of the lungs.

Central ray

- Perpendicular to the midline of the cassette and entering the patient on the midcoronal plane at the level of T7 or the inferior aspect of the scapula

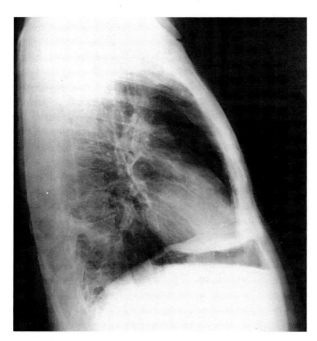

Fig. 10-37 Foreshortening.

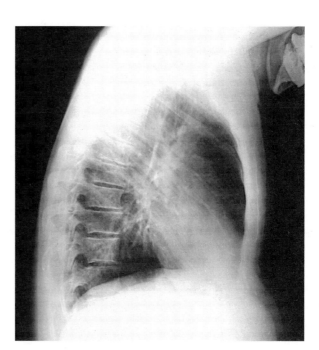

Fig. 10-38 Forward bending.

Structures shown

The preliminary left lateral chest position is used to demonstrate the heart, the aorta, and left-sided pulmonary lesions (Figs. 10-39 and 10-40). The right lateral chest position is used to demonstrate right-sided pulmonary lesions (Fig. 10-41). These lateral projections are employed extensively to demonstrate the interlobar fissures, to differentiate the lobes, and to localize pulmonary lesions.

EVALUATION CRITERIA

The following should be clearly demonstrated:
- Superimposition of the ribs posterior to the vertebral column
- Arm or its soft tissues not overlapping the superior lung field
- Long axis of the lung fields demonstrated in vertical position, without forward or backward leaning
- Lateral sternum with no rotation
- Costophrenic angles and the lower apices of the lungs
- Penetration of the lung fields and heart
- Open thoracic intervertebral spaces and intervertebral foramina, except in patients with scoliosis
- Sharp outlines of heart and diaphragm
- Hilum in the approximate center of the radiograph

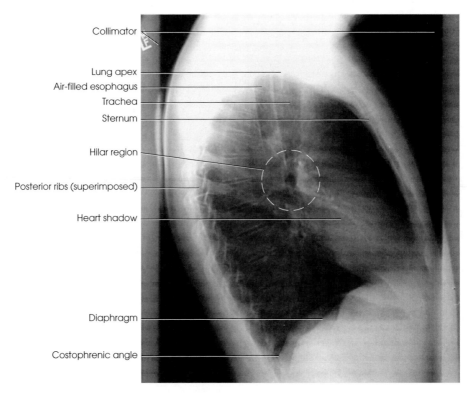

Fig. 10-39 Left lateral chest.

Collimator

Lung apex
Air-filled esophagus
Trachea
Sternum

Hilar region

Posterior ribs (superimposed)

Heart shadow

Diaphragm

Costophrenic angle

Cardiac studies with barium

The left lateral position is traditionally used during cardiac studies with barium. The procedure is the same as that described for the PA chest projection (see p. 527).

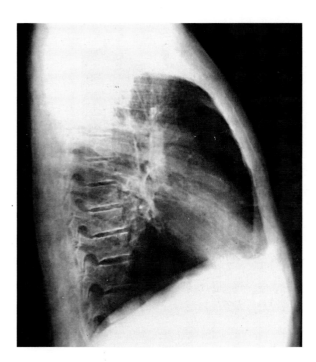

Fig. 10-40 Left lateral chest. (Compare the heart shadows with the radiograph of the same patient in Fig. 10-41.)

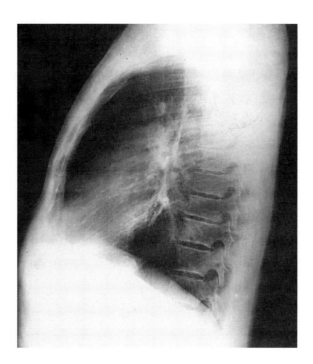

Fig. 10-41 Right lateral chest (same patient as in Fig. 10-40).

Lungs and Heart
♠ PA OBLIQUE PROJECTION
RAO and LAO positions

Image receptor: 35 × 43 cm (14 × 17 inches) lengthwise

SID: A minimum SID of 72 inches (183 cm) is recommended to decrease magnification of the heart and to increase recorded detail of the thoracic structures.

Position of patient
- Maintain the patient in the position (standing or seated upright) used for the PA projection.
- Instruct the patient to let the arms hang free.

- Have the patient turn approximately 45 degrees toward the left side for an LAO position and approximately 45 degrees toward the right side for an RAO position.
- Ask the patient to stand or sit straight. If the standing position is used, the weight of the patient's body must be equally distributed on the feet to prevent unwanted rotation.
- For PA oblique projections, the side of interest is generally the side *farther* from the cassette; however, the lung closest to the cassette is also imaged.
- The top of the cassette should be placed about 1½ to 2 inches (3.8 to 5 cm) above the vertebral prominens because the top of the shoulders may not be on the same plane.

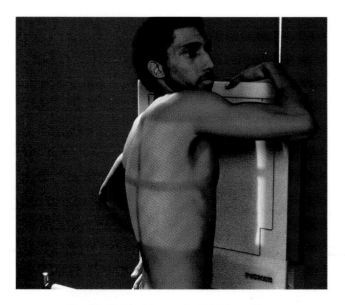

Fig. 10-42 PA oblique chest, LAO position.

Position of part

LAO position

- Rotate the patient 45 degrees to place the left shoulder in contact with the grid device, and center the thorax to the cassette. Ensure that both the right and left sides of the body are positioned to the cassette.
- Instruct the patient to place the left hand on the hip with the palm outward.
- Have the patient raise the right arm to shoulder level and grasp the side of the vertical grid device for support.

- Adjust the patient's shoulders to lie in the same horizontal plane, and instruct the patient to not rotate the head (Fig. 10-42).
- Use a 55- to 60-degree oblique position when the examination is performed for a *cardiac series*. This projection is usually performed with barium contrast medium. The patient swallows the barium just before the exposure.
- *Shield gonads.*
- *Respiration:* Full inspiration. The exposure is made after the *second* full inspiration to ensure maximum expansion of the lungs.

RAO position

- Reverse the previously described position, placing the patient's right shoulder in contact with the grid device and the left hand on the hip (Figs. 10-43 and 10-44).
- *Shield gonads.*
- *Respiration:* Full inspiration. The exposure is made after the *second* full inspiration to ensure maximum expansion of the lungs.

Central ray

- Perpendicular to the center of the cassette at the level of T7

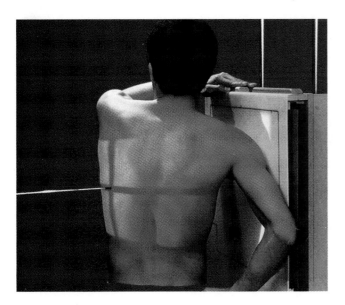

Fig. 10-43 PA oblique chest, RAO position.

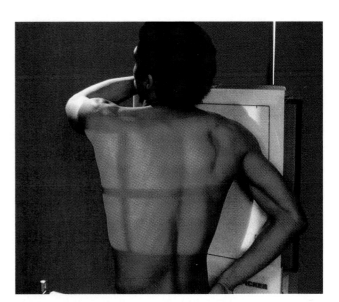

Fig. 10-44 PA oblique chest, RAO position.

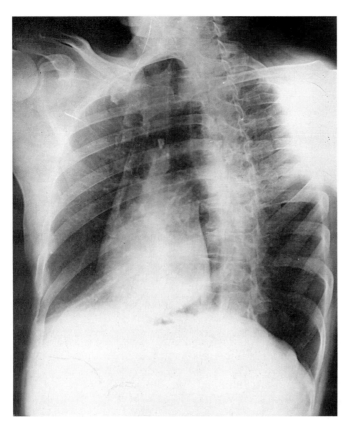

Fig. 10-45 PA oblique chest, LAO position.

Structures shown

LAO position

The maximum area of the right lung field (side farther from the cassette) is demonstrated. The anterior portion of the left lung is superimposed by the spine (Figs. 10-45 and 10-46). Also shown are the trachea and its bifurcation (the carina) and the entire right branch of the bronchial tree. The heart, the descending aorta (lying just in front of the spinae), and the arch of the aorta are also presented.

RAO position

The maximum area of the left lung field (side farther from the cassette) is demonstrated. The anterior portion of the right lung is superimposed by the spine (Figs. 10-47 and 10-48). Also shown are the trachea and the entire left branch of the bronchial tree. This position gives the best image of the left atrium, the anterior portion of the apex of the left ventricle, and the right retrocardiac space. When filled with barium, the esophagus is shown clearly in the RAO and LAO positions (see Fig. 10-48).

NOTE: The radiographs in this section, like the radiographs throughout this text, are printed as if the reader is looking at the patient's anterior body surface (see Chapter 1).

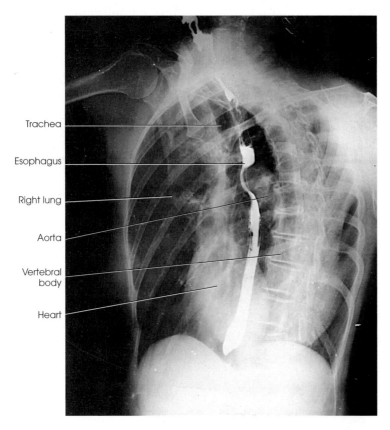

Trachea
Esophagus
Right lung
Aorta
Vertebral body
Heart

Fig. 10-46 PA oblique chest. The LAO position is 60 degrees with a barium-filled esophagus.

EVALUATION CRITERIA

The following should be clearly demonstrated:

- Both lungs in their entirety
- Trachea filled with air
- Visible identification markers
- Heart and mediastinal structures within the lung field of the elevated side in oblique images of 45 degrees

Barium studies

The RAO and LAO positions are routinely used during cardiac studies with barium. Follow the same procedure described in the PA chest section (see p. 527).

NOTE: A lesser-degree oblique position has been found to be of particular value in the study of pulmonary diseases. The patient is turned only slightly (10 to 20 degrees) from the RAO or LAO body position. This slight degree of obliquity rotates the superior segment of the respective lower lobe from behind the hilum and displays the medial part of the right middle lobe or the lingula of the left upper lobe free from the hilum. These areas are not clearly shown in the standard "cardiac oblique" of 45- to 60-degree rotation, largely because of superimposition of the spine.

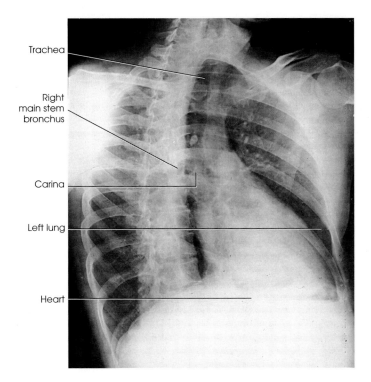

Trachea
Right main stem bronchus
Carina
Left lung
Heart

Fig. 10-47 PA oblique chest, RAO position.

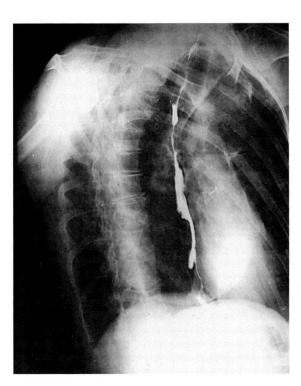

Fig. 10-48 PA oblique chest, RAO position.

Lungs and Heart
🔥 AP OBLIQUE PROJECTION
RPO and LPO positions

RPO and LPO positions are used when the patient is too ill to be turned to the prone position and sometimes as supplementary positions in the investigation of specific lesions. They are also used with the recumbent patient in contrast studies of the heart and great vessels.

One point the radiographer must bear in mind is that the *RPO corresponds to the LAO position* and the *LPO corresponds to the RAO position.* For AP oblique projections, the side of interest is generally the side *closest* to the cassette. The resulting image demonstrates the greatest area of the lung closest to the cassette. However, the lung farthest from the cassette is also imaged, and diagnostic information is often obtained for that side.

Image receptor: 35×43 cm (14×17 inch) lengthwise

SID: A minimum SID of 72 inches (183 cm) is recommended to decrease magnification of the heart and increase recorded detail of the thoracic structures.

Position of patient
- With the patient supine or facing the x-ray tube, either upright or recumbent, adjust the cassette so that the upper border of the cassette is about $1\frac{1}{2}$ to 2 inches (3.8 to 5 cm) above the vertebral prominens or about 5 inches (12.7 cm) above the jugular notch.

Position of part
- Rotate the patient toward the correct side, adjust the body at a 45-degree angle, and center the thorax to the grid.
- If the patient is recumbent, support the elevated hip and arm. Ensure that both sides of the chest are positioned to the cassette.
- Flex the patient's elbows and place the hands on the hips with the palms facing outward, or pronate the hands beside the hips. The arm closer to the cassette may be raised as long as the shoulder is rotated anteriorly.
- Adjust the shoulders to lie in the same transverse plane in a position of forward rotation (Figs. 10-49 and 10-50).
- *Shield gonads.*
- *Respiration:* Full inspiration. The exposure is made after the *second* full inspiration to ensure maximum expansion of the lungs.

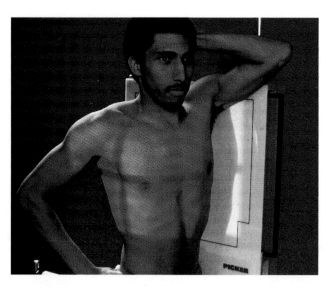

Fig. 10-49 Upright PA oblique chest, LPO position.

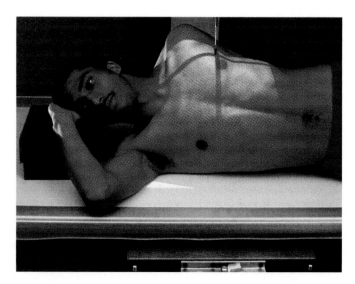

Fig. 10-50 Recumbent AP oblique chest, RPO position.

Central ray

- Perpendicular to the center of the cassette at a level 3 inches (7.6 cm) below the jugular notch (The central ray will exit at T7.)

Structures shown

This radiograph presents an AP oblique projection of the thoracic viscera similar to the corresponding PA oblique projection (Fig. 10-51). An RPO position is comparable to an LAO position. However, the lung field of the elevated side usually appears shorter because of magnification of the diaphragm. The heart and great vessels also cast magnified shadows as a result of being farther from the cassette.

The following should be clearly demonstrated:

- Both lungs in their entirety
- Trachea filled with air
- Visible identification markers
- The lung fields and mediastinal structures

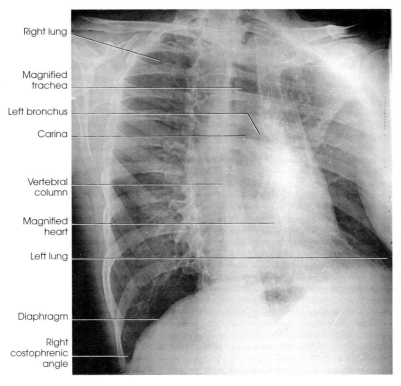 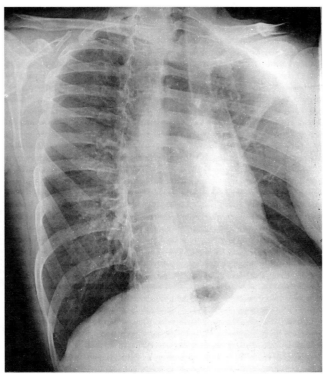

Right lung

Magnified trachea

Left bronchus

Carina

Vertebral column

Magnified heart

Left lung

Diaphragm

Right costophrenic angle

Fig. 10-51 AP oblique chest, LPO position.

AP PROJECTION[1]

The supine position is used when the patient is too ill to be turned to the prone position. It is sometimes used as a supplementary projection in the investigation of certain pulmonary lesions.

Image receptor: 35 × 43 cm (14 × 17 inches) lengthwise

SID: A SID of 72-inches (183 cm) or 60 inches (150 cm) SID is recommended if it can be attained using the equipment available.

Position of patient

- Place the patient in the supine or upright position with the back against the grid.

[1]See Chapter 30 for full description of *Mobile* AP.

Position of part

- Center the midsagittal plane of the chest to the cassette.
- Adjust the cassette so the upper border is approximately $1\frac{1}{2}$ to 2 inches (3.8 to 5 cm) above the relaxed shoulders.
- If possible, flex the patient's elbows, pronate the hands, and place the hands on the hips to draw the scapulas laterally. (Note, however, that this maneuver is often impossible because of the condition of the patient.)
- Adjust the shoulders to lie in the same transverse plane (Fig. 10-52).
- *Shield gonads.*
- *Respiration:* Full inspiration. The exposure is made after the *second* full inspiration to ensure maximum expansion of the lungs.

Central ray

- Perpendicular to the center of the cassette at a level 3 inches (7.6 cm) below the jugular notch

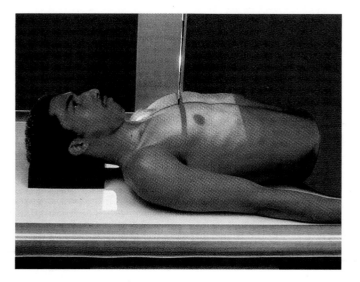

Fig. 10-52 AP chest.

Structures shown

- An AP projection of the thoracic viscera (Fig. 10-53) demonstrates an image somewhat similar to that of the PA projection (Fig. 10-54). Being farther from the cassette, the heart and great vessels are magnified, as well as engorged, and the lung fields appear shorter because abdominal compression moves the diaphragm to a higher level. The clavicles are projected higher, and the ribs assume a more horizontal appearance.

EVALUATION CRITERIA

The following should be clearly demonstrated:

- Medial portion of the clavicles equidistant from the vertebral column
- Trachea visible in the midline
- Clavicles lying more horizontal and obscuring more of the apices than in the PA projection
- Equal distance from the vertebral column to the lateral border of the ribs on each side
- Faint image of the ribs and thoracic vertebrae visible through the heart shadow
- Entire lung fields, from the apices to the costophrenic angles
- Pleural markings visible from the hilar regions to the periphery of the lungs

NOTE: Resnick[1] recommended an angled AP projection to free the basal portions of the lung fields from superimposition by the anterior diaphragmatic, abdominal, and cardiac structures. He reported that this projection also differentiates middle lobe and lingular processes from lower lobe disease. For this projection the patient may be either upright or supine, and the central ray is directed to the midsternal region at an angle of 30 degrees caudad. Resnick stated that a more suitable angulation may be chosen based on the preliminary films.

[1]Resnick D: The angulated basal view: a new method for evaluation of lower lobe pulmonary disease, *Radiology* 96:204, 1970.

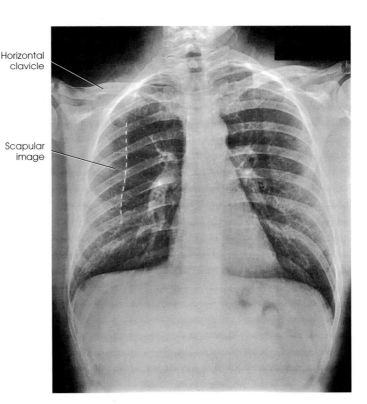

Horizontal clavicle

Scapular image

Fig. 10-53 AP chest.

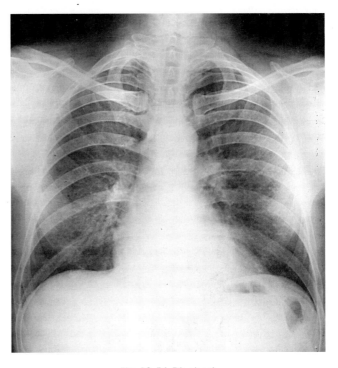

Fig. 10-54 PA chest.

Chest

♠ AP AXIAL PROJECTION
LINDBLOM METHOD
Lordotic position

Image receptor: 35 × 43 cm (14 × 17 inch) lengthwise

SID: A minimum SID of 72 inches (183 cm) is recommended to decrease magnification of the heart and to increase recorded detail of the thoracic structures.

Position of patient
- Place the patient in the upright position, facing the x-ray tube and standing approximately 1 foot (30.5 cm) in front of the vertical grid device.

Position of part
- Adjust the height of the cassette so that the upper margin is about 3 inches (7.6 cm) above the upper border of the shoulders when the patient is adjusted in the lordotic position.

Lordotic position
- Adjust the patient for the AP axial projection, with the midsagittal plane centered to the midline of the grid (Fig. 10-55).

Oblique lordotic positions—LPO or RPO
- Rotate the patient's body approximately 30 degrees away from the position used for the AP projection, with the affected side toward and centered to the grid (Fig. 10-56).
- With either of the preceding positions, have the patient flex the elbows and place the hands, palms out, on the hips.
- Have the patient lean backward in a position of extreme lordosis and rest the shoulders against the vertical grid device.
- *Shield gonads.*
- *Respiration:* Full inspiration. The exposure is made after the *second* full inspiration to ensure maximum expansion of the lungs.

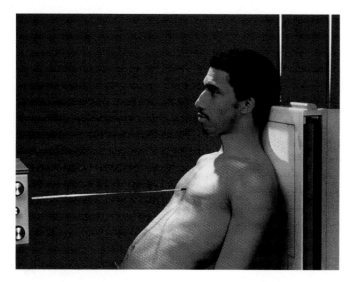

Fig. 10-55 AP axial pulmonary apices, lordotic position.

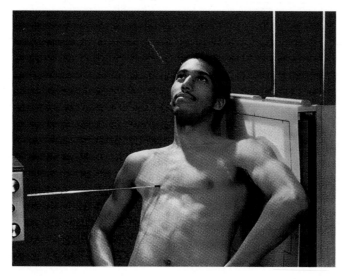

Fig. 10-56 AP axial oblique pulmonary apices, LPO lordotic position.

Thoracic viscera

Central ray

• Perpendicular to the center of the cassette at the level of the midsternum

COMPUTED RADIOGRAPHY

Collimation must be very close to keep unnecessary radiation from reaching the cassette phosphor.

Structures shown

The AP axial (Fig. 10-57) and AP axial oblique (Fig. 10-58) images of the lungs demonstrate the apices and conditions such as interlobar effusions.

EVALUATION CRITERIA

The following should be clearly demonstrated:

Lordotic position

■ Clavicles lying superior to the apices
■ Sternal ends of the clavicles equidistant from the vertebral column
■ Apices and lungs in their entirety
■ Clavicles lying horizontally with their medial ends overlapping only the first or second ribs
■ Ribs distorted with their anterior and posterior portions somewhat superimposed

Oblique lordotic position

■ Dependent apex and lung of the affected side in its entirety

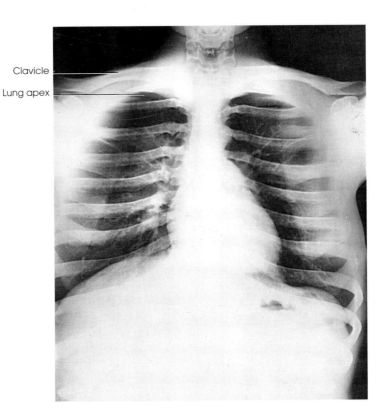

Fig. 10-57 AP axial pulmonary apices, lordotic position.

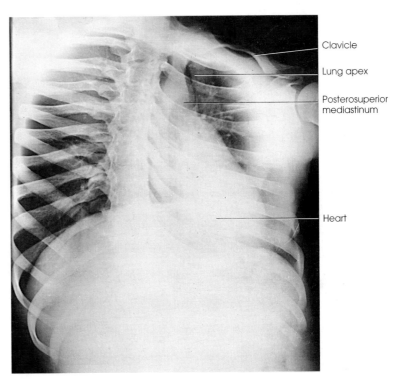

Fig. 10-58 AP axial oblique pulmonary apices, LPO lordotic position.

PA AXIAL PROJECTION

Image receptor: 24 × 30 cm (10 × 12 inch) or 30 × 35 cm (11 × 14 inch) crosswise

SID: A minimum SID of 72 inches (183 cm) is recommended to decrease magnification of the heart and to increase recorded detail of the thoracic structures.

Position of patient

• Position the patient, either seated or standing, before a vertical grid device. If the patient is standing, the weight of the body must be equally distributed on the feet.

Position of part

• Adjust the height of the cassette so that it is centered at the level of the jugular notch.
• Center the midsagittal plane of the patient's body to the midline of the cassette, and rest the chin against the grid device.
• Adjust the patient's head so that the midsagittal plane is vertical, then flex the elbows and place the hands, palms out, on the hips.
• Depress the patient's shoulders, rotate them forward, and adjust them to lie in the same transverse plane.
• Instruct the patient to keep the shoulders in contact with the grid device to move the scapulae from the lung fields (Fig. 10-59).
• *Shield gonads.*
• *Respiration:* Make the exposure at the end of *full inspiration* or optionally at *full expiration.* The clavicles are elevated by inspiration and depressed by expiration; the apices move little, if at all, during either phase of respiration.

Central ray
Inspiration
• Directed 10 to 15 degrees cephalad through T3 to the center of the cassette
Expiration (optional)
• Directed perpendicular to the plane of the cassette and centered at the level of T3

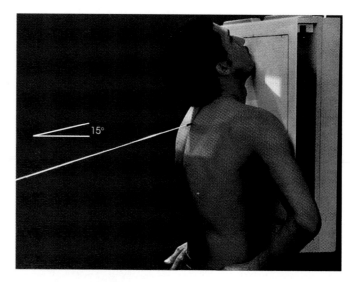

Fig. 10-59 PA axial pulmonary apices (inspiration).

Thoracic viscera

Structures shown

- The apices are projected above the shadows of the clavicles in the PA axial and PA projections (Figs. 10-60 and 10-61).

The following should be clearly demonstrated:

■ Apices in their entirety
■ Only the superior lung region adjacent to the apices
■ Clavicles lying below the apices
■ Medial portion of the clavicles equidistant from the vertebral column

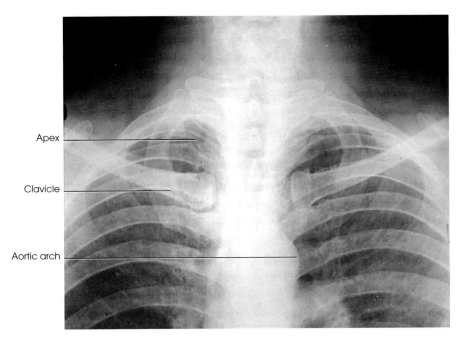

Fig. 10-60 PA axial pulmonary apices, inspiration with central ray angled.

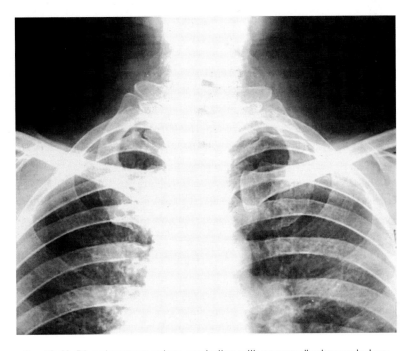

Fig. 10-61 PA pulmonary apices, expiration with perpendicular central ray.

AP AXIAL PROJECTION

Image receptor: 24 × 30 cm (10 × 12 inch) or 30 × 35 cm (11 × 14 inch) crosswise

SID: A minimum SID of 72 inches (183 cm) is recommended to decrease magnification of the heart and to increase recorded detail of the thoracic structures.

Position of patient
- Examine the patient in the upright or supine position.

Position of part
- Center the cassette to the midsagittal plane at the level of T2, and adjust the patient's body so that it is not rotated.
- Flex the patient's elbows and place the hands on the hips with the palms out, or pronate the hands beside the hips.
- Place the shoulders back against the grid and adjust them to lie in the same transverse plane (Fig. 10-62).
- *Shield gonads.*
- *Respiration:* Expose at the end of *full inspiration.*

Central ray
- Directed at an angle of 15 or 20 degrees cephalad to the center of the cassette and entering the manubrium

Structures shown
An AP axial projection demonstrates the apices lying below the clavicles (Fig. 10-63).

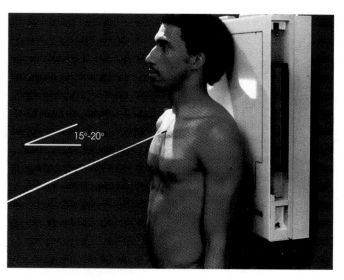

Fig. 10-62 AP axial pulmonary apices.

EVALUATION CRITERIA

The following should be clearly demonstrated:

- Clavicles lying superior to the apices
- Sternal ends of the clavicles equidistant from the vertebral column
- Apices in their entirety
- Superior lung region adjacent to the apices
- Clavicles lying horizontally with their medial ends overlapping only the first or second ribs
- Ribs distorted, with their anterior and posterior portions somewhat superimposed

NOTE: The AP axial projection is used in preference to the PA axial projection in hypersthenic patients and patients whose clavicles occupy a high position. The AP axial projection makes it possible to separate the apical and clavicular shadows without undue distortion of the apices.

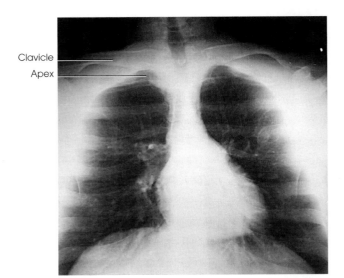
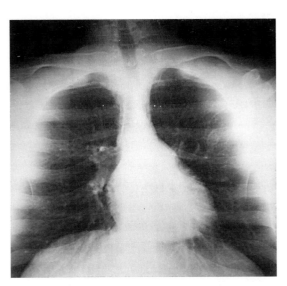

Clavicle

Apex

Fig. 10-63 AP axial pulmonary apices.

PA AXIAL PROJECTION
FLEISCHNER METHOD
Lordotic position

> **Image receptor:** 35 × 43 cm (14 × 17 inches) lengthwise

> **SID:** A minimum SID of 72 inches (183 cm) is recommended to decrease magnification of the heart and to increase recorded detail of the thoracic structures.

Position of patient

- Position the patient upright, facing the vertical grid device.

Position of part

- Adjust the height of the cassette so that the upper margin of the cassette is about 1 inch (2.5 cm) below the upper border of the shoulders *when the patient is standing upright.* With the patient in the lordotic position, the lungs will be correctly projected on the cassette.
- Center the midsagittal plane of the patient's body to the midline of the grid.
- Have the patient grasp the grid device, brace the abdomen against it, and then lean backward in a position of extreme lordosis. The thorax should be inclined posteriorly approximately 45 degrees (Figs. 10-64 and 10-65).
- *Shield gonads.*
- *Respiration:* Make the exposure at the end of *full inspiration.*

Central ray

- Perpendicular to the cassette at the level of T4

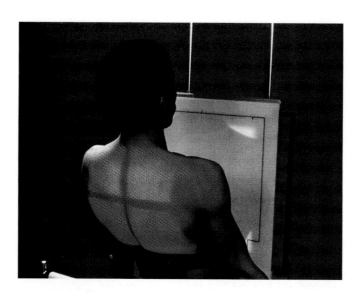

Fig. 10-64 PA axial pulmonary apices, lordotic position.

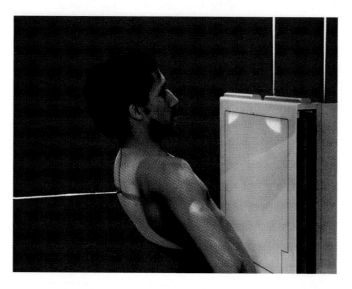

Fig. 10-65 PA axial pulmonary apices, lordotic position.

Structures shown

The PA axial projection demonstrates interlobar effusion and collapse of the right middle lobe. This positioning places the horizontal fissure parallel with the x-ray beam (Fig. 10-66). A similar radiograph can be obtained by adjusting the patient in the prone position and directing the central ray 45 degrees caudad (Fig. 10-67).

Kjellberg[1] recommended a prone position with a 30-degree caudal angulation of the central ray for the demonstration of minimal mitral disease.

EVALUATION CRITERIA

The following should be clearly demonstrated:
- Clavicles lying superior to the apices
- Sternal ends of the clavicles equidistant from the vertebral column
- Apices and lungs in their entirety
- Clavicles lying horizontally with their medial ends overlapping only the first or second ribs
- Ribs distorted, with their anterior and posterior portions somewhat superimposed

[1]Kjellberg SR: Importance of prone position in the roentgenologic diagnosis of slight mitral disease, *Acta Radiol* 31:178, 1949.

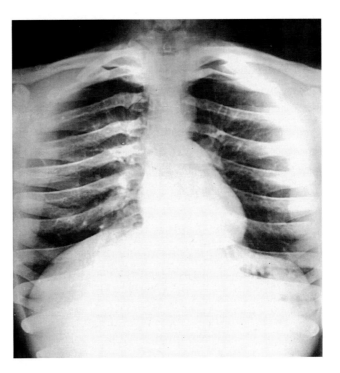

Fig. 10-66 Upright PA axial pulmonary apices, lordotic position.

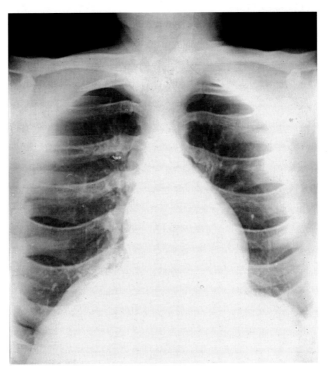

Fig. 10-67 Prone axial pulmonary apices with a 45-degree caudal central ray.

AP OR PA PROJECTION[1]
R or L lateral decubitus positions

Image receptor: 35 × 43 cm (14 × 17 inch) lengthwise

Position of patient
- Place the patient in a lateral decubitus position, lying on either the affected or the unaffected side, as indicated by the existing condition. A small amount of fluid in the pleural cavity is usually best shown with the patient lying on the affected side. With this positioning, the mediastinal shadows and the fluid will not overlap. A small amount of free air in the pleural cavity is generally best demonstrated with the patient lying on the unaffected side.
- Achieve the best visualization by allowing the patient to remain in the position for *5 minutes before the exposure.* This allows fluid to settle and air to rise.

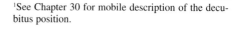

[1]See Chapter 30 for mobile description of the decubitus position.

Position of part
- If the patient is lying on the affected side, elevate the body 5 to 8 cm (2 to 3 inches) on a suitable platform or a firm pad.
- Extend the arms well above the head, and adjust the thorax in a true lateral position (Fig. 10-68).
- Place the anterior or posterior surface of the chest against a vertical grid device.
- Adjust the cassette so that it extends approximately 1½ to 2 inches (3.8 to 5 cm) beyond the shoulders.
- *Shield gonads.*
- *Respiration:* Full inspiration. The exposure is made after the *second* full inspiration to ensure maximum expansion of the lungs.

Central ray
- *Horizontal* and perpendicular to the center of the cassette at a level 3 inches (7.6 cm) below the jugular notch for the AP, and T7 for the PA

Structures shown
An AP or PA projection obtained using the lateral decubitus position demonstrates the change in fluid position and reveals any previously obscured pulmonary areas or, in the case of suspected pneumothorax, the presence of any free air (Figs. 10-69 to 10-71).

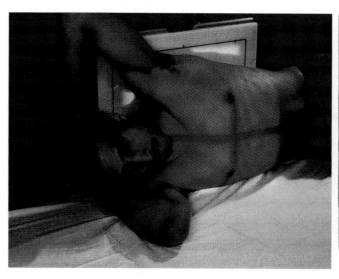

Fig. 10-68 AP projection, right lateral decubitus position.

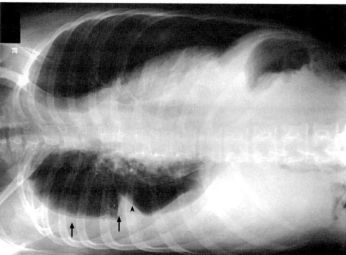

Fig. 10-69 AP projection, right lateral decubitus position, showing a fluid level *(arrows)* on the side that is down. Note the fluid in the lung fissure *(arrowhead).*

Thoracic viscera

EVALUATION CRITERIA

The following should be clearly demonstrated:

- No rotation of the patient from a true frontal position, as evidenced by the clavicles being equidistant from the spine
- Affected side in its entirety
- Apices
- Proper identification visible to indicate that decubitus was performed
- Patient's arms not visible in the field of interest

NOTE: An exposure made with the patient leaning directly laterally from the upright PA position is sometimes useful for demonstrating fluid levels in pulmonary cavities. Ekimsky[1] recommended this position, with the patient leaning laterally 45 degrees, for the demonstration of small pleural effusions. He reported that the inclined position is simpler to perform than the decubitus position and is equally satisfactory.

[1]Ekimsky B: Comparative study of lateral decubitus views and those with lateral body inclination in small pleural effusions, *Vestn Rentgenol Radiol* 41:43, 1966. (In Russian.) Abstract: *Radiology* 87:1135, 1966.

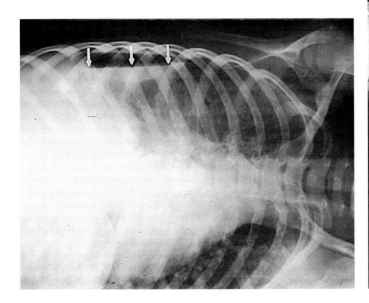

Fig. 10-70 AP projection, left lateral decubitus position, in same patient as in Fig. 10-71. The arrows indicate the air-fluid level (air on the side up).

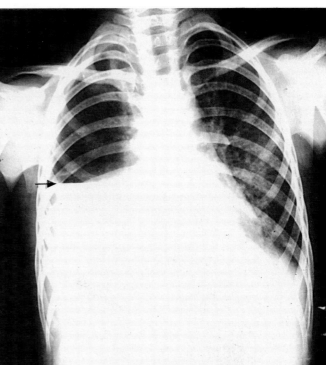

Fig. 10-71 Upright PA chest. The arrow indicates the air-fluid level.

☀ LATERAL PROJECTION
R or L position
Ventral or dorsal decubitus position

Image receptor: 35 × 43 cm (14 × 17 inch) lengthwise

Position of patient

- With the patient in a prone or supine position, elevate the thorax 2 to 3 inches (5 to 7.6 cm) on folded sheets or a firm pad, centering the thorax to the grid.
- Achieve the best visualization by allowing the patient to remain in the position for *5 minutes before the exposure.* This allows fluid to settle and air to rise.

Position of part

- Adjust the body in a true prone or supine body position, and extend the arms well above the head.
- Place the affected side against a vertical grid device, and adjust it so that the top of the cassette extends to the level of the thyroid cartilage (Fig. 10-72).
- *Shield gonads.*
- *Respiration:* Full inspiration. The exposure is made after the *second* full inspiration to ensure maximum expansion of the lungs.

Central ray

- *Horizontal* and centered to the cassette. The central ray enters at the level of the midcoronal plane and 3 to 4 inches (7.6 to 10.2 cm) below the jugular notch for the dorsal decubitus, and at T7 for the ventral decubitus.

COMPUTED RADIOGRAPHY

The kVp used for this projection requires that the collimation be very close. Scattered and primary radiation reaching the cassette phosphor may cause computer artifacts.

Structures shown

A lateral projection in the decubitus position shows a change in the position of fluid and reveals pulmonary areas that are obscured by the fluid in standard projections (Figs. 10-73 and 10-74).

EVALUATION CRITERIA

The following should be clearly demonstrated:

- Entire lung fields, including the anterior and posterior surfaces
- No rotation of the thorax from a true lateral position
- Upper lung field not obscured by the arms
- Proper marker identification visible to indicate the decubitus was performed
- T6 in the center of the cassette

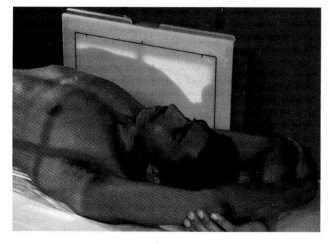

Fig. 10-72 Lateral projection, dorsal decubitus position.

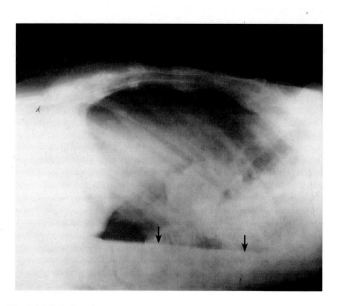

Fig. 10-73 Lateral projection, dorsal decubitus position. The arrows indicate the air-fluid level.

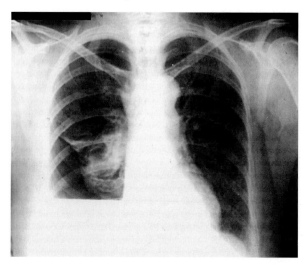

Fig. 10-74 Upright PA chest in same patient as in Fig. 10-73.

Bronchography*

Bronchography is the term applied to specialized radiologic examination of the lungs and bronchial tree with an opaque contrast medium introduced into the bronchi (Figs. 10-75 and 10-76). This examination has been used to investigate conditions such as hemoptysis, bronchiectasis, chronic pneumonia, bronchial obstruction, pulmonary tumors, cysts, and cavities, and bronchopleural-cutaneous fistulae.

At one time, bronchography was routinely performed in radiology departments. Today, however, it is performed only as a very specialized procedure, partly because of the availability of computed tomography, the improved diagnostic techniques available in nuclear medicine, and the development of the fiberoptic bronchoscope.

The fiberoptic bronchoscope has had a profound effect. In bronchography the lung can be imaged to the level of the fifth bronchial division. In fiberoptic bronchoscopy the bronchoscope can be placed in the trachea and advanced directly into the lung to level of the second division. The greatest advantage of the bronchoscope, however, is that lung tissue specimens can be obtained during bronchoscopy. Biopsy samples are not obtained during routine bronchography. Furthermore, some pulmonary masses that years ago would have required surgical removal are now successfully managed with antibiotics.

Numerous iodinated media, both aqueous and oily, are available for bronchography. However, the oily media are more generally used.

---

*This description of bronchography has been reduced from that in earlier editions. For those interested in an expanded description, please see volume 3 of the fourth or fifth edition of this text.

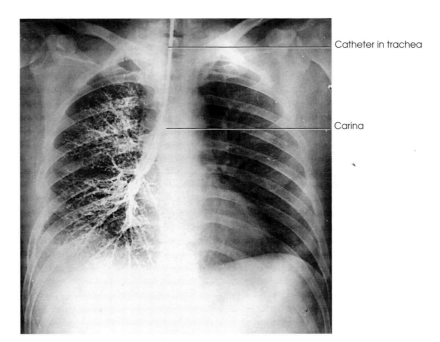

Catheter in trachea

Carina

Fig. 10-75 PA right lung.

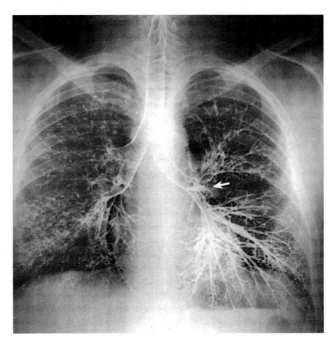

Fig. 10-76 PA showing obstruction of the main lingular branch bronchus in the left superior lobe *(arrow)*.

CONTRAST MEDIUM INSTILLATION

Several techniques can be used to instill contrast medium into the bronchial tree. In one technique, a local anesthetic is administered to the throat and larynx, and a catheter, or cannula, is used to drop the contrast medium onto the base of the anesthetized tongue. The contrast medium then flows into the bronchial tree without penetrating any patient surface. In the most often used technique a catheter is advanced across the larynx. The contrast medium may be injected into the superior trachea for a bilateral examination, or the catheter may be further advanced into the right or left main bronchus to examine the side of interest. In a seldom-used approach, the trachea is directly punctured, and the contrast medium is injected through a catheter, or cannula, with resultant distribution of contrast medium into one or both lungs.

Once the contrast medium has been introduced, distribution through the bronchial branches depends on gravity. Therefore, body position guides the direction of flow. Monitoring of the contrast medium generally occurs during fluoroscopy.

The resulting radiographic images may include the following: a supine AP projection, an upright PA projection (see Figs. 10-75 and 10-76), supine or upright oblique positions, a lateral position (Fig. 10-77), and images of small portions of interest (Figs. 10-78 and 10-79). Exposure factors must be increased from normal chest exposure technique to penetrate the contrast medium.

At the conclusion of the examination the patient coughs and expectorates as much of the contrast agent as possible. Any contrast medium remaining in the lungs is eventually excreted via the urinary system.

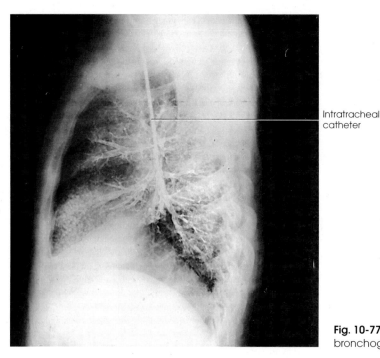

Fig. 10-77 Right lateral bronchogram.

Intratracheal catheter

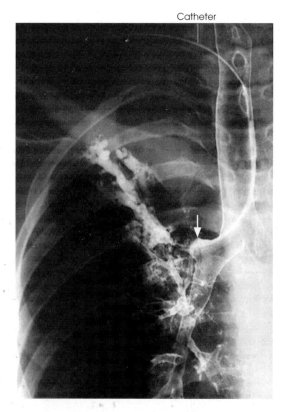

Catheter

Fig. 10-78 PA right superior lobe, showing partial occlusion of the bronchus in the lobe (*arrow*). Postobstructive bronchiectasis was found.

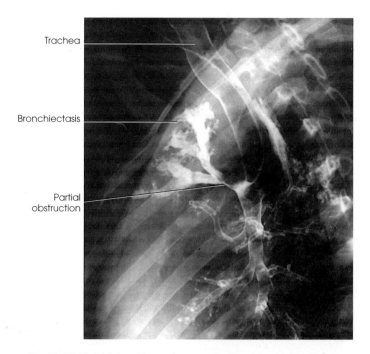

Trachea

Bronchiectasis

Partial obstruction

Fig. 10-79 Right lateral bronchogram in the same patient as in Fig. 10-78.

LONG BONE MEASUREMENT

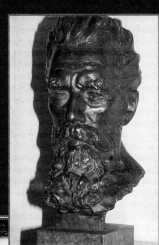

RIGHT: Bronze bust of Dr. Wilhelm C. Roentgen.

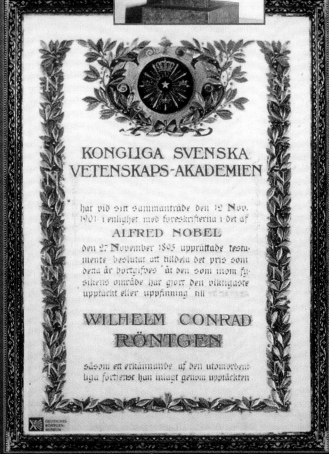

LEFT: The Nobel Prize award received by Dr. Roentgen. The gold medallion was reportedly melted down during World War I.

Radiography provides the most reliable means of obtaining accurate measurements of the length of long bones, specifically length differences between the two sides. Although studies are occasionally made of the upper limbs, radiography is most frequently applied to the lower limbs. This chapter considers only a few of the many radiographic methods that have been devised for long bone measurement.

Radiation Protection

Differences in limb length are not uncommon in children and may occur in association with a variety of disorders. Patients with unequal limb growth may require yearly radiographic evaluations. More frequent examinations may be necessary in patients who have undergone surgical procedures to equalize limb length. One treatment method controls bone growth on the normal side. This is usually accomplished by means of metaphysial-epiphysial fusion at the distal femoral or proximal tibial level. Another treatment technique is to increase the growth of the shorter limb. This is achieved by surgically cutting the femur and/or tibia-fibula. A frame is then placed around the cut ends and extended to the outside of the body. Gradual pressure on the frame separates the bone, extends the leg, and promotes healing at the same time.

Because patients with limb length differences require checkups at regular intervals over a period of years, gonad shielding is necessary to guard their well-being. In addition, careful patient positioning, secure immobilization, and accurate centering of a closely collimated beam of radiation are important to prevent unnecessary repeat exposures.

Position of Patient

Three exposures are made of each limb, with the accuracy of the examination depending on the patient not moving the limb or limbs even slightly. Small children must be carefully immobilized to prevent motion. If movement of the limb occurs before the examination is completed, all radiographs may need to be repeated.

- Place the patient in the supine position for all techniques, and examine both sides for comparison.
- When a soft tissue abnormality (swelling or atrophy) is causing rotation of the pelvis, elevate the low side on a radiolucent support to overcome the rotation, if necessary.

Position of Part

The limb to be examined should be positioned as follows:

- Adjust and immobilize the limb for an AP projection.
- If the two lower limbs are examined simultaneously, separate the ankles 5 to 6 inches (13 to 15 cm) and place the specialized ruler under the pelvis and extended down between the legs.
- If the limbs are examined separately, position the patient with a special ruler beneath each limb.
- When the knee of the patient's abnormal side cannot be fully extended, flex the normal knee to the same degree and support each knee on one of a pair of supports of *identical size* to ensure that the joints are flexed to the same degree and are equidistant from the cassette.

Localization of Joints

For the methods that require centering of the ray above the joints, the following steps should be taken:

- Localize each joint accurately, and use a skin-marking pencil to indicate the central ray centering point.
- Because both sides are examined for comparison and a discrepancy in bone length usually exists, mark the joints of each side after the patient is in the supine position .
- With the upper limb, place the marks as follows: for the *shoulder joint*—over the superior margin of the head of the humerus; for the *elbow joint*—$1/2$ to $3/4$ inch (1.3 to 1.9 cm) below the plane of the epicondyles of the humerus (depending on the size of the patient); and for the *wrist*—midway between the styloid processes of the radius and ulna.
- With the lower limb, locate the *hip joint* by placing a mark 1 to $1 1/4$ inches (2.5 to 3.2 cm) (depending on the size of the patient) laterodistally and at a right angle to the midpoint of an imaginary line extending from the anterior superior iliac spine to the pubic symphysis.
- Locate the *knee joint* just below the apex of the patella at the level of the depression between the femoral and tibial condyles.
- Locate the *ankle joint* directly below the depression midway between the malleoli.

In all radiographs made by a single x-ray exposure, the image is larger than the actual body part because the x-ray photons start at a very small area on the target of the x-ray tube and diverge as they travel in straight lines through the body to the cassette (Fig. 11-1). This magnification can be decreased by putting the body part as close to the cassette as possible and making the distance between the x-ray tube and the image receptor as long as possible (a procedure sometimes referred to as *teleoroentgenography*). However, a radiographic technique called *orthoroentgenology* can be used to determine the exact length of a child's limb bones.

For this radiographic technique, a metal measurement ruler is placed between the patient's lower limbs and three exposures are made on the same x-ray cassette. The following steps are observed:

- Using narrow collimation and careful centering of the limb parts to the upper, middle, and lower thirds of the cassette, make three exposures on one cassette.
- For all three exposures, place the central ray perpendicular to and passing directly through the specified joint (hence the term *orthoroentgenology*, from the Greek word *orthos*, meaning straight).
- Do not move the limb between exposures. Because the cassette is in the Bucky tray for all exposures, including that of the ankle, exposure factors must be modified accordingly.
- Position the x-ray tube directly over the patient's hip, and make the first exposure (Fig. 11-2, *A*).
- Move the x-ray tube to directly over the patient's knee joint, and make a second exposure (Fig. 11-2, *B*).
- Move the x-ray tube to directly over the patient's tibiotalar joint, and make a third exposure (Fig. 11-2, *C*).

If the child holds the leg perfectly still while the three exposures are made, the true distance from the proximal end of the femur to the distal end of the tibia can be directly measured on the image:

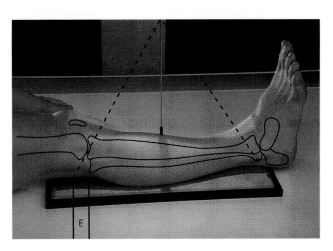

Fig. 11-1 Conventional radiographs are magnified (elongated) images. Proximal elongation in above example is equal to the distance (*E*). Similar elongation occurs distally.

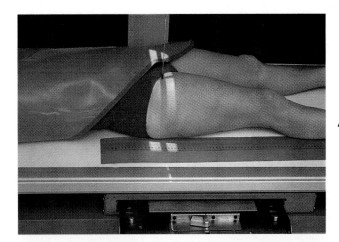

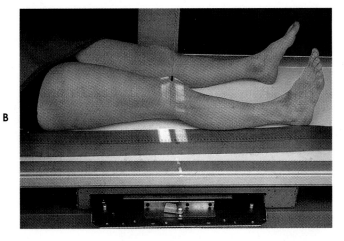

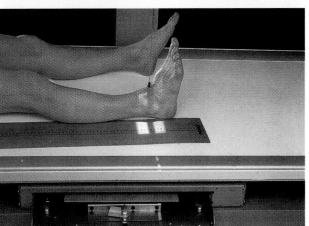

Fig. 11-2 Patient positioned for orthoroentgenographic measurement of lower limb. The central ray is centered over the hip joint (**A**), knee joint (**B**), and ankle joint (**C**). A metal ruler was placed near the lateral aspect of leg for photographic purposes. The ruler is normally placed between the limbs (see Fig. 11-4.)

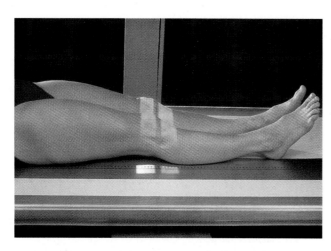

Fig. 11-3 Bilateral leg length measurement, with metal ruler placed beside leg for photographic purposes. (Proper placement of the ruler is shown in Fig. 11-4.)

- Place a special metal ruler (engraved with radiopaque centimeter or ¹/₂-inch (1.3-cm) marks that show when a radiograph is made) under the leg and on top of the table (see Fig. 11-2).
- If the cassette is placed in the Bucky tray and then moved between the exposures (see Fig. 11-2), calculate the length of the femur and tibia by subtracting the numerical values projected over the two joints obtained by simultaneously exposing the patient and the metal ruler.

Another method of measuring the lengths of the femurs and tibias is to examine both limbs simultaneously (Figs. 11-3 and 11-4):

- Center the midsagittal plane of the patient's body to the midline of the grid.
- Adjust the patient's lower limbs in the anatomic position (i.e., slight medial rotation).
- Tape the special metal ruler to the top of the table so that part of it is included in each of the exposure fields. This records the position of each joint.
- Place a cassette in the Bucky tray, and shift it for centering at the three joint levels without moving the patient.

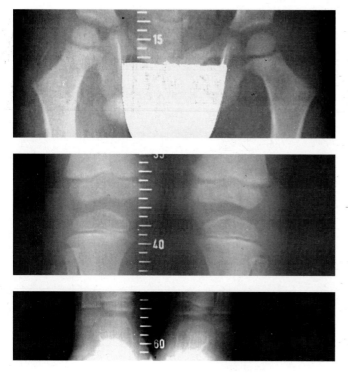

Fig. 11-4 Orthoroentgenogram for the measurement of leg length.

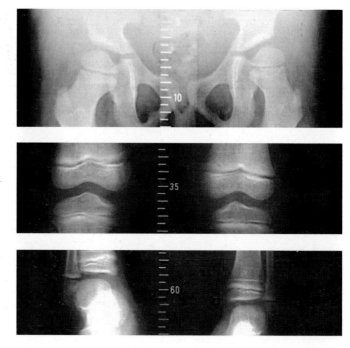

Fig. 11-5 Leg measurement showing that the right leg is shorter than the left leg.

- Center the cassette and the tube successively at the previously marked level of the hip joints, the knee joints, and the ankle joints for simultaneous bilateral projections.
- When a difference in level exists between the contralateral joints, center the tube midway between the two levels.
- Make the three exposures on one 35 × 43 cm (14 × 17 inch) or 30 × 35 cm (11 × 14 inch) cassette. Limb length can then be quickly determined.

The orthoroentgenographic method is reasonably accurate if the limbs are of almost the same length. When more than a slight discrepancy in limb length exists (Fig. 11-5), it is not possible to place the center of the x-ray tube exactly over both knee joints and make a single exposure or exactly over both ankle joints and make a single exposure. In such cases, the tube is centered midway between the two joints. However, this results in bilateral distortion because of the diverging x-ray beam. In Fig. 11-5 the measurement obtained for the right femur is somewhat less than the actual length of the bone, whereas the measurement of the left femur is somewhat greater than the true length. The following measure can be taken to correct this problem:

- Examine each limb separately (Fig. 11-6).
- Center the limb being examined on the grid, and place the special ruler beneath the limb.

- Make a closely collimated exposure over each joint. This restriction of the exposure field not only increases the accuracy of the procedure but also considerably reduces radiation exposure (most importantly, to the gonads).
- After making joint localization marks, position the patient and apply local gonad shielding.
- Adjust the collimator to limit the exposure field as much as possible.
- With successive centering to the localization marks, make exposures of the hip, knee, and ankle.
- Repeat the procedure for the opposite limb.
- Use the same approach to measure lengths of the long bones in the upper limbs (Fig. 11-7).

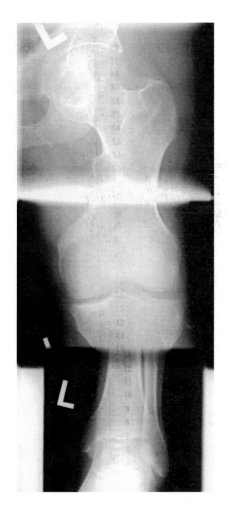

Fig. 11-6 Unilateral leg measurement.

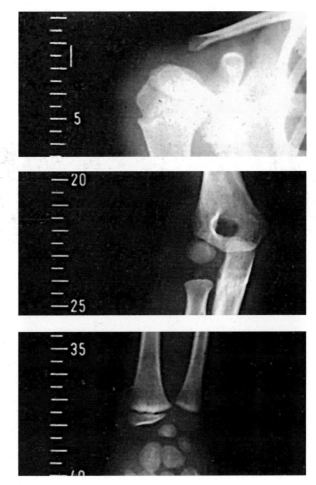

Fig. 11-7 Measurement of upper limb.

Computed Tomography Technique

Helms and McCarthy[1] reported a method for using computed tomography (CT) to measure discrepancies in leg length. Temme, Chu, and Anderson[2] compared conventional orthoroentgenograms with CT scans for long bone measurements. Both sets of investigators concluded that the CT scanogram is more consistently reproduced and that it causes less radiation exposure to the patient than the conventional radiographic approach. The CT approach is as follows:

- Take CT localizer or "scout" images of the femurs and tibias.
- Place cursors over the respective hip, knee, and ankle joints as described earlier in this chapter. To similarly study the upper limb, obtain scout images of the humerus, radius, and ulna.
- Place CT cursors over the shoulder, elbow, and wrist joints, and obtain the measurements. The measurements are displayed on the cathode ray tube (Figs. 11-8 to 11-10).

The accuracy of the CT examination depends on proper placement of the cursor. Helms and McCarthy[1] found that accuracy improved when the cursors were placed three times and the values obtained were averaged. These authors also reported that CT examinations used radiation doses that were 50 to 200 times less than those used with conventional radiography. CT examination requires about the same amount of time as conventional radiography.

[1] Helms CA, McCarthy S: CT scanograms for measuring leg length discrepancy, *Radiology* 252:802, 1984.

[2] Temme JB, Chu W, Anderson JC: CT scanograms compared with conventional orthoroentgenograms in long bone measurement, *Radiol Technol* 59:65, 1987.

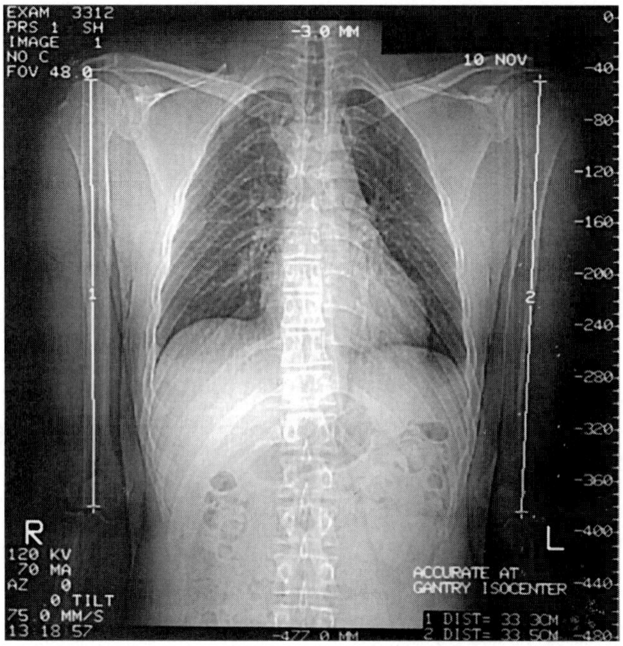

Fig. 11-8 Measurement of the arms using computed tomography (CT). Note the arm labels and measurements in the right lower corner.

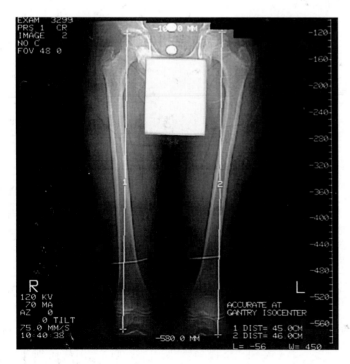

Fig. 11-9 CT measurements of femurs. The right femur is 1 cm shorter than the left femur in the same patient as in Fig. 11-8.

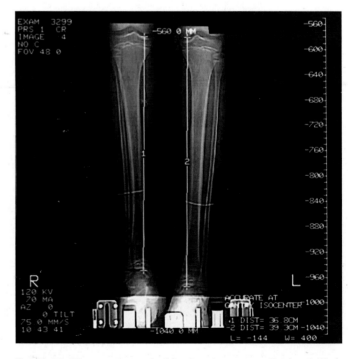

Fig. 11-10 CT measurement of the legs in same patient as in Figs. 11-8 and 11-9.

12

CONTRAST ARTHROGRAPHY

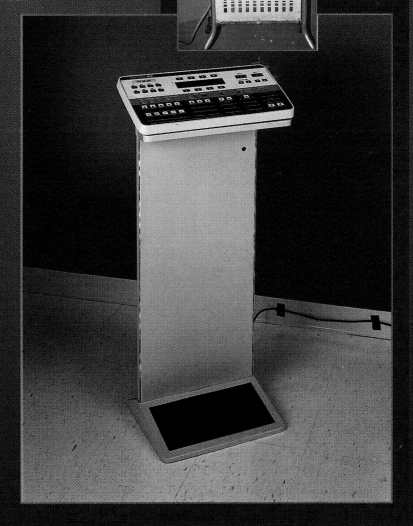

RIGHT: Marble-topped radiographic unit from 1920. Note the glass-insulating covers surrounding the electrical controls and protecting the operator from electric shock.

LEFT: High-frequency-generator radiographic control panel for the twenty-first century. The digital display console also contains anatomic programming and automatic exposure control.

(Courtesy TREX Medical Corp.)

Overview

The introduction and development of magnetic resonance imaging (MRI) have significantly reduced the number of arthrograms performed in radiology departments. Because MRI is a noninvasive imaging technique, the knee, wrist, hip, shoulder, temporomandibular joint (TMJ), and other joints previously evaluated by contrast arthrography are now studied using MRI (Fig. 12-1). As a result, radiographic contrast arthrography has increasingly specialized functions.

Arthrography (Greek *arthron,* meaning "joint") is radiography of a joint or joints. *Pneumoarthrography, opaque arthrography,* and *double-contrast arthrography* are terms used to denote radiologic examinations of the soft tissue structures of joints (menisci, ligaments, articular cartilage, bursae) after the injection of one or two contrast agents into the capsular space.

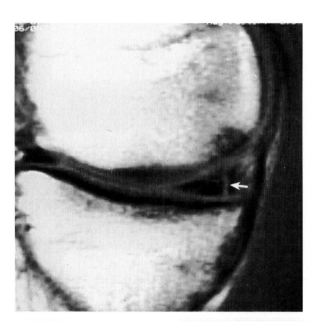

Fig. 12-1 Noninvasive MRI of knee, showing torn medial meniscus *(arrow).*

A gaseous medium is employed in pneumoarthrography, a water-soluble iodinated medium is used in opaque arthrography (Fig. 12-2), and a combination of gaseous and water-soluble iodinated media is used in double-contrast arthrography. Although contrast studies may be made on any encapsuled joint, the knee has been the most frequent site of investigation. Other joints examined by contrast arthrography include the shoulder, hip, wrist, and temporomandibular joints.

Arthrogram examinations are usually performed with a local anesthetic. The injection is made under careful aseptic conditions, usually in a combination fluoroscopic-radiographic examining room that has been carefully prepared in advance. The sterile items required, particularly the length and gauge of the needles, vary according to the part being examined. The sterile tray and the nonsterile items should be set up on a conveniently placed instrument cart or a small two-shelf table.

After aspirating any effusion, the radiologist injects the contrast agent or agents and manipulates the joint to ensure proper distribution of the contrast material. The examination is usually performed by fluoroscopy and spot images. Conventional radiographs may be taken when special images, such as an axial projection of the shoulder or an intercondyloid fossa position of the knee, are desired.

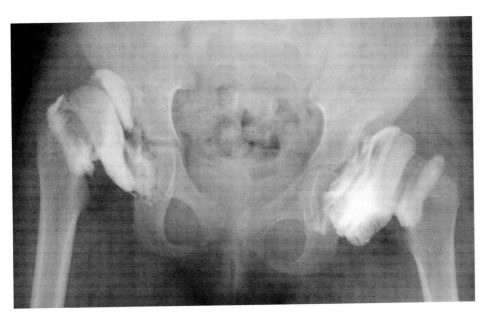

Fig. 12-2 Bilateral opaque arthrogram of bilateral congenital hip dislocations.

Contrast Arthrography of the Knee

VERTICAL RAY METHOD

Contrast arthrography of the knee by the vertical ray method requires the use of a stress device. The following steps are observed:

- Place the limb in the frame to widen or "open up" the side of the joint space under investigation. This widening, or spreading, of the intrastructural spaces permits better distribution of the contrast material around the meniscus.

- After the contrast material is injected, place the limb in the stress device (Fig. 12-3). To delineate the medial side of the joint, for example, place the stress device just above the knee; then laterally stress the lower leg.

- When contrast arthrograms are to be made by conventional radiography, turn the patient to the prone position, and fluoroscopically localize the centering point for each side of the joint. The mark ensures accurate centering for closely collimated studies of each side of the joint and permits multiple exposures to be made on one cassette. The images obtained of each side of the joint usually consist of an AP projection and a 20-degree right and left AP oblique projection.

- Obtain the oblique position by leg rotation or central ray angulation (Figs. 12-4 to 12-6).

- On completion of these studies, remove the frame and then perform a lateral and an intercondyloid fossa projection.

NOTE: Anderson and Maslin[1] recommended that tomography be used in knee arthrography. In addition, the technique can frequently be used for other contrast-filled joint capsules.

[1]Anderson PW, Maslin P: Tomography applied to knee arthrography, *Radiology* 110:271, 1974.

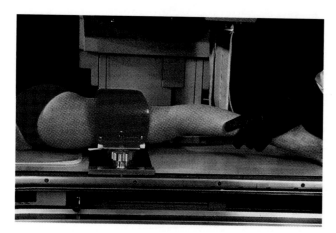

Fig. 12-3 Patient lying on lead rubber for gonad shielding and positioned in stress device on fluoroscopic table.

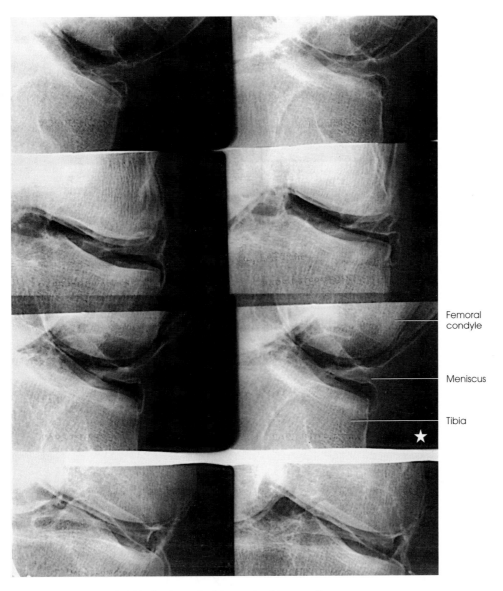

Femoral
condyle

Meniscus

Tibia

Fig. 12-4 Vertical ray double-contrast knee arthrogram.

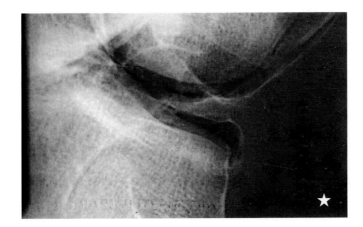

Fig. 12-5 Enlarged image of frame with star seen in Fig. 12-4.

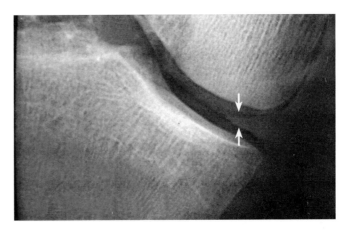

Fig. 12-6 Knee pneumoarthrogram showing normal lateral meniscus *(arrows)* surrounded with air above and below it.

563

Double-Contrast Arthrography of the Knee

HORIZONTAL RAY METHOD

The horizontal central ray method of performing double-contrast arthrography of the knee was described first by Andrén and Wehlin[1] and later by Freiberger, Killoran, and Cardona.[2] These investigators found that using a horizontal x-ray beam position and a comparatively small amount of each of the two contrast agents (gaseous medium and water-soluble iodinated medium) improved double-contrast delineation of the knee joint structures. With this technique, the excess of the heavy iodinated solutions drains into the dependent part of the joint, leaving only the desired thin opaque coating on the gas-enveloped uppermost part, the part then under investigation.

---

[1]Andrén L, Wehlin L: Double-contrast arthrography of knee with horizontal roentgen ray beam, *Acta Orthop Scand* 29:307, 1960.
[2]Freiberger RH, Killoran PJ, Cardona G: Arthrography of the knee by double contrast method, *AJR* 97:736, 1966.

Medial meniscus

- Adjust the patient in a semiprone position that places the posterior aspect of the medial meniscus uppermost (Figs. 12-7 and 12-8).
- To widen the joint space, manually stress the knee.
- Draw a line on the medial side of the knee, and then direct the central ray along the line and centered to the meniscus.
- With rotation toward the supine position, turn the leg 30 degrees for each of the succeeding five exposures.
- Direct the central ray along the localization line for each exposure, ensuring that it is centered to the meniscus.

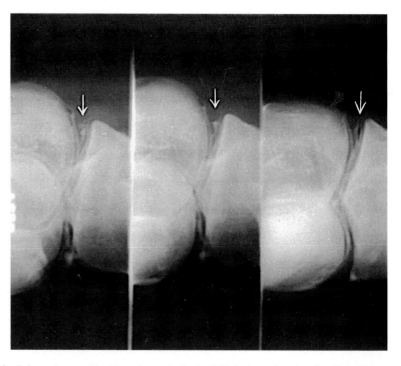

Fig. 12-7 Medial meniscus with a tear in posterior half. Note irregular streaks of positive contrast material within meniscal wedge *(arrows)*.

Lateral meniscus

- Adjust the patient in a semiprone position that places the posterior aspect of the lateral meniscus uppermost (Fig. 12-9).
- To widen the joint space, manually stress the knee.
- As with the medial meniscus, make six images on one cassette.
- With movement toward the supine position, rotate the leg 30 degrees for each of the consecutive exposures, from the initial prone oblique position to the supine oblique position.
- Adjust the central ray angulation as required to direct it along the localization line and center it to the meniscus.

NOTE: For demonstration of the cruciate ligaments after filming of the menisci is completed,[1] the patient sits with the knee flexed 90 degrees over the side of the radiographic table. A firm cotton pillow is placed under the knee and adjusted so that some forward pressure can be applied to the leg. With the patient holding a grid cassette in position, a closely collimated and slightly overexposed lateral projection is made.

---

[1]Mittler S, Freiberger RH, Harrison-Stubbs M: A method of improving cruciate ligament visualization in double-contrast arthrography, *Radiology* 102:441, 1972.

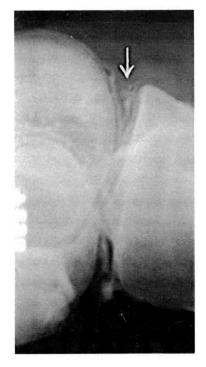

Fig. 12-8 Enlarged image showing tear in medial meniscus of the same patient as in Fig. 12-7.

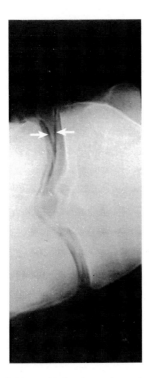

Fig. 12-9 Normal lateral meniscus (*arrows*) in the same patient as in Figs. 12-7 and 12-8.

Wrist Arthrography

The primary indications for wrist arthrography are trauma, persistent pain, and limitation of motion. After contrast material (approximately 1.5 to 4 ml) is injected through the dorsal wrist at the articulation of the radius, scaphoid, and lunate, the wrist is gently manipulated to disperse the medium. The projections most commonly used are the PA, lateral, and both obliques (Figs. 12-10 and 12-11). Fluoroscopy or tape recording of the wrist during rotation is recommended for the exact detection of contrast medium leaks.

Hip Arthrography

Hip arthrography is performed most often in children to evaluate congenital hip dislocation before treatment (see Fig. 12-2) and after treatment (Figs. 12-12 and 12-13). In adults the primary use of hip arthrography is to detect a loose hip prosthesis or confirm the presence of infection. The cement used to fasten hip prosthesis components has barium sulfate added to make the cement and the cement-bone interface radiographically visible (Fig. 12-14). Although the addition of barium sulfate to cement is helpful in confirming proper seating of the prosthesis, it makes evaluation of the same joint by arthrography difficult.

Because both the cement and contrast material produce the same approximate radiographic density, a subtraction technique is recommended—either photographic subtraction, as shown in Figs. 12-15 and 12-16 (see Chapter 26) or digital subtraction as shown in Figs. 12-17 and 12-18 (see Chapter 35). A common puncture site for hip arthrography is ³/₄ inch (1.9 cm) distal to the inguinal crease and ³/₄ inch (1.9 cm) lateral to the palpated femoral pulse. A spinal needle is useful for reaching the joint capsule.

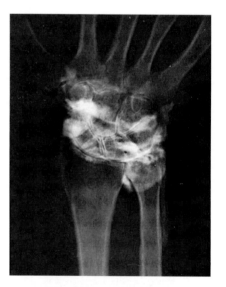

Fig. 12-10 Opaque arthrogram of wrist, demonstrating rheumatoid arthritis.

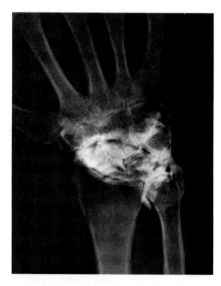

Fig. 12-11 PA arthrogram with wrist in radial deviation.

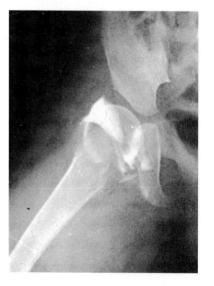

Fig. 12-12 AP opaque arthrogram showing treated congenital right hip dislocation in the same patient as in Fig. 12-2.

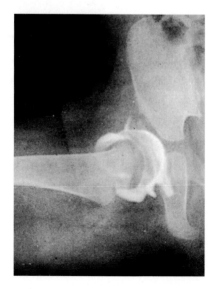

Fig. 12-13 Axiolateral "frog" right hip of patient treated for congenital dislocation of the hip.

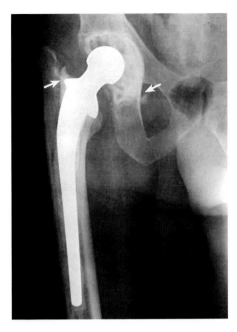

Fig. 12-14 AP hip radiograph showing radiopaque cement *(arrows)* used to secure hip prosthesis.

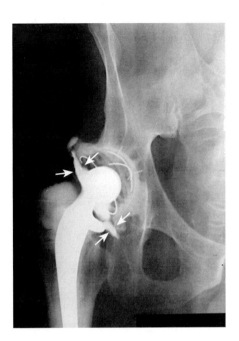

Fig. 12-15 AP hip arthrogram showing hip prosthesis in proper position. Cement with radiopaque additive is difficult to distinguish from contrast medium used to perform arthrography *(arrows)*.

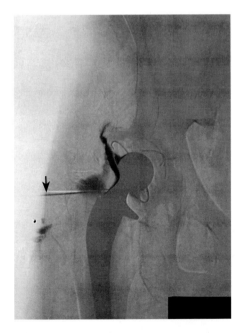

Fig. 12-16 Normal photographic subtraction AP hip arthrogram in same patient as in Fig. 12-14. Contrast medium *(black image)* is readily distinguished from the hip prosthesis by the subtraction technique. Contrast medium does not extend inferiorly below the level of the injection needle *(arrow)*. (See Chapter 26 for description of subtraction technique.)

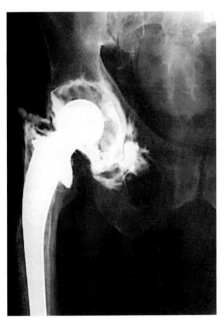

Fig. 12-17 AP hip radiograph after injection of contrast medium.

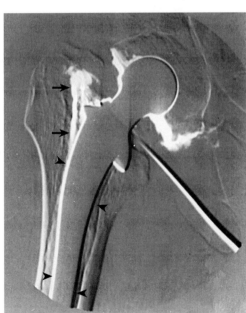

Fig. 12-18 Digital subtraction hip arthrogram in the same patient as in Fig. 12-17. Contrast medium around the prosthesis in the proximal lateral femoral shaft *(arrows)* indicates a loose prosthesis. Lines on the medial and lateral aspect of the femur *(arrowheads)* are a subtraction registration artifact caused by slight patient movement during the injection of contrast medium. (See Chapter 35 for description of subtraction technique.)

Shoulder Arthrography

Arthrography of the shoulder is performed primarily for the evaluation of partial or complete tears in the rotator cuff or glenoidal labrum, persistent pain or weakness, and frozen shoulder. A single-contrast technique (Fig. 12-19) or a double-contrast technique (Fig. 12-20) may be used.

The usual injection site is approximately $^1/_2$ inch (1.3 cm) inferior and lateral to the coracoid process. Because the joint capsule is usually deep, use of a spinal needle is recommended.

For a single-contrast arthrogram (Fig. 12-21), approximately 10 to 12 ml of positive contrast medium is injected into the shoulder.

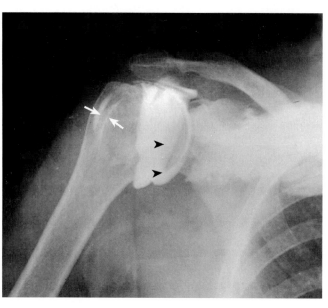

Fig. 12-19 Normal AP single-contrast shoulder arthrogram with contrast medium surrounding the biceps tendon sleeve and lying in the intertubercular (bicipital) groove *(arrows)*. The axillary recess is filled but has a normal medial filling defect *(arrowheads)* created by the glenoid labrum.

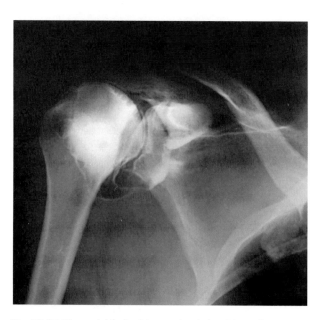

Fig. 12-20 Normal AP double-contrast shoulder arthrogram.

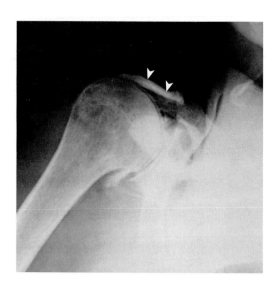

Fig. 12-21 Single-contrast arthrogram showing rotator cuff tear *(arrow)*.

For double-contrast examinations, approximately 3 to 4 ml of positive contrast medium and 10 to 12 ml of air are injected into the shoulder.

The projections most often used are the AP (both internal and external rotation), 30-degree AP oblique, axillary (Figs. 12-22 and 12-23), and tangential. (See Volume 1, Chapter 5, a description of patient and part positioning.)

After double-contrast shoulder arthrography is performed, computed tomography (CT) may be used to examine some patients. CT images may be obtained at each approximate 5 mm through the shoulder joint. In shoulder arthrography, CT has been found to be very sensitive and reliable in diagnosis. Radiographs and CT scans of the same patient are presented in Figs. 12-20 and 12-24.

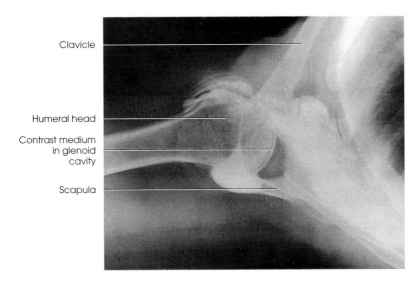

Fig. 12-22 Normal axillary single-contrast shoulder arthrogram.

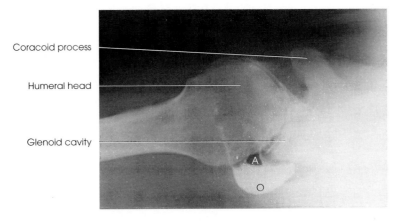

Fig. 12-23 Normal axillary double-contrast shoulder arthrogram projection of patient in supine position. Opaque medium (O) and air-created (A) density are seen anteriorly.

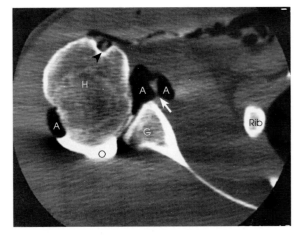

Fig. 12-24 CT shoulder arthrogram. The radiographic arthrogram in this patient was normal (see Fig. 12-20). However, the CT shoulder arthrogram shows a small chip fracture (arrow) on the anterior surface of the glenoid cavity. Head of humerus (H), air surrounding biceps tendon (arrowhead), air contrast medium (A), opaque contrast medium (O), and glenoid portion of scapula (G) are evident.

Temporomandibular Joint Arthrography

CT of the TMJ is often used instead of arthrography because CT is a noninvasive method of investigation. In many institutions, MRI has replaced CT, because MRI is also a noninvasive procedure with well-established diagnostic value (Fig. 12-25).

Contrast arthrography of the TMJ is useful in diagnosing abnormalities of the articular disk, the small, oval, fibrocartilaginous or fibrous tissue plate located between the condyle of the mandible and mandibular fossa. Abnormalities of this disk can be the result of trauma or a stretched or loose posterior ligament that allows the disk to be anteriorly displaced, causing pain.

Single-contrast opaque arthrography of the TMJ, although relatively uncomfortable for the patient, is easy to perform and requires 0.5 to 1 ml of contrast medium. The puncture site is approximately $^1/_2$ inch (1.3 cm) anterior to the tragus of the ear. The following steps are observed:

- Before the arthrogram is performed, take preliminary tomographic images with the patient's mouth in both the closed and open positions.
- After injection of the contrast medium, fluoroscopically observe the joint and take spot images to evaluate mandibular motion.

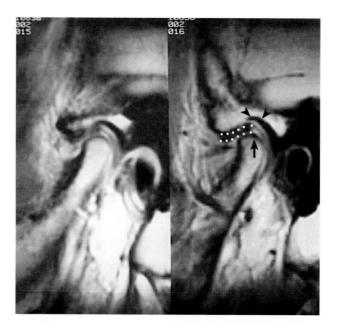

Fig. 12-25 Open-mouth lateral MRI of the TMJ, showing mandibular condyle *(arrow)*, mandibular fossa of temporal bone *(arrowheads)*, and articular disk *(dots)*.

- In general, obtain tomograms and/or radiographs (Fig. 12-26 and 12-27) with the patient's mouth in the closed, partially open, and fully open positions.

Other Joints

Essentially any joint can be evaluated by arthrography. However, the joints discussed in this chapter—the knee, shoulder, hip, wrist and TMJ—are the ones most often investigated.

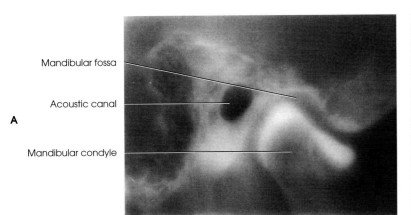

Mandibular fossa

Acoustic canal

A

Mandibular condyle

B

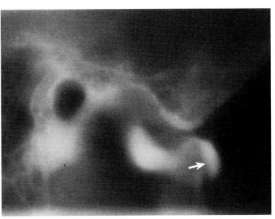

Fig. 12-26 Postinjection tomographic arthrogram of the TMJ taken with patient's mouth closed **(A)** and fully open **(B).** Positive contrast medium anterior to condyle *(arrow)* demonstrates anterior dislocation of the meniscus.

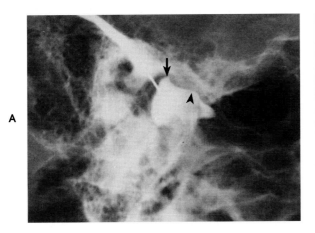

A

B

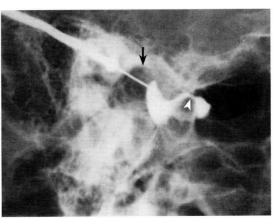

Fig. 12-27 Postinjection radiographs on same patient as in Fig. 12-26. Dislocated meniscus is shown with the mouth half open **(A)** and completely open **(B).** Mandibular fossa *(arrow)* and condyle *(arrowhead)* are shown.

FOREIGN BODY LOCALIZATION AND TRAUMA RADIOGRAPHY GUIDELINES

RIGHT: Pfeiffer-Comberg method of foreign body localization in which a leaded contact lens was placed directly over the cornea with this resulting image.

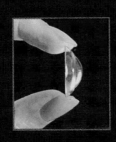

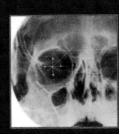

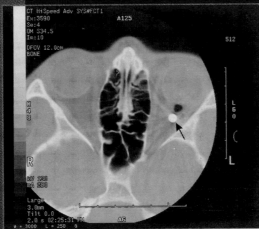

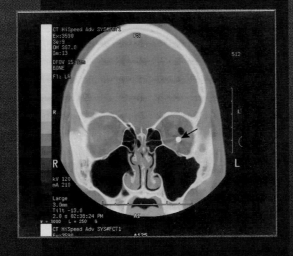

LEFT: Horizontal and coronal computed tomographic bone images show the location of a BB (arrow) in the eye of a 13-year-old boy who had been playing with a gun. The dense adjacent area is air. The boy now has monocular vision.

(Courtesy Mark H. Layne, R.T.)

An alien object that enters the body is called a *foreign body*. Foreign materials enter the body under many different circumstances—some by way of a puncture wound and others by way of a natural orifice (Figs. 13-1 to 13-3). A majority of these objects must be surgically removed.

The referring physician depends on the radiology department to verify the presence of a foreign body and to determine its nature and exact site. The physician then uses this information to determine the best procedure for removing the object.

This section describes the radiologic examinations most commonly used to detect and localize foreign bodies in regions other than the eye. (Information on radiology and ocular foreign bodies is provided in Chapter 20.) In civilian practice the most frequently encountered foreign bodies are those that have been aspirated or swallowed and those that have penetrated tissue (e.g., needles, broken glass, and wood and metal splinters). Children sometimes insert a foreign object into the nose, ear, or genital orifice. An object lodged in one of these areas can usually be removed without referring the patient to the radiology department. When referral is necessary, radiographs are made in at least two planes. In industrial areas and high-crime areas, foreign body traumas are frequently comparable to those sustained on battlefields. In these settings, high-velocity objects often cause extensive bone and/or soft tissue damage.

Aspirated and *swallowed foreign bodies* are discussed in this section because the examinations used to detect and localize objects entering through the mouth are limited to the two techniques involved (Figs. 13-4 to 13-6).

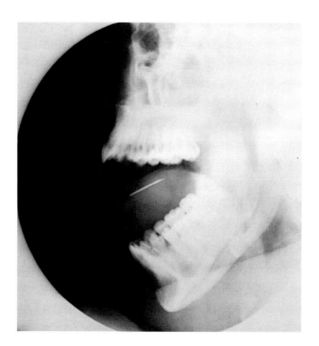

Fig. 13-1 Lateral open-mouth facial bones showing a pin in the tongue.

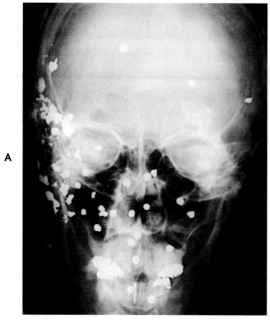
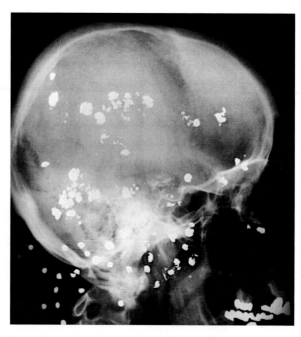

A

B

Fig. 13-2 PA skull radiograph **(A)** and lateral skull radiograph **(B)** demonstrating multiple shell fragments lodged in the superficial tissues of the cranium, face, and neck.

Foreign body localization and trauma radiography guidelines

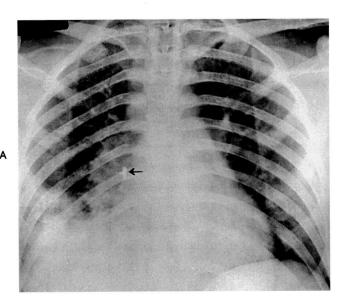

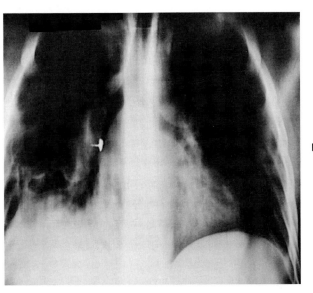

Fig. 13-3 Patient treated for chronic pneumonia with symptoms of cough, foul-smelling sputum, and intermittent fever. **A,** The frontal radiograph reveals pneumonia in the right lower lung and the presence of a foreign body *(arrow).* **B,** Computed tomography profiles a thumbtack lodged in the right lower lobe bronchus adjacent to the hilum. The thumbtack was removed bronchoscopically.

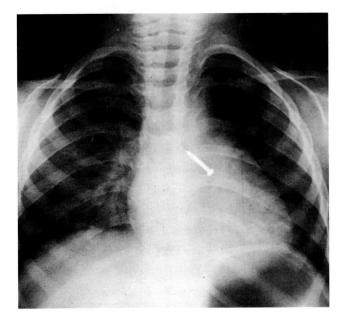

Fig. 13-4 Nail aspirated into left bronchus.

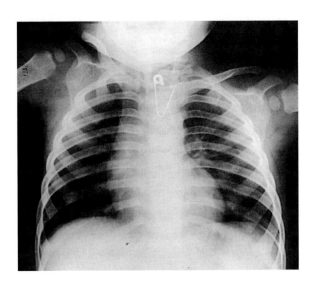

Fig. 13-5 Open safety pin lodged in esophagus of 13-month-old boy.

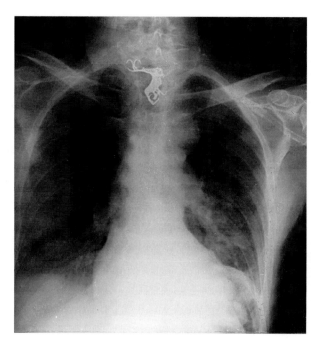

Fig. 13-6 Portable chest radiograph locating patient's missing dental partial.

Penetrating foreign bodies are localized using both radiographic and fluoroscopic techniques. Radiographic techniques are generally preferred because they provide a permanent record. Furthermore, after preliminary screening by the radiologist, the techniques can be performed by the radiographer (Fig. 13-7). During fluoroscopic screening the radiologist may place a mark on the skin surface, anteriorly or posteriorly, immediately over the center of the image of the foreign body. Then by turning the patient or by the parallax method, a mark may be placed on the body at the exact site of the object to indicate its depth. The radiographer can use a combination of these marks as centering points in positioning the patient, and the surgeon can use them as reference points for surgery.

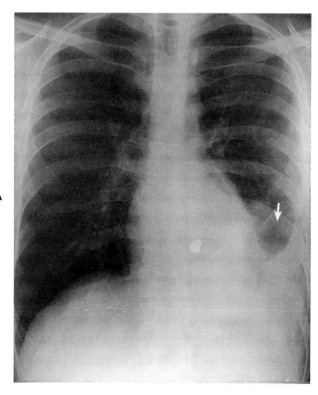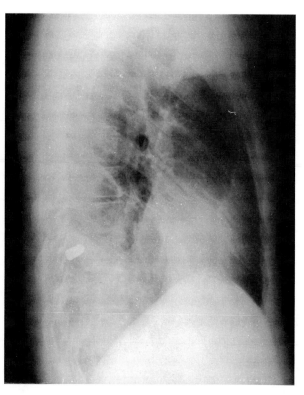

Fig. 13-7 Bullet in left chest, lateral to lower thoracic spine. No bone injury has occurred. **A,** PA projection showing left pleural effusion *(arrow)*. **B,** On the lateral image, fluid is seen mostly laterally and posteriorly.

Preliminary Considerations

Although careful attention to each of the factors affecting recorded radiographic detail is important in every examination, it is even more crucial when radiography is used to detect low-density foreign bodies. The following factors are of particular importance.

FOCAL SPOT

A small focal spot is necessary for maximum recorded detail. Pitting, cracking, and rippling of the anode are caused by overloading and overheating. These irregularities on the face of the target cause radiation to be emitted in all directions, resulting in serious loss of recorded detail. Use of the tube within the limits shown on its rating chart (the limits should be prominently displayed in every control booth) will prevent target damage.

SCREENS

Dust and other extraneous particles, nicks, scratches, and stains produce shadows that can simulate small foreign bodies. Imperfect intensifying-screen contact results in blurring similar to the blurring produced by motion. These imperfections can be caused by careless handling of cassettes and improper care of the contained screens.

EXPOSURE FACTORS

Exposure factors must be adjusted according to the tissue density of the part examined, and involuntary motion must be compensated for by the appropriate technique. A long scale of gray tones is generally desirable for demonstrating bony and soft tissue structures in thick parts.

Fragments of low-density materials such as plastic, wood, and glass are most frequently found in the superficial tissues. A short-scale contrast is generally needed to detect these materials. Thick surgical dressings should be removed for the x-ray exposures, leaving only a thin layer of sterile gauze. However, dressings should be removed only if permitted by the attending physician.

Detecting glass fragments is especially difficult. There are more than 70,000 types of glass, each with its own particular chemical composition. Many types of glass contain a high enough percentage of lime and/or metallic oxide (iron, gold, lead, copper, etc., added to obtain specific colors) to render them sufficiently opaque to cast a shadow through the surrounding tissues. Other types of glass are composed of a high percentage of silicon (silica glass) with a low lime and metallic content. Failure to detect this type of glass does not preclude its presence.

POSITIONING OF PATIENT

Patient positioning is of prime importance in foreign body localization because even slight rotation of the patient or body part can cause erroneous depth measurements. Positioning the patient for AP, PA, and lateral projections must be exact. Optimum oblique and tangential projections are usually determined using fluoroscopic control so that the radiologist can place the skin mark tangent to the cassette.

MOTION

Motion of the part—voluntary or involuntary—causes blurring and loss of recorded detail. As a result, objects of low density and/or small size may be obscured. For maximum recorded detail, every effort must be made to control the motion of body parts before an exposure is made. This must be done by methods other than compression because compression reduces tissue thickness, resulting in erroneous depth measurements. Length of exposure is the only way to overcome involuntary motion.

EQUIPMENT

Precision depth-measurement techniques require exact centering of the tube within its housing and the exact measurement of target-cassette and target-shift distances. The distance markings on the x-ray tube stand must be checked for accuracy so that exact compensation can be made for any discrepancy. The source-to-image receptor distance (SID) used for precision depth localization must be exact.

Penetrating Foreign Bodies

INITIAL EXAMINATION

The purpose of the initial examination is to verify the presence of suspected single or multiple foreign bodies and to determine their nature, size, shape, and location and the extent of bony and/or soft tissue trauma. In patients with severe injury, one or more initial radiographs may be all that can be obtained.

The smaller parts of the limbs do not usually require a preliminary radiograph. The foreign body is most often near the site of entry. The following steps are observed:

• Direct the central ray exactly through the foreign body.
• Obtain right-angle AP, PA, and lateral projections (Fig. 13-8).
• Indicate the site of the puncture wound by placing a lead marker on the cassette exactly opposite the wound.
• Obtain additional projections as indicated.

When the skull, chest, or abdominopelvic regions are involved, the initial examination may be performed using a preliminary radiograph or fluoroscopy (Figs. 13-9 to 13-11). Scout radiographs must be large enough to include the entire region being investigated. The angle of entrance of high-velocity objects such as bullets and fragments of metal must also be taken into consideration. High-velocity objects entering at an angle usually lodge at a distance from the puncture wound.

Preliminary screening expedites the examination because it enables the physician (1) to quickly locate radiopaque foreign bodies as being near or far from the site of entry, (2) to determine whether the object is located within deep structures or in the periphery of a rounded area where it is best shown by tangential projections, (3) to determine the localization technique best suited to the circumstances, and (4) to mark the skin overlying the shadow of the foreign body in two or more planes. When the foreign body is distant from natural reference points (joints or other bony parts), a metal marker may be attached to the skin as a reference point for the surgeon. Emergency radiology departments keep a supply of sterile wire rings and crosses for this purpose.

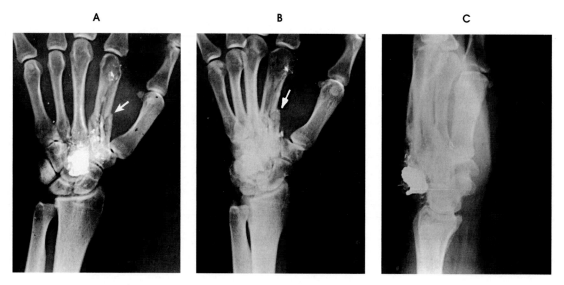

A   B   C

Fig. 13-8 Metallic foreign body (bullet) in dorsal aspect of wrist with comminuted fracture of second metacarpal *(arrow).*

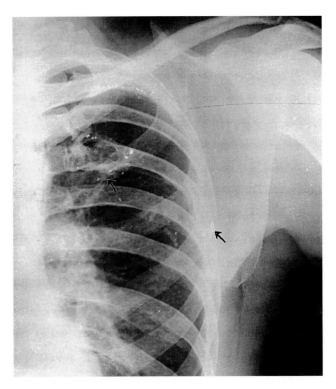

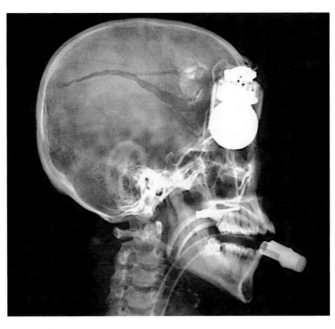

Fig. 13-9 Old, healed bullet wound fractures involving fifth rib laterally and posteriorly. Note track of lead deposits extending through soft tissues along path traveled by bullet *(arrows)*.

Fig. 13-10 Battlefield injury resulting in extensive bone and brain damage caused by hand grenade embedded in forehead.

A

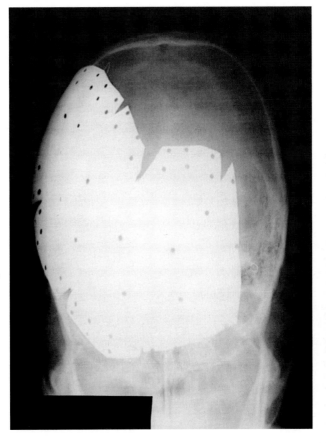

B

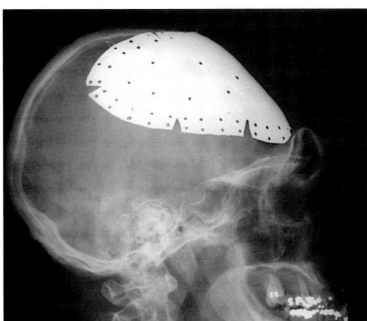

Fig. 13-11 Battlefield injury victim with cranial plate covering brain. **A**, Occipital (Towne method) radiograph. **B**, Lateral radiograph.

RADIOGRAPHIC LOCALIZATION TECHNIQUES

Radiographic localization techniques are as follows:
- Right-angle projections
- Oblique projections
- Tangential projections
- Single-image triangulation

Radiographic foreign body localization is performed after the surgeon has determined the route and body placement to be used for removing the foreign body. The localization images are then obtained with the patient adjusted in the body position to be used for surgery. The images must always be large enough to include natural reference points unless wire or other suitable markers have been attached to the skin or over a wound to serve this purpose.

Computed tomography is often used to localize foreign bodies. Magnetic resonance imaging is used *only* after the foreign body is known to be nonferrous in composition.

Right-angle projections

The right-angle technique of localization consists of taking exact right-angle AP, PA, and lateral projections with the central ray directed through the foreign body (Fig. 13-12). Thick parts, particularly the chest and abdominopelvic regions, require the following procedure:
- Adjust the patient in the body position to be used in the operating room to surgically remove the foreign body.
- Mark the skin overlying the site of the foreign body in both frontal and lateral planes.
- Direct the central ray through the center of the foreign body for accurate localization of the object. If the centering is not accurate, the shadow of the foreign body will be cast by divergent radiation emitted from the periphery of the x-ray tube target. The distance of the image displacement and the resultant error in localization depend on the distance between the foreign body and the image, the SID, and the distance that the body is "off-center."

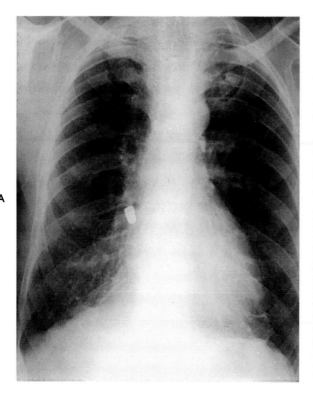
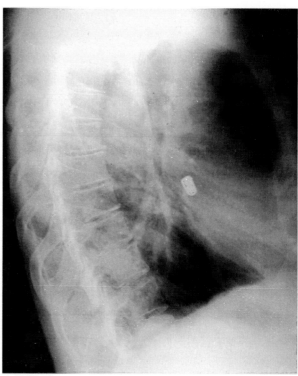

Fig. 13-12 A, AP projection. **B,** Lateral projection. Bullet in right chest of patient who has been asymptomatic for 15 years following shooting.

- Except for the hands and feet, obtain biplane projections whenever possible. This procedure is particularly important if the presence of a pointed or sharp-edged object is suspected, because movement of the patient could cause deeper penetration of the object and thus more soft tissue trauma. Biplane projections are also important when a foreign body is located in an area where a shift in its position is possible, as in the mediastinum and abdominopelvic areas.

When movement of a foreign body is possible because of its unstable location or because of movement of the patient during transfer from radiology to surgery, verify the location of the object with right-angle images in the operating room immediately before the operation.

The foregoing techniques are the simplest and most universally used procedures for the localization of penetrating foreign bodies.

Oblique projections

Oblique projections are used to separate overlapping structures in any region. They are particularly useful in determining the relationship of superimposed bone and foreign body images to demonstrate whether the object is embedded in the bone or is lodged in the adjacent soft tissues.

Tangential projections

Tangential projections are useful in foreign body detection when the physical configuration of the body part allows the central ray to "skim" between the foreign body and the primary body part. The projection is most useful for the evaluation of superficial foreign bodies in limbs.

Single-image triangulation

Single-image triangulation is a precise technique for depth localization and requires the following steps:
- Measure accurately and record the *exact* SID and tube-shift distance (TSD) used.
- Keep the patient and the cassette stationary for two exposures on one image.
- Measure accurately, and record the uppermost skin surface-to-cassette distance. The latter measurement is used in the final step of the depth calculation.

Any practical SID may be used—30, 36, or 40 inches (76 to 102 cm). The TSD may be 4, 6, 8, or 10 inches (10 to 15 cm). The greater the object-to-image receptor distance (OID), the greater the image shift distance (ISD). For this reason, a shorter TSD can be used for objects near the surface, whereas a longer TSD is more satisfactory for deep-seated objects because it ensures adequate separation of the images. The tube is shifted at right angles to the long axis of elongated objects. This prevents possible difficulty in measuring the exact image shift on partially superimposed shadows of slender or tapered objects.

Application of procedure

- Adjust the patient in an exact supine or prone body position as required to place him or her in the position to be used for the surgical removal of the foreign body.
- Center the central ray to the skin mark overlying the site of the foreign body.
- With the cassette in a Bucky tray, center it to the skin mark.
- Carefully measure the uppermost skin-to-image receptor distance in the plane of the foreign body, and record this measurement with the SID and TSD.
- Make the first exposure using half of the exposure time required for a conventional radiograph of the part.
- Shift the tube an *exact distance,* transversely or longitudinally as required, and, without disturbing the patient or cassette, make the second exposure using the same factors as for the first exposure. These two "half exposures" produce a radiographic density comparable to that obtained with a single full exposure of the region (Fig. 13-13). When a wide tube shift is used, adjust the collimator for the second (off-center) exposure to avoid a cutoff, as shown by the transverse line seen in Fig. 13-14. The upper right-hand corner cutoff was made by the gonad shield.
- Process the cassette in the usual manner.

Depth calculation

- From the same point on each image, measure the exact distance between the two images cast on the radiograph by the foreign body.
- Based on the three known factors (SID, TSD, and ISD), use the following formula to calculate the distance between the foreign body and the image receptor:

$$\frac{\text{SID} \times \text{ISD}}{\text{TSD} + \text{ISD}} = \text{Foreign body-image receptor distance}$$

For example, with an SID of 40 inches (102 cm), a TSD of 6 inches (15 cm), and an ISD of $1\frac{1}{2}$ inches (3.8 cm), calculate the foreign body-film distance as follows:

$$(40 \times 1.5) + (6 + 1.5) = 8 \text{ inches}$$

- Then calculate the depth of the foreign body below the skin surface by subtracting the foreign body-image receptor distance from the skin-image receptor distance. Assume the latter measurement to be 10 inches (24 cm). Using the result of the above example, $10 - 8 = 2$; this places the foreign body 2 inches (5 cm) below the skin surface.

- Record the measurement on a sheet of graph paper, using a scale of $\frac{1}{4}$ to 1 inch (0.6 to 2.5 cm), by drawing a set of triangles (Fig. 13-15) as follows:
  1. Draw a line representing the SID—line AB.
  2. Draw a line representing the TSD—line AC.
  3. Draw a line representing the ISD—line BD.
  4. Draw a line from C to D.
  5. Draw a line representing the skin surface—line SS.
  6. The location of the foreign body is where line CD intersects line AB.

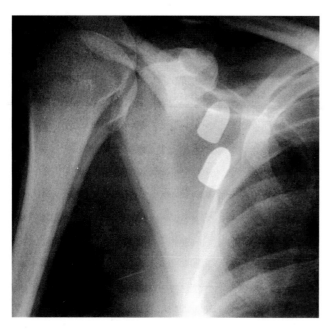

Fig. 13-13 Triangulation technique for locating a single bullet.

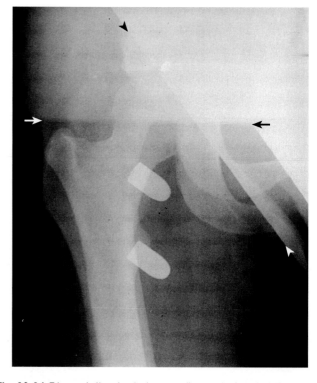

Fig. 13-14 Triangulation technique radiograph showing the line caused by intentionally off-centered collimated x-ray beam for second exposure *(arrows)* and diagonal lines *(arrowheads)* caused by gonad shield.

FLUOROSCOPIC LOCALIZATION TECHNIQUES

The fluoroscopic localization techniques include the following:

- Parallax method
- Right-angle method
- Profunda method

Because the fluoroscopic methods of foreign body localization can be performed quickly, they are used when circumstances indicate that speed is of greater importance than the permanent record afforded by the somewhat more time-consuming radiographic techniques.

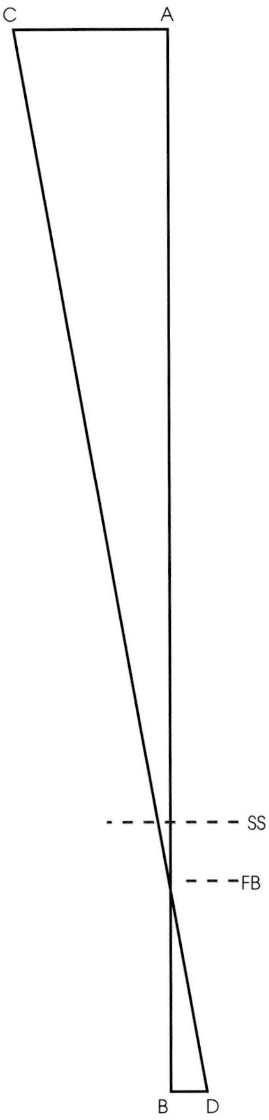

Parallax method

The parallax method is based on the principle that the images cast by two objects equidistant from the fluoroscopic screen will move together at the same amplitude when the fluoroscope and tube are simultaneously moved back and forth across them. A metal indicator is used for parallax localization of the depth of foreign bodies. (A round-headed screw in the end of a wooden rod or stick serves the purpose well.)

The fluoroscopist observes the following steps:

- After locating the foreign body, close the diaphragm shutters down to the size of the object to direct the central ray through its center.
- Mark the skin or tape with a suitable metallic marker in position to indicate the exact site of the foreign body in the frontal plane.
- Place the metal indicator against the side of the body. Hold the indicator in an exactly horizontal position, and move the screen back and forth while raising or lowering the indicator until the images of the foreign body and the indicator move at the same amplitude.
- Make a mark on the side of the body to indicate the depth of the foreign body.

The parallax method is the technique of choice for patients who cannot be turned for right-angle projections. It may also be used for depth localization in the shoulder, buttocks, and upper thigh regions.

Right-angle method

The right-angle method is applicable when movement is not precluded by the patient's condition or the nature or location of the foreign body. The following procedure is used:

- Locate and suitably mark the exact site of the foreign body in the frontal plane.
- Repeat the procedure with the patient in the lateral position.

Profunda method

The *profunda method* is defined as the removal of a foreign body under fluoroscopic guidance. The procedure can be time consuming. Because of the radiation dose to both patient and surgeon, the use of this method is generally discouraged.

Fig. 13-15 Graphic representation of location of foreign body. (*SS,* skin surface.)

Aspirated and Swallowed Objects

Infants and young children instinctively investigate things by taste, sight, and touch. Moreover, they put anything they can grasp into their mouths. Therefore foreign bodies are frequently aspirated or swallowed (Figs. 13-16 and 13-17).

In adults the most frequent foreign body traumas are fragments of bone (commonly fish or chicken bones), solid food boluses, and dental appliances (see Fig. 13-6). Adults are also prone to hold between their teeth such items as rings and open safety pins (see Figs. 13-18 and 13-19). Some craftsmen, most notably carpenters and those in the sewing trades,

find it expedient to hold such items as tacks, small nails, and pins in their mouths, to be fed out for rapid use in their work. Many mentally disturbed patients have a compulsion to ingest objects and sometimes manage to swallow surprisingly large items (Fig. 13-20).

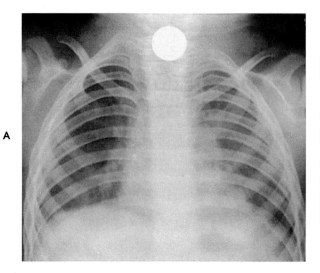
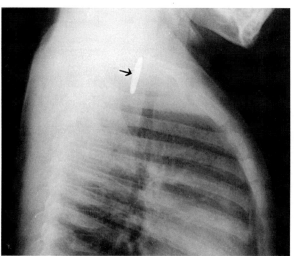

Fig. 13-16 Coin in lower cervical esophagus.

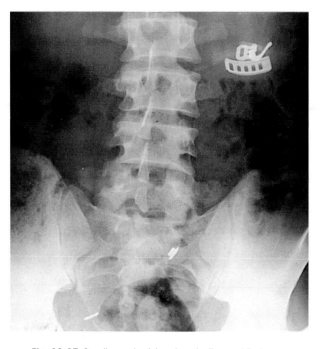

Fig. 13-17 Swallowed rubber boot clip and fastener.

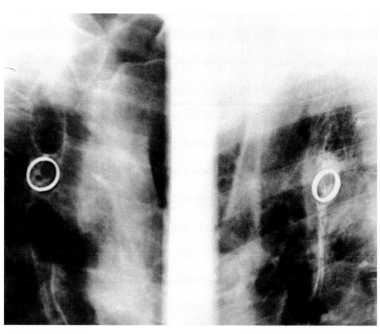

Fig. 13-18 Wedding ring in upper esophagus.

A foreign body that enters the mouth may initiate a gag reflex and be expelled immediately. If the object can be found and identified, the patient does not need to be examined.

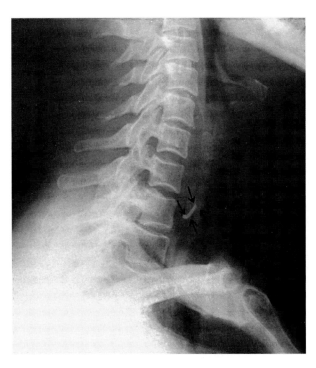

Fig. 13-19 Chicken bone in lower cervical esophagus.

A

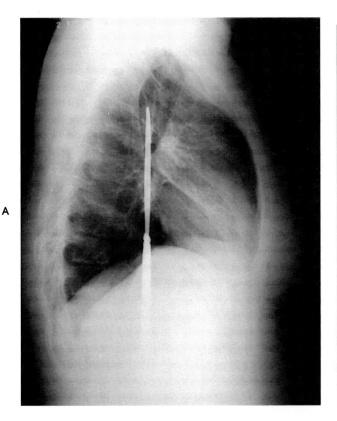

B

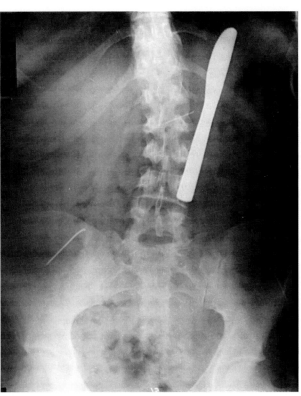

Fig. 13-20 A, Lateral chest showing table knife in esophagus. **B,** AP abdomen taken at a later date in the same patient as in **A**. The radiograph shows a different table knife and other small, straight foreign bodies.

More frequently, the foreign body is retained and is aspirated or swallowed (Fig. 13-21). Rarely the object is dislodged superiorly from the oral pharynx into the nasopharynx. If the foreign body is aspirated into air passages, it will be found above the diaphragm in the neck or chest (Fig. 13-22). If swallowed, the foreign body may pass beyond the oropharynx (Fig. 13-23) and possibly become lodged or impacted in the cervical or thoracic portion of the esophagus, or it may travel on into the stomach and intestines.

The patient's symptoms usually, but not always, indicate whether a foreign body has been aspirated or swallowed. If there is any doubt, particularly in an infant or a young child, the preliminary radiographic survey should include the patient's body from the level of the external acoustic meatuses to the level of the anal canal, thereby including the neck, chest, abdomen, and pelvis (i.e., images from the level of the highest external orifice to the level of the lowermost orifice). Once the location of the foreign body has been determined, accurate localization and follow-up radiographs to determine its progress depend on the object's size and shape and on the degree of impaction, if any.

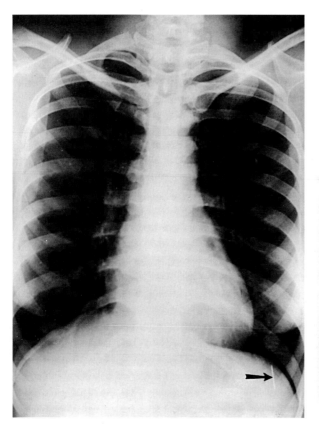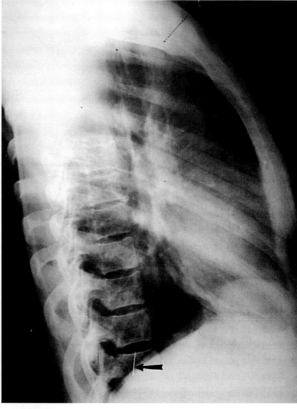

Fig. 13-21 Straight pin aspirated into posterior basal bronchus *(arrows).*

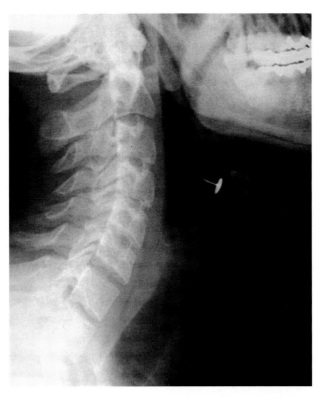

Fig. 13-22 Aspirated thumbtack lodged in epiglottis. The tack was spontaneously expelled when the patient coughed.

A   B   C

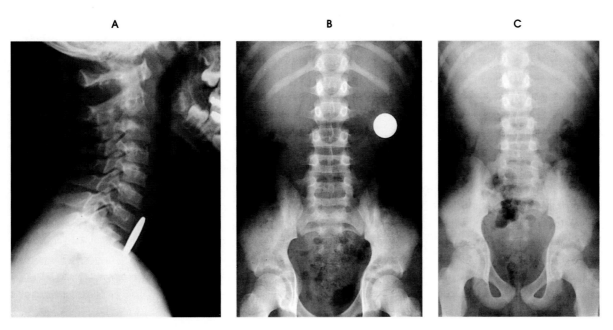

Fig. 13-23 A, Quarter in the lower cervical esophagus. **B,** Interval radiograph shows the coin in the stomach. **C,** Radiograph showing the quarter to have been expelled.

Control of involuntary motion usually is the only problem encountered in the detection of radiopaque foreign materials in the respiratory and alimentary tracts. Motion control requires patient cooperation and/or rapid exposure times.

Radiolucent foreign bodies require the use of a contrast medium to coat the object or localize the site of foreign body obstruction and to demonstrate the condition of the soft tissues at the site where the foreign body is lodged (Fig. 13-24).

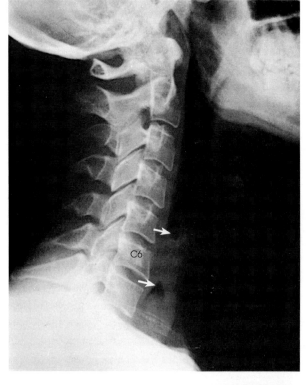

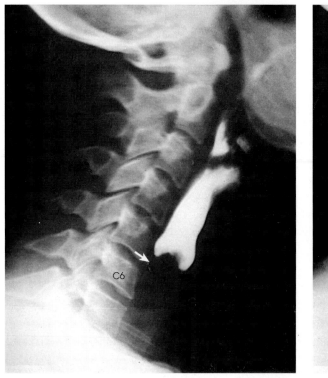

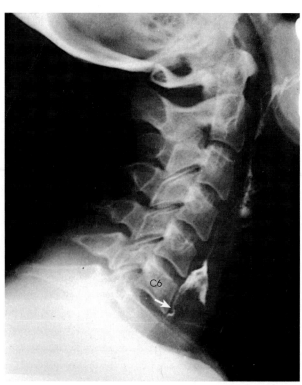

Fig. 13-24 A, Impacted, nonopaque meat bolus *(arrow)* has caused widening of the esophagus. **B,** Complete obstruction by meat bolus causes barium to stop at the site of the foreign body. **C,** Delayed radiograph shows small trickle of barium bypassing the foreign body posteriorly.

Aspirated Foreign Bodies

INFANTS AND YOUNG CHILDREN

Because an aspirated object can quickly be drawn into a distal branch of the airways, the initial radiographs of infants and young children should be large enough to include the entire respiratory system. The following steps are observed:

- Obtain an AP projection of the head and neck and a lateral image of the neck.
- Align the top border of the cassette at the level of the external acoustic meatuses to include the entire nasopharynx. This procedure is necessary for detecting an object that rarely is, but may possibly have been, explosively dislodged from a lower level only to become lodged in the nasopharynx.
- Ensure that the lower edge of the cassette used for the AP projection of the neck and chest extends below the level of the diaphragm.
- Place an infant in an upright immobilizing device or in a supine and immobilized position.
- If the infant is supine, obtain the lateral projection by the cross-table technique.
- Use the recommended infant technique, which is always based on the shortest possible exposure time. After reviewing the initial image, the physician will determine if more projections are needed.

OLDER CHILDREN AND ADULTS

Aspirated foreign bodies may lodge in the larynx, the trachea, a main bronchus (most frequently the right bronchus because of its larger diameter and more vertical direction). Small objects sometimes occlude one of the smaller bronchial branches. In this situation, exact localization of the site of obstruction may require bronchoscopy.

Larynx and upper trachea

Radiopaque foreign bodies lodged in the larynx and upper trachea are clearly shown on AP and lateral projections. The lateral projection of the trachea and mediastinum (see Chapter 10) is sometimes useful in patients with short necks and high shoulders. The following procedure is used:

- Center the cassettes and the central ray to the laryngeal prominence.
- Decrease the exposure technique to better visualize the soft tissue structures.
- The detection of radiolucent foreign bodies requires the use of a contrast medium. Laryngography is performed using fluoroscopic visualization, with spot images, conventional radiographs, and tomography being used as indicated.

Trachea and bronchial tree

Radiography of the intrathoracic respiratory system usually consists of two PA projections. The following steps are observed:

- Place a marker to indicate the correct phase of respiration on each image.
- Have the patient inspire deeply, and then obtain the first radiograph; obtain the second radiograph on maximum expiration.[1] Bronchial obstruction will reduce air flow in the affected segment of the lung.
- Compare the two images. Interference with air flow will be demonstrated by no change in the radiolucency of the lung in the affected area.
- When the affected side is determined, make a corresponding lateral image. Depending on the nature of the foreign body and its site, further studies and/or bronchoscopy may be indicated.

---

[1]Griffiths DM, Freeman NV: Expiratory chest x-ray examination in the diagnosis of inhaled foreign bodies, *Br Med J* 288:1074, 1984.

Swallowed Foreign Bodies

INFANTS AND YOUNG CHILDREN

Preliminary images of infants and young children should include the entire alimentary canal, irrespective of the time lapse between the accident and the radiography. The following steps are observed:

- Obtain a mandatory lateral projection of the neck and nasopharynx.
- Use the cross-table technique for ease of positioning and immobilization of small and/or uncooperative children.
- Use a 35 × 43 cm (14 × 17 inch) cassette for the AP projection of the neck and body of small infants. A smaller cassette is used for the lateral projection.
- Obtain two exposures—one for the neck and chest areas and one for the abdominopelvic areas—in larger children.
- Use the routine rapid-exposure infant technique for these studies.
- The radiologist determines the nature and site of nonopaque objects under fluoroscopic visualization. A contrast medium is administered to coat the object or to localize the site of obstruction.
- When a smooth-surfaced foreign body such as a coin or marble is swallowed, radiographs are usually obtained at 24-hour intervals to verify that the object clears the pylorus and the ileocecal valve. A final radiograph is obtained to confirm that the foreign object is no longer in the body. Radiographs are obtained at more frequent intervals when an object, such as an opened safety pin, has the potential to perforate an organ or other structure.

OLDER CHILDREN AND ADULTS

Pharynx and upper esophagus

Radiopaque foreign bodies lodged in the pharynx and upper esophagus can usually be clearly shown with one or two lateral soft tissue radiographs of the neck.

- In the preliminary examination, obtain one exposure on deep expiration to depress the shoulders and one at the height of deglutition to elevate the superior end of the esophagus. (See Volume 2, Chapter 15, for a more complete discussion of the lateral soft palate, pharynx, and larynx.)
- Obtain a lateral retrosternal projection to obtain delineation of the upper end of the esophagus in short-necked, high-shouldered subjects. (See Chapter 10, for a discussion of the transshoulder lateral projection using the Twining method to image the trachea and pulmonary apex.)
- As in infants and young children, use a contrast medium administered under fluoroscopic control to identify and localize nonopaque foreign bodies in this region. Then obtain radiographs if needed.

Esophagus, stomach, and intestines

When a foreign body is not found in the pharynx, it is customary to take a PA oblique projection of the esophagus in the right anterior oblique (RAO) position and an AP projection of the abdomen before performing fluoroscopy with a contrast medium. This precludes the possibility of obscuring a foreign object with the opaque medium.

One of the water-soluble iodinated media for the investigation of esophageal foreign bodies may be used. A water-soluble medium localizes the nonopaque foreign body by giving it an opaque coating, identifies the site of obstruction, and permits better evaluation of possible soft tissue trauma. The water-soluble medium does not adhere to the foreign body and therefore does not interfere with endoscopic removal of the object. In contrast, a barium suspension adheres to the foreign body, rendering it slippery and difficult for the physician to grasp and remove with an esophagoscope.

Foreign bodies that have reached the stomach but present no danger of perforation are followed with interval images to verify their passage through the pylorus and ileocecal valve. A final radiograph confirms that the object has been discharged from the body.

Patients who have experienced trauma are often referred to the radiology department for examination. The patient with a traumatic injury is often unable to assume the position necessary for routine radiographic examinations. After the patient has been evaluated by a physician, the radiographer who is responsible for performing the examination must move the radiographic and accessory equipment around the patient to avoid causing additional injury or discomfort. The radiographer must not move the patient in any manner that will cause additional injury.

Within the space of this text, it is not possible to describe all approaches and modifications needed to obtain radiographs of the critically injured patient. Each patient requires special attention and a slightly different approach, simply because each injured patient is unique. The following general trauma positioning guidelines must be considered:

- Do not move the patient unless competent medical personnel have deemed it safe to do so. If the patient has to be moved, ask qualified personnel for assistance.
- Obtain at least two radiographs for each body part. In general, try to obtain the radiographs at 90-degree angles to each other.

- If the patient is conscious and coherent, explain exactly what is going to be done *before* the patient is moved. If more than one approach can be used, ask the patient which would be more comfortable.
- Keep the routine central ray entrance and exit points as close together as possible for the body part being radiographed.
- Place the cassette (with or without a grid assembly) adjacent to the part being radiographed to center the part of interest to the cassette.
- When radiographing long bones, include both joints if possible. If this is not possible, include the joint closest to the injury, and obtain a separate radiograph of the other joint of the long bone.
- Do not remove splints or bandages unless instructed to do so. Removal of splints could lead to vascular or nerve injury by bone fragments.

Swallowed foreign bodies

Reversing or Modifying a Projection

The general trauma positioning guidelines emphasize the need to maintain the central ray's entrance and exit points as close together as possible. For example, a patient is brought to the trauma center after having sustained injury to the facial area. The patient is conscious, and an image of the facial bones is one of the radiographic examinations to be performed. Depending on the clinical condition and the cooperation offered by the patient, several radiographic approaches appear possible for completing the examination.

Most critically injured patients arrive in the trauma center in the *supine body position* and therefore are most often radiographed in that position. Reversing a position to obtain the diagnostic radiograph requires certain steps:

- The usual way of obtaining a Water's method, parietoacanthial projection (described in Chapter 21) is to align the midsagittal plane perpendicular to the plane of the cassette and have the orbitomeatal line form an angle of 37 degrees with the plane of the cassette (Figs. 13-25 and 13-26).
- If the patient is unable to assume the above *upright* position precisely, modify the approach.
- Mentally remove the cassette but maintain the central ray entrance and exit points as diagrammed in Fig. 13-27.
- If the patient is able to safely assume the upright body position represented in Fig. 13-28, the line representing the

central ray remains unchanged. Instead of angling the patient's head, angle the central ray to coincide with the entrance and exit points normally used.

- If the patient is brought to the radiographic room for the parietoacanthial projection in the *prone* position or if the patient is able to assume this position most comfortably, perform the radiograph normally (Fig. 13-29).
- If the patient is unable to assume this prone position with the chin extended, mentally remove the cassette as before (Fig. 13-30). A *similar* radiographic image is obtained if the entrance and exit points of the central ray and cassette alignment are maintained (Fig. 13-31).

As stated previously, most trauma patients are brought into the radiographic room in the *supine* position. The facial bones can be radiographically demonstrated (slightly magnified as a result of the increased OID) if the relationship of the central ray and the image receptor is maintained as described. The technique for obtaining a facial bone radiograph on the supine trauma patient is illustrated in Figs. 13-32 and 13-33. The following points should be kept in mind:

- Remember that most patients with traumatic injury of the facial bones may also have injuries of the cervical spine or other body area.
- Do not flex or extend the patient's neck to orient the central ray and the cassette. Instead, increase or decrease the central ray angulation to keep the same geometric arrangement.

It must be emphasized that the radiograph obtained with the different approaches will be similar but not identical. The preliminary radiograph is the basis for making the initial diagnosis. After the initial diagnosis, further evaluation may be performed if movement of the patient is allowed.

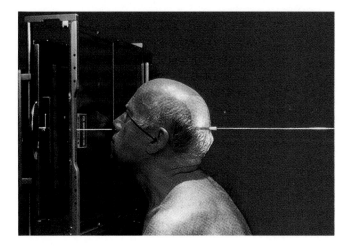

Fig. 13-25 Routine positioning to obtain a Water's method, parietoacanthial projection.

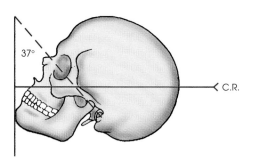

Fig. 13-26 Routine upright radiography.

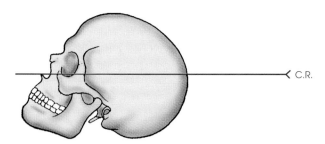

Fig. 13-27 Upright radiography with cassette line removed.

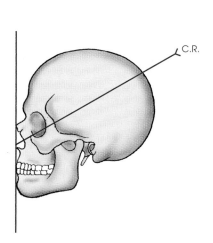

Fig. 13-28 Upright position with angled central ray.

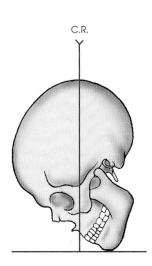

Fig. 13-29 Normal table radiography.

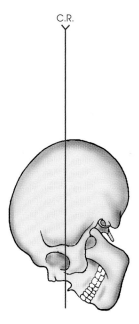

Fig. 13-30 Table radiography with cassette line removed.

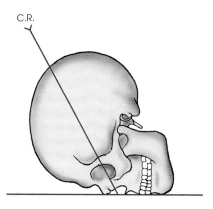

Fig. 13-31 Prone position requiring caudal central ray angulation.

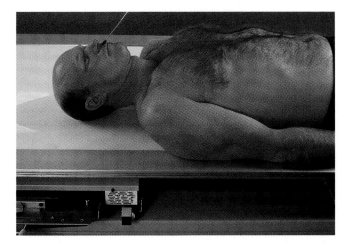

Fig. 13-32 Supine position requiring cephalic central ray angulation.

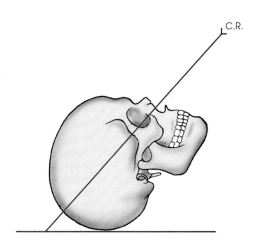

Fig. 13-33 Patient positioned for AP axial projection of facial bones.

Reversing or modifying a projection

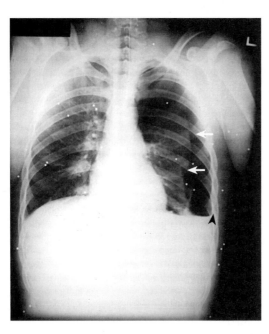

Fig. 13-34 PA chest radiograph of innocent bystander. Multiple buckshot caused hydropneumothorax. The *arrows* show the margin of collapsed lung with free air laterally; the *arrowheads* show fluid level at costophrenic angle of left lung.

Trauma Radiographs

NOTE: The authors extend special thanks to Sharon A. Coffey, MS, RT (R), for providing the excellent trauma radiographs shown throughout this chapter.

Figs. 13-34 to 13-53 illustrate the wide range of patient conditions that result from trauma. Patients must be individually evaluated and handled with extreme care, with radiographs often taken through the rescue-squad backboard. When working with trauma patients, the radiographer must make professional judgments and routinely modify the approach used to obtain the radiographs needed to make the diagnosis.

The general positioning guidelines presented in this chapter are intended to introduce the concept of adapting standard approaches to radiograph patients in the body position in which they arrive in the radiology department. Additional information on trauma radiography is presented in other chapters. For example, see Chapter 8 for specific information on radiography of a patient with trauma to the cervical spine.

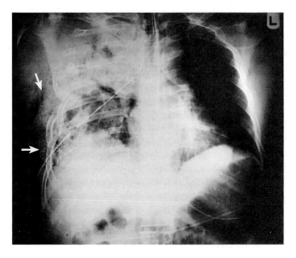

Fig. 13-35 AP chest radiograph of patient who received a crushing injury. Chest tube and multiple rib fractures are seen on the right side. Free air is also seen in soft tissue *(arrows)* lateral to the multiple rib fractures.

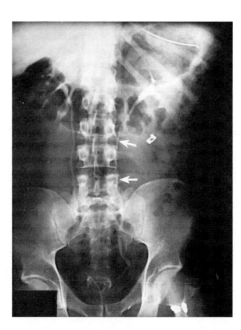

Fig. 13-36 Intravenous urogram of gunshot wound victim. The bullet entered the point marked by a surgical clip in upper left quadrant and stopped in the left hip area. Note medial displacement of the left hip area and medial displacement of the contrast-filled left ureter *(arrows)*, caused by retroperitoneal hemorrhage.

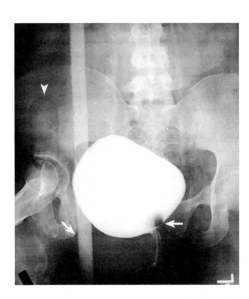

Fig. 13-37 AP projection with cystography of pelvis of auto accident victim. Note diastasis of pelvis (separation of pubic symphysis) (arrows). Vertical line and ovoid artifact (arrowhead) are the result of properly performing the examination on a rescue squad backboard.

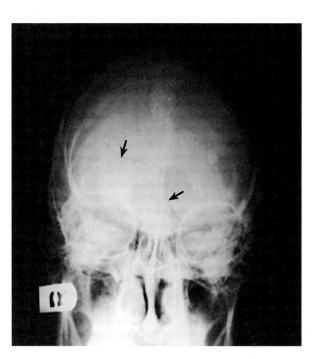

Fig. 13-38 AP projection of skull showing fracture extending from posterior to anterior surface (arrows).

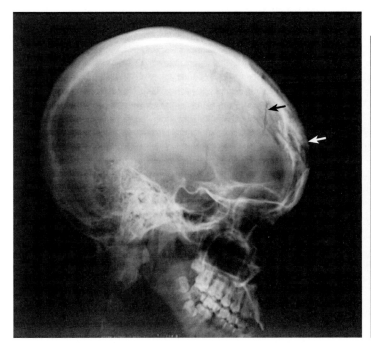

Fig. 13-39 Cross-table lateral skull of auto accident victim showing frontal skull fracture caused by contact with dashboard.

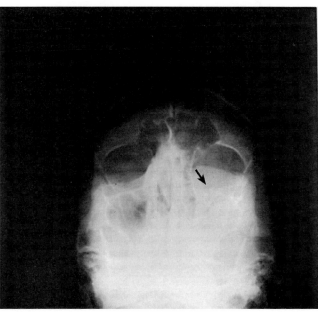

Fig. 13-40 Water's method, parietoacanthial projection, of supine patient. The patient was struck with a baseball bat in the left maxillary area. (This radiograph was obtained as demonstrated in Fig. 13-32.) Fracture of floor of left orbit is seen (arrow), along with related cloudiness of the maxillary sinus caused by fluid accumulation.

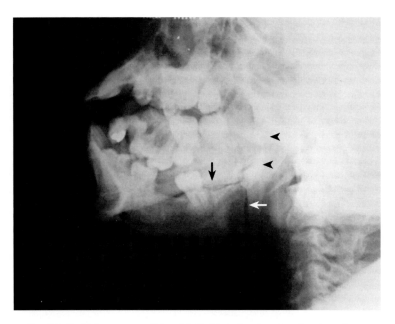

Fig. 13-41 Oblique mandible of fistfight victim showing fracture *(arrows)* extending from mandibular angle superiorly and anteriorly into the mandibular body. A tooth has also been fractured *(arrowheads)*.

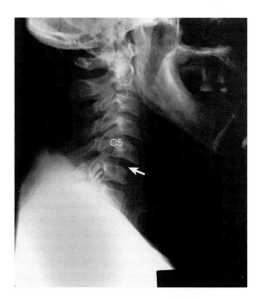

Fig. 13-42 Cross-table lateral cervical spine showing anterior subluxation *(arrow)* of C5 and C6 caused by patient diving into a shallow swimming pool.

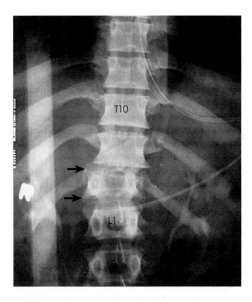

Fig. 13-43 AP thoracic spine of patient thrown from a horse. Compression fracture of T12 *(arrows)* and loss of alignment of spine at level of T11 and T12 are demonstrated. Contrast-filled kidneys are seen. Also noticeable is the vertical artifact caused by correctly taking radiographs of the patient while on rescue-squad backboard support.

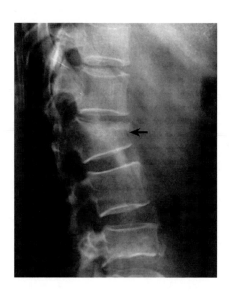

Fig. 13-44 Cross-table lateral lumbar spine showing compression fracture of the body of L2 *(arrow)*, caused by patient slipping and landing on backside.

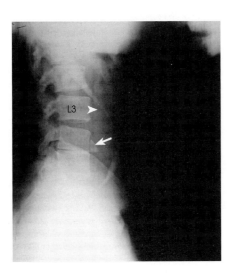

Fig. 13-45 Cross-table lateral lumbar spine of patient whose car was hit by a train, resulting in a compression fracture of L4 and L5 with an anteriorly displaced bone chip *(arrow)*. Bone chip caused localized swelling anteriorly, displacing the contrast-filled ureter *(arrowhead)*.

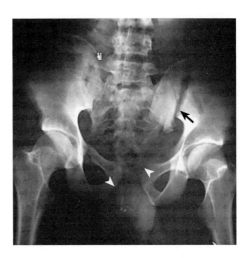

Fig. 13-46 AP projection of pelvis of teacher run over by a school bus. The projection demonstrates separation of the pubic bones *(arrowheads)* anteriorly and associated fracture of the ilium on the left *(arrow)*. The patient died as a result of hypovolemic shock, a common body response to such trauma.

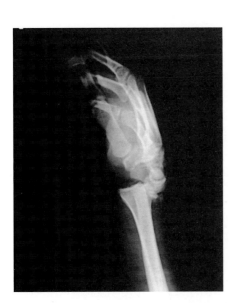

Fig. 13-47 Lateral wrist showing posterior carpal dislocation in a patient who was thrown from a motorcycle.

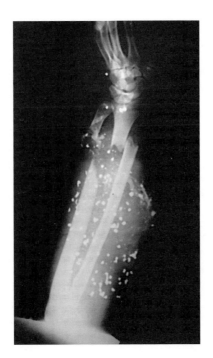

Fig. 13-48 Gunshot wound fracture of radius and ulna with extensive soft tissue damage.

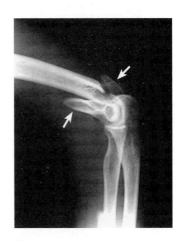

Fig. 13-49 Lateral elbow of patient who fell from a tree, fracturing the distal humerus and splitting the distal articular surface of the humerus *(arrows)*.

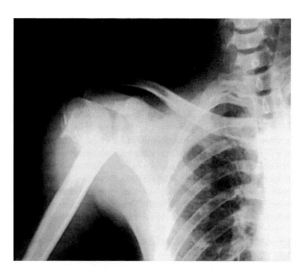

Fig. 13-50 AP shoulder of patient who fractured the surgical neck of the humerus in a fall.

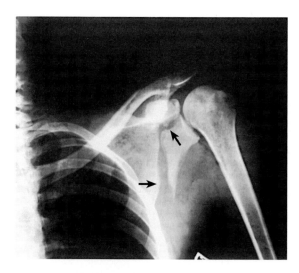

Fig. 13-51 AP projection of shoulder of auto accident victim. The patient had the arm out the window of the car at the time of the accident. Note fracture of the scapula through the glenoid cavity and extending inferiorly (*arrows*).

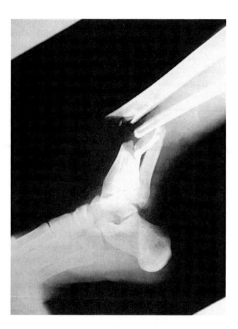

Fig. 13-52 Lateral image of a patient with a compound fracture of the tibia and fibula that was incurred in a skiing accident.

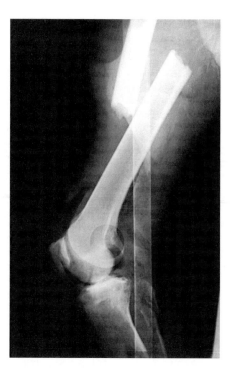

Fig. 13-53 Fracture of the femur that resulted from an industrial accident. The patient was radiographed on a rescue-squad backboard, and the proximal femur is seen in the AP projection. The fractured distal femur was rotated, resulting in the lateral image of the distal femur.

TERMINOLOGY CHANGES

To make using Volume One of this edition easier, the following summarizes the technical and anatomic terms that have changed since the eighth edition. The left column contains the *new term in italics,* and the right column contains the old term. If no old term is shown, the new term is introduced for the first time in the atlas.

Chapter 1
Preliminary Steps in Radiography

Image receptor	Film*
Cassette	Film*
Inspiration	Inhalation
Expiration	Exhalation
Universal precautions	
Source-to-skin distance (SSD)	
Computed radiography	

---

* Film is used only when referring to an actual sheet of film.

Chapter 3
General Anatomy and Radiographic Positioning Terminology
Body Planes

Midsagittal plane	Median sagittal plane
Midcoronal plane	Median coronal plane

Osteology

Axial skeleton	
Appendicular skeleton	
Spongy bone	Cancellous bone
Trabeculae	
Red marrow	
Yellow marrow	
Medullary cavity	Medullary canal
Nutrient foramen	
Nutrient artery	
Periostial arteries	

Arthrology
Epiphyseal line

Synovial Joints

Gliding	Plane
Hinge	Ginglymus
Pivot	Trochoid
Saddle	Sellar
Ball & socket	Spheroid

Bone Markings and Features

Line
Meatus
Notch

Fractures

Open
Closed
Nondisplaced
Displaced
Compound
Simple
Greenstick
Transverse
Spiral/oblique
Comminuted
Compression
Impacted

Anatomic Relationship Terms

Parietal
Visceral

Radiographic Body Projections

True projection

Radiographic Positions

Fowler's position
Lordotic position

Body Movement Terminology

Deviation

Chapter 4
Upper Limb
Wrist

Hook of the hamate	Hamulus
Median nerve	
Ulnar deviation	Ulnar flexion
Radial deviation	Radial flexion

Humerus
Humeral condyle

Fat Pads

Posterior fat pad
Anterior fat pad
Supinator fat pad

Chapter 6
Lower Limb
Calcaneous

Anterior facet	Anterior articular surface
Middle facet	Middle articular surface
Posterior facet	Posterior articular surface

Tibia

Tibial plateau
Anterior crest
Anterior tubercle
Fibular notch

Femur

Adductor tubercle

Knee joint

Posterior cruciate ligament
Anterior cruciate ligament
Tibial collateral ligament
Fibular collateral ligament

Chapter 7
Pelvis and Upper Femora
Pelvis
Pelvic girdle
Pubic symphysis   Symphysis pubis

Ilium
Iliac crest   Crest of ilium
Anterior inferior iliac spine
Posterior superior iliac spine
Posterior inferior iliac spine

Chapter 8
Vertebral Column
Thoracic vertebrae
Costal facet   Facet

Sacrum
Pelvic sacral foramina   Foramina
Sacral cornua   Sacral horn

Coccyx
Coccygeal cornua   Coccygeal horn

Chapter 9
Bony Thorax
Sternum
Manubrium   Manubrium sterni

Ribs
True ribs
False ribs
Facets
Vertebral end
Sternal end
Costal groove

Chapter 10
Thoracic Viscera
Respiratory System
Primary bronchi   Main bronchi
Secondary bronchi
Tertiary bronchi
Bronchioles
Bronchial tree

Lungs
Cardiac notch

INDEX

A

Abdomen
abdominal sequencing, **2:**46-47
anatomic definition of, **1:**55
bowel preparation, **1:**16
compression of, during alimentary canal evaluations, **2:**95
diagnostic ultrasound of, **3:**369-370
entrance skin exposure for, **1:**43t
magnetic resonance imaging of, **3:**354
mobile radiography projections of
AP, **3:**220-223
in left lateral decubitus position, **3:**222-223
in neonate
AP, **3:**232-235
lateral, **3:**236-237
in right or left dorsal decubitus position, **3:**236-237
PA, **3:**222-223
projections of
AP, **2:**42-45, **2:**47, **2:**53
description of, **2:**41
indications, **2:**41
lateral, **2:**48-51
in left dorsal decubitus position, **2:**50-51
in left lateral decubitus position, **2:**44-45
overview, **2:**34
PA, **2:**44-45
in right dorsal decubitus position, **2:**50-51
in right or left position, **2:**48-49
in upright position, **2:**44-45, **2:**47
quadrants, **1:**55
radiologic procedure
exposure technique, **2:**40
immobilization, **2:**41
preparation, **2:**40
radiologic protection, **2:**41
regions of, **1:**55
sectional anatomy of, **3:**126
Abdominal aortography, **3:**34-35
Abdominal cavity, **1:**54, **2:**35
Abdominal fistulae, radiologic procedure for, **2:**53
Abdominopelvic region, sectional anatomy of, **3:**112-127
Abduction, **1:**80
Absorbed dose, definition of, **1:**37, **3:**505
Acanthion, **2:**246
Acanthioparietal projection
of facial bones, **2:**320-321
for trauma, **2:**320
Accelerator, definition of, **3:**505

Accuracy, definition of, **3:**459
Acetabulum
Dunlap, Swanson, and Penner method, **1:**359
Judet method, **1:**358
projections for
AP axial oblique, **1:**358
axiolateral, **1:**359
overview, **1:**324t
PA axial oblique, **1:**358
in RAO and LAO position, **1:**358
in RPO and LPO position, **1:**358
radiologic imaging of, **1:**343
sectional anatomy of, **3:**123
Teufel method, **1:**358
Acini, **2:**429
Acoustic impedance, definition of, **3:**406
Acoustic properties, definition of, **3:**505
Acoustic shadow, definition of, **3:**406
Acquisition rate, **3:**327, **3:**333
Acromial extremity, **1:**155
Acromioclavicular articulation, **1:**211
Alexander method
for AP axial projection, **1:**192-193
for PA axial oblique projection, **1:**194
anatomy of, **1:**158, **1:**159
infraspinatus insertion, **1:**190
Pearson method, **1:**190-191
projections for
AP, **1:**190-191
AP axial, **1:**192-193
bilateral, **1:**190-191
overview, **1:**154t, **1:**180t
in RAO or LAO position, **1:**194
Acromion, **1:**156, **1:**205, **1:**209
Adam's apple; *see* Thyroid cartilage
Adduction, **1:**80
Adductor tubercle, **1:**225
Adipose capsule, **2:**160
Adrenal glands; *see* Suprarenal glands
Afferent arteriole, **2:**161
Afferent lymph vessel, definition of, **3:**90
Air calibration, definition of, **3:**304
Ala, **1:**381
Alexander method, for acromioclavicular articulations, **1:**180t
AP axial, **1:**192-193
PA axial oblique, **1:**194
Algorithm, definition of, **3:**304
Alignment, **3:**523
Alimentary canal
anatomy of, **2:**36, **2:**85
components of, **2:**85

Alimentary canal—cont'd
examination procedure
contrast media, **2:**92-94
equipment, **2:**95
examining room preparation, **2:**96
exposure time, **2:**96
radiologic apparatus, **2:**95
gastrointestinal transit, **2:**92
radiation protection, **2:**97
regions of, **2:**85
Allowable dose; *see* Recommended dose limit
Alpha particle, definition of, **3:**431
Alveolar process, **2:**246
Alveoli, anatomy of, **1:**508-509
American Society of Radiologic Technologists, ethics of, **1:**2
A-mode, definition of, **3:**406
Ampulla of Vater; *see* Hepatopancreatic ampulla
Anal canal, **2:**90
Analog, definition of, **3:**320, **3:**481
Analog-to-digital conversion, definition of, **3:**320
Anastomose, definition of, **3:**90
Anatomic position; *see also specific projections*
anteroposterior, **1:**8, **1:**9
definition of, **1:**6
illustration of, **1:**6, **1:**7
lateral, **1:**10
oblique, **1:**11
posteroanterior, **1:**8-1:**9, **1:**9
relationship terms, **1:**69
Anatomic snuffbox, **1:**86
Anatomy, definition of, **1:**52
Anechoic, definition of, **3:**406
Aneurysm, definition of, **3:**90
Angina pectoris, definition of, **3:**258
Angiography
arteriography; *see* Arteriography
catheterization, **3:**30-32
central nervous system use, **3:**13-14
cerebral
anatomic considerations, **3:**50-52
anterior circulation, projections of
AP axial, **3:**60-62
AP axial oblique, **3:**61-62
lateral projection, **3:**59
aortic arch angiogram, **3:**58
circulation time, **3:**54
definition of, **3:**90
equipment, **3:**55
examining room preparation, **3:**56
imaging program for, **3:**54
patient positioning for, **3:**56-57

Index

Index

Index

Index

Index

Xiphisternal joint
  anatomy of, **1:**469t
  description of, **1:**470
Xiphoid process, **1:**468
X-ray beam, collimation of, **1:**28, **1:**29
X-ray diffraction unit, **1:**39
X-ray grids, patient instructions regarding, **1:**19
X-rays
  discovery of, **1:**36
  early injuries associated with, **1:**36
X-ray units, quality assurance of
  beam alignment, **3:**515
  beam/light field congruence, **3:**515
  beam quality, **3:**516-517
  exposure reproducibility and linearity, **3:**518
  exposure time, **3:**515-516
  focal spot size, **3:**518
  kilovolts, **3:**518

Z
Zonography
  abdominal structures evaluated using, **3:**193
  definition of, **3:**179, **3:**205
Zoom, definition of, **3:**333
Z-scores, **3:**443, **3:**460
Zygapophyseal joints
  anatomy of, **1:**372, **1:**382
  of cervical vertebrae, **1:**375
  of lumbar region, **1:**379
  projections of
    AP oblique, **1:**423-425, **1:**434-435
    overview, **1:**369t
    PA oblique, **1:**423-425, **1:**436-437
    positioning rotations for, **1:**375t
    in RAO and LAO positions, **1:**423-425, **1:**436-437

Zygapophyseal joints—cont'd
  projections of—cont'd
    in recumbent position, **1:**424-425
    in RPO and LPO positions, **1:**423-425, **1:**434-435
    of thoracic vertebrae, **1:**377
Zygomatic arch
  description of, **2:**247
  May method, **2:**330-331
  modified Titterington method, **2:**332-333
  modified Towne method, **2:**334-335
  projections of
    AP axial, **2:**334-335
    overview, **2:**310t
    tangential, **2:**326-331
Zygomatic bones, **2:**247
Zygomatic process, **2:**242
Zygote, **2:**215

ISBN 0-8151-2651-4

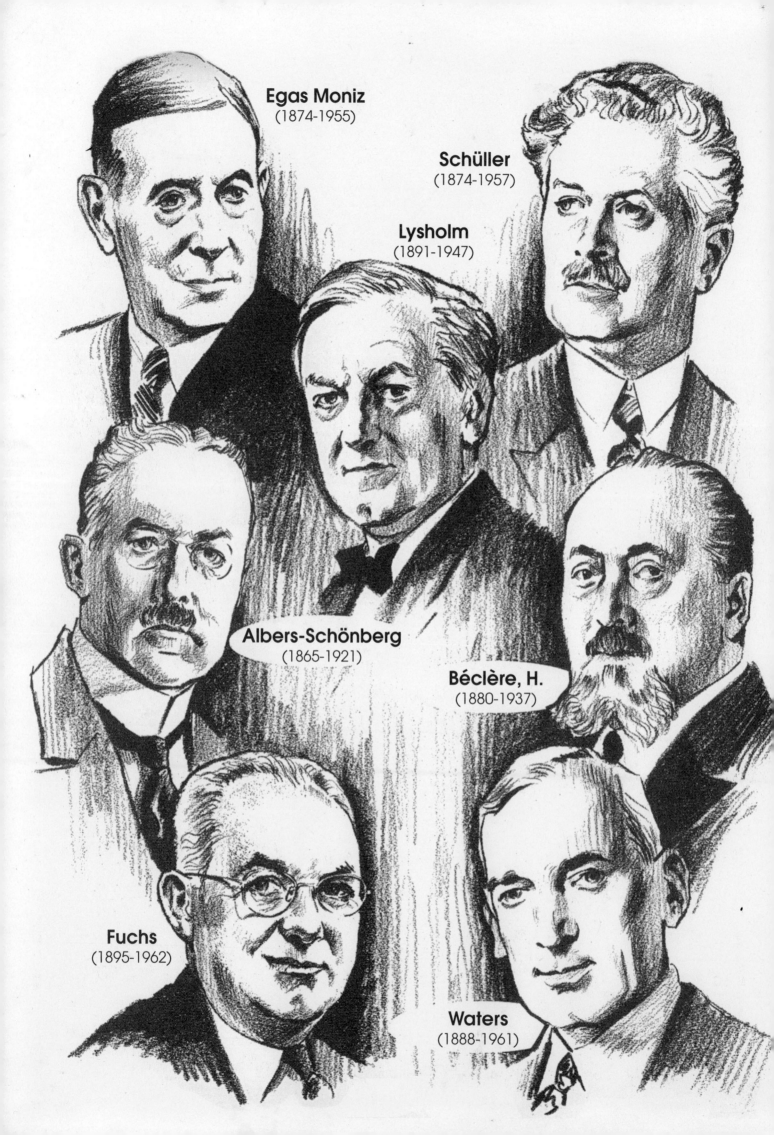

Egas Moniz
(1874-1955)

Schüller
(1874-1957)

Lysholm
(1891-1947)

Albers-Schönberg
(1865-1921)

Béclère, H.
(1880-1937)

Fuchs
(1895-1962)

Waters
(1888-1961)